Gerontological Nursing

THIRD EDITION

Charlotte Eliopoulos R.N.C., M.P.H., CDONA/LTC

Consultant, Lecturer, Author
Glen Arm, Maryland

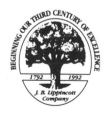

J. B. Lippincott Company
Philadelphia

Acquisitions Editor: Barbara Nelson Cullen
Coordinating Editorial Assistant: Jennifer E. Brogan
Project Editor: Molly E. Dickmeyer
Indexer: Sandi Schroeder
Design Coordinator: Christopher Laird
Interior Designer: Holly Reid McLaughlin
Cover Designer: William T. Donnelly
Production Manager: Caren Erlichman
Production Coordinator: Kevin Johnson
Compositor: G&S Typesetters, Inc.
Printer/Binder: R.R. Donnelly and Sons
Cover Printer: Lehigh Press, Inc.

Third Edition

6 5 4 3 2 1

Library of Congress Cataloging-in-Publication Data

Eliopoulos, Charlotte.
    Gerontological nursing / Charlotte Eliopoulos.—3rd ed.
        p.   cm.
    Includes bibliographical references and index.
    ISBN 0-397-54974-1 :
    1. Geriatric nursing.   I. Title.
    [DNLM: 1. Geriatric Nursing.   WY 152 E42g]
    RC954.E44   1993
    610.73'65—dc20
    DNLM/DLC
    for Library of Congress   92-2159
                                                        CIP

Any procedure or practice described in this book should be applied by the health-care practitioner under appropriate supervision in accordance with professional standards of care used with regard to the unique circumstances that apply in each practice situation. Care has been taken to confirm the accuracy of information presented and to describe generally accepted practices. However, the authors, editors, and publisher cannot accept any responsibility for errors or omissions or for any consequences from application of the information in this book and make no warranty express or implied, with respect to the contents of the book.

Every effort has been made to ensure drug selections and dosages are in accordance with current recommendations and practice. Because of ongoing research, changes in government regulations and the constant flow of information on drug therapy, reactions and interactions, the reader is cautioned to check the package insert for each drug for indications, dosages, warnings and precautions, particularly if the drug is new or infrequently used.

Gerontological Nursing

This book is dedicated to Manuel Eliopoulos, Jr.,
a new traveler down the path of aging.

Preface

A dozen years have passed since the publication of the first edition of *Gerontological Nursing*. During that time, this specialty has grown tremendously in depth, scope, and sophistication. In the '70s, the challenge for gerontological nurses was to ensure that the unique norms, needs, and rights of the elderly were recognized and incorporated into caregiving. The challenge in the '90s is to ensure that the momentum for specialty advancement continues and the health-care system supports the provision of the wide range of services needed by the ever-increasing and diverse older population.

While attempting to remain a basic introduction to the nursing of the elderly, *Gerontological Nursing*, in this third edition, has been revised and its content expanded to help nurses meet the challenges of providing services to elderly individuals with a variety of needs in a wide range of service settings. The book is still divided into four units: Unit I: Understanding the Aging Population; Unit II: Promoting Wellness and Self-Care; Unit III: Pathologies of Aging; and Unit IV: Geriatric Care Issues. Unit I includes current demographics that enable nurses to realistically discuss, analyze, and plan service needs. New findings regarding the aging process that reflect the continued evolution of our knowledge about normal aging have been included. Family caregiving has been given greater emphasis to reflect the increasing involvement of families in the long-term support and care of aging relatives. Unit II uses the self-care theory to lay a foundation for gerontological nursing practice and highlights nursing diagnoses that relate to self-care deficits. Specific, practical nursing measures that promote wellness and self-care are discussed. In response to nursing's increasing responsibility for comprehensive assessment, the nursing assessment chapter has been significantly expanded to include knowledge and specific procedures for assessment. Likewise, more specific direction is offered for care planning. Current knowledge about the unique manifestation and management of illness in old age is incorporated in Unit III. In-depth reviews of specific assessment skills related to individual systems are provided, along with menus of care plan goals and listings of resources to guide care activities. An expanded discussion of pharmacokinetics and pharmacodynamics has been added to the geriatric pharmacology chapter to reflect the continued unveiling of new insights into the complicated arena of drug therapy for the aged. Unit IV addresses ongoing concerns, such as helping older adults cope with chronic illness, protecting their rights, and facilitating a comfortable dying process. In addition, there is an examination

of issues that are receiving new emphasis, such as advance directives, the rationing of health care, and the subspecialization of gerontological nursing in diverse care settings.

Gerontological Nursing attempts to incorporate relevant research findings and new knowledge while remaining a practical, user-friendly resource to both students of the specialty and nurses caring for the elderly in a variety of service settings.

Charlotte Eliopoulos, R.N.C., M.P.H., CDONA/LTC

Preface to the Second Edition

When the first edition of *Gerontological Nursing* was published in 1979, it was among a few books dedicated to the specialty of providing nursing care for older adults. At that time it was sufficient for a gerontological nursing text to provide facts that would separate myths from realities and provide basic guidance to care delivery. The specialty was just getting accustomed to being a specialty, the certification process was only a few years old, the first journal for gerontological nurses had recently become established, and fewer puzzled expressions resulted from announcing that one was a gerontological nurse.

The growth in the sophistication and spread of gerontological nursing has been dramatic since the time that the first edition of this book appeared. Increasing numbers of the elderly are challenging nurses in virtually every practice setting. The nursing needs of the older population are becoming more diverse: gerontological nurses confront the need for new forms of wellness care from a healthier young-old population while facing highly complex physical and mental health problems of a growing old-old population. The novice to gerontological nursing soon learns that it is hardly "an easy specialty for nurses who can't make it in other settings" but rather one that demands highly skilled and knowledgeable professionals.

Gerontological Nursing has grown to address the challenges of today's gerontological nurse. Unit I, Understanding the Aging Population, lays the foundation by discussing facts about the older population, theories of aging, ethnicity, concerns of aging families, adjustments confronted by the elderly, and the normal aging process. The self-care theory is used as the structure for reviewing the impact of aging on normal daily life in Unit II, Promoting Wellness and Self-Care, and the nursing process comes alive in this section with specific guidelines for assessment and care planning and delivery. Unit III, Pathologies of Aging, approaches medical, surgical, and psychiatric problems with a nursing perspective and offers practical nursing actions. Included in Units II and III are tables that outline actual and potential nursing diagnoses related to specific problem areas that can aid in developing diagnostic statements and care plans. Special concerns in delivering services to older adults such as helping patients cope with chronic illness, legal risks, ethical dilemmas, matching services to needs, and trends are explored in Unit IV, Geriatric Care Issues. Sample assessment tools, age-adjusted laboratory values, organizations of interest to older adults, and other re-

sources are also included. The revision of existing content and the addition of relevant new material should make the second edition of *Gerontological Nursing* a useful basic resource for gerontological nursing practitioners and students.

Charlotte Eliopoulos, R.N.C., M.P.H.

Preface to the First Edition

The growing number of elderly persons in the population, and the more active role they are assuming, have increased society's awareness of the qualities, rights, and needs of its older members. Popular literature that dispels myths concerning the aging process proliferates. Government is demonstrating greater sensitivity to the problems of old age, as evidenced by legislation promoting increased security and care for the aged. The media expose the public to the often overlooked pleasures and problems of growing old in America. Society thus has a new concern for the aging population.

The increased numbers of the aged have influenced the helping professions to become more closely involved in the fields of gerontology and geriatrics. During the past few decades alone, tremendous strides have been made in conducting research, preparing specialists, developing educational programs, increasing literature, and providing clinical services in gerontology and geriatrics. Because of the complexities and challenges of working with the aged, greater numbers of professionals are entering this area of specialization.

The nursing profession is experiencing an outstanding attitudinal shift in its view of caring for the aged. Once viewed as the bottom rung of the nursing ladder—a stepchild specialty—gerontological nursing has blossomed into one of the most popular and expanding fields of practice. The sophisticated blend of knowledge and skill required to deliver appropriate gerontological care supports the fact that gerontological nurses must have special cognitive and clinical capabilities.

An introduction to the nursing care of aging persons is offered in this book. Characteristics of the older population are presented to help the reader differentiate myths from realities. There is a review of aging theories, emphasizing their strengths and weaknesses. Characteristics of the normal aging process will be identified and transferred into implications for the aged individual's daily life and the nursing care he or she may require. The unique knowledge and skill utilized in applying the nursing process to the aged will be discussed.

In addition to information pertaining to normal aging and health promotion in old age, it is important for the gerontological nurse to understand the special features of the aged's illnesses. A portion of this book reviews major problems that affect each body system and outlines differences in symptomatology, diagnosis, management, and related nursing care.

Currently popular issues in aging and geriatric care have special chapters devoted to them. Included among these topics are geriatric pharmacology, sexuality, the dying process, surgical care, sensory deficits, services for the aged, and mental health and illness.

This book is designed as an introduction to gerontology, geriatrics, and nursing care of the aged. It provides a basic framework upon which gerontological nursing practice can be developed. Rather than being all-inclusive, this book is a stepping-stone to assist the reader into a deeper exploration of gerontology literature.

The reader should note that the words *old, aged,* and *geriatric* are used throughout the text to describe older persons. Although a negative connotation is often associated with these words, it is the author's belief that the attitudes and behaviors demonstrated to older persons are far more significant than the labels they are given.

C. E.

Acknowledgments

No author writes a book alone; the ideas and support of persons too numerous to mention go into the birth of a book.

There are several persons to whom I'd like to express my gratitude. Donna Hilton of J. B. Lippincott provided support and encouragement during the revision of this book, as well as the freedom for me to follow my own style and instincts. My husband, Angelo Janouris, offered immeasurable support and patience. The many fine and caring gerontological nurses whom I've encountered through consultations and lectures throughout the country gave valuable feedback and insights that helped me to maintain that essential bridge between theory and the real world. Most of all, I am deeply indebted to the many older persons who taught me the wisdom, strength, and beauty of old age.

Contents

Gerontological Nursing

unit I

Understanding the Aging Population

1

Nursing and the Elderly

Older members of every society have always received some degree of attention, and many historical writings depict both the positive and the negative attributes of growing old. Confucius expressed a direct correlation between a person's age and the degree of respect to which that person was entitled. Taoism viewed old age as the epitome of life, and the ancient Chinese believed that attaining old age was an accomplishment that deserved the greatest honor. The early Egyptians, however, dreaded old age and experimented with a variety of potions and schemes to avoid growing old. Greek views were divided—myths portrayed many struggles between old and young and quests for immortality and fountains of youth, Plato promoted the aged as society's best leaders, and Aristotle denied the elderly any role in government matters. Ancient Romans had limited respect for their elders; in the nations that Rome conquered, the sick and the aged were customarily the first to be killed.

The Bible is laced with a theme of respect for the aged, although early Christian writings did little to elevate the status of the elderly. The Dark Ages were especially bleak for older persons; the Middle Ages did not bring considerable improvement. Strong feelings regarding the superiority of youth occurred during medieval times; these feelings were expressed in uprisings of sons against fathers. The art of this period, with its figures such as Father Time, also portrayed an uncomplimentary image of the aged. The elderly were also among the first to be affected by famine and poverty and the last to benefit during better times. Many gains in the treatment of the elderly that were made during the 18th and 19th centuries were lost because of the cruelties of the industrial revolution. Although child labor laws were developed to guard minors, the aged were left unprotected. Those unable to meet industrial demands were placed at the mercy of their offspring or forced to beg on the streets for sustenance.

Although Dr. I. L. Nascher, known as the father of geriatrics, wrote the first geriatric textbook in 1914, American literature during the first half of the 20th century reflects little improvement in the status of the aged. Most significant was the passage of the Federal Old Age Insurance Law under the Social Security Act in 1935, which provided some financial security for older persons. Only recent literature has viewed age with positivism rather than prejudice, intelligence rather than myth, and concern rather than neglect. The past few decades have brought a profound awakening of interest in older persons as their numbers in society have grown. A more humanistic attitude toward all people has also affected the aged, and improvements in health care and general living conditions ensure that more people have the opportunity to attain old age.

There has been a growing recognition that the unique needs and problems of older persons require separate attention, evidenced by the development of the American Geriatrics Society in 1942, the beginning of the Gerontological Society in 1944, the first National Conference on Aging in 1950, the founding of the Senior Citizens of America in 1954 and the American Society for the Aged in 1955, and

Table 1-1 *Life Expectancy at Birth From 1920–1988*

	US POPULATION		WHITE POPULATION			NONWHITE POPULATION		
Year	Total		Total	Men	Women	Total	Men	Women
1920	54.1		54.9	54.4	55.6	45.3	45.5	45.2
1930	59.7		61.4	59.7	63.5	48.1	47.3	49.2
1940	62.9		64.2	62.1	66.6	53.1	51.5	54.9
1950	68.2		69.1	66.5	72.2	60.8	59.1	62.9
1955	69.6		70.5	67.4	73.7	63.7	61.4	66.1
1960	69.7		70.6	67.4	74.1	63.6	61.1	66.3
1965	70.2		71.0	67.6	74.7	64.1	61.1	67.4
1970	70.9		71.7	68.0	75.6	65.3	61.3	69.4
1975	72.6		73.4	69.5	77.3	68.0	63.7	72.4
1980	73.7		74.4	70.7	78.1	69.5	65.3	73.6
1983	74.7		75.2	71.6	78.8	71.3	67.1	75.3
1988	74.9		75.6	72.3	78.9	69.2	64.9	73.4

Data from the US Department of Commerce. Statistical abstract of the US. 110th ed. Washington, DC: Bureau of the Census, 1990:72.

the establishment of a Federal Council on Aging in 1956. Concurrent efforts have been made to expand research, develop educational programs, and provide comprehensive services pertaining to aging individuals.

Facts About the Older Population

"Families forget their older relatives . . . most people become senile in old age . . . Social Security provides a good retirement income . . . a majority of the elderly reside in nursing homes . . . Medicare covers all health-care–related costs for older people. . . ." These and other myths are still perpetuated. Misinformation about the elderly is an injustice not only to this age group but also to persons of all ages who need accurate information to prepare realistically for their own old age. Gerontological nurses must know the facts about the older population to deliver effective services and educate the general public.

Growing Number of Older Adults

Persons older than 65 years of age represent more than 12% of the United States population. More people are surviving to their senior years than ever before. In 1930, slightly more than 6 million persons were age 65 years or older, and the average life expectancy was 59.7 years; the life expectancy in 1965 became 70.2 years, and the number of elderly exceeded 20 million. Life expectancy has reached 74.9 years, with over 30 million persons exceeding age 65 years (Table 1-1). It is predicted that growing

Table 1-2 *Increase in the "Old-Old" Population From 1960–1990 (in millions)*

AGE GROUP (Y)	1960	1970	1980	1990
Total 65+	16.7	20.1	25.7	30.3
65–69	6.3	7.0	8.8	9.9
70–74	4.8	5.5	6.8	8.0
75–79	3.1	3.9	4.8	5.9
80–84	1.6	2.3	3.0	3.6
85+	0.9	1.4	2.3	2.9

From US Department of Commerce. Statistical abstract of the US. 110th ed. Washington, DC: Bureau of the Census, 1990:16.

Table 1-3 *Race and Gender Differences in Life Expectancy (in years)*

| | MEN | | WOMEN | |
Total Population	White	Nonwhite	White	Nonwhite
74.9	72.3	64.9	78.9	73.4

From US Department of Commerce. Statistical abstract of the US. 110th ed. Washington, DC: Bureau of the Census, 1990:72.

numbers of persons will reach their senior years, with an anticipated 20% of the population being older than 65 years of age by the year 2020.

Not only are more people reaching old age, but they are living longer once they do—the number of people in their 70s and 80s has been steadily increasing and will continue to do so (Table 1-2). Advancements in disease control and health technology, the greater number of people able to survive the previously hazardous period of infancy and other dangers throughout the life span, improved sanitation, and better living conditions have helped to increase life expectancy for most Americans.

Older adults live in a variety of settings throughout the country, with the greatest numbers found in California, New York, Florida, Pennsylvania, and Texas. In terms of the percentage of a state's population older than 65 years of age, Florida takes the lead, followed by Pennsylvania, Iowa, Rhode Island, Arkansas, and West Virginia. In the past decade, the most dramatic increases in the percentage of elderly residents have occurred in Nevada, Alaska, Hawaii, and Arizona.

Gender and Race Differences

The differences in life expectancy between genders and races are shown in Table 1-3. From the late 1980s to the present, the gap between the life expectancy for whites and blacks has widened due to a decline in the life expectancy for the black population. The United States Department of Health and Human Services attributes the declining life expectancy of blacks to an increase in deaths from homicide and acquired immunodeficiency syndrome.

Throughout this century, the ratio of men to women has steadily declined to the point that there are fewer than 7 older men for every 10 older women (Table 1-4). The ratio declines with each advanced decade. The higher survival rates of women along with the practice of women marrying men older than themselves makes it no surprise that more than one half of women older than 65 years of age are widowed, and a majority of their male contemporaries are married (Table 1-5).

Table 1-4 *Gender Ratio in the Population 65 Years of Age and Older*

YEAR	NUMBER OF MEN PER 100 WOMEN
1910	101.1
1920	101.3
1930	100.5
1940	95.5
1950	89.6
1960	82.8
1970	72.1
1980	67.6
1985	67.9
1988	68.6

Data from the US Bureau of the Census. Based on US Census of Population: 1950, 1960, and 1970, part B; and Current Population Report. Series P-25, No. 949.

Table 1-5 *Marital Status of the Population 65 Years of Age and Older (in thousands)*

	MEN	WOMEN
Single	4.6	5.2
Married		
spouse present	75.1	39.9
spouse absent	2.5	1.6
Widowed	13.9	48.7
Divorced	3.9	4.5

From US Department of Commerce. Statistical abstract of the US. 110th ed. Washington, DC: Bureau of the Census, 1990:37.

Table 1-6 *Living Arrangements of People 65 Years of Age and Older*

	TOTAL	MEN	WOMEN
Living alone	30.4	16.2	40.6
Living with spouse	54.5	75.1	39.9
Living with other relative	12.8	6.7	17.2
Living with nonrelative	2.3	2.1	2.4

From US Department of Commerce. Statistical abstract of the US. 110th ed. Washington, DC: Bureau of the Census, 1990:37.

Most older adults live in a household with a spouse or other family member, although there are more than twice the number of women living alone than men in later life (Table 1-6). Most elderly have contact with their families and are not forgotten or neglected. Realities of the aging family are discussed in greater detail in Chapter 4.

Income and Employment

Although the percentage of the total population that the elderly represent is growing, they constitute a steadily declining percentage of workers in the labor force (Table 1-7). The percentage of older people below the poverty level has been declining concurrently, with less than 15% now falling in this category (Table 1-8). This is not to imply that the elderly are without financial problems. As Tables 1-8 and 1-9 show, women and minority groups have considerably less income than white men. The median net worth of older households was $60,300 in 1988, nearly twice the national average of $32,700.

Education

Slightly more than one-half of today's older population graduated from high school (Table 1-10), but within the next few decades the United States will

Table 1-7 *Percentage of Labor Force Participation for People 65 Years of Age and Older*

Employed	11.2
Unemployed	0.3
Not in labor force	88.5

From US Department of Commerce. Statistical abstract of the US. 110th ed. Washington, DC: Bureau of the Census, 1990:37.

witness a trend toward a more educated senior citizen group because of the significant increase in the number of persons completing high school during and since the 1940s. Elderly people with advanced degrees will be more prevalent than in the past.

Health Problems

The elderly experience fewer acute illnesses than younger age groups and have a lower death rate from these problems (Table 1-11). However, elderly people who do experience acute illnesses usually require longer periods of recovery and have more complications from these conditions.

Chronic illness is a major problem for the older population. Most elderly people have at least one chronic disease, and typically they have several chronic conditions that must be managed simultaneously (Table 1-12). Chronic illness causes some personal-care activity limitation in 49% of all older individuals, and 27% have difficulty with home-management activities. The older the age, the greater the likelihood of having difficulty with self-care activities and independent living (Table 1-13).

Chronic diseases are not only major sources of disability but are also the leading causes of death (Table 1-14). A shift in death rates from various causes of death has occurred—deaths from heart disease have declined, whereas those from cancer have increased over the past three decades.

Use of Resources

The growing number of persons older than 65 years of age has had an impact on the health and social service agencies that serve this group, and by association, on the government that is the source of payment for most of those services. The elderly have higher rates of hospitalization, surgery, and

Table 1-8 *Percentage of Persons 65 Years of Age and Older With Incomes Below the Poverty Level*

	1959	1970	1979	1982	1988
White	33.1	22.6	13.3	12.4	10
Black	62.5	47.7	36.3	38.2	32
Hispanic	NA	NA	26.8	26.6	22
Men	59.0	38.9	25.3	21.2	8
Women	63.3	49.8	30.5	28.7	15
Of total aged	35.2	24.6	15.2	14.6	12

NA, not available.
Data from the US Bureau of the Census. Current Population Report. Series P-60, No. 144.

physician visits than other age groups (Table 1-15), and this care is more likely to be paid by federal dollars than private insurers or the elderly themselves (Table 1-16).

Less than 5% of the older population is institutionalized at any given time, although about one in four older adults will spend some time in a nursing home during the last years of their lives. Most people who enter nursing homes as private-pay residents spend their assets by the end of one year and require government support for their care; most of the Medicaid budget is spent on long-term care.

As the percentage of the population who is elderly increases, society will face an increasing demand for the provision of and payment for services to this group. In this era of budget deficits, shrinking revenue, and increased competition for funding of other special interests, questions may arise as to the ongoing ability of the government to provide a wide range of services for older adults. There may be concern that the elderly are using a disproportionate amount of tax dollars and that limits

should be set. Gerontological nurses must ensure that they are actively involved in discussions and decisions pertaining to the rationing of services so that the rights of the elderly are expressed and protected. Likewise, gerontological nurses must assume leadership in developing cost-effective methods of care delivery that do not compromise the quality of services to older adults.

Development of Gerontological Nursing

Nurses, long interested in the care of the aged, seem to have assumed more responsibility than any other profession for people in this group. In 1904, the *American Journal of Nursing* printed the first nursing article on the care of the aged, presenting many principles that still guide gerontological nursing practice today:(Bishop, 1904)

You must not treat a young child as you would a grown person, nor must you treat an old person as you would one in the prime of life.

Table 1-9 *Annual Median Income of Households and Individuals 65 Years of Age and Older (in dollars)*

Households	
White	22,586
Black	13,541
Individuals	
Men	12,471
Women	7,103

From US Department of Commerce. Statistical abstract of the US. 110th ed. Washington, DC: Bureau of the Census, 1990:460.

Table 1-10 *Years of School Completed by Persons 65 Years of Age and Over*

YEARS OF SCHOOL COMPLETED	MALES	FEMALES
8 or less	31.7%	29.7%
1–3 y of high school	15.6	15.8
4 y of high school	33.0	35.5
1–3 y of college	9.8	10.5
4 y or more of college	13.5	8.5

From US Bureau of the Census. Current Population Reports. Series P-20, No. 433, 1990.

Table 1-11 *Rates of Acute Illness in Adults by Age (per 100 Population)*

	25–44 Y	45–64 Y	65+ Y
Infections and parasites	18.2	7.8	5.5
Upper respiratory	28.2	21.4	14.3
Other respiratory	46.0	28.3	20.4
Digestive system	5.0	3.3	6.8
Injuries	28.5	18.2	21.7

Data from US National Center for Health Statistics. Series 10 and unpublished data. 1988.

Interestingly, in that same year the same journal featured an article entitled "The Old Nurse," which emphasized the value of the aging nurse's years of experience:(DeWitt, 1904)

After the Federal Old Age Insurance Law was passed in 1935, many older persons had an alternative to alms houses and could independently pay for their room and board. Because many homes for the aged were opened by women who called themselves nurses, it is not coincidental that such residences later became known as nursing homes. For many years, care of the aged was an unpopular branch of nursing practice. A stigma was attached to geriatric nurses, implying that they were somewhat inferior in capabilities, not good enough for acute settings, or ready to "go to pasture." Geriatric facilities may have further discouraged many competent nurses from working in these settings by paying low salaries. Little was found to counter the negativism in educational programs, where experiences with older persons were inadequate in both quantity and quality, and focused on the sick rather than the well, who were actually more representative of the older population. Although nurses were among the few groups who were exposed to experiences with the aged, gerontology was nonexistent in most nursing curriculums until recently.

Frustration over the lack of value placed on geriatric nursing led to an appeal to the American Nurses Association (ANA) for assistance in promoting the status of this field. After years of study, in 1961 the ANA recommended that a specialty group for geriatric nurses be formed. In 1962, the ANA's Conference Group on Geriatric Nursing Practice held its first national meeting. This group became the Division on Geriatric Nursing in 1966, gaining full recognition as a nursing specialty. An important contribution by this group was the development in 1969 of Standards for Geriatric Nursing Practice, first published in 1970. Certification of nurses for excellence in geriatric nursing practice followed, with the first 74 nurses achieving this rec-

Table 1-12 *Rates of Chronic Illness in Adults by Age (per 1000 Population)*

	18–44 Y	45–64 Y	65–74 Y	75+ Y
Arthritis	52.8	273.3	463.6	511.9
Hypertension	61.8	252.0	392.4	337.0
Hearing impairments	54.1	135.6	264.7	348.0
Heart conditions	40.7	126.1	284.7	322.2
Chronic sinusitis	149.5	192.1	154.0	131.4
Visual impairments	29.3	47.3	56.3	111.2
Orthopedic problems	135.4	155.0	154.9	182.0
Diabetes	11.9	56.4	98.3	98.2
Varicose veins	26.8	54.1	82.5	64.8
Hemorrhoids	46.9	79.7	74.1	73.1

From US Department of Commerce. Statistical Abstract of the US. 110th ed. Washington, DC: Bureau of the Census, 1990:118.

Table 1-13 *Percentages of Older People Who Have Difficulty with Personal-Care and Home-Management Activities*

AGE GROUP (Y)	PERSONAL-CARE ACTIVITIES	HOME-MANAGEMENT ACTIVITIES
Total 65 +	23	27
65–74	17	21
75–84	28	33
85 +	49	55

From US Department of Health and Human Services. Vital and health statistics. series 13. no. 104. Hyattsville, MD: National Center for Health Statistics, 1990:4.

ognition in 1975. The birth of the *Journal of Gerontological Nursing*, the first professional journal to meet the specific needs and interests of gerontological nurses, also occurred in 1975.

Interest grew in changing the name of this professions from geriatric to gerontological nursing because geriatrics is concerned with the diseases of old age, whereas nurses working with the aged, in addition to caring for illnesses, have the broader goal of helping individuals maximize their capabilities throughout the aging process. In 1976, the Geriatric Nursing Division became the Gerontological Nursing Division. Landmarks in the growth of gerontological nursing appear in the following chronological listing:

1904—First nursing article on care of the aged published in the *American Journal of Nursing*
1961—ANA recommendation for formation of specialty group for geriatric nurses
1962—First national meeting of the ANA's Conference Group on Geriatric Nursing Practice held in Detroit
1966—Formation of Geriatric Nursing Division of the ANA
1969—Development of Standards for Geriatric Nursing Practice
1970—First publication of Standards for Geriatric Nursing Practice
1975—First nurses certified in geriatric nursing
1975—*Journal of Gerontological Nursing* first published
1976—Geriatric Nursing Division changes title to Gerontological Nursing Division.

The specialty of gerontological nursing has since witnessed profound growth. Only 32 articles on the topic of nursing care of the aged were listed in the *Cumulative Index to Nursing Literature* in 1956, and only twice that number appeared 10 years later. However, the number of articles published yearly doubled thereafter. Whereas only a few gerontological nursing texts existed in the 1960s, the number grew to a few dozen in the 1970s and has been significantly rising since then. Growing numbers of nursing schools are including gerontological nursing courses in their undergraduate programs and offering advanced degrees with a major in this area. Several hundred nurses annually achieve ANA certification in gerontological nursing. The spe-

Table 1-14 *Leading Causes of Death for Persons 65 Years of Age and Older (in thousands)*

CAUSE	65–74 Y	75–84 Y	85+ Y
Heart disease	180.8	239.0	199.3
Malignant neoplasms	146.8	116.6	44.7
Cerebrovascular diseases	28.4	52.0	48.9
Chronic obstructive pulmonary diseases	25.9	26.7	10.1
Pneumonia/influenza	10.2	22.0	28.7
Diabetes mellitus	10.3	11.0	5.9
Accidents and adverse effects	8.5	9.6	7.0
Chronic liver disease, cirrhosis	6.5	2.9	0.6
Suicide	3.4	2.3	0.6

From US Department of Commerce. Statistical abstract of the US. 110th ed. Washington, DC: Bureau of the Census, 1990:49.

Table 1-15 *Annual Number of Physician Visits
by Age*

AGE (Y)	ANNUAL PHYSICIAN VISITS
Under 6	6.7
6–16	3.3
17–24	4.4
25–44	4.8
45–64	6.4
65 and over	8.9

From US Department of Commerce. Statistical abstract of the US.
110th ed. Washington, DC: Bureau of the Census, 1990:103.

cialty has indeed advanced rapidly and will continue to blossom as the challenges of and demand
for specialized nursing of the elderly become more
apparent.

Standards

Professional nursing practice is guided by standards. Standards reflect the level and expectations
of care that are desired. They serve as a model
against which practice can be compared and
judged. Thus, standards aid in both guiding and
evaluating nursing practice.

Standards, or statements of expected levels of
care, that exist in practice settings come from vari-

Table 1-16 *Source of Payment for Hospital Care
of Older Adults*

PAYMENT SOURCE	PERCENT DISTRI-BUTION
Medicare	93.4
Private insurance	4.1
Medicaid	0.9
Worker's compensation	0.7
Self-pay	0.5
Other	0.2

From US Department of Commerce. Statistical abstract of the US.
110th ed. Washington, DC: Bureau of the Census, 1990:111.

ous sources. State and federal regulations outline
minimum standards of practice for various health-
care workers (*e.g.*, nurse practice acts) and agencies
(*e.g.*, skilled nursing facilities). The Joint Commission on Accreditation of Health-Care Organizations
has developed standards for services in various provider agencies. The ANA Standards for Gerontological Nursing Practice, as listed in Display 1-1, are the
only standards developed by and for gerontological
nurses and provide general guidelines for the nursing care of older adults. Nurses should regularly
evaluate their actual practices against these standards to ensure that their care reflects the highest
quality possible.

Nursing Diagnoses and Gerontological Nursing

In 1973 the National Group for the Classification of
Nursing Diagnosis, now called the North American
Nursing Diagnosis Association (NANDA), published
the first list of nursing diagnoses. The establishment of nursing diagnoses was a significant step,
enabling nursing to define its unique professional
contribution to care.

A nursing diagnosis is a way of describing a
problem, condition, or need that nurses can legiti-
mately identify and provide action for within the
realm of nursing practice. It differs from a medical
diagnosis that requires medical intervention and
direction. A nursing diagnosis can be actual or
potential in that the individual may already possess the problem or condition, or be at risk of
developing it. In the case of potential problems,
the diagnosis is begun with the term "High Risk
for." The diagnostic statement consists of two parts:
the health problem/condition/symptom noted and
the contributing or causative factor. These are
linked together with the phrase "related to," for
example:

> Social isolation related to death of spouse
> Fluid volume deficit related to vomiting
> Impaired physical mobility related to casted leg
> Self-care deficit: feeding related to altered
>   cognition.

The accepted nursing diagnoses are listed in
Display 1-2.

DISPLAY 1-1   Standards of Gerontological Nursing Practice

Standard I. Organization of Gerontological Nursing Services

All gerontological nursing services are planned, organized, and directed by a nurse executive. The nurse executive has baccalaureate or master's preparation and experience in gerontological nursing and administration of long-term care services or acute-care services for older patients.

Standard II. Theory

The nurse participates in the generation and testing of theory as a basis for clinical decisions. The nurse uses theoretical concepts to guide the effective practice of gerontological nursing.

Standard III. Data Collection

The health status of the older person is regularly assessed in a comprehensive, accurate, and systematic manner. The information obtained during the health assessment is accessible to and shared with appropriate members of the interdisciplinary health-care team, including the older person and the family.

Standard IV. Nursing Diagnosis

The nurse uses health-assessment data to determine nursing diagnoses.

Standard V. Planning and Continuity of Care

The nurse develops the plan of care in conjunction with the older person and appropriate others. Mutual goals, priorities, nursing approaches, and measures in the care plan address the therapeutic, preventive, restorative, and rehabilitative needs of the older person. The care plan helps the older person attain and maintain the highest achievable levels of health, well-being, and quality of life, as well as a peaceful death. The plan of care facilitates continuity of care over time as the client moves to various care settings and is revised as necessary.

Standard VI. Intervention

The nurse, guided by the plan of care, intervenes to provide care to restore the older person's functional capabilities and to prevent complications and excess disability. Nursing interventions are derived from nursing diagnoses and are based on gerontological nursing theory.

Standard VII. Evaluation

The nurse continually evaluates the client's and family's responses to interventions to determine progress toward goal attainment and to revise the data base, nursing diagnoses, and plan of care.

Standard VIII. Interdisciplinary Collaboration

The nurse collaborates with other members of the health-care team in the various settings in which care is given to the older person. The team meets regularly to evaluate the effectiveness of the care plan for the client and family and to adjust the plan of care to accommodate to the changing needs of the patient.

Standard IX. Research

The nurse participates in research designed to generate an organized body of gerontological nursing knowledge, disseminates research findings, and uses them in practice.

Standard X. Ethics

The nurse uses the code for nurses established by the American Nurses Association as a guide for ethical decision-making in practice.

Standard XI. Professional Development

The nurse assumes responsibility for professional development and contributes to the professional growth of interdisciplinary team members. The nurse participates in peer review and other means of evaluation to ensure the quality of nursing practice.

From American Nurses Association. Standards and Scope of Gerontological Nursing. Kansas City: American Nurses Association, 1987:3.

Pattern 1: Exchanging

Airway clearance, ineffective
Aspiration, high risk for
Body temperature, altered: high risk for
Bowel incontinence
Breathing pattern, ineffective
Cardiac output, altered: decreased
Constipation
Constipation, colonic
Constipation, perceived
Diarrhea
Disuse syndrome, high risk for
Dysreflexia
Fluid volume, altered: excess
Fluid volume deficit: actual
Fluid volume deficit: high risk for
Gas exchange, impaired
Hyperthermia
Hypothermia
Incontinence, functional/reflex/stress/total/urge
Infection, high risk for
Injury, high risk for
Nutrition, altered: less/more than body require-
    ments
Oral mucous membrane, altered
Poisoning, high risk for
Skin integrity, impaired: actual
Skin integrity, impaired: high risk for
Suffocation, high risk for
Thermoregulation, ineffective
Tissue integrity, impaired
Tissue perfusion, altered
Trauma, high risk for
Urinary elimination, altered
Urinary retention

Pattern 2: Communicating

Verbal communication, impaired

Pattern 3: Relating

Family processes, altered
Parental role conflict
Parenting, altered: actual
Parenting, altered: high risk for
Role performance, altered
Sexual dysfunction
Sexuality patterns, altered
Social interaction, impaired
Social isolation

Pattern 4: Valuing

Spiritual distress

Pattern 5: Choosing

Adjustment, impaired
Coping, defensive
Coping, ineffective family: compromised/disabling
Coping, ineffective individual
Decisional conflict (specify)
Denial, ineffective
Health-seeking behaviors (specify)
Noncompliance (specify)

Pattern 6: Moving

Activity intolerance, actual
Activity intolerance, high risk for
Breastfeeding, ineffective
Diversionary activity deficit
Fatigue
Growth and development, altered
Health maintenance, altered
Home maintenance management, impaired
Mobility, impaired physical
Self-care deficit (specify)
Sleep pattern disturbance
Swallowing, impaired

Pattern 7: Perceiving

Hopelessness
Neglect, unilateral
Powerlessness
Self-concept, disturbance in body image/personal
    identity, self-esteem
Self-esteem, chronic low/situational low
Sensory-perceptual alteration (specify)

Pattern 8: Knowing

Knowledge deficit (specify)
Thought processes, altered

Pattern 9: Feeling

Anxiety
Fear
Grieving, anticipatory/dysfunctional
Pain
Pain, chronic
Posttraumatic response
Rape trauma syndrome
Violence, high risk for: self-directed or directed at
    others

Principles Guiding Care

Scientific data regarding theories, life adjustments, and age-related changes combined with selected information from psychology, sociology, biology, and other physical and social sciences are used in providing specialized care to the older population. It is the responsibility of professional nurses to use these scientific data as the foundation for nursing practice and ensure through educational and supervisory means that others responsible for care also use this base of knowledge.

Data from a variety of disciplines are incorporated in the development of nursing principles—proven facts or theories that are accepted by society and direct nursing actions. In addition to the basic principles that guide the delivery of care to persons in general, specific principles are applied for the care of individuals in certain age groups or with particular health problems. Some of the principles guiding gerontological nursing practice appear in Display 1-3 and are described below.

DISPLAY 1-3   Principles Guiding Gerontological Nursing Practice

Aging is a natural process common to all living organisms.

Heredity, nutrition, health status, life experiences, environment, activity, and stress are factors that influence the aging process and demonstrate unique effects in each person.

Scientific data related to normal aging and unique psychobiosocial characteristics of older persons are combined with general nursing knowledge in the application of the nursing process to the older population.

Older adults share similar universal self-care demands with all other human beings, and each possesses unique capabilities and limitations in fulfilling those demands.

The focus of gerontological nursing is to take action in a planned, organized, and therapeutic manner to:

Strengthen self-care capacity

Eliminate or minimize self-care limitations

Provide direct-care services by acting for, doing for, or partially assisting when needs cannot be fulfilled independently.

Aging is a natural process common to all living organisms. Every living organism begins aging from the time of conception. The process of aging helps individuals achieve the mature cellular, organ, and system functioning necessary for the accomplishment of developmental tasks throughout life. Constantly and continuously, every cell of every organism ages. Despite the normality and naturalness of this experience, many people approach aging as though it is a pathological experience. It is not unusual to hear people describe aging as a period of any of the following:

- "getting senile"
- "looking gray and wrinkled"
- "losing health and independence"
- "becoming inflexible and demanding"
- "having less satisfaction from life"
- "returning to childlike behavior"
- "being useless."

These are hardly valid descriptions of the outcomes of aging for most people. Aging is not a crippling disease; although some limitations may be imposed as the body systems lose efficiency in function, aging itself does not reduce the opportunity for happiness, fulfillment, and independence. An increased understanding of the aging process may promote a more positive attitude toward old age.

A variety of factors influence the normal aging process. Heredity, nutrition, health status, life experiences, environment, activity, and stress demonstrate unique effects in each individual. Among the variety of factors either known or thought to affect the usual pattern of aging, inherited factors are believed by some researchers to produce chromosomal alterations that cause cells to age at a particular rate. Malnourishment can hasten the ill effects of the aging process, as can exposure to environmental toxins, diseases, and stress. Alternately, mental, physical, and social activity may reduce the rate and degree of declining function with age. Some of the theories of aging are described in Chapter 2.

Every person ages in an individualized manner, although some general characteristics may be evident among most people in a given age category. Just as we would not assume that all people 30 years of age are identical and would evaluate, approach, and communicate with each person in an

individualized manner, we must recognize that no two persons 60, 70, or 80 years of age are alike. Nurses must understand the multitude of factors that can influence the aging process and the unique outcomes for each individual.

Unique data and knowledge are used in applying the nursing process to the older population. In nursing the elderly, scientific data related to normal aging and the unique psychobiosocial characteristics of the older person are combined with a general knowledge of nursing. The nursing process provides a systematic approach to the delivery of nursing service, which integrates a wide range of knowledge and skills. The scope of nursing includes more than following a medical order or performing an isolated task; the nursing process involves a holistic approach to individuals and the care they require. The following four activities form the foundation of the nursing process:

1. Assessment
2. Planning
3. Implementation
4. Evaluation.

The physiological and psychological differences and unique socioeconomic problems of the elderly are considered in every step of the nursing process.

The elderly share similar universal self-care demands with all other human beings. As categorized by Dorothea Orem, these demands are as follows: (Orem, 1980)

- air
- water
- food

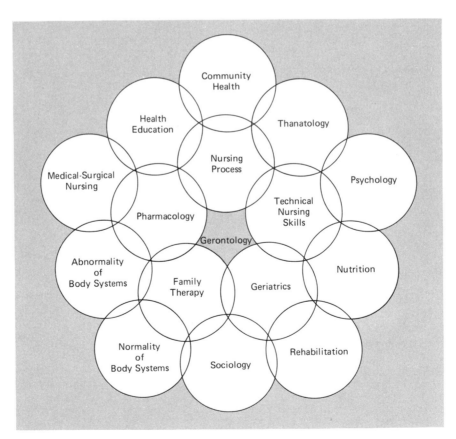

Figure 1-1. *Information system of the gerontological nurse.*

- excretion
- activity and rest
- solitude and social interaction
- avoidance of hazards to life and well-being
- being normal.

Through self-care practices, people usually perform activities independently and voluntarily to meet these life demands. When an unusual circumstance interferes with the individual's ability to meet these demands, nursing assistance may be warranted. The requirements for these needs and specific problems that the elderly may experience in fulfilling them are discussed in Unit II.

The focus of gerontological nursing is to take planned, organized, and therapeutic nursing action. Nursing actions are directed toward the following:

Strengthening the individual's self-care capacity.
Eliminating or minimizing self-care limitations.
Providing direct services by acting for, doing for, or assisting the individual when demands cannot be met independently.
Maintaining independence as much as possible. Although it may be more time consuming and difficult, allowing maximum independence of older persons in their care activities produces many advantages for their physical, mental, and social health.

These principles are basic to the nursing care of older adults and form a foundation for developing a specialized practice. A truly professional gerontological nurse demonstrates a distinct and effective blend of cognitive and technical skills to achieve excellence in gerontological care. Only by using sound valid data and independent problem solving for nursing issues can nurses surpass the technical level of practice and attain the realm of expert, professional care of the elderly.

Today a growing number of nurses are recognizing the complexities and challenges of gerontological nursing. Few other specialties provide an opportunity for nurses to blend knowledge and skills from so many disciplines (Fig. 1-1). The broad scope of gerontological nursing allows nurses to contribute to the care of the elderly in acute, community, and long-term care settings through direct clinical practice, education, research, and administrative or advocacy activities. Entering the specialty of gerontological nursing ensures a unique, challenging, and rewarding career for its practitioners.

References

Bishop LF. Relation of old age to disease with illustrative cases. Am J Nurs 1904;4(4):674.

DeWitt K. The old nurse. Am J Nurs 1904;4(4):177.

Orem D. Nursing: concepts of practice, 2nd ed. New York, McGraw-Hill, 1980.

Recommended Readings

American Nurses Association. Standards and scope of gerontological nursing practice. Kansas City, American Nurses Association, 1987.

Brock AM. Economics of aging. In: Murrow E, ed. Perspectives on gerontological nursing. Newbury Park, CA: SAGE, 1991:170.

Brower HT. Gerontological nursing: movement towards a paradigm state. J Prof Nurs 1988;1(6):328.

Dossey BM, Keegan L, Guzzetta CE, Kolkmeier LG. Holistic nursing: a handbook for practice. Rockville, MD: Aspen, 1988.

Dychtwald K, Flower J. Age wave: the challenges and opportunities of an aging America. Los Angeles: Jeremy P Tarcher, 1989.

Fowles D. A profile of older Americans. Washington, DC: American Association of Retired Persons, 1990.

Futrell M. Professional certification and gerontological nursing. J Gerontol Nurs 1990;16:3.

Peterson MD, White DL, eds. Health care of the elderly: an information source book. Newbury Park, CA: SAGE, 1989.

Rempusheski VF. Historical and futuristic perspectives on aging and gerontological nursing. In: Murrow E, ed. Perspectives on gerontological nursing. Newbury Park, CA: SAGE, 1991:3.

Specht JS. Nursing diagnosis: Key to improved care for the elderly (editorial). J Gerontol Nurs 1988;14(3):7.

2

Theories of Aging

For centuries people have been intrigued by the mystery of aging, some in hopes of achieving everlasting youth, others of discovering the key to immortality. Throughout history there have been numerous searches for a fountain of youth, the most famous being that of Ponce de León. Ancient Egyptian and Chinese relics show evidence of concoctions designed to prolong life or achieve immortality, and various other cultures have proposed specific dietary regimens, herbal mixtures, and rituals for similar ends. Ancient life-expanders, such as extracts prepared from tiger testicles, may seem ludicrous until they are compared with more modern-day measures such as injections of embryonic tissue and novocaine. Even persons who would not condone such peculiar practices may indulge in a specific brand of yogurt, megavitamins, cosmetic creams, and exotic spas that promise to maintain youth and delay the onset of old age.

No single known factor causes or prevents aging; the complexities of this process cannot be explained by one theory. Explorations into biological, psychological, and social aging continue, and although some of this interest focuses on achieving eternal youth, most sound research efforts are aimed toward gaining a better understanding of this process so people can age in a healthier fashion and postpone some of the negative consequences of growing old. In fact, there is a growing cry for research that promotes the compression of morbidity, whereby research and technology priorities shift from life-extension to postponement of the onset of chronic disease, that is, efforts to keep people healthy and active for a longer period of time rather than keeping them alive for a longer period of time.(Fries, 1988) Recognizing that aging theories offer varying degrees of universality, validity, and reliability, nurses can use this information to better understand the factors that may positively and negatively influence the health and well-being of persons of all ages.

Biological Theories

The process of biological aging not only differs from species to species but also from one human being to another. Some general statements can be made concerning anticipated organ changes, as described in Chapter 6; however, no two individuals will age identically. Varying degrees of physiological changes, capacities, and limitations will be found within a given age group. The rate of aging among different body systems within one individual may vary, with one system showing marked decline while another demonstrates no significant change. To explain biological aging, theorists have explored many factors, both internal and external to the human body.

Genetic Factors

Several theorists believe people inherit a genetic program that determines their specific life expectancy. In fact, various studies have shown a positive relationship between parental age and filial

life span. Studies of *in vitro* cell proliferation have demonstrated that various species have a finite number of cell divisions. Fibroblasts from embryonic tissue experienced a greater number of cell divisions than those derived from adult tissue, and among various species, the longer the life span, the greater the number of cell divisions. These studies support the belief that senescence is under genetic control and occurs at the cellular level.(Hayflick, 1983; Coni, Davison, and Webster, 1984)

Genetic mutations, described under the error theory, also are thought to be responsible for aging by causing organ decline as a result of self-perpetuating cellular mutations:

Mutation of DNA.
↓
Perpetuation of mutation
during cell division.
↓
Increasing number of mutant
cells in body.
↓
Malfunction of tissues,
organs, and systems.
↓
Decline in body functions.

Some theorists think that a growth substance fails to be produced, which results in the cessation of cell growth and reproduction, whereas others hypothesize that an aging factor responsible for development and cellular maturity throughout life is excessively produced, thereby hastening aging. Cross-linking of DNA strands is hypothesized by some to impair the cell's ability to function and divide. Although minimal research has been done to support this theory, aging may be a result of a decreased ability of RNA to synthesize and translate messages.

Cross-Linking

This theory proposes that cellular division is threatened as a result of a chemical reaction in which a cross-linking agent attaches itself to a DNA strand and prevents normal parting of the strands during mitosis. Over time, as these cross-linking agents accumulate, they form dense aggregates that impede intracellular transport; ultimately, the body's organs and systems fail. An effect of cross-linking on collagen (an important connective tissue

in the lungs, heart, vessels, and muscle) is the reduction in tissue elasticity associated with many age-related changes.

Free Radicals

Free radicals are highly reactive molecules generated from oxygen metabolism. These molecules can damage proteins, enzymes, and DNA by replacing molecules that contain useful biological information with faulty molecules that create genetic disorder. It is believed that these free radicals are self-perpetuating, in that they generate other free radicals. Physical decline of the body occurs as the damage from these molecules accumulates over time.

Lipofuscin

Considerable interest has been given to the role in the aging process of lipofuscin "age pigments," a lipoprotein byproduct of metabolism that can only be seen under a fluorescent microscope. Because lipofuscin is associated with oxidation of unsaturated lipids, it is believed to have a role similar to free radicals in the aging process. As lipofuscin accumulates, it interferes with the diffusion and transport of essential metabolites and information-bearing molecules in the cells. A positive relationship exists between an individual's age and the amount of lipofuscin in the body. Investigators have discovered the presence of lipofuscin in other species at amounts proportionate to the life span of the species (*e.g.,* an animal with one-tenth the life span of a human being accumulates lipofuscin at a rate approximately 10 times greater than human beings).

Autoimmune Reactions

The primary organs of the immune system are believed to be affected by the aging process. The immune response declines after young adulthood. The weight of the thymus decreases, as does the ability to produce T-cell differentiation. The bone marrow stem cells perform less efficiently. Some theorists believe that the reduction in immunologic activities leads to an increase in autoimmune response with age. One hypothesis regarding the role of autoimmune reactions in the aging process is that the body misidentifies aged, irregular cells as foreign agents and attacks them.

Cells undergo changes with age.
↓
Body perceives these cells as foreign substances.
↓
Antibodies are formed to attack and
rid body of foreign substances.
↓
Cells die.

Another reason for this reaction could be related to the breakdown of the body's immuno-chemical memory system, which causes it to misinterpret normal body constituents.

Cells are normal.
↓
Immunochemical memory system dysfunctions
and perceives cells as foreign substances.
↓
Antibodies are formed to attack
and rid body of foreign substances.
↓
Cells die.

Wear and Tear

This theory attributes aging to the wear and tear of the body as it performs its highly specialized functions over time. Like any complicated machine, the body will function less efficiently with prolonged use and numerous insults.

Stress

In recent years, the effects of stress on physical and psychological health have been widely discussed. Stresses to the body can have adverse effects and lead to conditions such as gastric ulcers, heart attacks, and thyroiditis. However, this theory is limited in its universality because individuals react differently to life's stresses—one person may be overwhelmed by a moderately busy schedule, whereas another may become uncomfortable when faced with a slow, dull pace.

Disease

Bacteria, fungi, viruses, and other organisms are thought to be responsible for certain physiological changes during the aging process. Although no conclusive evidence exists to link these pathogens with the body's decline, interest in this theory has been stimulated by the fact that human beings and animals have enjoyed longer life expectancies with the control or elimination of certain pathogens through immunization and the use of antimicrobial drugs.

Radiation

The relationship of radiation and age continues to be explored. Research with rats, mice, and dogs has shown a decreased life span results from nonlethal doses of radiation.(Lints, 1978) In human beings, repeated exposure to ultraviolet light is known to cause solar elastosis, the "old-age" type of skin wrinkling that results from the replacement of collagen by elastin; ultraviolet light also is a factor in the development of skin cancer. Radiation may induce cellular mutations that promote aging.

Nutrition

The importance of good nutrition at all ages is a theme hard to escape in our nutrition-conscious society. It is believed that what we eat has a significant influence on how we age. Experiments with underfed fish have shown their growth rate to be retarded, which results in an unusually longer life span.(Walford, 1986) Underfed rats also have proven to live longer than their overfed cohorts, who age at a faster rate.(Walford, 1986) Human obesity is said to shorten life, a view supported by insurance statistics and the high prevalence of certain diseases in overweight persons.

The quality of diet is as important as the quantity. Deficiencies of vitamins and other nutrients and excesses of nutrients such as cholesterol may cause various disease processes. Although the complete relationship between diet and aging is not well understood, enough is known to suggest that a good diet may minimize or eliminate some of the ill effects of the aging process.

Environment

Several environmental factors are known to threaten health and are thought to be associated with the aging process. The ingestion of mercury, lead, arsenic, radioactive isotopes, certain pesticides, and other substances can produce pathological changes in human beings. Smoking and breathing tobacco smoke and other air pollutants have adverse effects. Crowded living conditions,

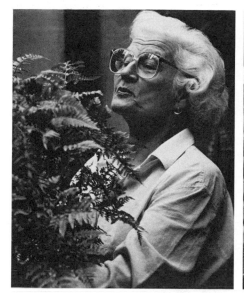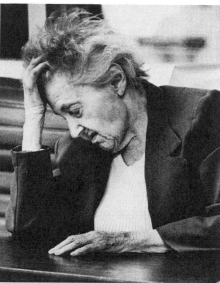

Aging is a highly individualized process, demonstrated by the differences between persons of similar ages. (Photograph by Eric Schenk.)

high noise levels, and other factors are thought to influence how we age.(Selye, 1976)

The number, diversity, and complexity of factors that potentially influence the aging process show that no one biological theory can adequately explain the cause of this phenomenon. Even when studies have been done with populations known to have a high life expectancy, such as the people of the Caucasus region in southern Russia, longevity has not been attributable to any single factor. These theories are significant to nursing. Nurses can adapt these theories by identifying elements known to influence aging and using them as a foundation to promote positive practices.

Psychosocial Theories

Psychological and social changes during the aging process are closely united, and they have a significant impact on each other. It is difficult to explain mental processes, behavior, and feelings without the perspective of social roles, positions, and norms. A purely social or psychological theory of aging would be most unusual; therefore, it is more useful to approach this discussion under the umbrella of psychosocial theories.

Disengagement Theory

One of the earliest, most controversial, and widely discussed theories is the disengagement theory, developed by Elaine Cumming and William Henry. (Cumming and Henry, 1961; Cumming, 1964) This theory views aging as a process whereby society and the individual gradually withdraw, or disengage, from each other, to the mutual satisfaction and benefit of both. The benefit to individuals is that they can reflect and be centered on themselves, having been freed from societal roles. The value of disengagement for society is that some orderly means is established for the transfer of power from the old to the young, making it possible for society to continue functioning after its individual members have died.

The theory does not indicate whether it is society or the individual who initiates the disengagement process, but several difficulties with this concept are obvious. Many older persons are highly satisfied to remain engaged and do not want their primary satisfaction to be derived from reflection on younger years. Senators, Supreme Court justices, and college professors are among those who commonly derive satisfaction and provide a valuable service for society by not disengaging. Because

the health of the individual, cultural practices, societal norms, and other factors influence the degree to which a person will participate in society during their later years, some critics of this theory claim that disengagement would not be necessary if society improved the health care and financial means of the aged and increased the acceptance, opportunities, and respect afforded them.

A careful examination of the population studied in the development of the disengagement theory hints at its limitations. The disengagement pattern that Cumming and Henry described was based on a study of 172 middle-class persons between 48 and 68 years of age. This group was wealthier, better educated, and of higher occupational and residential prestige than the general aged population. No blacks or chronically ill persons were involved in the study. Caution is advisable in generalizing findings for the entire aged population based on fewer than 200 persons who are generally not representative of the average aged person. Although nurses should appreciate that some older individuals may wish to disengage from the mainstream of society, this is not necessarily a process to be expected from all aged persons.

Activity Theory

At the opposite pole from the disengagement theory, the activity theory proclaims that an older person should continue a middle-aged life-style, denying the existence of old age as long as possible, and that society should apply the same norms to old age as it does to middle age and not advocate diminishing activity, interest, and involvement as its members grow old.(Havighurst, 1963) This theory suggests ways of maintaining activity in the presence of multiple losses associated with the aging process, including substituting intellectual activities for physical activities when physical capacity is reduced, replacing the work role with other roles when retirement occurs, and establishing new friendships when old ones are lost. Declining health, loss of roles, reduced income, a shrinking circle of friends, and other obstacles to maintaining an active life are to be resisted and overcome instead of being accepted.

This theory has some merit. Activity is generally assumed to be more desirable than inactivity because it facilitates physical, mental, and social well-being. Like a self-fulfilling prophecy, the expectation of a continued active state during old age may

be realized. Because of society's negative view of inactivity and acting old, it is probably best to encourage an active life-style among the aged to be consistent with societal values. Also supportive of the activity theory is the reluctance of many older persons to accept themselves as old, although one of its problems is the assumption that most older people desire and are able to maintain a middle-aged life-style. Some want their world to shrink to accommodate their decreasing capacities or their preference for less active roles. Many elderly people lack the physical, emotional, social, or economic resources to maintain active roles in society. Aged people who are expected to maintain an active middle-aged life-style on a retirement income of less than one-half that of middle-aged people may wonder if society isn't giving them conflicting messages. More must be learned regarding the effects on the elderly of not being able to fulfill expectations to remain active.

Continuity Theory

The continuity theory of aging, also referred to as the developmental theory, relates the factors of personality and predisposition toward certain actions in old age to similar factors during other phases of the life cycle.(Neugarten, 1964) Personality and basic patterns of behavior are said to remain unchanged as the individual ages. Activists at 20 years of age will most likely be activists at 70 years of age, whereas young recluses will probably not be active in the mainstream of society when they age. Concepts and patterns developed over a lifetime will determine whether individuals remain engaged and active or become disengaged and inactive. The recognition that the unique features of each individual allow for multiple adaptations to aging and that the potential exists for a variety of reactions give this theory validity and support. Aging is a complex process, and the continuity theory considers these complexities to a greater extent than most other theories. Although the implications and impact of this promising theory are uncertain because it is in an early stage of research, it should be closely followed.

Developmental Tasks

Several theorists have described the process of healthy psychosocial aging as resulting from the successful fulfillment of developmental tasks. De-

velopmental tasks are the challenges that must be met and adjustments that must be made in response to life experiences that are part of an adult's continued growth through the life span.

Erik Erikson described eight stages that human beings progress through from infancy to old age and the challenges, or tasks, that confront individuals during those stages (Table 2-1).(Erikson, 1963) The challenge of old age is to accept and find meaning in the life the person has lived; this gives the individual ego integrity that aids in adjusting and coping with the reality of aging and mortality. Feelings of anger, bitterness, depression, and inadequacy can result in inadequate ego integrity (*e.g.*, despair).

Robert Peck refined Erikson's description of old age tasks by detailing three specific challenges facing the elderly, which influence the outcome of ego integrity or despair:(Peck, 1968)

1. Ego differentiation versus role preoccupation: to develop satisfactions from one's self as a person rather than through parental or occupational roles.
2. Body transcendence versus body preoccupation: to find psychological pleasures rather than becoming absorbed with health problems or physical limitations imposed by aging.
3. Ego transcendence versus ego preoccupation: to achieve satisfaction through reflection on one's past life and accomplishments rather than to be preoccupied with the finite number of years left to live.

Robert Butler and Myrna Lewis have outlined the major tasks of later life to be the following:(Butler and Lewis, 1982)

- adjusting to one's infirmities
- developing a sense of satisfaction with the life that has been lived
- preparing for death.

Gerontological nurses play a significant role in assisting aging persons to find satisfaction and a sense of well-being in later life. In addition to specific measures that can assist the elderly in meeting their psychosocial challenges (Display 2-1), nursing staff must be sensitive to the tremendous impact their own attitudes toward aging can have on patients. Nursing staff who consider aging as a progressive decline ending in death may view old age as a depressing, useless period, and foster hopelessness and helplessness in older patients. On the other hand, staff who view aging as a process of continued development may appreciate old age as an opportunity to gain new satisfaction and understanding, thereby promoting joy and a sense of purpose in patients.

To an extent, the biological, psychological, and social processes of aging are interrelated and interdependent. Frequently, loss of a social role alters an individual's drives and speeds their physical decline. Poor health may force retirement from work, promoting social isolation and the development of a weakened self-concept. Although certain changes occur independently as separate events, most are closely associated with other age-related factors. It is impractical, therefore, to subscribe solely to one theory of aging. Wise nurses will be open minded in choosing the aging theories they will use in the care of older adults; they will also be cognizant of the limitations of these theories.

Table 2-1. *Erikson's Developmental Tasks*

STAGE	SATISFACTORILY FULFILLED	UNSATISFACTORILY FULFILLED
Infancy	Trust	Mistrust
Toddler	Autonomy	Shame
Early childhood	Initiative	Guilt
Middle childhood	Industry	Inferiority
Adolescence	Identity	Identity diffusion
Adulthood	Intimacy	Isolation
Middle age	Generativity	Self-absorption
Old age	Integrity	Despair

DISPLAY 2-1   *Assisting Individuals in Meeting the Psychosocial Challenges of Aging*

Overview

As individuals progress through their life span they face challenges and adjustments in response to life experiences called developmental tasks. These developmental tasks can be described as:

- coping with losses and changes
- establishing meaningful roles
- exercising independence and control
- finding meaning in life.

Satisfaction with oneself and the life one has lived is gained by successfully meeting these tasks; unhappiness, bitterness, and fear of one's future can result from not adjusting to and rejecting the realities of aging.

Goal

The aging persons will express a sense of ego integrity and psychosocial well-being.

Actions

Learn about patients' family backgrounds, work histories, hobbies, achievements, and life experiences. Encourage patients to discuss these topics and listen with sincere interest.

Build on lifelong interests and offer opportunities for patients to experience new pleasures and interests.

Accept patients' discussions of their regrets and dissatisfactions. Help them to put these in perspective of their total lives and accomplishments.

Encourage reminiscence activities between patients and their families. Help families and staff to understand the therapeutic value of reminiscence.

Use humor therapeutically.

If patients reside in an institutional setting, personalize the environment to the maximum degree possible.

Recognize the unique assets and characteristics of each patient.

References

Butler RN, Lewis MI. Aging and mental health. 3rd ed. St Louis: CV Mosby, 1982:142, 376.

Coni N, Davison W, Webster S. Aging: the facts. New York: Oxford, 1984.

Cumming E. New thoughts on the theory of disengagement. In: Kastenbaum R, ed. New thoughts on old age. New York: Springer-Verlag, 1964.

Cumming E, Henry E. Growing old: the process of disengagement. New York: Basic Books, 1961.

Erikson E. Childhood and society. 2nd ed. New York: WW Norton, 1963.

Fries JF. Aging, illness, and health policy: implications of the compression of morbidity. Perspect Biol Med Spring 1988;31:408.

Havighurst J. Successful aging. In: Williams RH, Tibbitts C, Donahue W, eds. Processes of aging. vol. 1. New York: Atherton Press, 1963:299.

Hayflick L. Theories of aging. In: Cape R, Coe R, Rossman I, eds. Fundamentals of geriatric medicine. New York: Raven, 1983:32.

Lints FA. Genetics and aging. Basel, Switzerland: S Karger, 1978.

Neugarten L. Personality in middle and late life. New York: Atherton Press, 1964.

Peck R. Psychological developments in the second half of life. In: Neugarten B, ed. Middle age and aging. Chicago: University of Chicago, 1968:88.

Selye H. The stress of life. New York: McGraw-Hill, 1976.

Walford RL. The 120 year diet: how to double your vital years. New York: PocketBooks, 1986.

Recommended Readings

Atchley R. Social forces in later life. Belmont, CA: Wadsworth, 1988.

Kent B, Butler RN, eds. Human aging research: concepts and techniques. New York: Raven, 1988.

Schultz R, Ewen RB. Adult development and aging: myths and emerging realities. New York: Macmillan, 1988.

Spence AP. Biology of human aging. Englewood Cliffs, NJ: Prentice-Hall, 1989.

3

Ethnicity

People from a variety of countries have ventured to America to seek a better life in a new land. To an extent, they assimilated and adopted the American way of life; however, the values and customs instilled in them by their native cultures were too deeply ingrained to be erased, and their language and biological heterogeneity were often obvious. The unique backgrounds of these newcomers to America influenced the way they reacted to the world around them and the manner in which that world reacted to them. To understand the uniqueness of each older adult encountered, consideration must be given to the influences of ethnic origin.

Members of an ethnic group share similar history, language, customs, and characteristics; they also hold distinct beliefs about aging and the elderly. Although individual differences within a given ethnic group exist and stereotypes should not be made, an understanding of the general characteristics of various ethnic groups can assist nurses in providing more individualized care.

Native Americans

Native Americans inhabited North America for centuries before Christopher Columbus explored the new world. An estimated 1 to 1½ million Native Americans populated America at the time of Columbus' arrival; many battles with the new settlers during the next four centuries reduced the Native American population to ¼ million. The Native American population has been steadily increasing, with the Census Bureau now showing nearly 1 million Native Americans who belong to the 493 recognized tribes in the United States. Approximately one-half of all Native Americans live on reservations, with the highest populations found in Arizona, Oklahoma, California, New Mexico, and Alaska. An estimated 250 different Native American languages are spoken, although most Native Americans claim English to be their first language. Approximately 5% of the Native American population is older than 65 years of age.

The Native Americans have a strong reverence for the Great Creator. They often link their state of health to good or evil forces or to punishment for their acts. Spiritual rituals, homemade drugs, and mechanical interventions such as suction cups may be used for the treatment of illness.

Close family bonds are typical among the Native American population. Family members may address each other by their family relationship rather than name (e.g., cousin, son, uncle, grandfather). Elders are respected and viewed as leaders, teachers, and advisors to the young, although younger and more "Americanized" members are starting to feel that the elders' advice is not as relevant in today's world and are breaking with this tradition. Native Americans strongly believe that individuals have the right to make decisions affecting their lives. The typical nursing assessment process may be offensive to the Native American patient, who may view probing questions, validation of findings, and documentation of responses as inappropriate

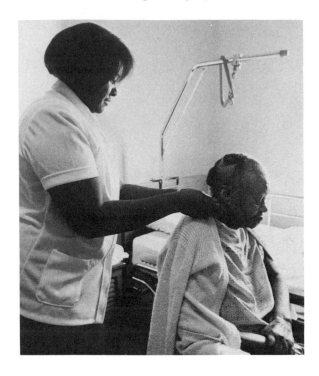

Although they possess a lower life expentancy than white Americans, black Americans can survive as long as their white counterparts once they reach old age. (Photo by Kathy Sloan.)

and disrespectful behaviors during the verbal exchange. The Native American patient may be ambivalent about accepting services from agencies and professionals. Such assistance has provided many social, health, and economic benefits to improve the life of the Native American, but it also conflicts with Native American beliefs of being useful, doing for oneself, and relying on spiritual powers to chart the course of life. Native American patients often will remain calm and controlled, even in the most difficult circumstances; it is important that providers not mistake this behavior for the absence of feeling, caring, or discomfort.

Various tribes may have specific rituals that are performed at death, such as burying certain personal possessions with the individual. Consulting with members of the specific tribe to gain insight into special rituals during sickness and at death would be advantageous for nurses working with Native American patients.

Black Americans

Approximately 12% of the United States population is black, and most of this group are of African descent. It is believed that a free black man, Pedro

Alonso Nino, accompanied Columbus on his 1492 voyage to America; however, most of the early experiences of blacks in this country occurred in the form of slavery. Displacement from families and tribes as they were sold into slavery, insults suffered through discrimination, and strong religious beliefs were major factors influencing the black population's deep commitment to the family and aged family members. The family could be depended on to aid and comfort its members in the face of the prejudices and hardships of society. Historically, black Americans have experienced a lower standard of living and less access to health care than their white counterparts. This is reflected in the lower life expectancies of black Americans (see demographics in Chap. 1). For black men, life expectancy has slightly decreased in recent years. However, once a black individual reaches the seventh decade of life, survival begins to equal that of similarly aged whites; this is referred to as the cross-over phenomenon.(National Institute on Aging, 1980)

To survive to old age is considered a major accomplishment that reflects strength, resourcefulness, and faith to this ethnic group; thus, old age is a personal triumph to blacks, not a dreaded curse.

Considering their history, it should not be surprising to find that black elderly:

Possess many health problems that have accumulated over a lifetime due to a poor standard of living and limited access to health-care services.

Hold beliefs and practice measures, which may be unconventional, to stay healthy and treat illness.

Look to family members for decision-making and care before using formal service agencies.

May have a degree of caution in interacting with and using health services, as a defense against prejudice.

Diverse subgroups within the black population, such as the Haitians, Tahitians, and Jamaicans, each possess their own unique customs and beliefs. Differences can be apparent even among black Americans from various regions of the United States. Nurses should be sensitive to the fact that the lack of awareness and respect for these differences can be interpreted as a demeaning or prejudicial sign.

Black skin color is the result of a high melanin content and can complicate the use of skin color for the assessment of health problems. To effec-tively diagnose cyanosis, for instance, examine the nail beds, palms, soles, gums, and under the tongue. The absence of a red tone or glow to the skin can indicate pallor. Petechiae are best detected on the conjunctiva, abdomen, and buccal mucosa.

Hypertension is a major health problem among black Americans and occurs at a higher rate than in the white population. One of the factors responsible for this problem is blunted nocturnal response. Only a minor decline in blood pressure occurs during sleep, which increases the strain on the heart and vessels; this is found to occur in the black population more than any other group. Blood pressure monitoring is an important preventive measure for black clients.

Despite the health problems of aged blacks, their rate of institutionalization is lower than that of the white population: only 12% of elderly blacks are in an institutional setting compared to 23% of elderly whites.

Jewish Americans

In the sense that they come from a variety of nations, with different customs and cultures, Jews are not an ethnic group *per se.* However, the strength of the Jewish faith forms a bond that

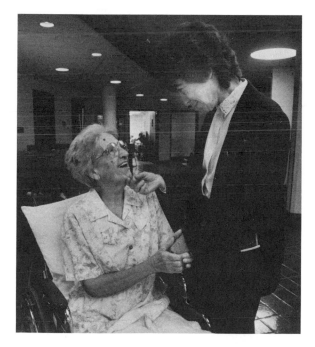

A message of sensitivity and caring is conveyed when nurses make an effort to recognize and support patients' ethnic backgrounds. (From Birchenall JM. Care of the Older Adult. 3rd ed. Philadelphia: JB Lippincott, 1993.)

crosses national origin and gives this group a strong sense of identity and shared beliefs.

Luis de Torres, a Jew, accompanied Columbus on his voyage to America; however, it was not until 1654 that a group of Sephardic Jews settled in New Amsterdam to formally develop the first Jewish community in America. Immigration continued after that time, with large numbers of German Jews entering America after the revolution of 1848, followed by even greater numbers of Yiddish-speaking Eastern European Jews arriving after the pogroms of 1881. Early life in America was not easy for these Jewish immigrants—they often were faced with employment in factories and homes in tenements, as well as prejudice from several quarters. Despite these rough beginnings, Jewish Americans have demonstrated profound leadership in business, arts, and sciences and have made positive contributions to American life. Scholarship is important in the Jewish culture: more than 80% of all Jewish Americans have attended college. Approximately 7 million Jews reside in the United States, with most living in urban areas of the mid-Atlantic states. It is estimated that one-half of the world's Jewish population resides in America.

Religious traditions are important to most Jews. Sundown Friday to sundown Saturday is the Sabbath, and medical procedures may be opposed during that time (exceptions may be made for seriously ill individuals). A belief that the head and feet should always be covered may be displayed by the desire to wear a skullcap and socks at all times. Orthodox Jews may oppose shaving. The Kosher diet (e.g., exclusion of pork and shellfish, prohibition of serving milk and meat products at the same meal or from the same dishes) is a significant aspect of Jewish religion and may be strictly adhered to by some. Fasting on holy days, such as Yom Kippur and Tisha Bab, and the replacement of matzo for leavened bread during Passover may occur.

Modern medical care is encouraged. Rabbinical consultation may be desired for decisions involving organ transplantation or life-sustaining measures. Certain rituals may be practiced at death, such as members of the religious group washing the body and sitting with it until burial. Autopsy is usually opposed.

Family bonds are strong among Jewish Americans; they have strong and positive feelings for the elderly. Jewish communities throughout the country have shown leadership in developing a network of community and institutional services for their aged, geared toward providing service while preserving Jewish tradition.

Chinese Americans

Although Chinese laborers probably lived in America for centuries before the mid-1800s, it was not until then that large-scale Chinese immigration occurred. During that time, more than 40,000 Chinese left their homes to escape the horrible drought that China was experiencing and to become part of the gold rush. They were welcomed as cheap labor for the transcontinental railroad construction; at that time 9 of every 10 railroad laborers were "coolies." Most of these Chinese laborers planned to earn large sums of money and then return home or send for their families to join them. Few were able to attain this goal, and they found that the poor economic conditions toward the end of the 19th century made them easy targets for prejudice by persons afraid that these "foreigners" were stealing their jobs; they were left in their new land alone and poor. This immigration pattern explains why older Chinese men in America outnumber older Chinese women. Prejudice and cultural differences promoted the development of "Chinatowns," which were a comfortable refuge for the Chinese in this country. The largest American Chinese populations are in San Francisco, New York, Los Angeles, Honolulu, and Chicago.

Care of the body and health are of utmost important to the Chinese. There is a belief in the balance of yin and yang—yin is the female negative energy that protects the inner body, and yang is the male positive energy that protects the body from external forces. Traditionally, the Chinese have used the senses for assessing medical problems (touching, listening to sounds, detecting odors) rather than machinery or invasive procedures. Herbs, acupuncture, acupressure, and other treatment modalities, which are just being recognized by the western world, continue to be treatments of choice for many Chinese individuals. These traditional treatments may be selected as alternatives or adjuncts to the use of modern treatment modalities. Ivory figurines of reclining women, now collectors' items, were used by female patients to point to the area of their problems because it was inappropriate for the male physician to touch

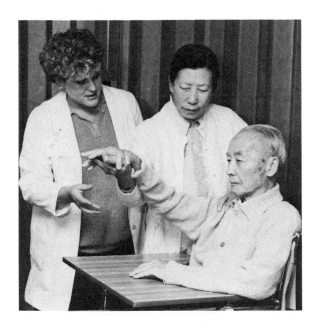

Asian Americans may subscribe to traditional health practices that are vastly different from western medical technology. (From Birchenall JM. Care of the Older Adult. 3rd ed. Philadelphia: JB Lippincott, 1993.)

a woman; although modern Chinese women may have forfeited this practice, they still may be embarrassed to receive a physical examination or health care from a man. Typically, disagreement or discomfort is not aggressively or openly displayed by Chinese persons. Nurses may need to observe more closely and ask specific questions (*e.g.*, Can you describe your pain? How do you feel about the procedure you are planning to have done? Do you have any questions?) to ensure that the quiet, compliant nature of the patient is not misinterpreted to imply that no problems exist.

To the Chinese, achieving old age is a blessing, and the elderly are held in high esteem. The old are respected and sought for advice. The family unit is expected to take care of its elder members; thus, there may be a reluctance to use service agencies for the elderly.

Japanese Americans

Although it is believed that Japanese sailors were washed ashore from their fishing ships in the late 18th century, it was not until 1850 that the first Japanese immigrant became naturalized. By the 1890s more than 25,000 Japanese immigrants lived in America, and the American workers' fear of losing their jobs to these newcomers resulted in prejudicial treatment and a restrictive immigration quota at the turn of the century. The prejudice continued with laws that forbid Japanese Americans to own property and discouraged the marriage of Japanese to native-born Americans. Perhaps the worst indignity suffered by this group occurred during World War II, when more than 70,000 American-born Japanese were confined to "relocation camps." Despite this treatment, Japanese Americans patiently struggled to improve their lot. Traditionally, many Japanese Americans have held jobs as gardeners and farmers, and they, like Chinese Americans, have a lower unemployment rate and higher percentage of professionals than the national average. Today, there are approximately 750,000 Japanese Americans, most of whom live in California and Hawaii.

Although the Japanese Americans have not tended to live in isolated pockets to the same extent as Chinese Americans, they have preserved many of their traditions, feel a close bond with one another, and highly value the family. The following terms describe each generation of Japanese American.

Issei   first generation (immigrant to America)
Nisei   second generation (first American-born)
Sansei   third generation
Yonsei   fourth generation

It is expected that families will take care of their elder members. As in the Chinese culture, the aged are viewed with respect.

The fact that Japanese men were discouraged from marrying American-born women led them to send for brides, often considerably younger than themselves, from their home country. Thus, we see a higher proportion of older Japanese widows in this country.

Similar to the Chinese, Japanese Americans may subscribe to traditional health practices and reject modern technology. They may not express their feelings openly or challenge the health professional; therefore, nursing sensitivity to covert needs is crucial.

Hispanic Americans

The term Hispanic encompasses a variety of Spanish-speaking persons in America, including Spaniards, Mexicans, Cubans, and Puerto Ricans. The peak immigration periods for each Hispanic subgroup differed. In 1513, Ponce de León discovered and claimed Florida for the King of Spain; in 1565, the Spanish founded the first permanent European colony in America in St. Augustine. The Spanish held claim to Florida for nearly two centuries, until they traded it for Cuba and the Philippines. Most Spanish immigrants settled in Florida and the southwest. Today there are approximately 250,000 Spanish Americans living in the United States. Although Mexicans inhabited the southwest for decades before the Pilgrims' arrival, most Mexican immigration occurred during this century as a result of the Mexican Revolution and the poor economic conditions in Mexico. The Mexican population in this country totals more than 8 million plus an estimated 3 to 5 million illegal immigrants; the majority reside in California and Texas.

Most Puerto Rican immigration occurred after the United States granted citizenship to all Puerto Ricans. After World War II, nearly one-third of all Puerto Rico's inhabitants immigrated to America; in the 1970s "reverse immigration" began as growing numbers of Puerto Ricans left the United States to return to their home island. An estimated 1 million Puerto Ricans live in New York City, where most of them have settled.

Most Cuban immigrants are recent newcomers to America; the majority of the greater than 1 million Cuban Americans fled Cuba after Castro seized power. More than one-fourth of the Cuban American population resides in Florida, with large pockets also found in New York and New Jersey. Among all Hispanics, Cubans are the most highly educated and have the highest earnings.

Many Hispanics view states of health and illness as the actions of God: by treating one's body with respect, living a good life, and praying, one will be rewarded by God with good health. Illness results when one has violated good practices of living or is being punished by God. Medals and crosses may be worn at all times to facilitate well-being, and prayer plays an important part in the healing process. Illness may be viewed as a family affair, with multiple family members involved with the care of the sick individual. Rather than using practitioners of Western medicine to treat their health problems, some Hispanics may prefer traditional practitioners such as the following.

Curranderos women who have special knowledge and charismatic qualities
Sobadoras persons who give massages and manipulate bones and muscles
Espiritualistas persons who analyze dreams, cards, premonitions
Brujos women who control witchcraft
Senoras older women who have learned special healing measures

Older relatives are held in high esteem by Hispanics. Old age is viewed as a positive time in which the aged person can reap the harvest of his life. It is expected that children will take care of their elder parents, and families try to avoid institutionalization at all costs; this group has a lower rate of nursing home utilization than the general population.

Nurses may find that English is a second language to Hispanics, which becomes particularly apparent during periods of illness when stress causes a retreat to the native tongue.

Numerous ethnic groups that have not been mentioned also possess unique histories, beliefs, and practices. Rather than viewing ethnic differences as being odd and forcing patients to conform to "American" traditions, nurses should respect the beauty of this diversity and make every effort to preserve it. Dietary preferences should be accommodated, adaptations made for special practices, and unique ways of managing illness understood. If nurses are unfamiliar with a particular ethnic group, they should invite family members to educate them or contact churches or ethnic asso-

ciations (*e.g.,* Polish American Alliance, Celtic League, Jewish Family and Children's Society, Slovak League of America) for interpreters or persons who can serve as cultural resources. A message of sensitivity and caring is conveyed when nurses make an effort to recognize and support patients' ethnic backgrounds. Nurses also will become enriched by gaining an appreciation and understanding of the many various interesting ethnic groups.

Reference

National Institute on Aging. Minorities and how they grow old. Bethesda, MD: National Institutes of Health, 1980:10.

Recommended Readings

Applewhite SR, ed. Hispanic elderly in transition: research, policy, and practice. New York: Greenwood Press, 1988.

Gunter LM. Cultural diversity among older Americans. In: Murrow E, ed. Perspectives on gerontological nursing. Newbury Park, CA: SAGE, 1991:215.

Jackson JS, Newton P, Ostfeld A, Savage D, Schneider EL, eds. The black American elderly: research on physical and psychosocial health. New York: Springer-Verlag, 1988.

Johnson FL, Foxall MJ, Kelleher E, Kentopp E, Mannlein EA, Cook E. Comparison of mental health and life satisfaction in five elderly ethnic groups. West J Nurs Res 1988;10:613.

4

The Aging Family

Aging is a family affair. Whether it is the retiree's concern about existing and supporting his family on a pension, or a middle-aged daughter's decision to accept her mother into her household, or a sister's attempt to care for her dying brother at home, the impact of one individual's aging process has a ripple effect on the entire family unit.

Who Is the Family?

Almost every individual is part of a family unit, although that family may not reflect the stereotypical nuclear family. In fact, one may find among the elderly a diversity of family structures, which could include the following:

- couples (married, unmarried, heterosexual, homosexual)
- couples with children (heterosexual, homosexual, married, unmarried)
- parent and child or children
- siblings
- groups of unrelated individuals
- multigenerations.

When interviewing older adults, it is important to explore all persons who are "significant others" to an individual and fulfill a family role, regardless of whether they are unrelated or reside in different households. For example, a widow can have a friend with whom she shares a close emotional tie or a cousin in a neighboring community who provides assistance and support.

The identification of family members can be more meaningful if one looks for those individuals who fulfill family functions. In aging families, family functions are somewhat modified to address the special needs of the elderly and focus on the following:

- ensuring fulfillment of physical needs
- providing emotional support and comfort
- maintaining links with family and community
- instilling a sense of meaning to life
- managing crises.

Significant persons who perform family functions for older adults can be identified by asking who:

- checks on them regularly?
- shops with or for them?
- escorts them to the clinic or physician?
- assists with or manages their problems?
- takes care of them when they are ill?
- helps them make decisions?

Those persons fulfilling significant family functions should be included in the plan of care of older adults.

Family Roles

Frequently, family members assume certain roles as a result of their socialization process and family needs and expectations. Possible roles include the following.(Eliopoulos, 1990)

Decision-maker   the person who is granted or assumes responsibility for making important decisions; may not be geographically close or involved in daily activities

Problem-solver   the crisis manager; may not be geographically close or involved in daily activities

Deviant   the "problem child" who has strayed from family norms; may be used to fulfill family need for scapecoat or provide sense of purpose

Dependent   an individual who relinquishes his or her own rights and responsibilities to the family

Victim   a person who forfeits his or her legitimate rights and may be physically, emotionally, socially, or economically abused by the family

The impact of these roles should be explored when assessing the family unit. Nurses must be sensitive to the fact that certain "negative" roles may not have the adverse effects on the family unit that would be anticipated and, likewise, "positive" roles may not be welcomed by the family. For example, the middle-aged son who drifts from town to town, chronically wiring his elderly parents for funds to pay off his latest indulgences, may not be representative of a responsible, mature adult, but he may bring an excitement and sense of being needed to his parents' lives, thereby having a positive effect. On the other hand, his brother who is financially secure and responsible and who takes care of his parents' affairs may be disliked because of his dullness and practicality.

Relationships

The dynamics among family members can have positive or negative effects on the elderly. In assessing the family unit it is useful to explore the following issues:

How family members feel about each other. Do they love but not like . . . admire . . . respect . . . enjoy each other? How do they express affection?

The manner of communication. Do they share daily events or have contact only on holidays? Is their style of interaction parent–child or adult–adult?

Their attitudes, values, and beliefs. Do they feel that the young should take care of the old or that children owe their parents nothing?

What are their expectations of family members, friends, and society?

Linkages with organizations and the community. How involved are they with persons external to the family unit? Is the family similar to others in the community?

As discussed in Chapter 1, the majority of elderly people are not abandoned by their children, and most do enjoy regular contact. Life-styles, housing, and societal expectations are not conducive to healthy parents and their adult children living together. Most elderly people want to live in their own residences, if possible, and the majority do. Approximately 10% of older women and 5% of older men live with their children and grandchildren.(Hendricks and Hendricks-Davis, 1981) The arrangement of generations living under separate roofs but within a 30-minute trip of each other is generally the most satisfactory. It is understood that parents and children will provide assistance and share a household if an unusual circumstance arises.

Grandparenting can be a positive experience for the elderly because they obtain the enjoyment, affection, and sense of purpose from caring for their grandchildren without the 24-hour stress of child-rearing responsibilities. Grandchildren can provide new interests and meaning to life. In turn, grandchildren usually receive the benefit of unconditional love and attention. As grandchildren grow into adulthood, their involvement with grandparents often lessens, but a strong bond continues to exist.

Next to that between parent and child, the relationship between siblings is stronger than any other relationship. The typical pattern is for siblings to drift apart during young and middle adulthood but then reestablish strong ties in later life. Socialization, emotional support, and financial and household assistance can be provided by siblings. Usually, earlier conflicts and differences become insignificant as siblings develop mutually supportive relationships in later life.

Elderly couples seldom divorce; even rocky marriages stabilize in later life as the couple faces a new interdependency. Spouses look to each other for security, support, and safety in an imperfect world. After years of experiencing and reinforcing each other's behaviors, the couple can understand, anticipate, and complement each other's actions. Spouses look after the care and welfare of

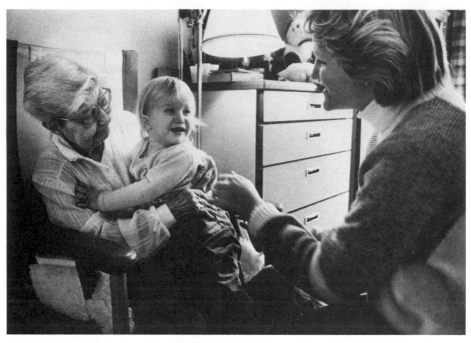

Aging is a family affair. (Photograph by Eric Schenk.)

their mates and derive security in having someone available to care about them.

Relationships in old age are affected by the forms of relationships experienced throughout life. Parents who ignored or abused their children early in life may produce children who want nothing to do with them in adulthood. Siblings who have unresolved anger over favoritism displayed by their parents may express their feelings by refusing to assist when the favored child is in need. Couples who never shared intimacy and friendship may exist in separate worlds under the same roof. Nurturing relationships at every stage of life are an investment in having meaningful, supportive relationships in later life.

Family Caregivers

A family is a strong chain of human experience that bonds its members through life's challenges and joys; however, that chain is only as strong as its weakest link. Effective gerontological nursing recognizes that the health of all family members must be maintained and promoted.

Maintaining independence facilitates normality in family relationships. Having to live with or be cared for by family members can threaten the status and roles of older persons and cause anger, resentment, and other feelings to develop (see Nursing Diagnosis Highlight). Sound health practices to prevent disease and disability are crucial to maintaining self-care ability and independence. If illness occurs, aggressive attention should be paid to avoiding complications and restoring the affected person to a healthy state. Interventions such as environmental modifications, financial aid, home-delivered meals, chore assistance, transportation for the handicapped, telephone reassurance, or a home companion can supplement deficits and strengthen the elderly's reserves for independent living.

If the caregiver is a spouse or sibling, chances are that he or she is an elderly person as well. Even the children of the elderly person can be aged themselves. The physical, emotional, and social health of the caregivers must be evaluated periodically to ensure they are competent to provide the required services and are not jeopardizing themselves in the process. Provisions must be made for what gerontological nurses refer to as their TLC:

T—Training in care techniques, safe medication use, recognition of abnormalities

L—Leaving the care situation periodically to obtain respite and relaxation and maintain their normal living needs

C—Care for themselves through adequate sleep, rest, exercise, nutrition, socialization, solitude, and health management.

Gerontological nurses should review the TLC needs of caregivers during every contact to ensure their continued effectiveness.

A particularly vulnerable group of caregivers is middle-aged daughters. After years of sacrificing and struggling with child-rearing, they are beginning to taste some freedom as their children gain independence and begin to leave home. They are concerned for their children's success and well-being and experience ambivalence over the less intense parental role. Increasing numbers of them are in the work force to resume delayed careers or assist with college costs or other family expenses. Perhaps they are coping with spouses who are experiencing midlife crises, having mixed feelings about their marriage, or reacting to undesirable changes in their physical appearance. They are clouded with the "superwoman" myth and desperately try to be the supportive parent, understanding wife, exciting lover, interesting friend, and aspiring employee, when all they really would like to do is climb into the nearest hole and cover their heads. At this point in life, the final straw may be dependent parents and their demands. These daughters feel that they certainly cannot deprive their parents, trust their care to strangers, or institutionalize them. However, what will this mean to their careers, income, marital relationships, friendships, leisure pursuits, and energy? As a growing number of middle-aged women confront this dilemma, special nursing intervention is warranted.

Nurses can aid family caregivers in the following ways:

Realistically viewing the situation. Maybe a leave of absence rather than resignation from a job is warranted to assist a parent or spouse through convalescence. Perhaps the needs are such that a lay caregiver (e.g., family member) will not be able to care for them adequately. Often, an objective outsider can guide the family in viewing the real situation and understanding the extent of care needs.

Supporting surfacing feelings. Raised with an abundance of "shoulds" and "oughts" regarding the treatment of older persons, families need to know that the guilt, anger, resentment, and depression they feel are neither uncommon nor bad.

Reviewing the total impact. Although caregivers may feel they alone are assuming responsibility for care, they need to examine the effects on the total family unit. How will their children's tuition be paid if they quit their jobs to care for a parent? Will someone have to forfeit a bedroom if the relative moves in? What is the relationship of the spouse with the in-laws? Who will help lift grandma into the tub? Will the family be able to take vacations and entertain at home? Is someone available to relieve them if they want to go out for a special occasion?

Exploring alternatives. Often, family members believe that care must be one of two extremes: institutionalization or total care provided in the caregiver's household. Although these are options, other possibilities exist within these extremes, including home health aides, live-in companions, geriatric day care, or shared family care in which the elder lives at specific times with various relatives, or relatives spend designated days at the elder's home. Caregivers also should be aided in identifying their limitations and the need for institutional care when necessary. See Chapter 40 for more information about services for the elderly and their caregivers.

Family Dysfunction

Many factors can threaten the healthy function of the family unit (see Nursing Diagnosis Highlight) and the gerontological nurse must be skilled at identifying and providing interventions for such problems. Family dysfunction occurs in many forms, ranging from an older parent's dominance and manipulation of an adult child to incestuous relationships. A lifelong history of dysfunction may exist, or the dysfunction may be a recent problem, associated with a wide range of factors (e.g., divorce, loss of income, increased dependency of elder, illness of caregiver). Families experiencing dysfunction may be:

- less able to fulfill the physical, emotional, socioeconomic, and spiritual needs of their members
- rigid in roles, responsibilities, opinions

- unable or unwilling to obtain and use help from others
- ineffective or inappropriate with their communication and behavior.

One form of dysfunction that has gained increased visibility in recent years is elder abuse. It is estimated that 5% of all older adults are abused each year, most by a close family member. Abuse occurs in all sorts of families, regardless of social, financial or ethnic background, and can present in many forms, including the following:

- inflicting pain or injury
- withholding food, money, medications, care
- confinement, physical or chemical restraint
- theft or intentional mismanagement of assets
- sexual abuse.

NURSING DIAGNOSIS HIGHLIGHT
Altered Family Processes

Overview

An alteration in family processes exists when the family's normal functions are disrupted. When this problem is present, the family may be unable to meet the physical, emotional, socioeconomic, or spiritual needs of its members, may deal with stress ineffectively, may communicate ineffectively of inappropriately, or may refuse to seek or accept help from others.

Causative or contributing factors

Illness or injury of family member, change in dependency level of member, change in role or function of family member, addition or loss of family member, relocation, reduced income, added expenses, social or sexual deviance by family member, break in religious or cultural practices by family members.

Goal

The family will demonstrate support and assistance to members in their fulfillment of physical, emotional, and socioeconomic needs; the family will seek and accept assistance from external sources as appropriate.

Interventions

- Collect a comprehensive family history that includes profile of family (include significant others who fill family functions as family members); age, health, and residence of members; roles and responsibilities of each member; typical patterns of communication, problem solving, and crisis management; recent changes in composition of the family and members' roles, responsibilities, and health statuses; new burdens; and the family's assessment of problem.
- Identify factors related to family dysfunction and plan appropriate interventions such as family therapy, financial aid, family conference, visiting nurse, or clergy visit.
- Facilitate open, honest communication among family members; assist in planning family conferences, promoting discussion by all members, developing realistic goals and plans, and allocating responsibility; provide privacy for family.
- When a member is receiving health services, explain care activities and expected outcomes, prepare for changes, and involve the family in care to the maximum extent possible.
- Provide caregiver education and support; help caregivers identify community resources; and emphasize the importance of respite for caregivers.
- Make the family aware of support and self-help groups that can assist them, such as Alzheimer's Disease and Related Disorders Association, American Cancer Society, Alcoholics Anonymous, and American Diabetes Association.

Not only is the actual commission of any of the above abuse, but the threat of committing the act is also considered abuse. The profile of the older adult at greatest risk for abuse is a disabled woman, older than 75 years of age, who lives with a relative and is physically, socially, or financially dependent on others. Most often, abuse stems from stressful caregiving situations; however, abuse can be associated with a family history of violence, emotional or cognitive dysfunction of the abused, or retaliation for a history of earlier abuse. A good family history can be helpful in gaining insight into the family dynamics that could contribute to abuse.

The older adult may be reluctant to report or admit to abuse. Nurses must manage this situation tactfully. Abused persons must have assurances that their plight will not be worsened by making the abuse public: they may prefer being verbally threatened or having their money taken to the alternative of living in an institution or foster home. The family needs empathy, not judgment, from the nurse. Although some individuals are consciously malicious and abusive for their own gain, most abusers are distressed persons who have lost their ability to cope effectively. Abuse may be stopped and family health salvaged by aiding the family in finding effective ways to manage their situation, such as through counseling or respite care.

A caring, interested family is one of the most valuable resources an individual can possess in old age. In turn, the love and richness of experiences offered by older persons adds a unique depth and meaning to the family. Gerontological nurses must view older adults in the perspective of their family units and structure care to enhance the functional capacity of all family members.

References

Eliopoulos C. Health assessment of the older adult. 2nd ed. Menlo Park, CA: Addison-Wesley, 1990:42.

Hendricks J, Hendricks-Davis C. Aging in mass society: myths and realities. 2nd ed. Cambridge, MA: Winthrop Publishers, 1981:306.

Recommended Readings

Bahr SJ, Peterson ET. Aging and the family, Lexington, MA: Lexington Books, 1989.

Baldwin B. Family caregiving: trends and forecasts. Geriatric Nurs 1990;11:172.

Bumogen VE, Hien KF. Helping the aging family: a guide for professionals. Glenview, IL: Scott, Foresman, 1990.

Janz M. Clues to elder abuse. Geriatric Nurs 1990; 11(5):220.

Klein S. Caregiver burden and moral development. Image: Journal of Nursing Scholarship 1989;21:94.

Lindgren CL. Burnout and social support in family caregivers. West J Nurs Res 1990;12:469.

McKenzie H. Caregiving. Washington, DC: National Council on Aging, 1990.

Rempusheski VF, Phillips LR. Elders versus caregivers: games they play. Geriatric Nurs 1998;9(1):30.

5

Adjustments in Aging

Growing old is not easy. Various changes during the aging process demand multiple adjustments requiring stamina, ability, and flexibility. Frequently, more simultaneous changes are experienced than during any other period of life. Many younger adults find it exhausting to keep pace with technological advances, societal changes, cost-of-living fluctuations, and labor market trends. Imagine how complex and complicated life can be for older individuals, who must also face retirement, reduced income, possible housing changes, frequent losses through deaths of significant persons, and a declining ability to function. To promote an awareness and appreciation of the complex and arduous adjustments involved, this chapter considers some of the factors that affect the successful management of the multiple changes associated with aging and the achievement of satisfaction and well-being during the later years. See the Nursing Diagnosis Highlight in this chapter for some nursing considerations associated with altered role performance.

Family Changes

The family unit is the major source of satisfaction for many older people and, contrary to the belief of many, most of the elderly have regular, frequent contact with family members. The love and companionship of a spouse, the rewards and pride derived as offspring develop into independent adults, the deepened—and often renewed—relationships with siblings, and the joy of grandchildren and great-grandchildren can be essential ingredients for a satisfying old age. The family can be a key source of support as well by cushioning the multiple losses and changes associated with aging while instilling hope and interest for a meaningful future.

The dynamic parental role frequently changes to meet the growth and development needs of both parent and child. During middle and later life, parents must adjust to the independence of their children as they become responsible adult citizens and leave home. The first child usually leaves home and establishes an independent unit 22 to 25 years after the parents were married. For persons who have invested most of their adult lives nurturing and providing for their offspring, a child's independence may have significant impact. Although parents who are freed from the responsibilities and worries of rearing children have greater time to pursue their own interests, they are also freed from the meaningful, purposeful, and satisfying activities associated with child-rearing, and this frequently results in a profound sense of loss.

A woman in late middle age or old age has been influenced by a historical period that emphasized the role of wife and mother. For instance, to provide job opportunities for men returning from World War II, women were encouraged to focus their interests on raising a family and to forfeit the scarce jobs to men. Unlike many of today's younger women, who combine (and in some situations equally value) employment and motherhood, these

women centered their lives on their families, from which they derived their sense of fulfillment. Having developed few roles from which to achieve satisfaction other than that of wife and mother, many of these older women feel a definite void when their children are grown and gone. To compound this problem, the highly mobile life-style of many young persons limits the degree of direct contact she has with her adult children and with her grandchildren.

The older man shares many of the same feelings as his wife. Throughout the years, he feels he has performed useful functions that made him a valuable member of society. He may have fought for his country in indisputably honorable wars. Most likely, he worked hard to support his wife and children, and his masculinity was reinforced with proof of his ability to beget and provide for offspring. With his children grown, he is no longer required to provide—a mixed blessing in which he may find both a sense relief and one of purposelessness. In addition, he learns that the rules have changed; his pride at being a war hero may have been shattered by antiwar advocates, his ability to support a family without the need for his wife to work is now viewed as oppressive by feminists, his efforts to replenish the earth are scorned by today's zero-population proponents, and his attempt to fill the masculine role for which he was socialized is considered macho or inane by today's standards.

Although the extended family was not as widespread or perfect as many thought, it was more prevalent in the past. It provided immediate support systems, shared responsibilities, economic benefits, and other advantages to young and old family members. Grandparenting was an active role that provided a sense of usefulness and satisfaction for the aged, who, in turn, could feel secure that the family unit would be responsible for their growing needs and increased requirements for assistance.

The emergence of today's nuclear family units changed the roles and functions of the individuals in a family. The elderly are expected to have limited input into the lives of their adult children. Children are not required to meet the needs of their aging parents for financial support, health services, or housing. Moreover, parents increasingly do not depend on their children for their needs, and the belief that children are the best old-age insurance is

fading. In addition, grandparenting, although satisfying, is not usually an active role, especially because grandchildren may be scattered throughout the country. These changes in family structure and function are not necessarily negative. Most children do not abandon or neglect their aging parents; they maintain regular contact. Separate family units may help the parent–child relationship develop on a more adult-to-adult basis, to the mutual satisfaction of young and old. Although the advantages of nuclear-family living are often seen primarily as a benefit to younger adults, older adults also enjoy the independence and freedom from responsibilities that nuclear-family life offers.

A common event that alters family life for the aged is the death of a spouse. The loss of that individual who has shared more love and life experiences, more joys and sorrows, may be intolerable. How, after many decades of living with another human being, does one adjust to the sudden absence of that person? How does one adjust to setting the table for one, to coming home to an empty house, or to not touching that warm, familiar body in bed? Adjustment to this significant loss is coupled with the demand to learn the new task of living alone.

Death of a spouse affects more women than men because most older men are married and most older women are widowed—a situation that is expected to continue in the future. Unlike many of today's younger women, who have greater independence through careers and changed norms, most of today's older women have led family-oriented lives and been dependent on their husbands. Their age, limited education, lack of skills, and long period of unemployment while raising their families are handicaps in a competitive job market. If these women can find employment, adjusting to the new demands of a work role may be difficult and stressful. On the other hand, the unemployed widow may learn that pensions or other sources of income may be reduced or discontinued when the husband dies, necessitating an adjustment to an extremely limited budget. In addition to financial dependence, the woman may have depended on her husband's achievements to provide her with gratification and identity. Frequently, the achievements of children serve this same purpose. Sexual desires may be unfulfilled because of lack of opportunity, fear of repercussion from children and society, or residual attitudes from early

teachings about sexual mores. If a woman's marriage promoted friendships with other married couples and only inactive relationships with single friends, the new widow may find that her number of single female friends is small.

For the most part, when the initial grief of the husband's death passes, most widows adjust quite well. The high proportion of older women who are widowed provides an availability of friends who share similar problems and life-styles, especially in urban areas. Old friendships may be revived to provide sources of activity and enjoyment. Some widows may discover that the loss of certain responsibilities associated with their partner's death, such as cooking, laundering, and cleaning for a husband, brings them a new and pleasant freedom. With alternative roles to develop, sufficient income, and choice over life-style, many women are able to make a successful adjustment to widowhood. The nurse may facilitate this adjustment by identifying sources of friendships and activities such as clubs, volunteer organizations, or groups of widows in the community, and by helping the widow understand and obtain all the benefits to which she is entitled. This may require reassuring her that enjoying her new freedom and desiring relationships with other men is no reason to feel guilty and supporting her as she learns to adjust to the loss of her husband and the new role of widow.

Retirement

One of the major adjustments to be made as an individual ages is the loss of a work role through retirement. For many, this is the first experience of the impact of aging. Retirement is especially difficult in our society, where worth is commonly judged by an individual's productivity. Work is often viewed as the dues required for active membership in a productive society. The attitude that unemployment, for whatever reason, is an undesirable state is adhered to by many of today's older persons, who were raised under the omnipresent cloud of the Puritan work ethic.

Occupational identity is largely responsible for an individual's social position and for the social role attached to that position. Although it is known that individuals function differently and uniquely in similar roles, some behaviors continue to be associated with certain roles, which promotes stereotypes. How frequently do certain stereotypes assigned to various roles continue to be heard— the tough construction worker, the wild go-go dancer, the fair judge, the righteous clergyman, the learned lawyer, and the healing doctor. The realization that these associations are not consistently valid does not prevent their propagation. Too frequently, individuals are described in terms of their work role rather than their personal characteristics, for example, "the nurse who lives down the road" or "my son the doctor." Considering the extent to which social identity and behavioral expectations are derived from the work role, it is not surprising that an individual's identity is threatened when retirement occurs. During childhood and adolescence, we are guided toward an independent, responsible adult role, and in academic settings, we are prepared for our professional roles; but where and when are we prepared for the role of retiree?

Gerontological nursing is concerned with the welfare of both the current aged population and future aged populations. A lifetime of poor health-care practices is a handicap that cannot be remedied in old age. Assisting aging individuals with their retirement preparations is preventive intervention, maximizing the potential for health and well-being in old age. As a part of such intervention, aging individuals should be encouraged to establish and practice good health habits such as following a proper diet; avoiding alcohol, drug, and tobacco abuse; and having regular physical examinations.

When one's work is one's primary interest, activity, and source of social contacts, separation from work leaves a significant void in one's life. Aging individuals should be urged to develop interests unrelated to work. Retirement is facilitated by learning how to use, appreciate, and gain satisfaction from leisure time throughout an employed lifetime. In addition, enjoying leisure time is a therapeutic outlet for life stresses throughout the aging process.

Gerontological nurses must understand the realities and reactions encountered when working with retired persons. Insight into this complicated process may be gained by considering the phases of retirement developed by Robert Atchley.(Atchley, 1975) Not all retirees go through all of the following phases.

Remote phase. Early in the occupational career, future retirement is anticipated, but rational preparation is seldom done.

Near phase. When the reality of retirement is evident, preparation for leaving one's job begins, as does fantasy regarding the retirement role.

Honeymoon phase. Following the retirement event, a somewhat euphoric period begins, in which fantasies from the preretirement phase are tested. Retirees attempt to do everything they never had time for simultaneously. A variety of factors (e.g., finances, health) limit this, leading to the development of a stable life-style.

Disenchantment phase. As life begins to stabilize, a letdown, sometimes a depression, is experienced. The more unrealistic the preretirement fantasy, the greater the degree of disenchantment.

Reorientation phase. As realistic choices and alternative sources of satisfaction are considered, the disenchantment with the new retirement routine can be replaced by developing a life-style that provides some satisfaction.

Stability phase. An understanding of the retirement role is achieved, and this provides a framework for concern, involvement, and action in the elderly person's life. Some enter this phase directly after the honeymoon phase, and some never reach it at all.

Termination phase. The retirement role is lost as a result of either the resumption of a work role or dependency due to illness or disability.

It is obvious that different nursing interventions may be required during each phase. Some of the preretirement planning recommendations discussed earlier can be used during the remote phase. Counseling regarding the realities of retirement may be part of the near phase, whereas helping retirees place their newfound freedom into proper perspective may be warranted during the honeymoon phase. Being supportive of retirees during the disenchantment phase without fostering self-pity and helping them identify new sources of satisfaction may facilitate the reorientation process. Appreciating and promoting the strengths of the stability phase may reinforce an adjustment to

retirement. For general nursing, many considerations are related to the phases of retirement. For example, when the retirement phase is terminated due to disease or disability, the tactful management of dependency and the respectful appreciation of losses are most important.

The nurses' evaluations of their own attitudes toward retirement are an essential part of their role in the retirement process. Does the nurse see retirement as a period of freedom, opportunity, and growth or of loneliness, dependency, and meaninglessness? Is the nurse intelligently planning for her own retirement or denying it by avoiding encounters with retirement realities? Nurses' views of retirement affect the retiree–nurse relationship. Gerontological nurses can provide especially good models of constructive retirement practices and attitudes.

Awareness of Mortality

Widowhood, death of friends, and the recognition of declining functions make older persons more aware of the reality of their own death. During their early years, individuals intellectually understand they will not live forever, but their behaviors deny this reality. The lack of a will and absence of burial plans may be indications of this denial. As the reality of mortality becomes acute with advancing age, interest in fulfilling dreams, deepening religious convictions, strengthening family ties, providing for the ongoing welfare of the person's family, and leaving a legacy are often apparent signs.

The significance of a life review in interpreting and refining our past experiences as they relate to our self-concept and help us understand and accept our life history has been well discussed. (Butler and Lewis, 1982) Rather than being a pathological behavior, discussing the past may be therapeutic and necessary for the elderly. The thought of impending death may be more tolerable if people feel that their life had depth and meaning. Unresolved guilt, unachieved aspirations, perceived failures, and other multitudinous aspects of "unfinished business" may be better understood and perhaps resolved. Although the condition of old age may provide limited opportunities for excitement and achievement, satisfaction may be gained in knowing that there were achievements, and many excitements as well, in other periods of life. The old

woman may be frail and wrinkled, but she can still delight in remembering how she once drove young men insane. The retired old man may feel that he is useless to society now, but he realizes his worth through the memory of wars he fought to protect his country and the pride he feels in knowing he supported his family through a depression.

The young can benefit from the reminiscences of the aged by gaining a new perspective on life as they learn about their ancestry. Imagine the impact of hearing about slavery, immigration, epidemics, industrialization, or wars from an older relative who has been part of making that history. What history book's description of the Great Depression can compare with hearing a grandparent describe events one's own family experienced, such as going to bed hungry at night? In addition to their place in the future, the young can fully realize their link with the past when the desire of the elderly to reminisce is appreciated and fostered.

Older persons should be encouraged to discuss and analyze the dynamics of their lives, and listeners should be receptive and accepting. Poems and autobiographies, as unsophisticated as they may be, should be recognized as significant legacies from the old to the young. One 71-year-old man started a family scrapbook for each of his children. Any photograph, newspaper article, or announcement pertaining to any family member was reproduced and included in every album. The family patiently tolerated this activity—reluctantly sending him copies of graduation programs and photographs for every scrapbook. The family viewed the main value of this activity as providing something benign to keep this old man occupied. It was not until years after his death that the significance of this great task was appreciated as a priceless gift. Such tangible items may serve as an assurance to both young and old that the impact of an aged relative's life will not cease at death.

Declining Function

The obvious changes in appearance and bodily function that occur during the aging process make it necessary for the aging individual to adjust to a new body image. Colorful soft hair turns gray and dry, flexible straight fingers become bent and painful, body contours are altered, and height decreases. Stairs once climbed several times daily de-

mand more time and energy to negotiate as the years accumulate. As subtle, gradual, and natural as these changes may be, they are recognized and, consequently, body image and self-concept are affected.

The manner in which individuals perceive themselves and function can determine the roles they play. A construction worker who has less strength and energy may forfeit his work role; a club member who cannot hear speech may forfeit membership; fashion models may forfeit that role when they perceive themselves as old. Interestingly, some persons well into their sixth and seventh decades refuse to join a senior citizen club and accept the role associated with being a member of such a club because they do not perceive themselves as being old. The nurse will gain insight into the self-concept of older persons by evaluating what roles they are willing to accept and what roles they reject.

It is sometimes difficult for the aging person to accept the declining efficiency of the body. Poor memory, slow response, easy fatigue, and altered appearance are among the many frustrating results of declining function, and they are dealt with in various ways. Some older people deny them and often demonstrate poor judgment in an attempt to make the same demands on their bodies as they did when younger. Others try to resist these changes by investing in cosmetic surgery, beauty treatments, miracle drugs, and other expensive endeavors that diminish the budget but not the normal aging process. Still others exaggerate these effects and impose an unnecessarily restricted lifestyle on themselves. Societal expectations frequently determine the adjustment individuals make to declining function.

Common results of declining function are illness and disability. As described in Chapter 1, most older people have one or more chronic diseases, and more than one-third have a serious disability that limits major activities such as work and housekeeping. The elderly often fear that their illness or disability may cause them to lose their independence. Becoming a burden to their family, being unable to meet the demands of daily living, and having to enter a nursing home are some of the fears associated with dependency. Children and parents may have difficulty exchanging dependent–independent roles. The physical pain arising

from an illness may not be nearly as intolerable as the dependency it causes.

Nurses should help aging persons understand and accept the normal physical decline associated with advanced age. Factors that can promote optimum function should be encouraged, including proper diet; paced activity; regular physical examination; early correction of health problems; and avoidance of alcohol, tobacco, and drug abuse. Assistance should be offered, with attention to preserving as much of the individual's independence and dignity as possible.

Reduced Income

Financial resources are important at any age because they affect our diet, health, housing, safety, and independence and influence many of our choices in life. The economic profile of many older persons is poor. Retirement income is less than one-half the income earned while fully employed. For a majority of the elderly, social security income, originally intended as a supplement, is actually the primary source of retirement income—and even it has not kept pace with inflation. Less than one-fifth of the older population has income from a private pension plan, and those who do often discover that the fixed benefits established when the plan was subscribed to have almost no value because of inflation. Among the workers who are currently active in the labor force, more than one-half will not have pension plans when they retire. More than one in six of all older adults live in poverty; only a minority are fully employed or financially comfortable. Few elderly persons have accumulated enough assets during their lifetime to provide financial security in old age.

A reduction in income is a significant adjustment for many older persons because it triggers other adjustments that must be made. An active social life and leisure pursuits may have to be markedly reduced or eliminated. Relocation to less expensive housing may be necessary, possibly forcing the aged to leave many family and community ties. Dietary practices may be severely altered, and health care may be viewed as a luxury over which other basic expenses, such as food and rent, take priority. If the older parent has to depend on children for supplemental income, an additional adjustment may be necessary.

The importance of making financial preparations for old age many years prior to retirement is clear. Nurses should encourage aging working people to determine whether their retirement income plans are keeping pace with inflation (Table 5-1). Older individuals need assistance in obtaining all the benefits they are entitled to and in learning how to manage their income wisely. Nurses should be aware of the impact of economic welfare on health status and should actively involve themselves in political issues that promote adequate income for all individuals.

Shrinking Social World

Loneliness and desolation emphasize all the misfortunes of people who are growing old. Children are grown and gone, friends and spouse may be deceased, and others who could allay the loneliness may avoid the older individual because they find it difficult to accept the changes they see or to face the fact that they too will be old some day. Location in a sparsely populated rural area can geographically isolate older persons, and when they live in an urban area, they may be fearful of going outdoors. Hearing and speech deficits and language differences, which present communication barriers, can also foster loneliness. Insecurity resulting from multiple losses can cause suspiciousness of others and lead to a self-imposed isolation. At a time of many losses and adjustments, personal contact, love, extra support, and attention are needed—not isolation. These are essential human needs. It is likely that a failure to thrive will occur in adults who feel unwanted and unloved just as it does in infants, who display anxiety, depression, anorexia, and behavioral and other difficulties when they perceive love and attention to be inadequate (Fig. 5-1).

Nurses should attempt to intervene when isolation and loneliness are detected in an elderly person. Various programs provide telephone reassurance or home visits as a source of daily human contact; the person's church may also provide assistance. Nurses can help the person identify and join social groups and sometimes even accompany the individual to the first meeting. A change in housing may be necessary to provide a safe environment conducive to social interaction. If the older person speaks a foreign language, relocation

Table 5-1 *Retirement Budget*

INCOME SOURCES	CURRENT MONTHLY INCOME	INCOME AFTER RETIREMENT
Salary		
Pension		
Second job		
Social security		
Spouse's income		
Other (*e.g.*, savings, rents, IRAs, investments)		
Total		

LIVING REQUIREMENTS	CURRENT MONTHLY EXPENSES	EXPENSES AFTER RETIREMENT
Living accommodations		
Mortgages or rent		
Utilities (*e.g.*, gas, electricity, water)		
Taxes		
Maintenance		
Telephone		
Food and other necessities		
Clothing		
Medical (*e.g.*, doctor, dentist, medicine)		
Insurance		
Life		
Health		
Automobile		
Other		
Loans and other credit		
Automobile expenses (*e.g.*, gas, oil, repairs)		
Entertainment		
Subtotal		
Other expenses (10% of subtotal)		
Total		
Net (income − expenses)	Current	After retirement

to an area in which members of the same ethnic group live can often remedy loneliness. Even pets are frequently significant and effective companions for the elderly.

It should be emphasized that being alone is not synonymous with being lonely. Periods of solitude are essential at all ages, providing us with the opportunity to reflect, analyze, and better understand the dynamics of our lives. Older individuals may want periods of solitude to reminisce and review their lives. Some individuals, young and old, prefer and choose to be alone and do not feel isolated or lonely in any way. Of course, attention should also be paid to the correction of hearing, vision, and other health problems that may be the cause of social isolation.

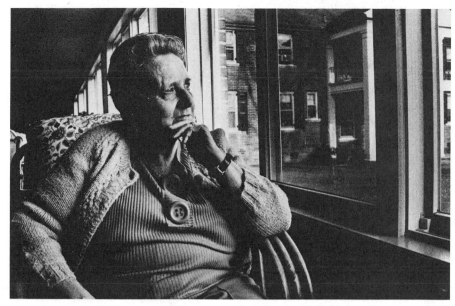

Figure 5-1. *Isolation and loneliness warrant intervention; however, periods of solitude are essential for all persons. (Photograph by Eric Schenk.)*

Societal Prejudice

It is not difficult to detect overt ageism in our society. Rather than showing appreciation for the vast contributions of the aged and their wealth of resources, society is beset with prejudices and lacks adequate provisions for them, thus derogating their dignity. The same members of society who oppose providing sufficient income and health-care benefits for the elderly enjoy an affluence and standard of living that was provided through the efforts of those older persons.

Although the elderly constitute the most diverse and individualized age-group within the entire population, they continue to be stereotyped by the following misconceptions:

Old people are sick and disabled.
Most old people are in nursing homes.
Senility comes with old age.
Old people are unhappy.
People either get very tranquil or very cranky as they age.

Old people have lower intelligence and are resistant to change.
Old people are not able to have sexual intercourse and are not interested in sex anyhow.
There are few satisfactions in old age.

For a majority of older persons, the above statements are not true. Increased efforts are necessary to make the members of society aware of the realities of aging. Groups such as the Gray Panthers have done an outstanding job of informing the public about the facts regarding aging and the problems and rights of older adults. More advocates for the elderly are needed.

Erik Erikson (1963) says that the last stage of the life cycle is concerned with integrity versus despair. Integrity results when the older individual derives satisfaction from an evaluation of his or her life. Disappointment with life and the lack of opportunities to alter the past bring despair. The experiences of our entire lifetime determine whether our old age will be an opportunity for freedom, growth, and contentment or a miserable imprisonment of our human potential.

NURSING DIAGNOSIS HIGHLIGHT
Altered Role Performance

Overview

An alteration in role performance exists when there is a change in the perception or performance of a role. This can be associated with a physical, emotional, intellectual, motivational, eduational, or socioeconomic limitation in the ability to fill the role, or restrictions in role performance imposed by others. There can be considerable distress, depression, or anger at not fulfilling the accustomed role and its associated responsibilities.

Causative or contributing factors

Illness, fatigue, pain, declining function, altered cognition, depression, anxiety, knowledge deficit, limited finances, retirement, lack of transportation, loss of significant other, ageism, restrictions imposed by others.

Goal

The client realistically appraises role performance, adjusts to changes in role performance, and learns to perform responsibilities associated with role.

Interventions

- Assess client's roles and responsibilities; identify deficits in role performance and reasons for deficits; review client's perception of role and feelings associated with altered role performance.
- Assist client in realistically evaluating cause of altered role performance and potential for improvement in role performance.
- Identify specific strategies to improve role performance (*e.g.*, instructing, negotiating with family members to allow client to perform role, counseling client to accept real limitations, referring to community resources, improving health problem, encouraging client to seek help with responsibilities, advising for stress management)
- Encourage client to discuss concerns with family members; assist client in arranging family conference.
- Refer client to assistive resources, as appropriate, such as support groups, occupational therapist, financial counselor, Over-60 Employment Service, visiting nurse, and social services.

References

Atchley RC. The sociology of retirement. Cambridge, MA: Schenkman, 1975.

Butler RH, Lewis MI. Aging and mental health. 3rd ed. St Louis: CV Mosby, 1982:58.

Erikson E. Childhood and society. 2nd ed. New York: WW Norton and Co., 1963.

Recommended Readings

Atchley R. Social forces in later life. Belmont, CA: Wadsworth, 1988.

Nkongho NO. Talk isn't cheap. Geriatric Nurs 1990; 11(6):282.

Koenig HG, Smiley M, Gonzales JAP. Religion, health and aging. New York: Greenwood, 1988.

Reker GT. Meaning and purpose in life and well-being: a life-span perspective. J Gerontol 1987;42(1):44.

Ross HK. Lesson of life. Geriatric Nurs 1990;11(6):274.

6

Common Aging Changes

Living is a process of continual change. Infants become toddlers, pubescent children blossom into young men and women, and dependent adolescents develop into responsible adult citizens. The continuation of change into later life is natural and expected.

The type, rate, and degree of physical, emotional, psychological, and social changes experienced during life are highly individualized. The types and degrees of these changes are influenced by genetic factors, environment, diet, health, stress, and numerous other elements. The result is not only individual variations among aged persons but also differences in the pattern of aging of various body systems within the same individual. Although some similar elements in the pattern of aging can be identified between individuals, the unique pattern of aging in each person must be recognized.

Physical Changes in Structure and Function

General Changes

Organ and system changes can be traced to changes at the basic cellular level. The number of cells is gradually reduced, leaving fewer functional cells in the body. Lean body mass is reduced, whereas fat tissue increases until the sixth decade of life. Cellular solids and bone mass are decreased. Extracellular fluid remains fairly constant, although intracellular fluid is decreased, resulting in less total body fluid. This makes the risk of dehydration significant in the elderly.

Some of the more noticeable effects of the aging process begin to appear after the fourth decade of life. It is then that men experience hair loss, and both sexes develop gray hair and wrinkles. As body fat atrophies, the body's contours gain a bony appearance along with a deepening of the hollows of the intercostal and supraclavicular spaces, orbits, and axillae. Elongated ears, a double chin, and baggy eyelids are among the more obvious manifestations of the loss of tissue elasticity throughout the body. Skin-fold thickness is significantly reduced in the forearm and on the back of the hands. The loss of subcutaneous fat content, responsible for the decrease in skin-fold thickness, also is responsible for a decline in the body's natural insulation, making older adults more sensitive to cold temperatures. Stature decreases, resulting in a loss of approximately two inches in height by 70 years of age. Body shrinkage is due to a loss of cartilage and thinning of the vertebrae, causing the long bones of the body, which do not shrink, to appear disproportionately long. Normal oral temperatures are lower in later life than in younger years. These changes are gradual and subtle. Further differences in structure and function can arise from changes to specific body systems (Fig. 6-1).

Cardiovascular System

Heart size does not change significantly with age; enlarged hearts are associated with cardiac disease, and marked inactivity can cause cardiac atrophy. Heart valves become thick and rigid as a result of sclerosis and fibrosis, compounding

% Change

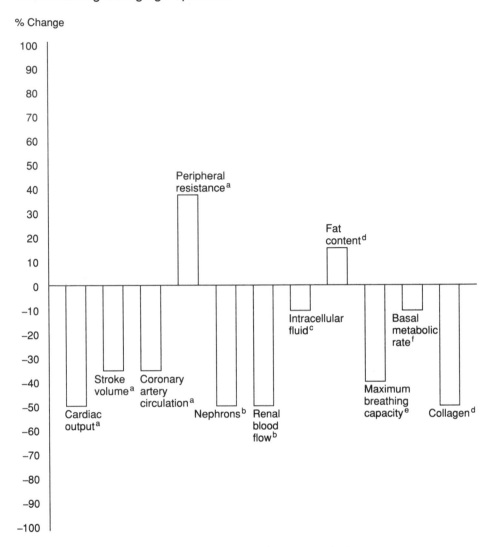

a (Data from Lakatta, EG. Normal changes of aging. In: Abrams WB, Fletcher AJ. The Merck
  manual of geriatrics. Rahway, NJ: Merck Sharp & Dohme Research Laboratories, 1990: 310.
b Rowe JW. Renal system. In: Abrams WB, Fletcher AJ. The Merck manual of geriatrics. Rahway,
  NJ: Merck Sharp & Dohme Research Laboratories, 1990: 598.
c Miller M. Disorders of water and sodium balance. In: Abrams WB, Fletcher AJ. The Merck
  manual of geriatrics. Rahway, NJ: Merck Sharp & Dohme Research Laboratories, 1990: 25.
d Kenney RA. Physiology of aging: A synopsis. Chicago: Yearbook, 1982.
e Krumpe P, Knudson R, Parson G, Reuser K. The aging respiratory system. Clin Geriatr Med,
  1985; 1:143.
f Cape RDT. Malnutrition, weight loss, and anorexia. In: Abrams WB, Fletcher AJ. The Merck
  manual of geriatrics. Rahway, NJ: Merck Sharp & Dohme Research Laboratories, 1990: 5.)

Figure 6-1. *Major age-related changes in body structure and function that occur by
70 years of age.*

the dysfunction associated with any cardiac disease that may be present. The aorta becomes dilated and elongated. The vessels lose their elasticity and accumulate calcium deposits, resulting in a narrowing of their lumen size. This reduced elasticity of the vessels coupled with thinner skin and less subcutaneous fat allows the vessels in the head, neck, and extremities to become more prominent.

Physiological changes in the cardiovascular system appear in a variety of ways. Throughout the adult years, the heart muscle loses its efficiency and contractile strength, resulting in a reduction in cardiac output by 1% per year. Stroke volume decreases by 0.7% yearly. The isometric contraction phase and relaxation time of the left ventricle are prolonged. Usually, adults adjust to this change quite well; they learn that it is easier and more comfortable for them to take an elevator rather than the stairs, to drive instead of walking a long distance, and to pace their activities. When unusual demands are placed on the heart (e.g., shoveling snow for the first time of the season, receiving bad news, running to catch a bus) the changes are realized. The same holds true for the elderly, who are not severely affected by less cardiac efficiency under nonstressful conditions. When older persons are faced with an added demand on their hearts, the difference is noted. Although the pulse rate may not reach the levels experienced by younger persons, tachycardia in the elderly will last for a longer time. Stroke volume may increase to compensate for this situation, which results in elevated blood pressure, although the blood pressure can remain stable as tachycardia progresses to heart failure in the elderly.

Resistance to peripheral blood flow increases by 1% each year. Decreased elasticity of the arteries is responsible for vascular changes to the heart, kidney, and pituitary gland.

The increased rigidity of vessel walls and their narrower lumen necessitate that more force be used to pump blood through the vessels (i.e., systolic and diastolic pressures rise). The level at which the normal elevation becomes hypertension that requires treatment is a source of controversy in geriatric medical circles. Some physicians adhere to conservative practices and treat individuals with blood pressures exceeding 140 mmHg systolic and 90 mmHg diastolic pressure; others would not treat higher levels if no symptoms or damages are apparent (Fig. 6-2). Reduced sensitivity of the blood-pressure–regulating baroreceptors increases problems with orthostatic hypotension.

Respiratory System

Various structural changes in the chest reduce respiratory activity. The calcification of costal cartilage makes the rib cage more rigid; the anterior–posterior chest diameter increases, often demonstrated by kyphosis; and thoracic inspiratory and expiratory muscles are weaker. Alveoli are reduced in number and stretched due to a loss of elasticity. The lungs become more rigid and have less recoil. These changes cause less lung expansion, insufficient basilar inflation, and decreased ability to expel foreign or accumulated matter. The lungs exhale less effectively, thereby increasing the residual volume. As the residual volume increases, the vital capacity is reduced; maximum breathing capacity also decreases. If respiratory activity is reduced under normal circumstances, one can imagine the profound effects of immobility on the respiratory system. With less effective gas exchange and lack of basilar inflation, the elderly are at high risk for developing respiratory infections (Fig. 6-3).

Gastrointestinal System

Although not as life-threatening as cardiovascular or respiratory problems, gastrointestinal symptoms are of more bother and concern to older persons. This system is altered by the aging process at all points. Tooth loss is not a normal consequence of growing old, but poor dental care, diet, and environmental influences contributed to most of today's older population being edentulous. After 30 years of age, periodontal disease is the major reason for tooth loss. Most of the elderly must rely on dentures, which may not be worn regularly because of discomfort or poor fit. If natural teeth are present, they often are in poor condition, having flatter surfaces, stains, and varying degrees of erosion and abrasion of the crown and root structure. Dentin production is decreased, the root pulp experiences shrinkage and fibrosis, the gingiva retracts, and bone density in the alveolar ridge is lost. The tooth brittleness of some older people creates the possibility of aspiration of tooth fragments.

Taste sensations become less acute with age because the taste buds atrophy; chronic irritation (as

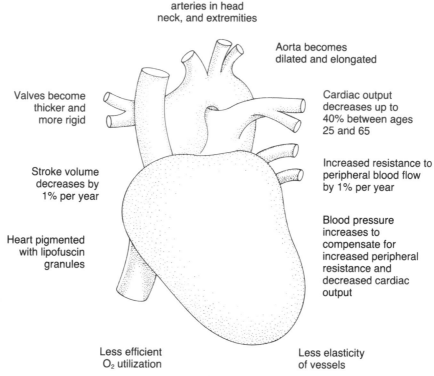

More prominent
arteries in head
neck, and extremities

Aorta becomes
dilated and elongated

Valves become
thicker and
more rigid

Cardiac output
decreases up to
40% between ages
25 and 65

Stroke volume
decreases by
1% per year

Increased resistance to
peripheral blood flow
by 1% per year

Blood pressure
increases to
compensate for
increased peripheral
resistance and
decreased cardiac
output

Heart pigmented
with lipofuscin
granules

Less efficient
O_2 utilization

Less elasticity
of vessels

Figure 6-2. *Cardiovascular changes that occur with aging.*

from pipe smoking) can reduce taste efficiency to a greater degree than that experienced through aging alone. The sweet sensations on the tip of the tongue tend to suffer a greater loss than the sensations for sour, salt, and bitter flavors. Excessive seasoning of foods may be used to compensate for taste alterations and could lead to health problems for the elderly. Loss of papillae and sublingual varicosities on the tongue are common findings.

Approximately one-third of the amount of saliva is produced in old age as in younger years. Salivary ptyalin is decreased, interfering with the breakdown of starches.

Esophageal motility is decreased and the esophagus tends to become slightly dilated. Esophageal emptying is slower, which can cause discomfort because food remains in the esophagus for a longer time. Relaxation of the lower esophageal sphincter may occur; when combined with the elderly's weaker gag reflex and delayed esophageal emptying, aspiration becomes a risk.

The stomach is believed to have reduced motility, along with decreases in hunger contractions and emptying time. The gastric mucosa atrophies. Lesser amounts of hydrochloric acid, pepsin, lipase, and pancreatic enzymes are produced, creating many of the indigestion problems experienced by older adults. Fat absorption is slower, and dextrose and xylose are more difficult to absorb. Absorption of vitamin B, vitamin B_{12}, calcium, and iron is faulty.

Some atrophy occurs throughout the small and large intestines, and fewer cells are present on the absorbing surface of intestinal walls. Constipation is promoted by decreased colonic peristalsis. Neural impulses that sense the signal to defecate are slower and duller, which can cause the need to be postponed, resulting in constipation or impaction. The internal anal sphincter loses its tone with age.

With advancing age, the liver becomes smaller and consequently has less storage capacity. Less

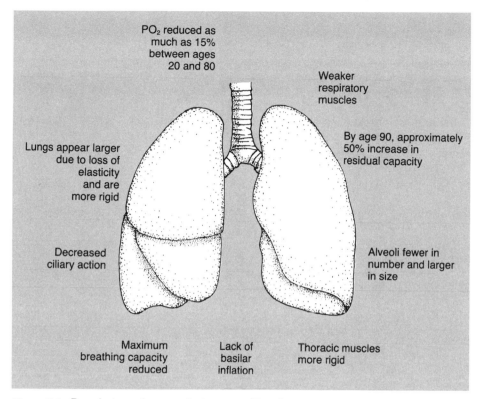

PO₂ reduced as much as 15% between ages 20 and 80

Weaker respiratory muscles

Lungs appear larger due to loss of elasticity and are more rigid

By age 90, approximately 50% increase in residual capacity

Decreased ciliary action

Alveoli fewer in number and larger in size

Maximum breathing capacity reduced

Lack of basilar inflation

Thoracic muscles more rigid

Figure 6-3. *Respiratory changes that occur with aging.*

efficient cholesterol stabilization and absorption cause an increased incidence of gallstones (Fig. 6-4). The pancreatic ducts become dilated an distended, and often the entire gland prolapses.

Genitourinary System

The renal mass becomes smaller with age, which is attributable to a cortical loss rather than a loss of the renal medulla. Renal tissue growth declines, and atherosclerosis may promote atrophy of the kidney. These changes can have a profound effect on renal function. Approximately a 50% decrease in renal blood flow and the glomerular filtration rate occurs between the ages of 20 and 90 years. Tubular function decreases, causing less effective concentration of urine—the maximum specific gravity at age 80 years has been shown to be 1.024, whereas at younger ages it was 1.032. This decrease in function also causes decreased reabsorption of glucose from the filtrate, which can

cause 1+ proteinurias and glycosurias to not be of major diagnostic significance. Decreased renal functioning is further displayed by declines in daily urinary creatinine excretion and creatinine clearance, and an average blood urea nitrogen value of 21.2 mg/dl at age 70 years. From ages 30 to 40 years, the average is 12.9 mg/dl.

Urinary frequency, urgency, and nocturia accompany bladder changes with age. Bladder muscles weaken and bladder capacity decreases. Emptying of the bladder is more difficult; retention of large volumes of urine may result. The micturition reflex is delayed. Although urinary incontinence is not a normal outcome of aging, some stress incontinence may occur because of a weakening of the pelvic diaphragm, particularly in multiparous women (Fig. 6-5).

Prostatic enlargement occurs in most elderly men. The rate and type vary between individuals. Three-fourths of men age 65 years and older have some degree of prostatism, which causes problems

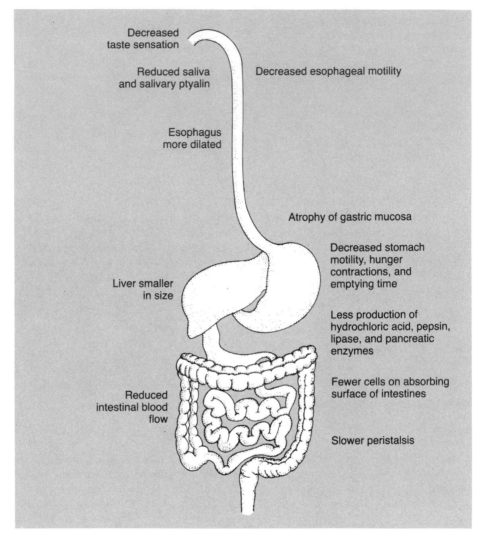

Decreased
taste sensation

Reduced saliva
and salivary ptyalin

Decreased esophageal motility

Esophagus
more dilated

Atrophy of gastric mucosa

Decreased stomach
motility, hunger
contractions, and
emptying time

Liver smaller
in size

Less production of
hydrochloric acid, pepsin,
lipase, and pancreatic
enzymes

Fewer cells on absorbing
surface of intestines

Reduced
intestinal blood
flow

Slower peristalsis

Figure 6-4. *Gastrointestinal changes that occur with aging.*

with urinary frequency. Although most prostatic enlargement is benign, it does pose a greater risk of malignancy and requires regular evaluation. The older man does not lose the physical capacity to achieve erections or ejaculations.

The female genitalia demonstrate many changes with age, including atrophy of the vulva from hormonal changes, accompanied by the loss of subcutaneous fat and hair and a flattening of the labia. The vagina of the older woman appears pink and dry with a smooth, shiny canal because of the loss of elastic tissue and rugae. The vaginal epithelium becomes thin and avascular. The vaginal environment is more alkaline in older women and is ac-

companied by a change in the type of flora and a reduction in secretions. The cervix atrophies and becomes smaller; the endocervical epithelium also atrophies. The uterus shrinks and the endometrium atrophies; however, the endometrium continues to respond to hormonal stimulation, which can be responsible for incidents of postmenopausal bleeding in older women on estrogen therapy. The fallopian tubes atrophy and shorten with age, and the ovaries atrophy and become thicker and smaller. Despite these changes, the older woman does not lose the ability to engage in and enjoy intercourse or other forms of sexual pleasure (Fig. 6-6).

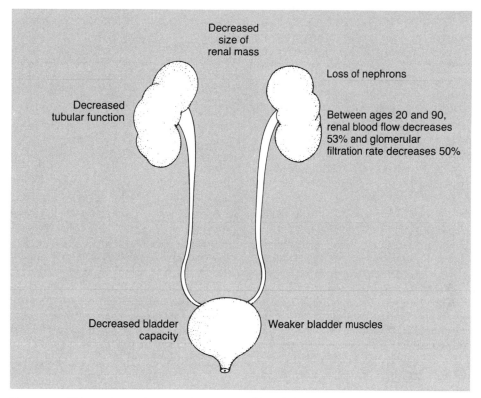

Figure 6-5. *Urinary tract changes that occur with aging.*

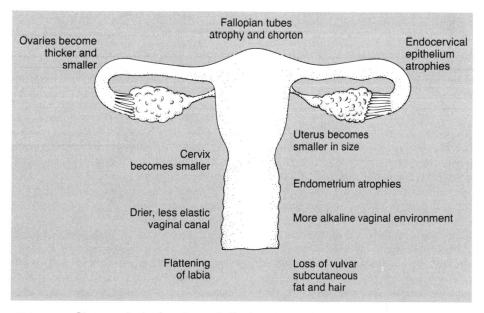

Figure 6-6. *Changes in the female genitalia that occur with aging.*

Musculoskeletal System

The kyphosis, enlarged joints, flabby muscles, and decreased height of many elderly persons announce the variety of musculoskeletal changes occurring with age. Along with other body tissue, muscle fibers atrophy and decrease in number, with fibrous tissue gradually replacing muscle tissue. Overall muscle mass, muscle strength, and muscle movements are decreased; the arm and leg muscles, which become particularly flabby and weak, display these changes well. The importance of exercise to minimize the loss of muscle tone and strength cannot be emphasized enough. Muscle tremors may be present and are believed to be associated with degeneration of the extrapyramidal system. The tendons shrink and harden, which causes a decrease in tendon jerks. Reflexes are lessened in the arms and are nearly totally lost in the abdomen, but are maintained in the knee. For various reasons, muscle cramping frequently occurs.

Bone mineral and mass are reduced, contributing to the brittleness of the bones of older people, especially older women. There is a gradual reabsorption of the interior surface of the long bones and a slower production of new bone on the outside surface. These changes make fractures a serious risk to the elderly. Although long bones do not significantly shorten with age, thinning disks and shortening vertebrae reduce the length of the spinal column, causing a reduction in height with age. Height may be further shortened because of varying degrees of kyphosis, a backward tilting of the head, and some flexion at the hips and knees. A deterioration of the cartilage surface of joints and the formation of points and spurs may limit joint activity and motion (Fig. 6-7).

Nervous System

It is difficult to identify with accuracy the exact impact of aging on the nervous system because of the dependence of this system's function on other body systems. For instance, cardiovascular problems can reduce cerebral circulation and be responsible for cerebral dysfunction. Declining nervous system function may be unnoticed because changes are often nonspecific and slowly progressing. A reduction in nerve cells and cerebral blood flow and metabolism are known to occur. The nerve conduction velocity is lower. These changes are manifested by slower reflexes and delayed response to multiple stimuli. Kinesthetic sense lessens. Because the brain affects the sleep–wake cycle, changes in the sleep pattern occur, with stages III and IV of sleep becoming less prominent. Frequent awakening during sleep is not unusual, although only a minimal amount of sleep is actually lost (Fig. 6-8).

Sensory Organs

Vision

Each of the five senses becomes less efficient with advanced age, interfering in varying degrees with safety, normal activities of daily living, and general well-being. Perhaps the greatest of such interferences results from changes in vision. Presbyopia, the inability to focus properly, is characteristic of older eyes and begins in the fourth decade of life. This vision problem causes most middle-aged and older adults to need corrective lenses. The visual field narrows, making peripheral vision more difficult. The pupil is less responsive to light because the pupil sphincter hardens and pupil size decreases. The light perception threshold increases and vision in dim areas or at night is difficult; older individuals require more light than younger persons to see adequately. Yellowing of the lens and altered color perception make the elderly less able to differentiate the low tone colors of the blues, greens, and violets. Depth perception becomes distorted, causing problems in correctly judging the height of curbs and steps. Dark and light adaptation takes longer. Less efficient reabsorption of intraocular fluid increases the older person's risk for developing glaucoma. The appearance of the eye may be altered; reduced lacrimal secretions can cause the eyes to look dry and dull, and a partial or complete glossy white circle may develop around the periphery of the iris (arcus senilis). Corneal sensitivity is diminished, which can increase the risk of injury to the cornea. In the posterior cavity, bits of debris and condensation become visible and may float across the visual field; these are commonly called floaters.

Hearing

Presbycusis is progressive hearing loss that occurs as a result of aging, and it is the most serious problem affecting the inner ear and retrocochlear. High-frequency sounds are the first to be lost; middle

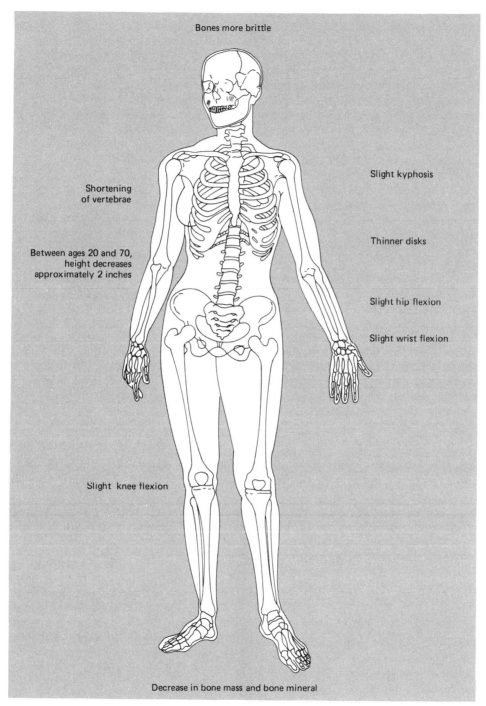

Bones more brittle

Slight kyphosis

Shortening
of vertebrae

Thinner disks

Between ages 20 and 70,
height decreases
approximately 2 inches

Slight hip flexion

Slight wrist flexion

Slight knee flexion

Decrease in bone mass and bone mineral

Figure 6-7. *Skeletal changes that occur with aging.*

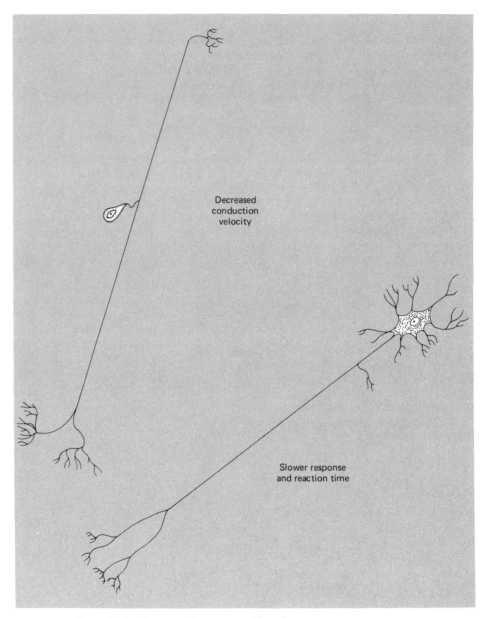

Figure 6-8. Neurologic changes that occur with aging.

and lower frequencies may also be lost as the condition progresses. A variety of factors, including continued exposure to loud noise, may contribute to the occurrence of presbycusis. This problem causes speech to sound distorted as some of the high-pitched sounds (s, sh, f, ph, ch) are filtered from normal speech. This change is so gradual and subtle that affected persons may not realize the extent of their hearing impairment. Hearing can be further jeopardized by an accumulation of cerumen in the middle ear; the higher keratin content of cerumen as one ages contributes to this problem. In addition to hearing problems, equilibrium can be altered because of degeneration of the vestibular structures and atrophy of the cochlea, organ of Corti, and stria vascularis.

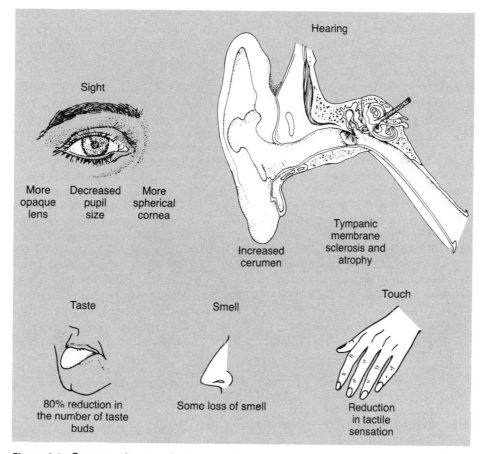

Figure 6-9. *Sensory changes that occur with aging.*

Taste

Although various flavors can be differentiated, taste in the elderly is less acute because the number of functioning taste buds is reduced and they become inefficient in relaying flavors.

Smell

The sense of smell is reduced with age because of a decrease in the number of sensory cells in the nasal lining and fewer cells in the olfactory bulb of the brain.

Touch

Tactile sensation is reduced, as observed in the elderly's reduced ability to sense pressure and pain and differentiate temperatures. These sensory changes can cause misperceptions of the environment and, as a result, profound safety risks (Fig. 6-9).

Endocrine System

With age, the thyroid gland undergoes fibrosis, cellular infiltration, and increased nodularity. The resulting decreased thyroid gland activity causes a lower basal metabolic rate, reduced radioactive iodine uptake, and less thyrotropin secretion and release. Protein-bound iodine levels in the blood do not change, although total serum iodide is reduced. The release of thyroidal iodide decreases with age, and excretion of the 17-ketosteroids declines. The thyroid gland progressively atrophies, and the loss of adrenal function can further decrease thyroid activity. The thyroid-stimulating hormone (TSH) secretion and serum concentration of thyroxine (T_4) do not change. Overall, thyroid function remains adequate.

Much of the secretory activity of the adrenal cortex is regulated by adrenocorticotropic hor-

mone (ACTH), a pituitary hormone. As ACTH secretion decreases with age, secretory activity of the adrenal gland decreases also. Although the secretion of ACTH does not affect aldosterone secretion, it has been shown that less aldosterone is produced and excreted in the urine of older persons. The secretion of glucocorticoids, 17-ketosteroids, progesterone, androgen, and estrogen, also influenced by the adrenal gland, are reduced as well.

The pituitary gland decreases in volume by approximately 20% in older persons. Somatotropic growth hormone remains present in similar amounts, although the blood level may be reduced with age. Decreases are seen in ACTH, TSH, follicle-stimulating hormone, luteinizing hormone, and luteotropic hormone to varying degrees. Gonadal secretion declines with age, including gradual decreases in testosterone, estrogen, and progesterone. With the exception of alterations associated with changes in plasma calcium level or dysfunction of other glands, the parathyroid glands maintain their function throughout life.

There is a delayed and insufficient release of insulin by the beta cells of the pancreas in the elderly, and there is believed to be a decreased sensitivity to circulating insulin. The older person's ability to metabolize glucose is reduced, and sudden concentrations of glucose cause higher and more prolonged hyperglycemia levels; therefore, it is not unusual to detect higher blood glucose levels in nondiabetic older persons.

Immune System

The depressed immune response of older adults causes infections to be a significant risk for this age group. After midlife, thymic mass is lost steadily, to the point that serum activity of thymic hormones is almost undetectable in the aged. T-cell activity declines, and more immature T cells are present in the thymus. A significant decline in cell-mediated immunity occurs, and T lymphocytes are less able to proliferate in response to mitogens. Changes in the T cells contribute to the reactivation of varicella-zoster and *Mycobacterium tuberculosis* infections that are witnessed in many older individuals. Serum immunoglobin concentration is not significantly altered; the concentration of IgM is lower, whereas the concentrations of IgA and IgG are higher. Responses to influenza, parainfluenza, pneumococcus, and tetanus vaccines are less effective (although vaccination is recommended for the elderly). Inflammatory defenses decline and, often, inflammation presents atypically in the elderly (*e.g.*, low-grade fever, minimal pain).

Integumentary System

Diet, general health, activity, exposure, and hereditary factors influence the normal course of aging of the skin. This system's changes are often the most bothersome because they are obvious and clearly reflect advancing years. Flattening of the dermal–epidermal junction, reduced thickness and vascularity of the dermis, and a degeneration of elastin fibers occurs. As the skin becomes less elastic and more dry and fragile and as subcutaneous fat is lost, lines, wrinkles, and sagging become evident. Skin becomes irritated and breaks down more easily. Melanocytes cluster, causing skin pigmentation commonly referred to as age spots; these are more prevalent in areas of the body exposed to the sun. Scalp, pubic, and axilla hair thins and grays; hair in the nose and ears becomes thicker. The growth of facial hair may occur in older women. Fingernails grow more slowly and are hard and brittle. Perspiration is slightly reduced because the number and function of the sweat glands are lessened.

Psychological Changes

Psychological changes during the aging process cannot be isolated from concurrent physical and social changes. Sensory organ impairment can impede interaction with the environment and other people, thus influencing psychological status. Feeling useless and socially isolated may obstruct optimum psychological function. Psychological changes can be influenced by general health status, genetic factors, educational achievement, and activity. Recognizing the variety of factors potentially affecting psychological status and the range of individual responses to those factors, some generalizations can be discussed.

Personality

Drastic changes in basic personality normally do not occur as one ages. The kind and gentle old person was most likely that way when young; likewise, the cantankerous old person probably was not mild and meek in earlier years. Excluding patho-

logical processes, the personality will be consistent with that of earlier years; possibly it will be more openly and honestly expressed. The alleged rigidity of older persons is more a result of physical and mental limitations rather than a personality change. An older person's insistence that her furniture not be rearranged may be interpreted as rigidity, but it may be a sound safety practice for someone coping with poor memory and visual deficits. Changes in personality traits may occur in response to events that alter self-attitude, such as retirement, death of a spouse, loss of independence, income reduction, and disability. No personality type describes all older adults. Morale, attitude, and self-esteem tend to be stable throughout the life span.

Memory

Retrieval of information from long-term memory can be slowed, particularly if the information is not used or needed on a daily basis. Healthy older women have been found to have a greater ability to recall nouns presented in a list than their male counterparts.(Bleeker, 1988) Some age-related forgetfulness can be improved by the use of memory aids (mnemonic devices) such as associating a name with an image, making notes or lists, and placing objects in consistent locations.

Intelligence

In general, it is wise to interpret the findings related to intelligence and the elderly with much caution, because results may be biased from the measurement tool or method of evaluation used. Early gerontological research on intelligence and aging was guilty of such biases. Sick old people cannot be compared with healthy persons; people with different educational backgrounds cannot be compared; and one group of individuals who are skilled and capable of taking an IQ test cannot be compared with those who have sensory deficits and may not have ever taken this type of test. Longitudinal studies that measure changes in a specific generation as it ages and that compensate for sensory, health, and educational deficits are relatively recent, and they serve as the most accurate way of determining intellectual changes with age. It has been shown that basic intelligence is maintained; one does not become less bright or wiser with age. The abilities for verbal comprehension

and arithmetic operations are unchanged. Crystallized intelligence, which arises from the dominant hemisphere of the brain, is maintained through the adult years; this form of intelligence enables the individual to use past learning and experiences for problem-solving. Fluid intelligence, emanating from the nondominant hemisphere, controls emotions, retention of nonintellectual information, creative capacities, spatial perceptions, and aesthetic appreciation; this is believed to decline in later life. Some decline in intellectual function occurs in the moments preceding death.

Learning

Although learning ability is not seriously altered with age, other factors can interfere with the older person's ability to learn, including motivation, attention span, delayed transmission of information to the brain, perceptual deficits, and illness. Older persons may display less readiness to learn and depend on previous experience for solutions to problems rather than experiment with new problem-solving techniques. Differences in the intensity and duration of the elderly's physiological arousal may make it more difficult to extinguish previous responses and acquire new material. The early phases of the learning process tend to be more difficult for older persons than younger individuals; however, after a longer early phase, they are then able to keep equal pace. Learning occurs best when the information is related to previously learned information. Although little difference is apparent between the old and young in verbal or abstract ability, older persons do show some difficulty with perceptual motor tasks. Some evidence indicates a tendency toward simple association rather than analysis. Because it is generally a greater problem to learn new habits when old habits exist and must be unlearned, relearned, or modified, elderly persons with many years of history will have difficulty in this area.

Attention Span

Older adults demonstrate a decrease in vigilance performance (*i.e.*, the ability to retain attention longer than 45 minutes). They are more easily distracted by irrelevant information and stimuli and are less able to perform tasks that are complicated or require simultaneous performance.

(Text continues on page 60)

Table 6-1 *Nursing Actions Related to Age-Related Changes*

AGE-RELATED CHANGE	NURSING ACTION
Reduction in intracellular fluid	Prevent dehydration by ensuring fluid intake of at least 1500 ml daily
Decrease in subcutaneous fat content, decline in natural insulation	Ensure adequate clothing is worn to maintain body warmth; maintain room temperatures between 70°F (21°C) and 75°F (24°C)
Lower oral temperatures	Use thermometers that register low temperatures; assess baseline norm for body temperature when patient is well to be able to identify unique manifestations of fever
Decreased cardiac output and stroke volume; increased peripheral resistance	Allow rest between activities, procedures; recognize the longer time period required for heart rate to return to normal following a stress on the heart and evaluate presence of tachycardia accordingly; ensure blood pressure level is adequate to meet circulatory demands by assessing physical and mental function at various blood pressure levels
Decreased lung expansion, activity, and recoil; lack of basilar inflation; increased rigidity of lungs and thoracic cage; less effective gas exchange and cough response	Encourage respiratory activity; recognize that atypical symptoms and signs can accompany respiratory infection; monitor oxygen administration closely, keep oxygen infusion rate under 4 ml unless otherwise prescribed
Brittleness of teeth; retraction of gingiva	Encourage daily flossing and brushing; ensure patient visits dentist annually; inspect oral cavity for periodontal disease, jagged edged teeth, other pathologies
Reduced acuity of taste sensations	Observe for overconsumption of sweets and salt; be sure foods are served attractively; season foods
Drier oral cavity	Offer fluids during meals; have patient drink before swallowing tablets and capsules, and examine oral cavity after administration to ensure drugs have been swallowed
Decreased esophageal and gastric motility; decreased gastric acid	Assess for indigestion; encourage 5–6 small meals rather than 3 large ones; advise patient not to lie down for at least 1 h following meals
Decreased colonic peristalsis; duller neural impulses to lower bowel	Encourage toileting schedule to provide time for bowel elimination; monitor frequency, consistency, and amount of bowel movements
Decreased size of renal mass, number of nephrons, renal blood flow, glomerular filtration rate, tubular function	Ensure age-adjusted drug dosages are prescribed; observe for adverse responses to drugs; recognize that urine testing for glucose can be unreliable, urinary creatinine excretion and creatinine clearance are decreased, and blood urea nitrogen level is higher
Decreased bladder capacity	Assist patient with need for frequent toileting; ensure safety for visits to bathroom during the night

Table 6-1 *Nursing Actions Related to Age-Related Changes (Continued)*

AGE-RELATED CHANGE	NURSING ACTION
Weaker bladder muscles	Observe for signs of urinary tract infection; assist patient to void in upright position
Enlargement of prostate gland	Ensure patient has prostate examined annually
Drier, more fragile vagina	Advise patient in safe use of lubricants for comfort during intercourse
Increased alkalinity of vaginal canal	Observe for signs of vaginitis
Atrophy of muscle; reduction in muscle strength and mass	Encourage regular exercise; advise patient to avoid straining or overusing muscles
Decreased bone mass and mineral content	Instruct patient in safety measures to prevent falls and fractures; encourage good calcium intake and exercise
Less prominent stages III and IV of sleep	Avoid interruptions at night; assess quantity and quality of sleep
Decreased visual accommodation; reduced peripheral vision; less effective vision in dark and dimly lit areas	Ensure patient has ophthalmologic exam annually; use nightlights; avoid drastic changes in level of lighting; ensure objects used by patient are within visual field
Yellowing of lens	Avoid using shades of greens, blues, and violets together
Decreased corneal sensitivity	Advise patient to protect eyes
Presbycusis	Ensure patient has audiometric exam if problem exists; speak to patient in loud, low-pitched voice
Reduced capacity to sense pain and pressure	Ensure patient changes positions before tissue reddens; inspect body for problems that patient may not sense; recognize unique responses to pain
Reduced immunity	Prevent persons who have infectious diseases from coming in contact with patient; promote positive health practices; identify unique manifestations of infection early; recommend pneumococcal, tetanus, and annual influenza vaccinations; promote good nutritional status to improve host defenses
Slower metabolic rate	Advise patient to avoid excess calorie consumption
Altered secretion of insulin and metabolism of glucose	Advise patient to avoid high carbohydrate intake; observe for unique manifestations of hyper- and hypoglycemia
Flattening of dermal–epidermal junction; reduced thickness and vascularity of dermis; degeneration of elastin fibers	Use principles of pressure ulcer prevention
Skin drier	Recognize need for less frequent bathing; avoid use of harsh soaps; use skin softeners
Slower response and reaction time	Allow adequate time for patient to respond, process information, perform tasks

Nursing Implications

An understanding of common aging changes is essential to ensure competent gerontological nursing practice. Such knowledge can aid in promoting practices that enhance wellness, reducing risks to health and well-being, and identifying pathology in a timely manner. Table 6-1 lists some of nursing actions related to age-related changes.

Gerontological nurses must realize that despite the numerous changes commonly experienced with age, most older adults function admirably well and live normal, satisfying lives. Although nurses should acknowledge factors that can alter function with aging, they should also emphasize the capabilities and assets possessed by older adults and assist persons of all ages in achieving a healthy aging process.

Reference

Bleeker M, Bolla-Wilson AJ, Meyers D. Age-related sex differences in verbal memory. J Clin Psychol 1988;44(3):403.

Recommended Readings

Berman R, Haxby JV, Pomerantz RS. Physiology of aging. Part I: normal changes. Patient Care 1988;22:20.

Bolin AK, Kligman AM. Aging and the skin. New York: Raven, 1988.

Bortz WM. Redefining human aging. J Am Geriatr Soc 1989;37(11):1092.

Evans DW. Renal function in the elderly. American Family Practice 1988;38:147.

Fenske NA, Clifford CW. Skin changes of aging. Geriatrics 1990;45(3):26.

Forbes GB. Human body composition: growth, aging, nutrition, and composition. New York: Springer-Verlag, 1987.

Jackson RA, Hawa MI, Roshania RD, Sim BM, DiSilvio L, Jaspan JB. Influence of aging on hepatic and peripheral glucose metabolism in humans. Diabetes 1988;37:119.

Lonergan ET. Aging and the kidney: adjusting treatment to physiologic change. Geriatrics 1988;43(3):27.

Kart CS, Metress EK, Metress SP. Aging, health and society. New York: Jones & Barlett, 1988.

Morris JC, McManus DQ. The neurology of aging: normal vs. pathologic change. Geriatrics 1991;46(8):47.

Rosenthal J. Aging and the cardiovascular system. Gerontology 1987;33(suppl 1):3.

Shock NW, Greulich RC, Andres R, et al. Normal human aging: The Baltimore Longitudinal Study of Aging. Bethesda, MD: National Institutes of Health, 1984.

Whitbourne SK. The aging body: physiological changes and psychological consequences. New York: Springer-Verlag, 1985.

Promoting Wellness and Self-Care

7

Facilitating Self-Care

Surviving to old age is a tremendous accomplishment. Basic life requirements such as obtaining adequate nutrition, keeping oneself relatively safe, and maintaining the body's normal functions must have been met with some success. The hurdles of coping with crises, adjusting to change, and learning new skills have been confronted and overcome to varying degrees. Throughout their lives, the elderly have faced many important decisions such as the following:

Should they leave the old country to make a fresh start in America?

Should they stay in the family business or seek a job in the local factory?

Should they risk their lives to fight in a war they believe in?

Should they invest their entire savings in a business of their own?

Should they allow their children to continue their education when the children's employment would ease a serious financial hardship?

The elderly have had to be strong and resourceful to navigate the stormy waters of life.

Too often, nurses initiate interventions from other sources to meet the needs of the elderly and overcome their weaknesses rather than by helping the elderly do so themselves. The elderly then become passive participants in their care. After a lifetime of taking care of themselves and others, making their own decisions, and meeting life's most trying challenges, it may be difficult for the elderly to accept less involvement in their care. They may become angry or depressed at being forced to forfeit their decision-making functions to others. They may unnecessarily develop feelings of dependency, uselessness, and powerlessness. Gerontological nurses must recognize the strengths and capabilities of older people so that they can be participants in rather than objects of care. Tapping the resources of the elderly in their own care promotes normalcy, independence, and individuality; it aids in avoiding secondary problems related to the reactions of older adults to an unnecessarily imposed dependent role.

Self-Care Theory

Sound nursing practice is based on a theoretical framework—an organized statement of principles to guide actions. Theoretical frameworks can make nursing care easier and more effective by offering systematic approaches that can be used for every patient. Among the various theories available to nurses, Orem's self-care theory is particularly relevant to gerontological care.(Orem, 1980) Orem's theory states that:

All human beings have to meet certain needs or life demands such as air, food, water, excretion, activity, rest, solitude, social interaction, avoidance of hazards to life and well-being, and maintaining normalcy.

Each individual has unique capacities and limitations regarding the ability to fulfill these demands.

Self-care capacity exists when individuals are able to be independent and take responsibility for meeting these needs.

A self-care limitation exists when an individual's ability to fulfill a demand is partially or totally restricted.

Nursing actions focus on promoting capacity and reducing limitations of the individual so that care can be provided for oneself as independently as possible.

Self-Care Model and Gerontological Nursing

Using the basic principles of Orem's theory, a self-care model for gerontological nursing practice can be developed. Figure 7-1 demonstrates how the self-care model flows. It can be described as follows:

Universal life demands. Older individuals share similar universal life demands with all other human beings. These are basic requirements for the optimum and integrated functioning of the total individual. Age, illness, and disability may interfere with the ability to meet any of

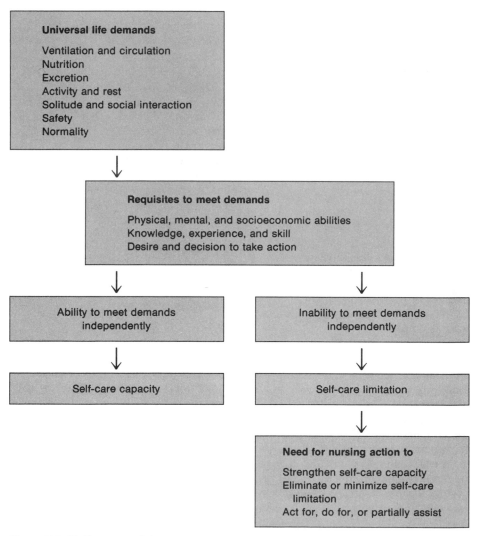

Figure 7-1. *Self-care model.*

these demands. Assistance may be required, perhaps in the form of nursing services.

Requisites to meet demands. The ability of the elderly to meet universal life demands depends on several factors.

Physical, mental, and socioeconomic abilities. Aged individuals may be able to remain active and involved in life if they have adequate financial resources. Individuals will be able to prevent contractures if they are physically able to have unrestricted motion. On the other hand, if individuals lack the finances to obtain necessary health-care services, the energy to ambulate and feed themselves, or the mental faculties to cross a street safely, self-care will be limited.

It is the nurses' responsibility to minimize or reduce limitations imposed by physical, mental, and socioeconomic restrictions. Nursing services that assist in the reduction of limitations are discussed in Chapter 18.

Knowledge, experience, and skills. Limitations exist when the knowledge, experience, or skills required for a given self-care action are inadequate or nonexistent. An individual with a wealth of social skills is capable of a normal, active life that includes friendships and other social interaction. People who have knowledge of the hazards of cigarette smoking will be more capable of protecting themselves from health problems associated with this habit. On the other hand, an older man who is widowed may not be able to cook and provide an adequate diet for himself if he depended on his wife for meal preparation. The diabetic person who lacks skill in self-injection of insulin may not be able to meet the therapeutic demand for insulin administration. Specific nursing considerations for enhancing self-care capacities will be offered in other chapters.

Desire and decision to take action. The value a person sees in performing the action, as well as the person's knowledge, attitudes, beliefs, and degree of motivation, influence the desire and decision for action. Limitations result if a person lacks desire or decides against action. If an individual is not interested in preparing and eating meals because of social isolation and loneliness, a dietary deficiency may develop. A hypertensive individual's lack of desire and decision to forfeit potato chips and pork products in the diet because of a belief that it is not worth the effort may create a real health threat. The person who is not informed of the importance of physical activity may not realize the need to arise from bed during an illness and consequently may develop complications. Dying individuals, viewing death as a natural process, may decide against medical intervention to sustain life and may not comply with prescribed therapies.

Values, attitudes, and beliefs are deeply established and not easily altered. Although the nurse should respect the right of individuals to make decisions affecting their lives, if limitations restrict their ability to meet self-care demands, the nurse can help by explaining the benefit of a particular action, providing information, and developing motivation. In some circumstances, as with an emotionally ill or mentally incompetent person, desires and decisions may have to be superseded by professional judgments.

Self-care capacity. If the individual is successful in fulfilling life demands, there is no need for nursing intervention except to reinforce the capability for self-care.

Self-care limitation. The inability to meet demands independently creates a need for nursing intervention. Nursing actions are directed toward strengthening self-care capacities, eliminating or minimizing self-care limitations, and providing direct services by acting for, doing for, or assisting the individual when demands cannot be independently fulfilled.

Self-Care Model and Geriatric Nursing

Frequently, nursing's involvement with the elderly is associated with intervening when health-care problems exist. When individuals are ill, new demands frequently arise, such as administering medications, observing for symptoms, and performing special treatments. In geriatric nursing, consideration must be given to assessing the impact of the illness on the individual's self-care capacity and

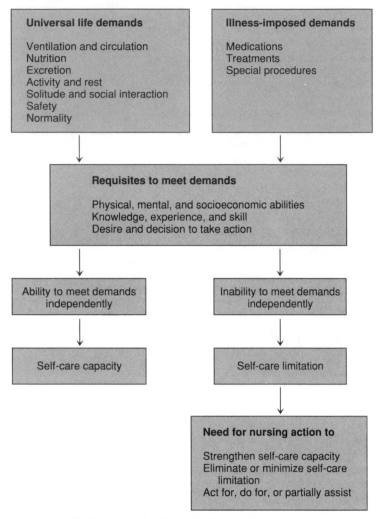

Figure 7-2. *Self-care model for geriatric nursing.*

identifying appropriate nursing interventions to ensure that both the universal life demands and the demands imposed by illness are adequately met.

Figure 7-2 demonstrates how the self-care model becomes operational in geriatric nursing practice. During the assessment the nurse identifies the specific illness-imposed demands that are present.

Mr. R has been a long-term diabetic who administers insulin daily and follows a diabetic diet. Because of a recent urologic problem, he may now need to take antibiotics daily and perform intermit-

tent self-catheterization. During the assessment, the nurse identifies the presence of these illness-imposed demands.

After the primary assessment has revealed the presence of these illness-imposed demands, the nurse will evaluate how well these demands are met.

The nurse finds that Mr. R performs self-catheterization according to procedure, is administering his antibiotics as prescribed, but is not adhering to his

diabetic diet and alters his insulin dosage based on "how he feels that day."

The next level of assessment must seek the reasons for deficits in meeting the illness-imposed demands.

Mr. R has knowledge of the diabetic diet and wants to comply, but had depended on his wife to prepare meals and now that she is deceased, he has difficulty cooking nutritious meals independently. He denies ever being informed of the need for regular doses of his insulin and states that he has relied on the advice of his brother-in-law, also a diabetic, who told him "to take an extra shot of insulin when he eats a lot of sweets."

Once the skill and knowledge deficits behind the patient's deficits in meeting these illness-imposed demands are identified, specific nursing care plan actions can be developed.

The Self-Care Theory and the Nursing Process

The self-care theory interfaces well with the nursing process. It can be described as follows:

Assessment. Through the assessment process, information is gained about the structure and function of the individual. In reviewing the data, the nurse can determine the ability of the person to meet universal life demands. For example, a person may have teeth in poor condition, which could affect the life demands of:
Nutrition: altered intake of food
Social interaction: embarrassment at appearance of teeth
Safety: risk of aspirating a dislodged tooth
Normalcy: poor self-concept
The reasons for the poor dental status must be determined and could include the following:
Physical inability to care for teeth because of arthritic fingers
Mental inability to remember steps in brushing teeth
Inadequate bathroom facilities to brush and floss teeth
Lack of knowledge of good dental practices
Too depressed to care about dental hygiene

Once the reasons for the deficit are specifically identified, a nursing diagnosis can be derived (see Nursing Diagnoses). For example:
Alteration in nutrition: less than body requirement, related to painful teeth and inability to chew
Pain related to poor condition of teeth and gums
Disturbance in self-concept related to unattractive teeth
Planning. Nursing actions are planned to strengthen self-care capacity, remove or minimize limitations, or care for or partially assist the individual in meeting demands.
Implementation. The nursing plans are put into action.
Evaluation. A determination is made as to how effectively the demands are being fulfilled and if any change has occurred in the fulfillment of previously satisfied demands.

Figure 7-3 exemplifies the relationship of the self-care model to the nursing process.

Case Example

The following case demonstrates how this model can work.

The Case of Mrs. D

Mrs. D, 78 years of age, was admitted to a hospital service for acute conditions with the identified problems of a fractured neck of the femur, malnutrition, and a "disposition problem." Initial observation revealed a small-framed, frail-looking lady, with obvious signs of malnutrition and dehydration. She was well oriented to person, place, and time and was able to converse and answer questions coherently. Although her memory for recent events was poor, she seldom forgot to inform anyone who was interested that she neither liked nor wanted to be in the hospital. Her previous and only other hospitalization had been 55 years earlier.

Mrs. D had been living with her husband and an unmarried sister for more than 50 years when her husband died. For the 5 years following his death, she depended heavily on her sister for emotional support and guidance. Then her sister died, which

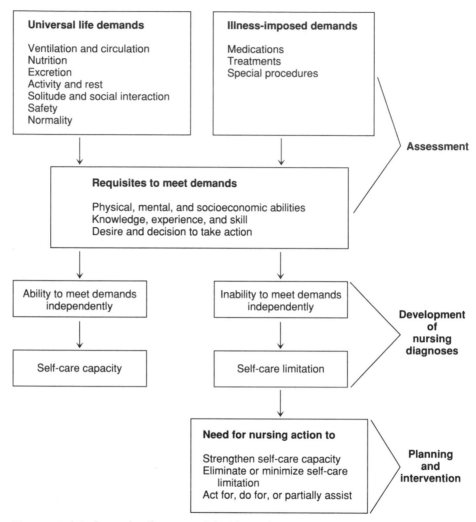

Figure 7-3. *Interface of self-care model with nursing process.*

promoted feelings of anxiety, insecurity, loneliness, and depression. Living alone, she cared for her six-room home in the county with no assistance other than that from a neighbor who did the marketing for Mrs. D and occasionally provided her with transportation. A year later, on the day of her admission to the hospital, Mrs. D fell on her kitchen floor, weak from her malnourished state. Discovering her hours later, her neighbor called an ambulance, which transported Mrs. D to the hospital. Once the diagnosis of fractured femur was established, plans were made to perform a nailing procedure, to correct her malnourished state, and to find a new living arrangement because her home demanded more energy and attention than she was capable of providing.

Based on Mrs. D's self-care capacities and limitations, the following nursing diagnoses, based on universal life demands, were identified and related actions planned.

Universal Life Demand: Ventilation and Circulation

Nursing Diagnoses

Impaired physical mobility related to fracture
Impaired gas exchange related to immobility

Goals

Facilitate adequate ventilation
Prevent respiratory distress and infection
Prevent obstructions to circulation

Related Nursing Action	*Type of Action*
1. Maintain normal respirations	
Prevent blockage of airway or any other interference with normal breathing	Partially assisting
Observe for and detect respiratory problems early	Partially assisting
2. Promote active and passive exercises	
Teach and encourage turning, coughing, and deep-breathing exercises	Strengthening self-care capacity
Encourage active exercises, such as using blow bottles and deep-breathing	Strengthening self-care capacity
Perform passive range-of-motion exercise	Doing for
3. Avoid external interferences with respiration	
Provide good room ventilation	Doing for
Avoid restrictive clothing, linens, or equipment	Doing for
Position in manner conducive to best respiration	Partially assisting
Prevent anxiety-producing situations, such as delays in answering call bell	Doing for

Universal Life Demand: Nutrition

Nursing Diagnoses

Altered nutrition: less than body requirements related to depression and loneliness

Goals

Consumption of at least 1500 ml of fluids and 1800 calories of nutrients daily
Increase weight to 125 pounds

Continued on next page

Related Nursing Action	**Type of Action**
1. Stimulate appetite	
Plan diet according to person's preferences, consistent with therapeutic requirements	Partially assisting
Provide a quiet, pleasant environment that allows for socialization with others	Doing for
Stimulate appetite through appearance and seasoning of foods	Minimizing self-care limitation
2. Plan meals	
Read menu selection to patient	Partially assisting
Guide choice of high-protein, carbohydrate, and vitamin- and mineral-rich foods	Minimizing self-care limitation
Assess food preferences and include them in menu selections	Acting for
3. Assist with feeding	
Conserve energy and promote adequate intake by preparing food tray, encouraging rest periods, and feeding when necessary	Strengthening self-care capacity, doing for, and partially assisting
4. Prevent complications	
Do not leave solutions, medications, or harmful agents in location where they may be mistakenly ingested (especially when assessment indicates visual limitations)	Acting for
Check temperature of foods and drinks to prevent burns (especially when assessment indicates decreased cutaneous sensation)	Acting for
Assist in the selection of foods conducive to bone healing and correction of malnutrition	Partially assisting
Observe fluid intake and output for early detection of imbalances	Minimizing self-care limitation
Assess general health status frqeuently to detect new problems or improvements that have resulted from changes in nutritional status (*e.g.,* weight changes, skin turgor, mental status, strength)	Acting for and minimizing self-care limitation

Universal Life Demand: Excretion

Nursing Diagnoses

Constipation related to immobility
High risk for infection related to malnutrition and interferences with normal bathing

Goals

Prevent infection
Establish regular bowel elimination schedule
Prevent constipation
Promote and maintain positive hygienic practices

Related Nursing Action	*Type of Action*
1. Promote regular elimination of bladder and bowels	
Guide the selection of a diet high in roughage and fluids	Partially assisting
Observe and record elimination pattern	Acting for and minimizing self-care limitation
Assist with exercises to promote peristalsis and urination	Partially assisting
Arrange schedule to provide regular time periods for elimination	Acting for
Assist with hygienic care of body surfaces	Partially assisting
Provide privacy when bedpan is used	Acting for
2. Develop good hygienic practices	
Teach importance and method of cleansing perineal region after elimination	Strengthening self-care
3. Prevent social isolation	
Prevent, detect, and correct body odors resulting from poor hygienic practices	Acting for, minimizing self-care limitation

Universal Life Demand: Activity and Rest

Nursing Diagnoses

Activity intolerance related to malnutrition and fracture

Impaired physical mobility related to fracture

Sleep pattern disturbance related to hospital environment and movement limitations associated with fracture

Goals

Prevent sleep deprivation and fatigue

Maintain or improve range of motion of joints

Prevent complications secondary to immobility

Related Nursing Action	*Type of Action*
1. Adjust hospital routines to individual's pace	Strengthening self-care capacity
Space procedures and other activities	Acting for
Allow longer periods for self-care activities	Minimizing self-care limitation
2. Provide for energy conservation	
Promote security and relaxation through the avoidance of frequent changes of personnel	Acting for
Allow for short rest periods several times a day	Strengthening self-care capacity
Control environmental noise, light, and temperature	Acting for
3. Prevent complications associated with immobility (such as decubiti, constipation,	

Continued on next page

renal calculi, contractures, hypostatic
pneumonia, thrombi, edema, and lethargy)

Encourage frequent change of position	Minimizing self-care limitation
Motivate and reward activity	Strengthening self-care capacity
Teach simple exercises to prevent complications and improve motor dexterity	Strengthing self-care capacity
Plan activities to increase independence progressively	Acting for and strengthening self-care capacity

Universal Life Demand: Solitude and Social Interaction

Nursing Diagnoses

Anxiety, fear, hopelessness, and powerlessness related to hospitalization and health state
Impaired social interaction related to hospitalization

Goals

Promote and maintain social interaction
Prevent emotional distress

Related Nursing Action	*Type of Action*
1. Control environmental stimuli	
Schedule the same personnel to care for person	Acting for
Maintain a regular daily schedule	Strengthening self-care capacity
Arrange for a roommate with similar interests and background	Acting for and strengthening self-care capacity
Regulate the amount of visitors	Acting for
Space activities and procedures	Acting for and minimizing self-care limitation
2. Promote meaningful social interactions	
Instruct others to speak clearly and sufficiently loud while facing the person	Strengthening self-care capacity
Plan activities in which person can be involved	Strengthening self-care capacity
Promote and maintain an oriented state	Strengthening self-care capacity and minimizing self-care limitation
Display interest in person's social interactions and encourage their continuation	Strengthening self-care capacity
Initiate contacts with community agencies to develop relationships that can continue after discharge	Acting for and minimizing self-care limitation
Assist with grooming and dressing	Partially assisting and minimizing self-care limitation
3. Provide opportunities for solitude	
Provide several preplanned time periods during the day in which person can be alone	Acting for
Provide privacy by pulling curtains around bed and making use of facilities such as chapel	Minimizing self-care limitation and partially assisting

Universal Life Demand: Safety

Nursing Diagnoses

Sensory–perceptual alterations (visual, auditory, olfactory, tactile) related to advanced age

High risk for injury related to sensory deficits

High risk for impaired skin integrity related to immobility, malnutrition, and decreased sensations

Impaired home maintenance management related to altered health state, convalescence

Goals

Prevent injury

Maintain skin integrity

Compensate for sensory deficits through the use of assistive devices, eyeglasses, hearing aids (as prescribed)

Identify and arrange for safe, acceptable living arrangements postdischarge

Related Nursing Action	*Type of Action*
1. Compensate for poor vision	
Read to person	Doing for and minimizing self-care limitation
Write information and label with large letters and color coding when possible	Minimizing self-care limitation
Remove obstacles that could cause accidents, such as foreign objects in bed, clutter on floor, and solutions that could be mistaken as water	Minimizing self-care limitation and acting for
Communicate this problem to other personnel	Acting for
Initiate an ophthalmology referral	Acting for
2. Compensate for decreased ability to smell	
Prevent and correct odors resulting from poor hygienic practices	Partially assisting and minimizing self-care limitations
Detect unusual odors early (may be symptomatic of infection)	Acting for
3. Compensate for hearing loss	
Speak clearly and loudly while facing person	Minimizing self-care limitation
Use feedback techniques to make sure person has heard and understood	Minimizing self-care limitation
Initiate referral to ear, nose, and throat clinic	Acting for
4. Maintain good skin condition	
Inspect for rashes, reddened areas, and sores	Doing for
Assist with hygienic practices	Partially assisting
Give back rubs, change person's position	Doing for
frequently, and keep person's skin soft and dry	Partially assisting and minimizing self-care limitation
5. Prevent falls	
Support person who is ambulating or being transported	Partially assisting
Maintain muscle tone	Strengthening self-care capacity

Continued on next page

Keep bed rails up and support person in wheelchair	Doing for
Provide rest periods between activities	Strengthening self-care capacity and minimizing self-care limitation
Place frequently used objects within easy reach	Partially assisting
6. Maintain proper body alignment	
Use sandbags, trochanter rolls, and pillows	Minimizing self-care limitation and partially assisting
Support person's affected limb when it is lifted or moved	Partially assisting and minimizing self-care limitation
7. Seek safe living arrangements in preparation for person's discharge	
Evaluate patient's preferences, capacities, and limitations to suggest appropriate arrangements	Acting for and partially assisting
Initiate referral to social worker	Acting for

Universal Life Demand: Normality

Nursing Diagnoses

Self-esteem disturbance related to health problems and life situation

Goals

Restore preinjury level of physical activity
Promote maximum degree of independent self-care

Related Nursing Action	*Type of Action*
1. Improve physical limitations where possible	
Assist with reeducation for ambulation	Partially assisting and strengthening self-care capacity
Exercise body parts to maintain function	Partially assisting and minimizing self-care limitation
Encourage patient to consume an adequate diet	Strengthening self-care capacity
Initiate referral for audiometric examination to explore utility of hearing aid	Acting for Minimizing self-care limitation
Initiate ophthalmology referral to explore utility of corrective lenses	Acting for and minimizing self-care limitation
2. Maintain familiar components of life-style	
Adjust hospital routine to person's home routine as much as possible	Acting for and minimizing self-care limitation
Encourage person to wear own clothing	Minimizing self-care limitation
Provide person with personal items from home, pillow, blanket, photographs, and tea cup	Minimizing self-care limitation
Provide leisure activities person is accustomed to	Minimizing self-care limitation and strengthening self-care capacity

3. Promote active participation

Provide person with opportunities to make own decisions whenever possible	Strengthening self-care capacity
Involve person in care	Strengthening self-care capacity
Stimulate and encourage communication	Strengthening self-care capacity

Reference

Orem D. Nursing: concepts of practice. 2nd ed. New York: McGraw-Hill, 1980.

Recommended Readings

Burnside I. Nursing and the aged: a self-care approach. 3rd ed. New York: McGraw-Hill, 1988.

Walker SN. Wellness and aging. In: Murrow E, ed. Perspective on gerontological nursing. Newbury Park, CA: SAGE, 1991:41.

8

Ventilation and Circulation

The exchange of carbon dioxide with oxygen in the lungs (*i.e.*, ventilation) and in all blood-carrying vessels throughout the body (*i.e.*, circulation) is essential to life. These acts, of which we are seldom conscious in earlier life, can become major foci of attention in later years because of the impact of age-related changes (Table 8-1). It is crucial that actions be planned to prevent and address some of the potential nursing problems related to ventilation and circulation.

Tissue Health

Good tissue health depends on adequate tissue perfusion (*i.e.*, the circulation to and from a body part). To ensure good tissue perfusion, arterial blood pressure must be maintained within a normal range. Factors that can alter tissue perfusion include the following:

Cardiovascular disease: arteriosclerotic heart disease, hypertension, congestive heart failure, varicosities

Other diseases: diabetes mellitus, cancer, renal failure

Blood dyscrasias: anemia, thrombus, transfusion reactions

Hypotension: arising from anaphylactic shock, hypovolemia, hypoglycemia, hyperglycemia, orthostatic hypotension

Medication side-effects: antihypertensives, vasodilators, diuretics, antipsychotics

Other conditions: edema, inflammation, prolonged immobility, hypothermia, malnutrition.

The adequacy of tissue circulation should be assessed in older adults by reviewing the individual's health history, evaluating vital signs, inspecting the tissues, and noting signs or symptoms. Display 8-1 lists indications of altered tissue perfusion.

Because the elderly possess age-related changes and a high prevalence of health conditions that increase their risk of altered tissue perfusion, gerontological nurses should promote interventions that improve tissue circulation, such as the following:

Ensure blood pressure is maintained within an acceptable range (recognizing that older adults may require higher blood pressure levels to provide adequate tissue perfusion than do younger persons).

Prevent and eliminate sources of pressure on the body.

Remind or assist patients to change positions frequently.

Prevent pooling of blood in the extremities.

Encourage physical activity.

Prevent hypothermia, maintaining body warmth (particularly of the extremities).

Massage the body.

Monitor drugs for the side-effect of hypotension.

Educate to reduce risks (*e.g.*, avoiding excess alcohol ingestion, cigarette smoking, obesity, inactivity).

Periodically evaluate physical and mental health to identify signs and symptoms of altered tissue perfusion.

Tips on pressure ulcer prevention can be found in Chapter 29, which offers guidance in keeping

Table 8-1 *Aging and Risks to Adequate Ventilation and Circulation*

AGE-RELATED FACTOR	POTENTIAL NURSING DIAGNOSIS
Ventilation	
Reduced elastic recoil of lungs during expiration	Impaired gas exchange
Increase in residual capacity	Ineffective breathing pattern
Decrease in vital capacity	Altered respiratory function
Decrease in maximum breathing capacity	High risk for infection
Reduced number and elasticity of alveoli	Ineffective airway clearance
Increased diameter of bronchioles and alveolar ducts	Activity intolerance due to decreased respiratory efficiency
Reduced ciliary activity	
Loss of skeletal muscle strength in thorax and diaphragm	
Increased rigidity of thoracic muscles and ribs	
Increased diameter of anteroposterior chest	
Less efficient cough response	
Circulation	
Decreased elasticity of blood vessels	Altered tissue perfusion
Increased resistance of peripheral vessels	
Less efficient cardiac oxygen usage	Activity intolerance
Reduced proportion of oxygen extracted from arterial blood by tissues	Altered tissue perfusion
	Impaired gas exchange

skin healthy and intact. An often overlooked measure to promote tissue circulation is the maintenance of an adequate blood pressure level. Hypotension can reduce cerebral circulation and subsequently decrease the amount of oxygenation of that tissue; this is an important consideration for the elderly taking antihypertensive drugs. What may be a high blood pressure for a 40-year-old person can be normal for an older adult.

Effective Breathing

To ensure adequate ventilation, respiratory infection must be prevented. In addition to the precautions any adult would take, older persons need to be particularly attentive to obtaining influenza and pneumonia vaccines and avoiding exposure to individuals who have respiratory infections. The susceptibility of older people to drafts necessitates that indirect room ventilation be used—fibrosis, common in the elderly, can be aggravated by chilling and drafts. The elderly should be advised to seek medical attention promptly if any sign of a respiratory infection develops. Frequently, older people do not experience the chest pain associated with pneumonia to the same degree as younger adults, and their normally lower body temperature can cause an atypical appearance of fever (*i.e.*, at lower levels than would occur for younger persons). Thus, by the time symptoms are

DISPLAY 8-1   Indications of Altered Tissue Perfusion

Hypotension
Tachycardia, decreased pulse quality
Claudication
Edema
Loss of hair on extremities
Tissue necrosis
Dyspnea, increased respirations
Pallor, coolness of skin
Cyanosis
Decreased urinary output
Delirium (altered cognition and level of consciousness)
Restlessness
Memory disturbances

visible to others, pneumonia can be in an advanced stage. The elderly should be taught to report changes in the character of sputum, which could be associated with certain disease processes. For example, the sputum will be tenacious, translucent, and grayish white with chronic obstructive pulmonary disease; it is purulent and foul smelling with a lung abscess or bronchiectasis; and it is red and frothy with pulmonary edema and left-sided heart failure.

Approximately 80% of the elderly population has some degree of chronic obstructive pulmonary disease; people with this disorder tend to retain a higher amount of carbon dioxide in their lungs. The nurse should teach deep breathing exercises to all older persons and encourage that they be done regularly (Fig. 8-1). To aid in making these exercises a habit in daily routine, they can be linked to other routines, for example, before meals or every time the person sits down to watch the news. Carbon dioxide retention increases the risk of developing the serious complication of carbon dioxide narcosis during the administration of oxygen therapy. Oxygen should be used prudently with the elderly; blood gases should be monitored and the patient should be observed for symptoms of carbon dioxide narcosis. These include confusion, muscle twitching, visual defects, profuse perspiration, hypotension, progressive degrees of circulatory failure, and cerebral depression, which may be displayed as increased sleeping or a deep comatose state.

Although it may appear to be a relatively minor consideration, hair in the nostrils becomes thicker with age and may readily accumulate a greater amount of dust and dirt particles during inspiration. Unless these particles are removed and the nasal passage is kept patent, there may be an interference with the normal inspiration of air. Blowing the nose and mild manipulation with a tissue may adequately rid the nostrils of these particles. When particles are difficult to remove, a cotton-tipped applicator moistened with warm water or saline solution may help loosen them. Caution should be taken not to insert the cotton-tipped applicator too far into the nose because trauma can easily result. Any nasal obstruction not easily removed should be brought to a physician's attention. Some considerations for promoting effective breathing can be found in the Nursing Diagnosis Highlight.

Promoting Mobility

A variety of highly prevalent health problems can make normal movement difficult and painful. For instance, arthritic joints can be uncomfortable to

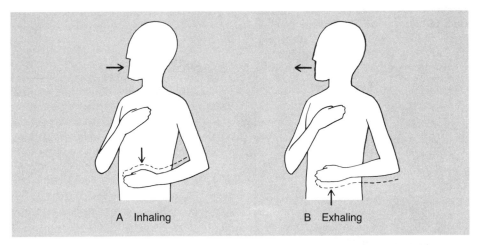

| A Inhaling | B Exhaling |

Figure 8-1 *Breathing exercises should emphasize forced expiration. (**A**) With one hand on the stomach (below the ribs) and the other over the middle anterior chest, the patient should inhale to the count of one. The hand over the stomach should fall as the stomach moves downward; the hand over the chest should not move. (**B**) Expire air to the count of three. The hand over the stomach should rise as the stomach moves upward; the hand over the chest should not move.*

NURSING DIAGNOSIS HIGHLIGHT
Ineffective Breathing Pattern

Overview

In late-life there is a high prevalence of conditions that limit the ability to adequately inflate the lungs or rid them of sufficient amounts of carbon dioxide. Signs such as dyspnea, shortness of breath, abnormal arterial blood gases, cyanosis, pursed-lip breathing, retraction of respiratory muscles during breathing, and shallow respirations could be associated with this diagnosis.

Causative or contributing factors

Weakness, fatigue, pain, paralysis, immobility, altered mental status, respiratory or musculoskeletal disease.

Goal

The patient displays an effective breathing pattern, is free from signs of ineffective breathing, and possesses normal arterial blood gases.

Interventions

- Instruct patient in breathing exercises (see Fig. 8-1).
- Control symptoms (*e.g.,* pain) that could threaten effective respirations.
- Raise head of bed at least 30° when patient is lying down, unless contraindicated.
- Instruct patient to turn, cough, and deep breathe at least once every 2 hours.
- Monitor rate, depth, and rhythm of respirations; coloring; coughing pattern; blood gases; and mental status.

move, medications can create drowsiness, and shortness of breath may lead individuals to live a sedentary life. Elderly persons are more likely to possess problems that can reduce their mobility, and their ventilatory and circulatory functions suffer serious consequences. Secretions can pool in the lungs and lead to serious infections, breathing will be shallow and lead to ineffective gas exchange, and tissue circulation can be impaired.

A basic component of health education for the elderly and their caregivers is the warning that immobility should be avoided at all costs. Well-intentioned caregivers may believe they are being kind by encouraging the older person to rest or stay in bed; elderly persons may hold the misconception that when one is sick one should go to bed. They need to understand the serious harm and further discomfort that can result from immobility. Movement of each body part several times daily and frequent position changes are essential to good health. Chapter 11 describes various exercises that promote an active state.

Recommended Readings

Acee S. Helping patients breathe more easily . . . noninvasive nursing measures. Geriatr Nurs 1984;5(6):230.

deVries HA. Exercise. In: Cassel CK, Walsh JR, eds. Geriatric medicine. vol. 2. New York: Springer-Verlag, 1984:175.

Ebersole P, Hess P. Toward healthy aging: human needs and nursing response. 3rd ed. St Louis: CV Mosby, 1990:155.

Hitzhusen JC. The elderly heart: special signs and symptoms to watch for. Geriatrics 1984;39(6):38.

McConnell ES. Nursing diagnoses related to physiological alterations. In: Matteson MA, McConnell ES, eds. Gerontological nursing: concepts and practice. Philadelphia: WB Saunders, 1988:331.

Orem SE. Assessment of the cardiovascular system. In: Eliopoulos C, ed. Health assessment of the older adult. Menlo Park, CA: Addison-Wesley, 1984:47.

Sigmon HD. Assessment of the respiratory system. In: Eliopoulos C, ed. Health assessment of the older adult. Menlo Park, CA: Addison-Wesley, 1984:81.

9

Nutrition

The impact of nutrition on health and functional capacity is profound. The ability to defend the body against disease, maintain anatomical and structural normality, think clearly, and possess the energy and desire to engage in social activity is determined by one's nutritional status. Numerous age-related changes, often subtle and gradual, can progressively jeopardize the ability of the elderly to maintain good nutritional status; these changes demand special nursing attention (Table 9-1).

Although the body's needs for basic nutrients are consistent throughout life, the required amount of specific nutrients may vary. One of the most significant differences in nutrient requirements among people of different ages involves caloric intake. Several factors contribute to the elderly's reduced needs for calories.

The older body has less body mass and a relative increase in adipose tissue. Adipose tissue metabolizes more slowly than lean tissue and does not burn calories as quickly.

The activity level for most older adults is usually lower than it was during their younger years.

The diet of the elderly should reflect a lower quantity and higher quality of food. Fewer carbohydrates and fats are required in the diets of older adults. The decreased ability of the older person to maintain a regular blood glucose level emphasizes the need for a reduced carbohydrate intake. A high carbohydrate diet can stimulate an abnormally high release of insulin in the elderly. This can cause hypoglycemia, which can first present in the elderly as a confusional state. At least 1 g protein per kilogram body weight is necessary to renew body protein and protoplasm and to maintain enzyme systems. Several protein supplements are available commercially and may be useful additives to the older person's diet. Although the ability to absorb calcium decreases with age, calcium is still required in the diet to maintain a healthy musculoskeletal system as well as to promote the proper functioning of the body's blood-clotting mechanisms. The use of calcium supplements may benefit older persons but should first be discussed with the physician to ensure that other medical problems do not contraindicate them.

It is recommended that older women reduce their caloric intake to 1800 calories until age 75 years and to 1600 calories thereafter; for older men, 2400 calories, reduced to 2050 calories after age 75 years, is advised. It must be emphasized that these calorie requirements serve as general guidelines—each person will have a unique calorie need based on individual body size, metabolism, health status, and activity level. Tables 9-2, 9-3, and 9-4 present averages for body composition for the elderly population.

Because fewer calories will be ingested in later life, those calories should be of higher quality to

Table 9-1 *Aging and Risks to Nutritional Status*

AGE-RELATED FACTOR	POTENTIAL NURSING DIAGNOSIS
Teeth have various degrees of erosion, abrasions of crown and root structure, high prevalence of tooth loss	Altered nutrition: less than body requirements related to limited ability to chew foods Pain related to poor condition of teeth
Reduction in saliva to approximately one-third volume of earlier years	Altered nutrition: less than body requirements related to less efficient mixing of foods
Inefficient digestion of starch due to decreased salivary ptyalin	Altered nutrition; less than body requirements related to reduced breakdown of starches
Atrophy of epithelial covering in oral mucosa	Altered oral mucous membrane
Increased taste threshold; approximately one-third the number of functioning taste buds per papilla of earlier years	Sensory–perceptual alterations: gustatory Altered nutrition: more than body requirements related to excessive intake of salts and sweets to compensate for taste alterations
Decreased thirst sensations; reduced hunger contractions	Altered nutrition: less than body requirements related to reduced ability to sense hunger Fluid volume deficit related to decreased thirst sensations
Weaker gag reflex; decreased esophageal peristalsis; relaxation of lower esophageal sphincter; reduced stomach motility	High risk for injury from aspiration Altered nutrition: less than body requirement related to self-imposed restrictions to avoid discomfort
Less hydrochloric acid, pepsin, and pancreatic acid produced	Altered nutrition: less than body requirement related to ineffective breakdown of food
Less fat tolerance	Altered comfort: pain related to indigestion
Decreased colonic peristalsis; reduced sensation for signal to defecate	Altered nutrition: less than body requirement related to reduced appetite and self-imposed restrictions related to constipation
Less efficient cholesterol stabilization and absorption	High risk for infection related to risk of gallstone formation
Increased fat content of pancreas; decreased pancreatic enzymes	Altered nutrition: less than body requirements related to problems in normal digestion

ensure an adequate intake of other nutrients. Table 9-5 lists the recommended daily allowances, also known as RDAs, for older adults.

Nutritional Assessment

A wide range of physical, mental, and socioeconomic factors affect nutritional status in later life. Because these factors can change, regular nutritional assessment is necessary. Effective nutritional assessment involves the collaboration of the physician, nurse, nutritionist, and social worker. The basic components of the nutritional assessment are described in Display 9-1.

Hydration

With age, intracellular fluid is lost, resulting in decreased total body fluids. This reduces the margin of safety for any fluid loss; a reduced fluid intake or increased loss that would be only a minor problem in younger persons could be life-threatening to the elderly. Special measures must be taken to ensure a minimum fluid intake of 1500 ml daily. The el-

Table 9-2 *Comparison of the Weight-for-Height Tables from Actuarial Data (Build Study): Non-Age-Corrected Metropolitan Life Insurance Company and Age-Specific Gerontology Research Center Recommendations**

Height (ft–in)	METROPOLITAN 1983 WEIGHTS (LBS) FOR AGES 25–59†		GERONTOLOGY RESEARCH CENTER WEIGHT RANGE FOR MEN AND WOMEN (LBS)‡				
	Men	Women	Age 25	Age 35	Age 45	Age 55	Age 65
4–10	—	100–131	84–111	92–119	99–127	107–135	115–142
4–11	—	101–134	87–115	95–123	103–131	111–139	119–147
5–0	—	103–137	90–119	98–127	106–135	114–143	123–152
5–1	123–145	105–140	93–123	101–131	110–140	118–148	127–157
5–2	125–148	108–144	96–127	105–136	113–144	122–153	131–163
5–3	127–151	111–148	99–131	108–140	117–149	126–158	135–168
5–4	129–155	114–152	102–135	112–145	121–154	130–163	140–173
5–5	131–159	117–156	106–140	115–149	125–159	134–168	144–179
5–6	133–163	120–160	109–144	119–154	129–164	138–174	148–184
5–7	135–167	123–164	112–148	122–159	133–169	143–179	153–190
5–8	137–171	126–167	116–153	126–163	137–174	147–184	158–196
5–9	139–175	129–170	119–157	130–168	141–179	151–190	162–201
5–10	141–179	132–173	122–162	134–173	145–184	156–195	167–207
5–11	144–183	135–176	126–167	137–178	149–190	160–201	172–213
6–0	147–187	—	129–171	141–183	153–195	165–207	177–219
6–1	150–192	—	133–176	145–188	157–200	169–213	182–225
6–2	153–197	—	137–181	149–194	162–206	174–219	187–232
6–3	157–202	—	141–186	153–199	166–212	179–225	192–238
6–4	—	—	144–191	157–205	171–218	184–231	197–244

*Values in this table are for height without shoes and weight without clothes. To convert inches to centimeters, multiply by 2.54; to convert pounds to kilograms, multiply by 0.455.
†The weight range is the lower weight for small frame and the upper weight for large frame.
‡Data from Andres R. Mortality and obesity: the rationale for age-specific height-weight tables. In: Andres R, Bierman EL, Hazzard WR, eds. Principles of geriatric medicine. New York: McGraw-Hill, 1985:311.
From Andres R, Elahi D, Tobin JD, Muller DC, Brant L. Impact of age on weight goals. Ann Intern Med 1985:103(6):1032.

Table 9-3 *Percentiles for Triceps Skinfold Thickness (in mm)*

Age	95%		50%		5%	
	Men	Women	Men	Women	Men	Women
65	27.0	33.0	13.8	21.6	8.6	13.5
70	26.1	32.0	12.9	20.6	7.7	12.5
75	25.2	31.0	12.0	19.6	6.8	11.5
80	24.3	30.0	11.2	18.6	6.0	10.5
85	23.4	29.0	10.3	17.6	5.1	9.5
90	22.6	28.0	9.4	16.6	4.2	8.5

A skinfold measurement below the 5th percentile can indicate a calorie deficiency; a measurement above the 95th percentile can be associated with obesity.
Courtesy of Ross Laboratories, Columbus, OH.

Table 9-4 *Percentiles for Midarm Muscle Area (in cm²)*

Age	95%		50%		5%	
	Men	*Women*	*Men*	*Women*	*Men*	*Women*
65	77.1	66.4	59.4	44.5	43.2	33.5
70	75.3	65.9	57.7	44.1	41.4	33.0
75	73.5	65.5	55.9	43.6	39.6	32.6
80	71.7	65.1	54.1	43.2	37.8	32.2
85	69.9	64.7	52.3	42.8	36.0	31.8
90	68.2	64.2	50.5	42.4	34.3	31.3

A protein deficiency can be associated with midarm muscle area below the 5th percentile.
Courtesy of Ross Laboratories, Columbus, OH.

derly should be evaluated for factors that can cause them to consume less fluid, such as the following:

- age-related reductions in thirst sensations
- fear of incontinence
- lack of accessible fluids

Table 9-5 *Recommended Dietary Allowances for People Over 50 Years of Age*

	MEN	WOMEN
Protein (g)	56	44
Vitamin A (μg RE*)	1000	800
Vitamin D (μg)	5	5
Vitamin E (mg α-TE†)	10	8
Vitamin C (mg)	60	60
Thiamin (mg)	1.2	1
Riboflavin (mg)	1.4	1.2
Niacin (mg NE‡)	16	13
Vitamin B$_6$ (mg)	2.2	2
Folacin (μg)	400	400
Vitamin B$_{12}$ (μg)	3	3
Calcium (mg)	800	800
Phosphorus (mg)	800	800
Magnesium (mg)	350	300
Iron (mg)	10	10
Zinc (mg)	15	15
Iodine (μg)	150	150
Calories	2400	1800
after age 76	2050	1600

*Retinol equivalents
†α-Tocopherol equivalents
‡Niacin equivalents
Recommended dietary allowances. 9th ed. Washington, DC: National Academy of Sciences, 1980.

- inability to obtain or drink fluids independently
- lack of motivation
- altered mood or cognition
- nausea, vomiting, gastrointestinal distress.

When such factors are present or there is any suspicion as to the adequacy of fluid intake, fluid intake and output should be recorded and monitored. The Nursing Diagnosis Highlight discusses the nursing diagnosis relating to this problem.

Fluid restriction not only predisposes the elderly to infection, constipation, and decreased bladder distensibility, but also can lead to serious fluid and electrolyte imbalances. Dehydration, a life-threatening condition to older persons because of their already reduced amount of body fluid, is demonstrated by dry, inelastic skin; dry, brown tongue; sunken cheeks; concentrated urine; blood urea value elevated above 60 mg/dl; and, in some cases, confusion. At the other extreme, the elderly are also more sensitive to overhydration caused by decreased cardiovascular and renal function. Overhydration is a consideration if intravenous fluids are needed therapeutically.

Oral Health

Painless, intact gums and teeth will promote the ingestion of a wider variety of food. The ability to meet nutritional requirements in old age is influenced by basic dental care throughout one's lifetime. Poor dental care, environmental influences, inappropriate nutrition, and changes in gingival tissue commonly contribute to severe tooth loss in older persons. After the third decade of life, peri-

DISPLAY 9-1   *Components of the Nutritional Assessment*

History

- Review health history and medical record for evidence of diagnoses or conditions that can alter the purchase, preparation, ingestion, digestion, absorption, or excretion of foods.
- Review medications for those that can affect appetite and nutritional state.
- Patient's description of diet, meal pattern, food preferences and restrictions.
- Diary of all food intake for a week.

Physical Examination

Inspect hair: hair loss or brittleness can be associated with malnutrition.

Inspect skin: note persistent "goose bumps" (vitamin-B_6 deficiency), pallor (anemia), purpura (vitamin-C deficiency), brownish pigmentation (niacin deficiency), red scaly areas in folds around eyes and between nose and corner of mouth (riboflavin deficiency), dermatitis (zinc deficiency), fungus infections (hyperglycemia).

Test skin turgor. Skin turgor, although poor in many older adults, tends to be best in the areas over the forehead and sternum; therefore, these are preferred areas to test.

Note muscle tone, strength and movement. Muscle weakness can be associated with vitamin and mineral deficiencies.

Inspect eyes. Ask about changes in vision, night vision problems (vitamin-A deficiency).

Note the patient's percentile rank (see Table 9-4).

Biochemical Evaluation

Obtain blood sample for screening of total iron binding capacity, transferrin saturation, protein, albumin, hemoglobin, hematocrit, electrolytes, vitamins, prothrombin time.

Obtain urine sample for screening of specific gravity.

Inspect oral cavity. Note dryness (dehydration), lesions, condition of tongue, breath odor, condition of teeth or dentures.

Ask about signs and symptoms: sore tongue, indigestion, diarrhea, constipation, food distaste, weakness, muscle cramps, burning sensations, dizziness, drowsiness, bone pain, sore joints, recurrent boils, dyspnea, anorexia, appetite changes.

Cognition and Mood

Test cognitive function.

Note alterations in mood, behavior, cognition level of consciousness. Be alert to signs of depression (can be associated with deficiencies of vitamin B_6, magnesium, or niacin).

Ask about changes in mood or cognition.

Anthropometric Measurement

Measure and ask about changes in height and weight. Use age-adjusted weight chart for evaluating weight (see Table 9-2). Note weight losses of 5% within the past 1 month and 10% with the past 6 months.

Determine triceps skinfold measurement. To do so, grasp a fold of skin and subcutaneous fat halfway between the shoulder and elbow and measure with a caliper. Note the patient's percentile rank (see Table 9-3).

Measure the midarm circumference with a tape measure (using centimeters) and use this to calculate midarm muscle mass with formula:

$$\frac{MC - \dfrac{3.14 \times TSM^2}{10}}{12.56} = MMA$$

MC, midarm circumference; MMA, midarm muscle area; TSM, triceps skin-fold measurement.

---

odontal disease becomes the first cause of tooth loss; by 70 years of age, most people have lost all their teeth. Obviously, a lifetime of poor dental care cannot be reversed. Geriatric dental problems need to be prevented early in a person's life. Although the specialty of geriatric dentistry is growing, many persons do not have access to this service nor do they always possess the financial means to avail themselves of this care.

Through education, the nurse should make the public aware of the importance of good, regular dental care and oral hygiene at all ages, as well as the fact that aging alone does not necessitate the loss of teeth. The use of a toothbrush is more effec-

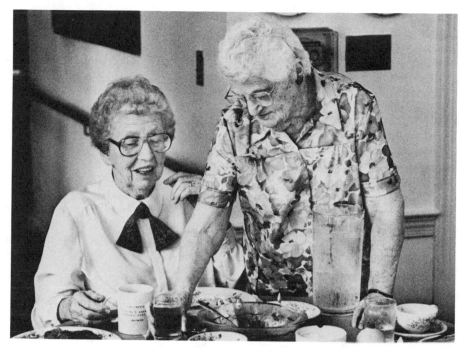

Although they usually need to ingest fewer calories than younger persons, older adults' diets must include a high quality of nutrients. (Photograph by Eric Schenk.)

tive in improving gingival tissues and removing soft debris from the teeth than are swabs or other soft devices. However, care should be taken not to traumatize the tissues because they are more sensitive, fragile, and prone to irritation in the elderly. Dental problems can affect virtually every system of the body; therefore, they must be corrected promptly. Loose teeth should be extracted to prevent them from being aspirated and causing a lung abscess.

Many older adults believe that having dentures eliminates the necessity for dental care. The nurse must correct this misconception and encourage continued dental care for the individual with dentures. Lesions, infections, and other diseases can be detected by the dentist and corrected to prevent serious complications from developing. Changes in tissue structure may have affected the fit of the dentures and require readjustment. Poorly fitting dentures need not always be replaced; sometimes they can be lined to ensure a proper fit. This should be made known to the elderly who may resist correction out of concern for the expense involved. Most importantly, dentures should be used

and not kept in a pocket or dresser drawer! Wearing dentures will allow proper chewing and encourage the elderly to introduce a wider variety of foods in their diets.

Threats to Good Nutrition
Poor Appetite

A poor appetite resulting from decreased taste sensation can have adverse effects on the elderly's nutritional status. Taste receptors are lost with age because of taste bud atrophy, chronic irritation, or general wear. The receptors on the tip of the tongue lose the most sensation, including those for sweet and salt. The taste buds for bitter and sour tastes remain, contributing to the elderly's perception that many foods taste unpleasant. Those working with the elderly should recognize this factor and understand the reason for older adults adding excessive amounts of salt and sugar to their food. These taste deficiencies compound the difficulties in adjusting to a limited sodium or sugar diet, fre-

quently prescribed for the elderly. The use of sugar and salt substitutes and other flavoring such as lemon should be considered to compensate for taste alterations. Appetite also can be stimulated by serving food attractively and perhaps with a small glass of wine.

Indigestion and Food Intolerance

Indigestion and food intolerance are common among the elderly because of decreased stomach motility, less gastric secretion, and a slower gastric-emptying time. Older persons frequently attempt to manage these problems by using antacids or limiting food intake—both potentially predispose them to other risks. Other means to manage these problems should be explored, such as the following:

Eating several small meals rather than three large ones. This not only provides a smaller amount of food to be digested at one time but also aids in maintaining a more stable blood glucose level throughout the day.

Avoiding or limiting fried foods. It is easier to digest broiled, boiled, or baked food.

Identifying and eliminating specific foods from the diet to which an intolerance exists. Often the elderly need help identifying problem foods, particularly if they have included those foods in their diets throughout their entire lives.

Sitting in a high Fowler position while eating and for one-half hour following meals. Sitting upright increases the size of the abdominal and thoracic cavities, provides more room for the stomach, and facilitates swallowing and digestion.

Ensuring adequate fluid intake and activity to assist the motility of food through the digestive tract.

Constipation

Constipation is a common problem among the elderly because of slower peristalsis, inactivity, and less bulk and fluid in the diet. If food intake is reduced to relieve discomfort, nutritional status can be threatened. Laxatives, another relief measure, can result in diarrhea, leading to dehydration; if oil-based laxatives are used, fat-soluble vitamins (*e.g.*, A, D, K, and E) can be drained from the body, leading to vitamin deficiencies. Constipation must be recognized as a frequent problem for the elderly, and preventive measures should be encouraged. Plenty of fluids, fruits, vegetables, and activity are advisable, as is providing a regular and adequate time allowance for a bowel movement. Fiber is important but must be used with care. Excessive fiber intake can cause bowel obstruction, diarrhea, or the formation of bezoars, which are dense masses of seeds, skins, and other fiber-containing components of plants that form in the stomach. (Yen, 1991) The lower gastric acidity contributes to bezoar development, which is demonstrated by nausea, vomiting, fullness, abdominal pain, and diarrhea.(Yen, 1991) Laxatives should be considered only after other measures have proven unsuccessful, and when necessary should be used with great care.

Malnutrition

Because malnourishment is a potential and serious threat to the elderly, it should be closely monitored. The variety of factors contributing to this problem include decreased taste and smell sensations, reduced mastication capability, slower peristalsis, decreased hunger contractions, reduced gastric-acid secretion, and less absorption of nutrients because of reduced intestinal blood flow and a decrease in cells of the intestinal absorbing surface. Socioeconomic factors contributing to malnutrition must be considered. The appearance of the elderly can be misleading and delay the detection of a malnourished state. Some of the clinical signs of malnutrition include the following:

- weight loss greater than 5% in the past month or 10% in the past 6 months
- weight 10% below or 20% above ideal range
- serum albumin level lower than 3.5 g/100 ml
- hemoglobin level below 12 g/dl
- hematocrit value below 35%.

Of course, other problems can indicate malnutrition, such as dermatitis, hair loss, lethargy, and fatigue. It is crucial that keen assessment skills be used to recognize early malnourishment in the elderly and that good nutritional practices be encouraged to prevent its occurrence.

NURSING DIAGNOSIS HIGHLIGHT
Fluid Volume Deficit

Overview

Fluid volume deficit refers to a state of dehydration in which intracellular, extracellular, or vascular fluid is less than that required by the body. This condition can be indicated by increased output, reduced intake, concentrated urine, weight loss, hypotension, increased pulse, poorer skin turgor, dry skin and mucous membranes, increased body temperature, weakness, and elevated serum creatinine, blood urea nitrogen, and hematocrit.

Causative or contributing factors

Vomiting, diarrhea, polyuria, excessive drainage, profuse perspiration, increased metabolic rate, insufficient intake due to physical or mental limitation, inaccessible fluids, medications (*e.g.,* diuretics, laxatives, sedatives).

Goal

The patient possesses an intake and output balance within 200 ml and has cause of problem identified and corrected.

Interventions

- Perform a comprehensive assessment to identify underlying cause of fluid volume deficit; obtain treatment for underlying cause as appropriate.
- Maintain a strict record of intake and output.
- Closely monitor vital signs, urine specific gravity, skin turgor, mental status.
- Monitor the patient's weight daily until problem corrected.
- Force fluids, at least 2000 ml during a 24-hour period unless contraindicated; offer foods that are high in fluid content (*e.g.,* gelatin, sherbets, soup); keep fluids easily accessible.
- Consult with physician regarding need for intravenous fluid replacement; if prescribed, monitor carefully because of high risk of overhydration in elderly persons.
- Assist with or provide good oral hygiene.
- Identify persons at high-risk for dehydration and closely monitor their intake and output.

Reference

Yen, PK. The dark side of fiber. Geriatr Nurs 1991;12(1):43.

Recommended Readings

Garry PJ, Rhyne RL, Halioua L, Nicholson C. Changes in dietary patterns over a 6 year period in an elderly population. In: Murphy C, Cain WS, Hegsted DM, eds. Nutrition and the chemical senses in aging. Ann NY Acad Sci 1989;561:104.

Geriatrics Panel Discussion: Practical nutritional advice for the elderly. Geriatrics 1990;45(11):47.

Hoffman NB. Dehydration in the elderly: insidious and manageable. Geriatrics 1991;46(6):35.

Kunkel ME. Nutrition and aging. In: Murrow E, ed. Perspectives on gerontological nursing. Newbury Park, CA: SAGE, 1991:323.

Yen PK: The picture of malnutrition. Geriatr Nurs 1989;10(3):159.

10

Excretion

To maintain a healthy state, the body must rid itself of waste material and that eliminated material must be properly disposed. Excretory processes are seldom given considerable thought; they are automatic and natural. With age, however, these processes are less efficient and demand more conscious thought and assistance to be performed satisfactorily (Table 10-1).

Bladder Elimination

Changes in the urinary tract with age may cause various elimination problems. One of the greater annoyances is caused by decreased bladder capacity. The bladders of some older people may have the capacity for only 200 ml or less of urine; frequency is common in older adults as a result. This factor should be kept in mind when individuals who are unable to ambulate independently are placed in wheelchairs; they will not be able to sit all day without needing to void, and unnecessary incontinence may result if toileting is not provided. Trips and activities should be planned to allow bathroom breaks at frequent intervals. Not only do older people find more frequent voiding necessary during the day, but night frequency may be a bothersome problem also. Often, kidney circulation improves when a recumbent position is assumed, and voiding may be required a few hours after the individual lies down and at other times during the night.

With the increased light-perception threshold of the elderly making night vision difficult, nocturia could predispose them to accidents and threaten their safety. Night-lights should be used to improve visibility during trips to the bathroom, and any clutter or environmental hazards that could cause a fall should be removed. Reducing fluids immediately before bedtime may help, although they should not be significantly restricted. If multiple episodes of nocturia occur nightly, medical evaluation may be warranted to ensure that no urinary tract problem is present. The elderly and their caregivers should be advised that longer-acting diuretics such as the thiazides, even when administered in the morning, can cause nocturia.

Bladder muscles weaken with age, which may promote the retention of large volumes of urine. The most common cause of retention in women is a fecal impaction; prostatic hypertrophy, present to some degree in most older men, is the primary cause in men. Symptoms of retention include the following:

- urinary frequency
- straining
- dribbling
- palpable bladder
- feeling that the bladder has not been emptied.

Retention can predispose older individuals to the development of a urinary tract infection. Good fluid intake and efforts to enhance voiding should be emphasized, including the following:

Table 10-1 *Aging and Risks to Normal Excretion of Wastes*

AGE-RELATED FACTOR	POTENTIAL NURSING DIAGNOSIS
Loss of nephrons; approximately 50% decrease in glomerular filtration rate	Altered health maintenance related to ineffective filtration of drugs, wastes from blood
Decreased resorption of glucose from filtrate; less concentration of urine	Altered health maintenance related to unreliable urine specimen findings on which to identify health deviations
Weaker bladder muscles; decreased bladder capacity; slower micturation reflex; prostate enlargement	Altered patterns of urinary elimination: urgency, frequency, nocturia related to age-related changes
Decreased colonic perstalsis; duller neural impulses for signal to defecate	Altered bowel elimination: constipation related to age-related changes
Weaker respiratory muscles; inefficient cough response	High risk for infection related to ineffective breathing patterns, causing reduced ability to expel material

- voiding in upright position
- massaging bladder area
- rocking back and forth
- running water
- soaking hands in warm water.

The filtration efficiency of the kidneys decreases with age, which is an important factor in the elimination of drugs. The nurse should observe the patient for signs of adverse drug reactions resulting from an accumulation of toxic levels of medications. Higher blood urea nitrogen levels may occur duc to reduced renal function, causing lethargy, confusion, headache, drowsiness, and other symptoms. Decreased tubular function may cause problems in the concentration of urine; the maximum specific gravity at 80 years of age has been shown to be 1.024, whereas at younger ages it is 1.032. Reduced ability to concentrate and dilute urine in response to water or sodium excess or depletion occurs. Decreased reabsorption from the filtrate makes a proteinuria of 1.0 usually of no diagnostic significance in the elderly. An increase in the renal threshold for glucose is a serious concern, because the elderly can be hyperglycemic without evidence of glycosuria. False-negative results in diabetic urine testing can occur for this reason.

The inability to control the elimination of urine (*i.e.,* incontinence) is not a normal occurrence with advanced age. Incontinence reflects a physical or mental disorder and demands a thorough evaluation. Some stress incontinence may be present, particularly in women who have had multiple pregnancies or in persons who postpone voiding after they sense the urge. More information on incontinence can be found in Chapter 25.

Bowel Elimination

Bowel function is often a major concern of the elderly, many of whom were raised with the belief that anything other than a single daily bowel movement is abnormal. Slower peristalsis, inactivity, reduced food and fluid intake, and the ingestion of less bulk food are responsible for the high incidence of constipation in the elderly (see Nursing Diagnosis Highlight). Decreased sensory perception may cause the signal for bowel elimination to go unnoticed, which can promote constipation. There also is a tendency toward incomplete emptying of the bowel at one voiding; 30 to 45 minutes after the initial movement, the remainder of the bowel movement may need to occur and, if not heeded, problems may develop.

Laxative abuse as a reaction to real or anticipated constipation is common among the elderly. These drugs are not benign substances, as many people believe, and their habitual use should be discouraged. The problems associated with chronic laxative use include the following:

Dehydration: diarrhea can occur and deplete fluids rapidly.

Electrolyte imbalances: the high amounts of sodium and other substances in laxative preparations can alter blood levels of electrolytes.

Digestion disturbances: magnesia-based preparations can reduce the already lowered amount of gastric acid.

Vitamin depletion: fat-soluble vitamins A, D, K, and E can dissolve in oil-based laxatives and be excreted.

Education is important to help the elderly and their caregivers understand that daily bowel elimination is not crucial. As long as the bowels move on some regular basis (*e.g.*, every few days) without strain, the stools are not hard and dry, and no abdominal swelling or discomfort occurs, no concern is necessary.

A good fluid intake, a diet rich in fruits and vegetables, activity, and the establishment of a regular time for bowel elimination can be beneficial in maintaining a regular elimination pattern in the elderly. Because of the tendency for incomplete emptying of the bowel at one voiding, opportunity should be provided for full emptying and for repeated attempts at elimination at subsequent times. Sometimes, an older person's request to be taken to the bathroom or to have a bedpan for bowel elimination shortly after a movement occurred is viewed as an unnecessary demand and ignored; it is then wondered why fecal incontinence results. It is useful for older adults to attempt a bowel movement following breakfast because the morning activity and ingestion of food and fluid following a period of rest stimulate peristasis. Suppositories occasionally may be necessary to stimulate elimination, and they should be administered one-half hour before bowel elimination is desired. Fecal softeners are commonly prescribed to promote elimination in older persons.

Itching and discomfort around the rectum may result from poor hygienic practices, hemorrhoids, or dryness caused by reduced secretions of the mucous membrane. Scratching and dryness can irritate the tissue and lead to skin breaks and infection. Regular, thorough cleansing with mild soap and water, followed by the application of a small amount of a lubricant, can minimize this problem. Coarse toilet tissue always should be avoided.

Flatulence

Flatulence, common in the elderly, is caused by constipation, irregular bowel movements, certain foods, and poor neuromuscular control of the anal sphincter. Achieving a regular bowel pattern and avoiding flatus-producing foods may relieve this problem, as may the administration of specific medications intended for this purpose.

Discomfort associated with the inability to expel flatus may occur occasionally. Increased activity can provide relief, as may a knee-chest position, if possible. A flatus bag consisting of a rectal tube with an attached plastic bag that prevents the entrance of air into the rectum can be beneficial (Fig. 10-1).

Fecal Impaction

Prevention of constipation aids in avoiding fecal impaction. Observation of the frequency and character of bowel movements may aid in detecting the development of an impaction; a defecation record is essential for older people in a hospital or nursing home. Indications of a fecal impaction include:

- distended rectum
- abdominal and rectal discomfort
- oozing of fecal material around the impaction; often mistaken as diarrhea
- palpable, hard fecal mass

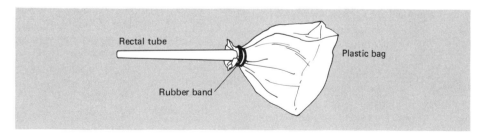

Rectal tube

Plastic bag

Rubber band

Figure 10-1. *A flatus bag can be made by attaching a plastic bag to a rectal tube.*

Fecal impactions should be corrected promptly and with care. Sometimes an oil retention enema will soften the impaction and facilitate its passage. If this initial procedure is not effective, it may be essential to break up the impaction with a lubricated gloved finger. Inserting 60 ml hydrogen peroxide before the digital attempt at removal sometimes will assist in breaking the impaction. This procedure should be done only after confirming that no lower gastrointestinal problems exist and consulting with the physician.

Excretion Through the Skin

The cleansing process of waste excretion through the skin is different in advanced age because of age-related changes. Perspiration and oil production are decreased, making less frequent bathing necessary. Reduced hydration and vascularity of the dermis make the skin less elastic and more delicate. Consequently, dryness, itching, and breakage of the skin can result from too much bathing. Unless some problem warrants a different

---

NURSING DIAGNOSIS HIGHLIGHT
Constipation

Overview
Constipation is a condition in which there is an infrequent passage of dry, hard stools. Some of the findings consistent with constipation include: decreased frequency of bowel movements (as compared to patient's normal pattern), straining to have bowel movement, hard, dry stools, abdominal distention and discomfort, palpable mass and sense of pressure or fullness in rectum, poor appetite, back ache, headache, reduced activity level, and request for or use of laxatives or enemas.

Causative or contributing factors
Age-related decrease in peristalsis, inactivity, immobility, hemorrhoidal pain, poor dietary intake of fiber and fluids, dehydration, surgery, dependency on laxatives or enemas, side-effects of medications (e.g., antacids, calcium, anticholinergics, barium, iron, narcotics).

Goal
The patient establishes a regular pattern of bowel elimination and passes normal consistency stool without straining or experiencing discomfort.

Interventions
- Establish and maintain record of frequency and characteristics of bowel movements.
- Ensure patient consumes at least 1500 ml fluids daily (unless contraindicated).
- Review dietary pattern with patient and educate as needed regarding the inclusion of high-fiber foods in diet; monitor dietary intake.
- Assist patient in developing a program to increase activity level as appropriate.
- Assist patient in developing a regular schedule for toileting; provide toileting assistance as needed; ensure privacy is provided during toileting; if bedpan must be used, be sure patient is in upright position, unless contraindicated, and made comfortable.
- Administer laxatives as prescribed; avoid long-term use of laxatives unless patient's condition warrants otherwise.
- Monitor for fecal impaction.
- Assess patient's use of laxatives and enemas; if dependency on laxatives or enemas for bowel elimination exists, educate patient about hazards associated with this dependency and develop a plan to gradually taper patient from laxative or enema use (abrupt discontinuation is contraindicated).
- Educate patient as to nonpharmacological means to stimulate bowel movement.

pattern, complete bathing is not required more than every third or fourth day. Daily partial sponge baths to the face, axillae, and perineum should be sufficient to prevent odor and irritation. Neutral or superfatted soaps and bath oils should be used for bathing, followed by the application of skin softeners and moisturizers. Tub baths are not only effective for good cleansing but also enhance circulation and provide an opportunity to exercise stiff joints. Showers also may be enjoyed by the elderly; the use of shower chairs, lifts, hand-controlled shower heads, and other appliances can assist with this activity. The individual's unique bathing habits, schedule, and preferences should be appreciated and respected, as should the right to privacy and protection from exposure during bathing activities. To reduce the risk of burns, bath water temperature should range from 100°F to 105°F.

Recommended Readings

Lonergan ET. Aging and the kidney: adjusting treatment to physiologic change. Geriatrics 1988;43(3):27.

Murray FE. Geriatric constipation: brief update and a common problem. Geriatrics 1991;46(3):64.

11

Activity

A multitude of physical, psychological, and social benefits are gained through regular activity. Physical activity aids respiratory, circulatory, digestive, excretory, and musculoskeletal functions. Mental activity helps to maintain the mind's functions and promotes a sense of normality. Multiple health problems such as atherosclerosis, joint immobility, pneumonia, constipation, decubiti, depression, and insomnia can be avoided when an active state is maintained. However, as Table 11-1 describes, outcomes of the aging process challenge the older person's ability to remain active and demand special attention by gerontological nurses.

Physical Activity

Maintaining a physically active state is an increasingly difficult task not only for the elderly but also for most of the adult population. Fewer and fewer occupations require hard physical labor, and those that still do often use technological inventions to perform the more strenuous tasks. Television viewing and spectator sports are popular forms of recreation. Automobiles, taxicabs, and buses provide transportation to destinations once conveniently reached by walking. Elevators and escalators minimize stair climbing. Modern appliances have considerably eased the physical energy expended in household chores. Growing numbers of Americans find that they must schedule jogging or trips to the gym to remain in good physical condition.

Because many real obstacles get in the way of being physically active in later life, special efforts

are demanded by the elderly and those caring for them to compensate for this problem. An important basic measure is educating the public, especially caregivers, about the importance of physical activity for older adults. Sometimes families believe they are assisting their older relatives by allowing them to be sedentary. Often, assisting with household responsibilities not only enhances good functioning of the body's systems but also promotes a sense of worth by providing an opportunity for productivity. Although physical activity may be more uncomfortable or demanding than inactivity, future health problems and disability may be spared by its regular practice. Motivation may be necessary to stimulate interest in physical activity. For instance, encouraging membership in a senior-citizen's club can motivate many types of activity in that the individual will have a reason to perform the following tasks, among others:

- get out of bed
- prepare and eat breakfast
- bathe
- dress
- comb their hair
- travel to the club
- negotiate a new environment
- interact with others
- participate in activities
- travel home
- undress.

Those involved with the care of the elderly can provide motivation by demonstrating a sincere interest in their activities, for example, asking what

Table 11-1 *Aging and Risks to Maintaining an Active State*

AGE-RELATED FACTOR	POTENTIAL NURSING DIAGNOSIS
Decreased cardiac output	Activity intolerance related to less efficient management of stress
Reduced breathing capacity and efficiency	Activity intolerance related to shortness of breath
Delayed oxygen diffusion	Altered tissue perfusion related to delayed oxygen diffusion
Decrease in muscle mass, strength, and movements	Activity intolerance related to muscle weakness and fatigue
Demineralization of bone; deterioration of cartilage, surface of joints	Impaired physical mobility related to decreased range of motion High risk for injury related to brittleness of bones Pain related to stiff joints
Poorer vision and hearing	Impaired social interactions related to sensory deficit Social isolation related to sensory deficit Impaired verbal communication related to sensory deficit
Wrinkling of skin; thinning, loss, and change in color of hair	Disturbance in self-concept related to age-related changes to appearance
Lower basal metabolic rate	Impaired physical mobility related to slower functions High risk for injury and infection related to decreased bodily functions during resting/sleeping states
Higher prevalence of chronic, disabling disease	Activity intolerance related to chronic disease Impaired physical mobility related to chronic disease Pain related to chronic disease Social isolation related to chronic disease
Reduced income	Diversional activity deficit related to fewer funds available for leisure pursuits Disturbance in self-concept related to decreased income Social isolation related to fewer funds available for transportation, entertainment, leisure pursuits

they did, admiring crafts they made, or listening to the details of a trip. Recognizing housekeeping efforts, using their handmade gifts, and commenting on a well-groomed appearance are small but meaningful ways to reinforce the older person's positive efforts toward being active.

Exercise

The fitness craze continues in our society, and the elderly are not untouched by this movement. Exercise can improve body tone, circulation, appetite, digestion, elimination, respiration, sleep, and self-concept. Opportunities for socialization and recreation can be enhanced through participation in exercise programs. Growing numbers of older adults

understand the benefits of and are engaging in exercise programs. Although exercise is highly beneficial to the elderly, it can cause problems if adjustments are not made for their advanced age. Display 11-1 describes some of the guidelines that could assist older adults in obtaining maximum benefit from exercise programs.

Exercise programs are best followed if they match the individual's interests and needs. A wide range of options should be considered in planning activities, such as brisk walking, dancing, swimming, yoga, and aerobic exercises.

Some older individuals may be unable to participate in formal exercise programs. For these persons, less aggressive exercises should be built into their daily activities, and effort should be made to promote their activity during routine care activities.

DISPLAY 11-1   Exercise Program Guidelines for Older Adults

Ensure that a recent physical examination has been done to detect conditions that could affect or be affected by an exercise program (*e.g.*, heart disease, diabetes). If health conditions are present, consult with the physician as to restrictions or modifications to the exercise program.

Assess the patient's current activity level, range of motion, muscle strength and tone, and response to physical activity. In collaboration with the patient, develop an exercise program that recognizes interests, capacities, limitations, and realistic potential.

Exercises that focus on good speed and rhythm (*e.g.*, low weights, high reps) should be emphasized. "Resistance" exercises should be kept at a low level and isometric exercises avoided.(Hunt, 1990)

Determine the training heart rate and evaluate heart rate during exercise to ensure that the rate stays within a safe range. To determine an age-adjusted training heart rate, start with the figure of 220 and subtract the person's age from that, multiply that answer by 70%.(Hunt, 1990) This calculates the maximum rate that will provide vascular and other benefits without causing deleterious effects. The resting heart rate can serve as the lower level and the training heart rate as the upper level for a safe heart rate range during exercise. The physician should be consulted as to the appropriateness of the exercise program for persons who have a resting heart rate exceeding 100.

Perform warm-up exercises (*e.g.*, stretching), for at least 10 minutes before engaging in full exercise program.

Provide for a period of cooling down after exercises.

Begin with a conservative exercise program and gradually increase activity. Monitor vital signs and symptoms at various activity levels. Note arrhythmias, significant changes in blood pressure, dyspnea, shortness of breath, fatigue, angina, and intermittent claudication.

Suggest that the patient do foot, leg, shoulder, and arm circling while watching television.

Instruct the patient to do deep breathing and limb exercises in the period between awakening and rising from bed.

Encourage the patient to wash dishes or light laundry by hand to exercise the fingers with the benefit of warm water.

When greeting a patient in the hall, ask the person to raise both arms as high as possible and wave.

When giving a medication, ask the patient to bend each extremity several times.

During bathing activities, ask the patient to flex and extend all body parts.

Figure 11-1 depicts several exercises that can easily be incorporated into the older adult's daily activities.

Exercises should be paced throughout the day, and fatigue from exercising should be avoided because of potential muscle pain and cramping. Morning exercise loosens stiff joints and muscles, which encourages activity, whereas bedtime exercises promote relaxation and encourage sleep. If an older person is not accustomed to a great deal of physical activity, exercises should be introduced gradually and increased according to individual progress. Some tachycardia normally may occur during the exercises and continue for as long as several hours thereafter in the elderly. Longer periods must be allowed for the older person to perform exercises, and rest periods should follow activity. Warm water and warm washcloths or towels wrapped around the joints may ease joint motion and facilitate exercising.

The thinner, weaker, and more brittle bones of the elderly lend themselves to easy fracturing. Exercises that stress an immobilized joint, strenuous sports, and running and jumping exercises must be avoided to prevent trauma. Older adults with cardiac or respiratory problems should seek advice from their physician about the amount and type of exercise best suited for their unique capacities and limitations. At times, older persons may need partial or complete assistance with exercises. The nurse or other caregivers will find it useful to remember the following points:

Exercise all body joints through their normal range of motion at least three times daily. Re-
(*Text continues on page 98*)

Exercises to Do While In Bed

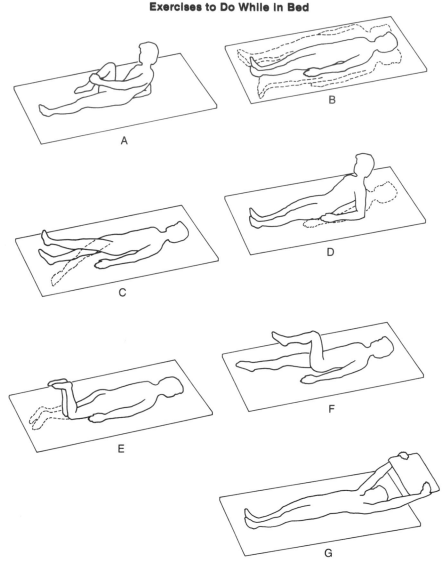

Figure 11-1 Exercises to do while in bed: (**A**) *Flexing the knee with the opposite hand holding the foot for assistance.* (**B**) *Rolling from side to side.* (**C**) *Scissorlike crossing of the legs.* (**D**) *Raising the chest.* (**E**) *Flexing the knees while lying on the abdomen.* (**F**) *Bicycling.* (**G**) *Lifting a pillow over the head with the arms straight.*

Exercises to do while sitting: (**A**) *Circling motion of the shoulder joint with the arm at the side.* (**B**) *Circling the arms.* (**C**) *Rotating the head.* (**D**) *Flexing and extending the neck.* (**E**) *Pushing up in a chair with the use of the arms.* (**F**) *Kicking the legs while sitting.* (**G**) *Rolling the foot on a can.*

All exercises can be built into regular activities. Exercises to do anytime: (**A**) *Rolling a pencil on a hard surface.* (**B**) *Flexing the fingers around a pencil.* (**C**) *Exaggerating chewing motions.* (**D**) *Rubbing the back with a towel.* (**E**) *Tightening the rectoperineal muscles.* (**F**) *Holding the stomach in to tighten the abdominal muscles.*

(continued)

Exercises to Do While Sitting

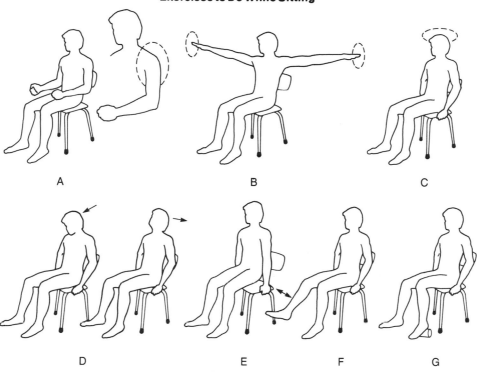

A   B   C

D   E   F   G

Exercises to Do Anytime

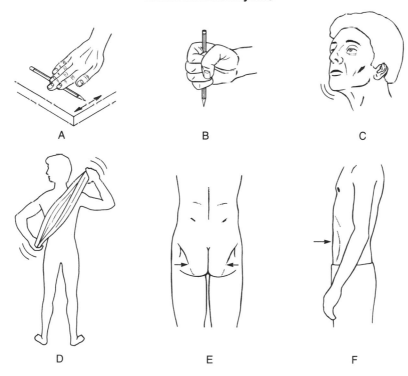

A   B   C

D   E   F

Figure 11-1 (continued)

fer to Chapter 17 for the normal range of motion for various joints.

Support the joint and distal limb during the exercise.

Do not force the joint past the point of resistance.

Some of the assistive devices that can aid the elderly in being active are reviewed in Chapter 34.

Mental Stimulation

Psychological activity is as vital to the total well-being of the elderly as physical activity. Stimulation and challenges help the older mind maintain lucid functioning. Barring the existence of health problems, the personality and interests will remain consistent through an individual's lifetime. The assertive, independent young woman will most likely resent not having an active role in decisions involving her and being addressed in a patronizing manner when she grows old. The couple who enjoyed nightclub entertainment throughout the years will not suddenly cease this activity when they begin to be labeled "old." The individual who preferred privacy and solitude when young will probably not live gregariously in later life. Activities for older adults must be planned according to the unique interests of the given individuals and could include arts, crafts, travel, classes, gardening, auto repair, dancing, listening to music, people-watching, and collecting. Pets are frequently a source of interest, activity, and companionship for the elderly. Old age can be the time for the development of new hobbies and interests.

Therapeutic recreation is structured leisure with a specific goal in mind, for example, working with clay to exercise fingers, painting to express feelings, and cooking classes to restore or maintain roles. Specialists in recreation, music, art, or dance therapy can provide valuable assistance in matching activities to the unique needs, interests, and capacities of older persons.

With any activity, adequate time and patience are necessary. Slower passage of impulses through the nervous system, sensory deficits, and the vast storehouse of information being triggered and sorted in response to psychological stimuli are just a few of the factors that interfere with rapid reactions in older people.

Inactivity

Maintaining an active state can be challenging for the elderly. Age-related changes in muscle strength and endurance, reduced opportunities for activity, and fatigue, pain, dizziness, dyspnea, and other symptoms associated with health problems prevalent in later life can reduce activity levels.

Inactivity can have many deleterious effects on older adults, some of which are listed in Display 11-2. Every effort must be made to maximize the activity level of the elderly. Learning about interests can assist in identifying activities that will be familiar and enjoyable to patients. Patients should be made aware of local resources that can aid in promoting activity, such as senior centers, exercise classes, educational and recreational programs at local schools or colleges, volunteer opportunities, and local clubs. In addition, activity can be promoted by arranging transportation that can aid the elderly in attending activities. For homebound eld-

---

DISPLAY 11-2   *Deleterious Effects of Inactivity*

Changes in physiological function

- reduced pulse rate
- decreased chest expansion and ventilation
- reduced muscle strength, tone, and endurance
- demineralization of bones, increased ease of fractures
- slower gastrointestinal motility
- slower metabolism

Increased risk of complications

- postural hypotension
- hypostatic pneumonia
- pressure ulcers
- poor appetite
- constipation
- urinary tract infection
- joint stiffness, limited range-of-joint motion

Changes in mood and self-concept

- increased feelings of helplessness, depression
- perception of self as incapable, frail

Increased dependency
Reduced opportunities for socialization

erly, special services offered by libraries, vision associations, Pets on Wheels, social service organizations, and other agencies can assist in providing resources and companionship that promote activity. Refer to the listing of resources at the end of Chapter 34 for agencies that address specific needs. Additional interventions for promoting mobility are described in the Nursing Diagnosis Highlight.

Self-Fulfilling Prophecy

An older adult's unique capacities and limitations will dictate the appropriate activities for that individual. Some older persons may derive psychological satisfaction from discussing a football game with friends at a local tavern, yet others may seek satisfaction from completing a college degree at the local university. Individual differences, prefer-

---

NURSING DIAGNOSIS HIGHLIGHT
Impaired Physical Mobility

Overview
Impaired physical mobility is a state in which movement is limited. Some degree of mobility limitation will be observed, ranging from the use of special equipment for movement to total dependency on others for movement. Other signs associated with this diagnosis could include decreased muscle strength or control, restricted range of motion, impaired coordination, altered gait, decreased level of consciousness, pain, paralysis, and imposed restrictions on movement.

Causative or contributing factors
Arthritis, malnutrition, neuromuscular disease, sensory deficits, edema, missing limb, cardiovascular disease, pulmonary disease, obesity, side-effects of medications, altered mood or cognition.

Goal
The patient will increase mobility to optimal level possible and be free from complications associated with impaired mobility.

Interventions
- Assess muscle strength and tone, active and passive range of motion, and mental status. Review history for conditions that can limit mobility or require alteration in level of mobility. Consult with physician as to restrictions on mobility and any necessary modifications for exercises.
- Develop an individualized exercise program, which could include: passive or active range-of-motion exercises, structured exercise classes, walking programs.
- Assist patient in maintaining good body alignment and hourly position changes.
- Promote a good nutritional status. Consult with nutritionists as needed.
- If necessary, refer for canes, walkers, wheelchairs, braces, traction devices, and other aids to increase mobility. Provide related health teaching as needed.
- Collaborate with physical therapist, occupational therapist, recreational therapist, and other health team members to develop a program to increase the patient's mobility.
- Encourage family and significant others to assist in efforts to increase the patient's mobility.
- Provide diversional activities based on the patient's interests and level of function.
- Observe for complications associated with immobility and seek prompt correction. Instruct patient in recognition of complications.

ences, and abilities must be considered and appreciated. Stereotyping the elderly by assuming they all will enjoy exactly the same activities violates the underlying nursing principle of individualized care and severely limits the opportunities available for older persons. If it is expected that the elderly will be dull, disinterested, and confused, and if they are treated in this manner, they most likely will fulfill these expectations. On the other hand, if they are expected to keep oriented and involved with the world around them, they have a better probability of remaining alert, aware, and mentally active.

Recommended Readings

Heexhen SJ. Getting a handle on patient mobility. Geriatr Nurs 1989;10(3):146.

Hunt HF. Geriatric exercise programs require careful design. Geriatrics 1990;45(10):20.

Stevenson JS, Topp R. Effect of moderate and low intensity long-term exercise by older adults. Res Nurs Health 1990;13:209.

Wheat ME, Lowenthal DT. Exercise. In: Abrams WB, Berkow R, eds. The Merck manual of geriatrics. Rahway, NJ: Merck Sharp & Dohme Research Laboratories, 1990:278.

12

Rest

All human beings must retreat from activity and stimulation to renew their reserves. Several periods of relaxation throughout the day and 5 to 7 hours of sleep aid in promoting a healthy pattern of rest; however, conditions experienced in later years can interfere with the ability to achieve adequate rest (Table 12-1). Astute assessment is necessary to ensure that rest requirements are being fulfilled and to identify obstacles to rest for which intervention is warranted.

Activity and Rest

Satisfying, regular activity promotes rest and relaxation. Greater amounts of rest are required by older people and should be interspersed with periods of activity throughout the day. On awakening, the elderly should spend several minutes resting in bed and stretching their muscles, followed by several more minutes of sitting on the side of the bed before rising to a standing position. This will reduce morning stiffness of the muscles and prevent dizziness and falls resulting from postural hypotension. Many older adults focus all their activity in the early part of the day so that they will have the evening free. For instance, the early morning hours may be used for household cleaning, marketing, club meetings, gardening, cooking, and laundering; the evening hours may then be spent watching television, reading, or sewing. This pattern may be an outgrowth of decades of employment, whereby one worked during the day and relaxed in the evening. Older people need insight into the advantages of pacing activities throughout the entire day and providing ample periods for rest and naps between activities. The nurse may find it useful to review the older person's daily activities hour by hour and assist in developing patterns that more equally distribute activity and rest throughout the day.

Sleep

Although more rest is required by older persons, the length of time required for sleep is reduced. As mentioned earlier, 5 to 7 hours of sleep a night is sufficient for the elderly; longer periods may be harmful to their physical and mental functioning. Older people sleep less soundly, and stage IV of their sleep is absent or decreased (Display 12-1).

Sleep is frequently interrupted by muscle cramps and tremors, environmental interferences, and nocturia. It is common for older people to be initially disoriented and confused when they waken in a dark room; this, combined with visual deficiencies and postural hypotension, may predispose them to accidents. A night-light should be provided in the bedroom and, if possible, bathroom lighting should be on throughout the night. Clutter and furniture should not obstruct the pathway from the bedroom to the bathroom. It may be beneficial to provide a urinal, bedpan, or commode in the bedroom if the bathroom is on a different floor of the home.

The attachment of side rails to the bed may be a beneficial protective measure for the older person at home. This prevents falls from bed, assists

Table 12-1 *Aging and Risks to the Ability to Achieve Rest*

AGE-RELATED FACTOR	POTENTIAL NURSING DIAGNOSIS
Increased awakening during sleep; sleep stages III and IV less prominent	Sleep pattern disturbance related to less prominent sleep stages
Increased incidence of nocturia	Sleep pattern disturbance related to nocturia
Altered perception of night environment, resulting from visual and hearing deficits	Anxiety and fear related to difficulty in falling asleep
Increased incidence of muscle cramps during resting states	Pain related to muscle cramps

DISPLAY 12-1. Stages of Sleep

Stage I
  Begins nodding off
    Can be easily awakened
    If undisturbed, will reach next stage in a
      few minutes
Stage II
  Deeper stage of relaxation reached
  Some eye movement noted through closed
    lids
  Can be easily awakened
Stage III
  Early phase of deep sleep
  Reduced temperature and heart rate
  Muscles relaxed
  More difficult to be awakened
Stage IV
  Deep sleep and relaxation
  All body functions reduced
  Considerable stimulation needed to be
    awakened
  Insufficient amount of this stage of sleep can
    cause emotional dysfunction
REM sleep
  Rapid eye movement (REM) occurs
  Increased vital signs (sometimes irregular)
  Will enter REM sleep approximately once
    every 90 minutes of stage IV sleep
  Certain drugs can decrease REM sleep, in-
    cluding alcohol, barbiturates, and pheno-
    thiazine derivatives
  Insufficient REM sleep can cause emotional
    dysfunction, including psychosis

with movement, and provides a means of orientation to place. It is important that the person feel confident that they can remove these rails to get out of bed or that someone will be readily available to help them do so when necessary. Occasionally, hospital or nursing home patients will resist having side rails because of fear of staff delays in helping them from bed. These patients need verbal and behavioral reassurance that they are not trapped and unable to leave their beds. Falls resulting from attempts to climb over the side rails may be prevented by prompt staff response to calls for assistance.

Vision and hearing limitations of the elderly produce difficulties for care providers who need to communicate necessary questions, warnings, or directions during the night. Whispering to avoid awakening other sleeping individuals may be missed by the older person who has a reduced ability to hear or whose hearing aid is removed, and lipreading is difficult in dimly lit bedrooms. Focusing a flashlight on the lips of the speaker can help the individual read lips, and cupping the hands over the ear and speaking directly into it can aid hearing. A stethoscope also can be used to amplify conversation by placing the earpieces into the individual's ear and speaking into the bell portion. It is a good idea to explain this procedure and practice during the day so that the patient will understand your actions during the night.

The elderly often have difficulty falling asleep. Unfortunately, the first means frequently used to encourage sleep is the administration of a sedative. Although medications are reviewed later in this

book, it is worthwhile to mention here that sedatives must be used with utmost care. Barbiturates are general depressants, especially to the central nervous system, and they can significantly depress some vital body functions, lowering basal metabolic rate more than it already is and decreasing blood pressure, mental activity, and peristalsis to the extent that other problems may develop. These serious effects, combined with a greater susceptibility to adverse reactions, warrant that barbiturates be used with extreme caution. Nonbarbiturate sedatives also create problems, and they should be used only when absolutely necessary. Because of the prolonged half-life of medications in the elderly, the effects of sedatives may exist into the daytime and result in confusion and sluggishness. Sometimes these symptoms are treated with medications, further complicating the situation. Occasionally, sleeping medications will reverse the normal sleep rhythm. All sedatives may decrease body movements during sleep and predispose the older person to the many complications of reduced mobility.

Alternatives to sedatives should be used to induce sleep whenever possible. The activity schedule of the elderly should first be evaluated. If they have been inactive in a bed or wheelchair all day, most likely they will not be sleepy at bedtime. Including more stimulation and activity during the day may be a solution. The amount of time allotted for sleep must be evaluated. With a reduced demand for sleep, it cannot be expected that the older person who goes to bed at 8 P.M. should be able to sleep until 8 A.M. the following day. A warm bath at bedtime can promote muscle relaxation and encourage sleep, as can a back rub, a comfortable position, a glass of warm milk, and the alleviation of pain or discomfort. A quiet environment at a temperature preferred by the individual should be provided. Electric blankets and flannel sheets can promote comfort and relaxation.

Changes in sleep patterns may indicate signs of other problems in the elderly (see Nursing Diagnosis Highlight). Although early morning rising is not unusual for the elderly, a sudden change to earlier awakening or insomnia may be symptomatic of an emotional disturbance. Sleep disturbances also may arise from cardiac or respiratory problems, which produce difficulties such as orthopnea and pain related to poor peripheral circulation. Restlessness and confusion during the night may indicate an adverse reaction to a sedative. Nocturnal frequency may be a clue to the presence of diabetes. It is important that the quality and quantity of sleep be assessed.

Stress Management

Stress is a normal part of life. Most individuals confront a variety of physical and emotional stressors daily such as the following:

- changes in temperature
- pollutants
- viruses
- injury
- time pressures
- fear
- receiving bad news
- facing an unpleasant or difficult task.

Many real or perceived threats to our physical, emotional, and social homeostasis can create stress. Pressures and activity levels are not necessarily correlated with stress; a busy schedule or numerous responsibilities to juggle may be less stressful than a boring, monotonous existence. Regardless of the source of the stress, the body reacts in a similar manner in that the sympathetic nervous system is stimulated. This causes stimulation of the pituitary gland; the release of adrenocorticotropic hormone, also known as ACTH; and an increase in the body's adrenaline supply. The following series of changes occur:

Mental alertness increases.
Fingers, hands, and toes become cold as more blood goes to the body's muscles.
Glycogen converts to glucose.
Heart rate and respirations increase.
Pupils dilate.
Hearing becomes more acute.
Blood-clotting activity increases.
Sexual interest and drive is reduced, menstrual irregularities occur, testosterone level is lowered.
Ability to concentrate decreases, causing more errors and irrational decisions.
Anxiety, fear, or a sense that "something isn't right" occur.

Life is a series of stress and recovery episodes that produce no harmful effects. However, chronic stress without recovery can produce serious con-

sequences, including heart disease, hypertension, cerebrovascular accident, cancer, ulcers, skin eruptions, complications of existing illnesses, and a variety of social and emotional problems. It is important, therefore, to prevent chronic stress from developing. The key to stress control is not avoiding stress but managing it by learning compensatory measures.

Respond to stress in a healthy manner. Good nutrition, rest, exercise, and other sound health practices strengthen the body's ability to con-

---

NURSING DIAGNOSIS HIGHLIGHT
Sleep Pattern Disturbance

Overview

A sleep pattern disturbance exists when the quantity or quality of sleep causes disruption to daily function. This disturbance can be displayed by problems falling or staying asleep, nighttime sleep of less than 4 hours, daytime drowsiness, frequent yawning, lack of energy or motivation to engage in activities, dark circles under eyes, weakness, and disturbances in mood or cognition.

Causative or contributing factors

Age-related decrease in stage IV sleep, nocturia, muscle cramps, orthopnea, dyspnea, angina, poor peripheral circulation, cough, incontinence, diarrhea, insufficient activity or exercise, immobility, pain, new environment, depression, confusion, anxiety, medications (*e.g.,* antidepressants, antihypertensives, tranquilizers), noise, interruptions.

Goal

The patient will obtain 5 to 8 hours of sleep daily and be free from symptoms and signs associated with sleep pattern disturbance.

Interventions

- Assess sleep pattern. Ask the patient about number, length and quality of naps, activity pattern, bedtime, quality of sleep, awakening time, symptoms and interruptions to sleep. Attempt to identify and correct factors associated with sleep disturbance.
- Increase daytime activity; limit naps.
- Maintain bedroom temperature between 70°F (21°C) and 75°F (24°C); control interruptions; provide a nightlight.
- Assist patient with toileting at bedtime. Be aware that renal circulation improves when one lies down; therefore, the patient may need to toilet shortly after going to bed.
- Use measures that are known to stimulate sleep, such as soft music, television, drinking warm milk.
- Offer backrubs, P.M. care, and other comfort measures to relax the patient and induce sleep.
- Instruct patient in measures to improve sleep.
- If sedatives are necessary, use those that are least disruptive to sleep cycle and monitor 24-hour effects from the drug.
- Reduce the potential for injury by having bed in lowest position, using side rails, providing nightlight, adjusting lighting so that patient does not have to travel from dark bedroom to bright bathroom, encouraging patient to ask for assistance with transferring and ambulating as needed.
- Record or have patient record sleep pattern (*e.g.,* time to bed, time when asleep, times awakened during the night, signs and symptoms during sleep, rising time, self-assessment of restfulness).

front stress. When in a stressful situation, adherence to these principles continues to be important. It is beneficial to learn to remain calm when faced with stress; reacting in an unhealthy manner worsens the situation.

Manage life-style. Little in the lives of most people would bring the world to a halt if not completed at a certain time or in a specific manner. Things should be put in perspective; for example, what difference will it really make if the clothes are not washed today or if one is 10 minutes late? Whenever possible, anticipate the consequences of a situation so that the stress of an unpredictable situation can be reduced.

Relax. Be it a good book, swimming, weaving, travel, music, or woodcarving, find something in which to get absorbed so that there is some respite from life's demands. Yoga, meditation, and relaxation exercises can be effective.

Recommended Readings

Ancoli-Israel S. Epidemiology of sleep disorders. In: Roth T, Roehrs T, eds. Clinics in geriatric medicine. Philadelphia: WB Saunders, 1989.

Herrera CO. Sleep disorders. In: Abrams WB, Berkow R, eds. The Merck manual of geriatrics. Rahway, NJ: Merck Sharp & Dohme Research Laboratories, 1990:128.

Hoch CC. Sleep in old age. In: Murrow E, ed. Perspectives on gerontological nursing. Newbury Park, CA: SAGE, 1991:59.

Hoch CC, Reynolds CF. Sleep disturbances and what to do about them. Geriatr Nurs 1986;7:24.

Hoch CC, Reynolds CF, Houck PR. Sleep patterns in Alzheimer, depressed, and healthy elderly. West J Nurs Res 1988;10:239.

Kedas A, Lux W, Amodeo S. A critical review of aging and sleep research. West J Nurs Res 1989;11:196.

North A. The effect of sleep on wound healing. Ostomy/Wound Management 1990;27:56.

13

Solitude and Social Interaction

Human growth and satisfaction are enhanced by periods of solitude and social interaction. Social interaction provides opportunities for us to experience a range of feelings, stay in touch with the mainstream of culture, and develop the social and emotional facets of our lives. Solitude gives us the time to retreat from the numerous stimuli in our social world, reflect, and refresh our social and psychological selves. As we grow older, various changes interfere with the ability to interact and obtain solitude (Table 13-1). Assistance must be provided to aid the elderly in achieving a healthy balance of solitude and social interaction.

Communication

The axiom that people are social beings holds true for the elderly as well. Through social interaction we share our joys and burdens, derive feelings of normalcy, validate our perceptions, and maintain a link with reality. The ability to communicate is an essential ingredient for social interaction, but because of a variety of intrinsic and extrinsic factors, older persons may face unique obstacles in their attempts to interact with others.

Hearing Deficits

Presbycusis may cause speech to be inaudible or distorted, as can impacted cerumen, a common problem in the elderly. Older people may be self-conscious of this limitation and avoid situations in which they must interact. In turn, others may avoid them because of this difficulty. Telephone conversation can be affected by this problem, limiting social contact even further for the individual who may be socially isolated for other reasons. Approximately one-tenth of the elderly have some difficulty hearing telephone conversation. Corrective measures for hearing problems should be explored. The first step to managing or correcting hearing problems is to assess the underlying problem through professional evaluation, including an audiometric examination.

Hearing aids can benefit persons with some hearing disorders, but they are not effective for all hearing problems. An audiometric evaluation can determine if the specific hearing problem can be improved by the use of a hearing aid. A hearing aid should never be purchased without being specifically prescribed. Sometimes elderly persons will attempt to improve hearing by purchasing an aid through a private party or a mail order catalog, which often results in disappointment and a waste of money from an already limited budget. Nurses should educate the public about the realities of hearing aid use.

Even when a hearing aid may be appropriate, problems can arise with its use. Inability to adjust to the presence of the aid and the distortion of sound caused by the amplification of environmental noise along with speech sounds may make the

Table 13-1 *Aging and Risks to Solitude and Social Interaction*

AGE-RELATED FACTOR	POTENTIAL NURSING DIAGNOSIS
Loss of subcutaneous fat, causing deepening of hollows of orbits, axillae, and intercostal and supraclavical spaces; skin wrinkling; decrease in muscle mass; high prevalence of arthritic joints; increase in prevalance of "age spots"; hair loss and graying	Disturbance in self-concept, impaired social interactions, and social isolation related to altered appearance
Increased prevalence of needing to live in multigenerational household or institutional setting due to health and financial limitations	Anxiety and powerlessness related to limited opportunity for privacy
Poor vision and hearing	Impaired verbal communication related to sensory deficit Impaired social interactions related to sensory deficit
Reduced ability to travel independently in community	Impaired social interactions related to inteference with independent travel
Reduced financial and physical resources available for entertainment and recreation	Social isolation related to limited finances

patient reject its use. New hearing aid users need support during the adjustment phase and should be advised to wear the aid for progressively longer periods each day until comfort is gained and to avoid its use in noisy environments such as airports, train stations, and stadiums. The aid must be checked regularly to ensure that the earpiece is not blocked with cerumen and that the battery is working. This appliance may easily correct a hearing problem and reintroduce the older individual to a socially active world.

If a hearing aid cannot correct the problem, efforts should be made to speak clearly and distinctly, in a low frequency but at an audible level, while facing the individual. Shouting should be avoided because it raises the high-frequency sounds that older persons already have difficulty hearing, causing even greater hearing problems. Cupping the hands over the less deficient ear and talking directly into the ear may be helpful. Using gestures and pictures and pointing to items while talking about them can assist in communication. Other considerations for communicating with hearing-impaired people are discussed in Chapter 27.

The nurse should examine an older adult's ears frequently for cerumen accumulation. The ear should be gently irrigated with warm water or a hydrogen peroxide and water solution; commer-cial preparations also are available. It is wise for older persons to have assistance when irrigating ears, because dizziness often occurs during the procedure. Even allowing water to run in the ears during showers or shampoos can aid in loosening cerumen. Cotton-tipped applicators should not be used for cerumen removal because they can push the cerumen back into the ear canal and cause an impaction.

It is beneficial for nurses to provide health education about the effects of environmental noise on hearing and general health. Nurses also should take an active role in advocating legislation to control noise pollution and the enforcement of that legislation.

Visual Deficits

The ability to see is equally important in communication. Most elderly people require some form of corrective lenses, and approximately one-half of all individuals identified as legally blind each year are 65 years of age or older. Visual limitations can make communication problematic because facial expressions and gestures, which are as important as the words themselves, may be missed or misinterpreted. Lipreading to compensate for hearing deficits may be difficult and written correspondence may be limited because independent read-

ing and writing become almost impossible tasks. Remaining aware of current events through newspapers and socialization through playing cards and other games may be hampered.

For visual deficits, one of the first assistive measures is a thorough eye examination, including tonometry, by an ophthalmologist. The importance of an annual eye examination, not only to detect vision changes and needs for alterations in corrective lenses but also for early discovery of problems such as cataracts, glaucoma, and other disease processes, must be stressed. The financial ability of the individual to afford an eye examination and glasses must be evaluated because health insurance seldom covers this important service; community resources or the negotiation of special payment plans may assist the elderly in acquiring the necessary aid.

To compensate for visual limitations, one should face the individual and exaggerate gestures and facial expressions when speaking. To compensate for poor peripheral vision common in older people, one should approach these individuals from the front and ensure that seating allows for full sight of persons or objects with which they are interacting. Ample lighting is important and should be provided by several soft indirect lights rather than a single, bright, glaring source. Interaction can be promoted by using large print games and playing cards, telephone dials with enlarged numbers that glow in the dark, and cassette recorders. Books and magazines with large print and recordings of current events and popular literature can provide a source of recreation and a means of keeping informed.

Socialization

Because of declining physical function, the older person may have less energy to invest in social interaction. Urinary frequency and incontinence make people reluctant to engage in social activities, as do stiff, painful joints and other discomforts. Changes in appearance may alter the individual's self-concept and interfere with the motivation for and quality of social interaction. Although many of these problems cannot be eliminated, nursing intervention can help reduce the limitations they cause. Education of younger adults regarding the normal aging process can enhance their sensitivity and patience and help them understand the socialization handicaps that elderly persons face, perhaps thereby also helping them learn how to minimize and manage these limitations as they grow old. Assuring the elderly that their problems are

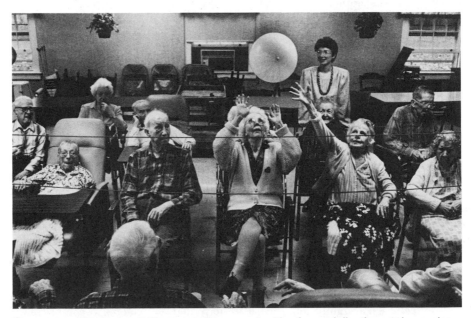

Figure 13-1. *Planned activities can offer opportunities for socialization and exercise. (Photograph by Eric Schenk.)*

shared by many others and that some of their limitations are a natural part of aging may help them feel "normal" and thus promote social interaction (Fig. 13-1).

Using good common sense in nursing care will facilitate social activity. The nurse can review and perhaps readjust the person's schedule to conserve energy and maximize opportunities for socialization. Medication administration should be planned so that, during periods of social activity, analgesics will provide relief, tranquilizers will not sedate, diuretics will not reach their peak, and laxatives will not begin working. Likewise, fluid intake and bathroom visits before activities begin should be planned to reduce the fear or actual occurrence of incontinence; activities for the elderly should include frequent break periods for visits to the bathroom. The control of these minor obstacles can often facilitate social interaction.

Given the capacity to interact socially and manage their problems independently, the elderly must then confront social factors over which they have no control. Their circle of friends and relatives may become smaller through deaths, and a limited budget may necessitate giving food and shelter priority over social functions. A youth-oriented, fast-paced society may not provide an atmosphere conducive to active social involvement. If segments of society disengage from the elderly, the ability to socially interact is lessened. Fortunately, as described in

NURSING DIAGNOSIS HIGHLIGHT
Social Isolation

Overview

Social isolation exists when the patient is alone and desires contact with others but is unable to make that contact. This is not the same as solitude, which is the voluntary choice to be alone for rest or personal renewal. Patients experiencing social isolation may be observed to be alone much of the time, demonstrate mood or behavior changes (*e.g.,* anger, depression, irritability, dull affect), have alterations in sleep and eating patterns, and verbalize feelings of boredom, abandonment, insecurity, and poor self-concept.

Causative or contributing factors

Loss of significant other, relocation, institutionalization, disability, incontinence, pain, hearing or vision deficit, lack of transportation, limited finances, unsafe neighborhood, inappropriate or annoying behavior of person.

Goal

The patient will have cause of social isolation corrected, if possible; will establish meaningful social contacts and express satisfaction with the quality and frequency of those contacts.

Interventions

- Explore factors causing or contributing to social isolation and reduce or eliminate these factors as appropriate.
- Assess roles and interests of the patient and use this information in helping patient develop opportunities for increased socialization.
- Refer patient to resources that can provide socialization (*e.g.,* senior centers, adult day care, volunteer groups, churches, alternate housing options such as life care communities, telephone reassurance programs).
- Mobilize family, neighbors, and friends to increase social contact for patient.
- Identify needs for assistive or prosthetic devices and services that can improve patient's normality of appearance and function (*e.g.,* adult briefs for incontinence, enterostomal therapist for advice on controlling ostomy odors, physical therapist for prescription and instruction on use of cane, cosmetic consultant for camouflage of scars, hearing aids for deafness).
- Assist patient in arranging transportation for social activities.
- As appropriate, recommend house sharing, pets, and friendly visitors.

Chapter 4, families become a strong source of socialization to the elderly. Nurses need to promote social activity among the elderly, including helping persons of all ages see the attributes of the unique human being housed within the aged body (see Nursing Diagnosis Highlight).

Being Alone

Solitude is important for most individuals. It offers a rest from the many stimuli and interactions to which we are regularly exposed and provides for introspection, whereby insights into ourselves, others, and our environment are gained. Reflecting on and analyzing our life's events help us to understand life. Periods of solitude are therapeutic to the elderly. Unresolved feelings from earlier years may be contemplated and resolved, resulting in personal satisfaction. In reminiscing, evaluating, and understanding the dynamics of life's earlier events and achievements, older persons can find a satisfaction with the quality of their lives that helps compensate for their multiple losses. They can also gain a new perspective on themselves and others. The death of friends, a spouse, and others and the realization of one's own mortality necessitate thought regarding the reality of death and dying.

Time should be provided daily in which no interruptions interfere with solitude. How often are meaningful thoughts and resolutions of unfinished business interrupted by a care provider who wants to distribute a medication or take the individual to the dayroom or change bed linens? Often, busy care providers with a multitude of tasks to complete are not sensitive to the fact that elderly persons who appear to be doing nothing are performing a psychological task as important as any other activity that could be performed for them a that time. Private designated areas, such as the corner of a dayroom or a bedroom, should be provided and respected.

It must be emphasized that solitude and loneliness are not synonymous. The nurse may discover that some older adults enjoy and value sitting alone in the park for hours and may prefer a quiet evening at home to a party. To choose solitude differs from being socially isolated and not having opportunities for social activity.

Recommended Readings

Atchley R. Social forces in later life. Belmont, CA: Wadsworth, 1988.

McGuire FA, Boyd R. Leisure in later life. In: Murrow E, ed. Perspectives on gerontological nursing. Newbury Park, CA: SAGE, 1991;95.

14

Sexuality

Despite the physical ability to maintain a sexually active state in old age, various factors threaten the elderly person's ability to remain sexually active (Table 14-1). To ensure wellness and normality, sensitive attention to the maintenance and promotion of sexual function and identity is important.

For many years, sex was a major conversational taboo in our country. Discussion and education concerning this natural, normal process were discouraged and avoided in most circles. Literature on the subject was minimal and usually secured under lock and key. An interest in sex was considered sinful and highly improper. Although there was an awareness that sexual intercourse had more than a procreative function, the other benefits of this activity were seldom openly shared; sexual expression outside of wedlock was viewed as disgraceful and indecent. The reluctance to accept and intelligently confront human sexuality led to the propagation of numerous myths, the persistence of ignorance and prejudice, and the relegation of sex to a vulgar status.

Fortunately, attitudes have changed over the years, and sexuality has come to be increasingly understood and accepted as natural and pleasurable. Education has helped erase the mysteries of sex for both adults and children, and magazines and books on the topic flourish. Sex courses, workshops, and counselors throughout the country are helping people gain greater insight about and enjoyment of sex. Not only has the stigma attached to premarital sex been greatly reduced, but increasing numbers of unmarried couples are living together with society's acceptance. To a large degree, sex is now viewed as a natural, good, and beautiful shared experience.

Natural, good, and beautiful—seldom are these terms used to describe the sexual experiences of aged individuals. When the topic of sex and the aged is confronted, many ignorances and prejudices concerning sex reappear. Education about the sexuality of old age is minimal; literature abounds on the sexuality of all individuals in the society except the elderly. Any signs of interest in sex or open discussions of sex by older persons are discouraged and often labeled as lecherous. The same criteria that makes a man a "playboy" at 30 years of age make him a "dirty old man" at 70 years of age. Unmarried young and middle-aged adults who engage in pleasurable sexual experiences are accepted, but widowed grandparents seeking the same enjoyment are often viewed with disbelief and disgust. Myths run rampant. How many times do we hear that women lose all desire for sex after menopause, that older men cannot achieve an erection, that older people are not interested in sex? The aged are neutered—mostly by the lack of privacy afforded them; by the lack of credence given to their sexuality; and by the lack of acceptance, respect, and dignity granted to their continued sexual expression. The myths, ignorance, and vulgar status previously associated with sex in general have been conferred on the sexuality of the aged.

Such misconceptions and prejudices are an injustice to persons of all ages. They reinforce any fears and aversion the young have to growing old.

Table 14-1 *Aging and Risks to Sexuality*

AGE-RELATED FACTOR	POTENTIAL NURSING DIAGNOSIS
Wrinkling and sagging of tissues; age spots; graying and loss of hair; arthritic joints; loss of muscle tone; high prevalence of tooth loss; increased incidence of disabling disease	Disturbance in self-concept and sexual dysfunction related to altered appearance
Increased physical stimulation required to achieve erection and lubricate vagina	Sexual dysfunction related to inadequate preparation for intercourse
Increased prevalence of chronic disabling diseases	Sexual dysfunction related to discomfort, preoccupation with health, or positional restrictions
Higher ratio of women to men in advanced years	Sexual dysfunction related to unavailability of a sexual partner
Ageism	Sexual dysfunction related to belief that sex in old age is inappropriate

They impose conformity on the aged, which requires that they either forfeit warm and meaningful sexual experiences or suffer feelings of guilt and abnormality. Nurses can play a significant role in educating and counseling about sexuality and the aged; they can encourage attitudinal changes by their own example. A good perspective regarding sexuality is required because sex encompasses much more than a physical act. It includes love, warmth, caring, and sharing between people, seeing beyond gray hair, wrinkles, and other manifestations of aging, and the exchange of words and touches by sexual human beings. Feeling important to another and wanted by that person promotes security, comfort, and emotional well-being. With the multiple losses of roles and functions that the aged experience, the comfort and satisfaction derived from a meaningful relationship are especially significant.

Sexuality also includes expressing oneself as and being perceived as a man or a woman, although many persons are currently attempting to eliminate masculine and feminine stereotypes. Today's aged were socialized into masculine and feminine roles—the aged have had a lifetime of experience with the understanding that men are to be aggressive, independent, and strong and that women are to be pretty, dainty, and dependent on their male counterparts. It is difficult and equally unfair to try to alter the roles of aged persons as it is to try to convince today's liberated woman that she is limited to the roles of wife and mother. The socialization of today's older population and their role ex-

pectations must be recognized and respected. Yet nurses may witness subtle or blatant violations of respect to the aged's sexual identity. Examples of such a lack of respect include the following:

Belittling the aged's interest in clothing, cosmetics, and hairstyles

Dressing men and women residents of an institution in similar and asexual clothing

Denying a woman's request for a female aide to bathe her

Forgetting to button, zip, or fasten clothing when dressing the elderly

Unnecessarily exposing aged individuals during examination or care activities

Discussing incontinent episodes when the involved individual's peers are present

Ignoring a man's desire to be cleaned and shaved before his female friend visits

Not recognizing attempts by the aged to look attractive

Joking about two aged persons' interest in and flirtation with each other.

Why is it so difficult to understand that a recognition of sexual identity is important to the aged? It is not unusual for a 30-year-old to be interested in the latest fashions, for two 35-year-olds to be dating, or for a 20-year-old woman to prefer a female gynecologist. Almost any younger woman would panic if a new date saw her before she had time to adjust her cosmetics, hair, and clothing. Chances are that no care provider would walk into the room of a 25-year-old in traction and undress and bathe

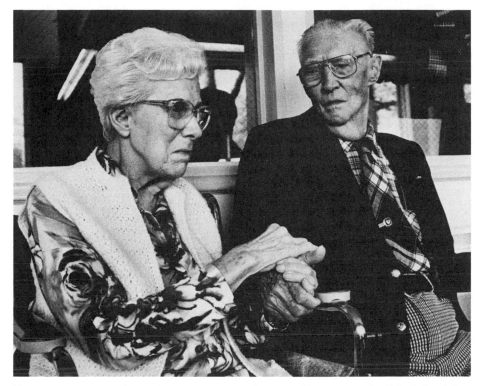

Human contact remains an important need in later life. (Photograph by Eric Schenk.)

him in full view of other patients in the room. The aged require the same dignity and respect and appreciate the same recognition as sexual human beings that is afforded to persons of other ages. The aging process does not neuter the aged person, nor does it alter the significance of sexual identity to that individual.

Sexual Intercourse

With the exception of the outstanding work by Kinsey (1948) and Masters and Johnson (1966), there had been minimal exploration into the realities of sex in old age until recent years. Possibly contributing to the lack of research and information are the following factors:

The acceptance and expansion of sexology has been relatively recent.

Impropriety was formerly associated with open discussions of sex.

There is a misconception on the part of many professionals, the aged, and the general public that the aged are neither interested in nor capable of sex.

Practitioners lack experience in and do not have an inclination for discussing sex with any age group. Even today, medical and nursing assessments frequently do not reflect inquiry into sexual history and activity.

Nurses should be aware of recent interest and research in the area of sex in old age and communicate these research findings to colleagues and clients in an effort to promote a more realistic understanding of the aged's sexuality. Research has disproven the belief that aged persons are not interested in or capable of engaging in sex; older individuals can and do enjoy the pleasures of sexual foreplay and intercourse. Because the general pattern of sexual behavior is basically consistent throughout life, individuals who were disinterested in sex and had infrequent intercourse throughout their lifetime will not usually develop a sudden insatiable desire for sex in old age. On the other hand, a couple who has maintained an interest

in sex and continued regular coitus throughout their adult life will most likely not forfeit this activity at any particular age. Homosexuality, masturbation, a desire for a variety of sexual partners, and other sexual patterns also continue into old age. Sexual styles, interests, and expression must be placed in the perspective of the individual's total life experience.

Although clinical data are minimal and additional research is necessary, some general statements can be made about sex in the older person.

There tends to be a decrease in sexual responsiveness and a reduction in the frequency of orgasm.(Masters and Johnson, 1981)

Older men are slower to erect, mount, and ejaculate.

Older women may experience dyspareunia as a result of less lubrication, decreased distensibility, and thinning of the vaginal walls.

Many older women gain a new interest in sex, possibly because they no longer have to fear an unwanted pregnancy or because they have more time and privacy with their children grown and gone.

Although individual differences occur in the intensity and duration of sexual response in older people, regular sexual expression for both sexes is important in promoting sexual capacity and maintaining sexual function. With good health and the availability of a partner, sexual activity can continue well into the seventh decade and beyond.

The findings from Masters and Johnson's clinical investigations into the sexual responses of older persons are presented in their fine book *Human*

Table 14-2 *Human Sexual Response Cycle and the Elderly*

PHASE	OLDER WOMEN	OLDER MEN
Excitement: results from stimulation from any source	Same clitoral response and nipple erection as younger woman; sex flush (vasocongestive skin response) occurs less frequently; less muscle tension elevation in response to sexual stimuli; unlike in younger women, labia majora does not separate, flatten, and elevate; reduced reactions of labia minora; less secretory activity of Bartholin's gland; less vaginal lubrication and wall expansion	Takes two to three times longer for erection to be achieved (although once achieved, it can be maintained for a longer period before ejaculation); significant reduction in vasocongestive response of scrotum; less sex flush
Plateau: sexual tensions intensified; if they reach an extreme, orgasm will be achieved; if tension level drops, resolution phase will be entered	Reduced intensity; less degree of engorgement of areolae	Slower; full erection may not occur until just prior to ejaculation
Orgasm: lasts a few seconds; sexual stimuli released; although entire body is involved to varying degrees, primarily concentrated in genitalia	Same vaginal contractions as younger woman but of shorter duration; similar slight degree of involuntary distention of external urinary meatus	Similar response as younger man, only slower; during ejaculation, more of a seepage of semen rather than a forceful emission; orgasm may not occur with every intercourse, especially if it is frequent
Resolution: sexual tensions subside	Nipple erection can continue for hours; urinary symptoms may be present	Longer duration

Sexual Response (1966). Because only a brief summary is presented in this text (Table 14-2), the nurse is encouraged to review their work for more specific information.

Sexual Problems

Various physical, emotional, and social variables threaten the elderly person's ability to remain sexually active (Table 14-3 and Nursing Diagnosis Highlight). Comprehensive nursing assessment should include a sexual history, which can reveal these problems. Sensitive attention to the maintenance of sexual function and identity is significant in promoting wellness and normality.

Availability

A practical interference with sexual function in later life is the lack of a partner, particularly for older women. Consider the following obstacles:

By 65 years of age there are only 7 men to every 10 women; by 85 years of age the ratio becomes 1:5.

There is a tendency for men to marry women younger than themselves—one-third of men older than 65 years of age have wives younger than 65 years of age; therefore, most older men are married and most older women are widowed.

Even when an older person has a spouse or partner, that person may be too infirm to remain sexually active and, in some cases, may be institutionalized.

Psychological Barriers

The elderly are not immune to the attitudes around them. As they hear comments about the inappropriateness of older people engaging in sex and watch television shows that portray sex among the elderly in a condescending or ridiculing manner, they may feel foolish or unnatural in having sexual desires and activity. If they happen to have sexual partners who are disinterested in sex and negatively label their advances, the problem is intensified. As the impact of others' reactions is internalized, there may be a reluctance or inability to engage in sexual activity, and this function may be forfeited unnecessarily. Nurses can aid by educating persons of all ages in the realities and impor-

tance of sexual function in later life and ensuring that nursing care does not reinforce negative attitudes about sex.

It is not unusual for older men occasionally to have difficulty achieving an erection; erections also may be easily lost if there is an interruption (e.g., a telephone ringing or a partner who leaves the bed to use the bathroom). These factors may lead older men to believe they are losing their sexual capabilities. A cycle of problems can then be triggered, whereby an episode of impotence causes anxiety over the potential loss of sexual function permanently, and this anxiety interferes with the ability to become erect, which heightens anxiety. Aging persons need realistic explanations—preferably before the situation arises—that occasional impotency is not unusual nor an indication that one is "too old for sex." Open discussions and reassurance are beneficial. The partner needs to be included in this process and made aware of the importance of patience and sensitivity in helping the man deal with this problem. The couple should be encouraged to continue their efforts and, if erection is occasionally a problem, compensate with other forms of sexual gratification. Of course, chronic impotency can indicate a variety of disorders and deserves a thorough evaluation.

Body image and self-concept may discourage sexual activity. In a society in which beauty is judged by youthful figures, older persons may believe that their wrinkles, gray hair, and sagging torsos make them physically unappealing. This can be particularly difficult for single elderly people who must deal with baring their bodies to new partners. The fear of being unattractive and rejected may cause older adults to avoid encountering such situations and assume a sexually inactive role.

For single older people, developing a sexual relationship can be difficult. Older women were socialized during a period when sex was considered appropriate only in wedlock, and to some persons, only for the purpose of procreation. The thought of seeking sexual gratification with a partner to whom one is not married creates anxiety and guilt in many older women. The older man, socialized in the aggressor role, may not have had to practice his courtship skills for years if he has been monogamous for a long period, and he may feel insecure in his ability to seduce a partner or find one who understands his individual preferences. He, too, may be emotionally uncomfortable in establishing a sexual relationship. The hurdle of building new

Table 14-3 *Physical Conditions Interfering With Sexual Function*

CONDITION	PROBLEM CREATED	INTERVENTION
Men		
Prostatitis	Discomfort, interference with ejaculation	Treat infection; prostatic massage
"Open" type prostatectomy	Disturbed function of internal sphincter, causing impotency	Penile prosthesis
Peyronie's disease	Painful, dorsal bending of penis from fibrous scarring associated with inflammatory process	Local injections of corticosteroids Surgery
Infections of genitalia	Pain, inhibition of erection, scarring that narrows urethral outlet	Treat infection Surgical dilation of narrowed outlet
Arteriosclerosis	Testicular cellular function disturbed, leading to decline in male sex hormone	Testosterone therapy
Parkinsonism	Decrease in sexual interest secondary to loss of potency	Levodopa therapy
Cord compression from arthritic changes	Impotency	Surgery may not restore potency if reflex arc is permanently broken Penile prosthesis
Women		
Decreased level of estrogen	Excessive vaginal dryness	Local estrogens
Virginity	Thick or large hymen	Surgery Dilation
Infection of genitalia	Discomfort, itching	Treat infection and underlying cause (poor hygiene, hyperglycemia)
Prolapsed uterus	Pain, difficulty with penile penetration	Pessary Surgery
Cyctocele	Discomfort, dribbling urine	Surgery
Both Sexes		
Cardiovascular, respiratory disease	Shortness of breath, coughing, discomfort, fear of heart attack or death during sex	Counseling on realistic restrictions necessary Instruction in alternative positions to avoid strain Advise to avoid large meals for several hours before, relax, plan medications for effectiveness during sex
Arthritis	Limited movement	Instruction on alternative positions
Diabetes mellitus	Local genital infection	Treat infection
	Failure of erection due to inhibition of parasympathetic nervous system	Penile prosthesis
	Absence of orgasm (women)	Instruction in alternative forms of sexual expression
Stroke	Decreased libido	Counseling
	Fear	Instruction in alternative positions
Alcoholism	Decreased potency Delayed orgasm (women)	Counseling and treatment for alcoholism

sexual relationships can be so great that many older people may find it easier to repress their sexual needs.

Married elderly also may experience problems with sex. Not all marriages enjoy fulfilling sex. Some women have conceded to sex because it was a "wife's duty," yet they never achieved satisfaction from this intimate experience. Some spouses may have become bored with the same partner or form of sex. Perhaps physical changes or an inattention to appearance causes dissatisfaction with the partner. Love and caring may have been lost from the marriage. Elderly couples experience sexual problems for many of the same reasons that younger couples do.

Misconceptions are often responsible for creating obstacles to a fulfilling sex life in old age and can include the following:

Erections are not possible after prostatectomy.
Penile penetration can be harmful to a woman after a hysterectomy.
Menopause eliminates sexual desire.
Sex is bad for a heart condition.
After a hip fracture, intercourse can refracture the bone.
Sexual ability and interest are lost with age.

Straightforward explanations and public education can aid in correcting these misconceptions, as can realistic descriptions of how illness, surgery, and drugs do and do not affect sexual function.

Physical Barriers

A variety of physical conditions can affect sexual function in later life, many of which can respond to treatment (see Table 14-3). Thorough evaluation is crucial in determining a realistic approach to aiding the elderly with these problems. Interventions of value to younger people also can benefit the elderly, including penile prostheses, lubricants, surgery, and sex counseling. Nurses should communicate their understanding of the importance of sexual functioning to the elderly and a willingness to assist them in preserving sexual capabilities.

Drugs

Frequently, medications prescribed to the elderly affect potency, libido, orgasm, and ejaculation. Some of these drugs include the following:

- clonidine
- guanethidine
- haloperidol
- phenothiazines
- reserpine
- sedatives
- thiazide diuretics
- tranquilizers
- tricyclic antidepressants.

It is important to prepare older people for the potential changes in sexual function that drugs can produce. Imagine what it does to a newly diagnosed hypertensive when he experiences drug-related impotency and begins to feel anxious about the sudden changes in both health and sexual function. Drugs should be reviewed when new sexual dysfunction occurs and, whenever possible, nondrug treatment modalities should be used to manage health problems.

Cognitive Impairment

The sexual behavior of demented individuals tends to be more difficult for those around them than for the affected persons. Inappropriate behavior such as undressing and masturbating in public areas and grabbing and making sexual comments to strangers can occur. The spouse may be accused of being a stranger improperly trying to share their bed, and care procedures (e.g., baths, catheterization) may be confused as sexual advances. Sometimes touching and statements such as "How's my sweetheart?" or "Are you going to give me a big hug?" can be misinterpreted as invitations to become sexually intimate. Family members and caregivers need to understand that this is a normal feature of the illness. Rather than become upset or embarrassed, they need to learn to respond simply, for example, by taking the individual to a private area when masturbating or stating "I'm not a stranger, I'm Mary, your wife."

Promoting Sexuality

The nurse can foster sexuality in the elderly in various ways, some of which have already been discussed. Basic education can help the elderly and persons of all ages understand the effects of the aging process on sexuality by providing a realistic framework of sexual functioning. A willingness on

the nurse's part to discuss sex openly with older people demonstrates recognition, acceptance, and respect for their sexuality. A sexual history as part of the nursing assessment provides an excellent framework for launching such discussions. Physi-cal, emotional, and social threats to the elderly's sexuality should be identified, and solutions should be sought for problems—whether caused by the disfigurement of surgery, obesity, depression, poor self-concept, fatigue, or lack of privacy.

NURSING DIAGNOSIS HIGHLIGHT
Sexual Dysfunction

Overview
Sexual dysfunction implies a problem in the ability to derive sexual satisfaction. This con-dition can be identified through the patient's history (*e.g.*, complaints of impotency, dys-pareunia, lack of interest in sex, changes in relationship with partner), physical findings (*e.g.*, genital infection, prolapsed uterus, dia-betes mellitus), or behavior (*e.g.*, depression, anxiety, self-deprecation). Sometimes changes in the patient's life can give clues as to the presence of sexual dysfunction problems, such as recent widowhood, onset of a new health problem, or moving to a child's home.

Causative or contributing factors
Age-related dryness and fragility of vaginal canal, vaginal infection, venereal disease, neurological disease, cardiovascular disease, diabetes mellitus, decreased hormone pro-duction, pulmonary disease, arthritis, pain, prostatitis, prolapsed uterus, cyctocele, rec-tocele, medications, overeating, obesity, fa-tigue, alcohol consumption, fear of worsen-ing health problem, lack of partner, unwilling/unable partner, boredom with part-ner, fear of failure, guilt, anxiety, depression, stress, negative self-concept, lack of privacy, religious conflict, altered appearance.

Goal
The patient will express satisfaction with sexual function.

Interventions
- Obtain a sexual history from the patient. Note availability of and quality of relation-ship with partner, lifelong pattern of sexual function, recent changes to sexual function, signs and symptoms of sexual dysfunction, knowledge and attitudes about sex, medical problems, drugs used, mental status, myths and misinformation, feelings about sexual dysfunction.
- If the cause of sexual dysfunction is not readily available through the history, refer patient for comprehensive physical exami-nation.
- Identify causative or contributing factors to sexual dysfunction and plan interventions to correct them.
- Refer to sexual counselor or therapist as needed.
- Clarify misconceptions (*e.g.*, cannot have sex after a heart attack).
- Provide education as to normal sexual func-tion, measures to promote sexual function, how to minimize impact of health prob-lems on sexual function (Heart Association, Arthritis Foundation, and other disease-specific organizations provide literature on promoting sexual function in presence of disease).
- Assist patient in having good appearance and improving self-concept as needed.
- Advise in health practices that will promote sexual function, such as regular gynecologi-cal examinations, alcohol use in modera-tion, good diet, exercise.
- Ensure staff are nonjudgmental about pa-tient's unique means of sexual expression.
- If patient hospitalized or institutionalized, provide privacy for sexual expression.

Consideration must be given to the sexual needs of older persons in institutional settings. Too often, couples admitted to the same facility are not able to share a double bed, and frequently they are not even able to share the same room if they require different levels of care. It is unnatural, unreal, inhumane, and unfair to force a person to travel to another wing of a building to visit a spouse who has intimately shared 40, 50, or 60 years of their life. There are few or no places in most institutional settings where two such individuals can find a place to share intimacy where they will not be interrupted or are in full view of others. Older people in institutional settings have a right to privacy that goes beyond lip service. They should be able to close and lock a door, feeling secure that this action will be honored. They should not be made to feel guilty or foolish by their expressions of love and sexuality. They should not have to have their sexuality sanctioned, screened, or severed by any other person.

"Petting rooms," "courting rooms," and other areas designated for couples to have privacy have been in vogue periodically. Although the intent in providing privacy is positive, the artificiality of these structures must be examined. How many couples could relax and enjoy sex in a room specifically labeled for such a purpose, knowing that everyone outside the room knew why they were there? Is privacy really provided when curious minds realize a couple is in this room and fantasize about the activities behind the closed doors? Perhaps it would be more natural and beneficial to respect elderly people's privacy in their own bedrooms and to designate periods of the day when residents know they will not be disturbed unless an emergency develops. Nursing staff in facilities should never overlook the basic courtesy of knocking on a person's door before entering a room.

Masturbation often is beneficial in releasing sexual tensions and maintaining continued function of the genitalia. Nurses can convey their acceptance and understanding of the value of this activity by providing privacy and a nonjudgmental attitude. An open view can prevent the elderly from developing feelings of guilt or abnormality related to masturbation.

Nurses must recognize, respect, and encourage sexuality in the elderly. Nurses, as role models, can foster positive attitudes. Improved understanding, increased sensitivity, and humane attitudes can help the older population of today and tomorrow realize the full potential of sexuality in their later years.

References

Kinsey A. Sexual behavior in the human male. Philadelphia: WB Saunders, 1948.

Masters W, Johnson V. Human sexual response. Boston: Little Brown, 1966.

Masters W, Johnson V. Sex and the aging process. J Am Geriatr Soc 1981;9:385.

Recommended Readings

Steinke EE. Older adults' knowledge and attitudes about sexuality and aging. Image: Journal of Nursing Scholarship 1988;20:93.

Steinke EE. Sexuality in aging. In: Murrow E, ed. Perspectives on gerontological nursing. Newbury Park, CA: SAGE, 1991;78.

Walz T, Blum N. Sexual health in later life. Lexington, MA: D.C. Health, 1987.

15

Safety

Throughout life, human beings confront threats to their lives and well-being such as acts of nature, pollutants, communicable diseases, accidents, and crime. Normally, adults take preventive action to avoid these hazards and attempt to control them, should they occur, to minimize their impact. Older persons face the same hazards as any adult, but their risks are compounded by age-related factors that reduce their capacity to protect themselves from and increase their vulnerability to safety hazards. Gerontological nurses need to identify safety risks during the assessment of older adults and provide interventions that will address existing and potential threats to safety, life, and well-being.

Aging and Risks to Safety

Except for middle-aged adults, the elderly have an overall lower rate of injury than other age groups (Table 15-1). Older women have a higher rate of injuries than any adult female age group, whereas the rate among men declines through adult years. The death rate from accidents is lower among the older population than other adult age groups (Table 15-2); accidents rank as the sixth leading cause of death for the elderly.

Age-related changes, altered antigen–antibody response, and the high prevalence of chronic disease cause older persons to be highly susceptible to infections. Pneumonia and influenza rank as the fourth leading cause of death in this age group, and pneumonia is the leading cause of infection-related death. Older adults have a threefold greater

incidence of nosocomial pneumonia as compared to younger age groups; the elderly experience gastroenteritis caused by *Salmonella* species more frequently than persons younger than 65 years of age; and urinary tract infections increase in prevalence with age.(Bush and Kaye, 1990) The elderly account for more than half of all reported cases of tetanus, endocarditis, cholelithiasis, and diverticulitis. Atypical symptomatology often results in delayed diagnosis of infection, contributing to the elderly's higher mortality rate from infections; for instance, older persons are 10 times more likely to die from appendicitis than younger persons and have a 7% mortality from cholecystitis compared with less than 2% in the general population.(Bush and Kaye, 1990)

Altered pharmacokinetics, self-administration problems, and the high volume of drugs consumed by older individuals can lead to considerable risks to safety. It is estimated that 5% to 30% of geriatric admissions to hospitals are associated with inappropriate drug administration.

Table 15-3 lists the various age-related factors that can pose risks to the safety and well-being of older adults and potential nursing problems associated with these risks.

Reducing Risks

Good preventive practices form the foundation for safety. In addition to the usual practices that would promote safety for persons of any age, additional measures must be promoted for older

Table 15-1 *Incidence of Injuries for Various Age Groups*

AGE (y)	PERSONS INJURED (IN MILLIONS)			RATE/100 POPULATION		
	Total	Men	Women	Total	Men	Women
Total	62.1	33.6	28.4	26.0	29.1	23.1
< 5	4.8	2.7	2.1	26.1	28.9	23.2
5–17	14.4	8.4	6.0	31.9	36.4	27.3
18–44	29.0	16.7	12.2	28.3	33.5	23.5
45–64	8.0	4.0	4.0	17.9	18.7	17.2
65 and older	6.0	1.9	4.1	21.1	15.9	24.8

From US Department of Commerce. Statistical abstract of the U.S. 110th ed. Washington DC: Bureau of the Census, 1990.

adults. These measures not only aid in avoiding injury and illness, but also can increase self-care capacity in older adults. These considerations include the following:

Sufficient fluid intake. Adequate fluid intake can be difficult for the elderly, particularly if they are depressed, demented, or physically incapable of maintaining good fluid and food intake. Thirst perception declines with age, causing older persons to be less aware of their fluid needs. Sometimes a self-imposed fluid restriction is a means of managing urinary frequency; in other situations the mental capacity to respond to the thirst sensation may be lacking. The result is insufficient fluid intake, which causes the body's already reduced tissue fluid reserves to be tapped. Un-

less contraindicated, the elderly should ingest at least 1500 ml of fluids each day. Many sources other than plain water can provide this requirement, including soft drinks, coffee, juices, Jello, ices, and fresh citrus fruits.

Adequate nutrition. Poor oral health, gastrointestinal symptoms, altered cognition, depression, and dependency on others for food can lead to poor food intake. Even healthy elderly people may have difficulty ingesting a proper diet because of factors such as limited funds, problems in shopping for food, and lack of motivation to prepare healthy meals. The fatigue, weakness, dizziness, and other symptoms associated with a poor nutritional status can predispose the elderly to accidents and illness. An appropriate quality and quantity of food intake can increase the body's resistance to such problems. See Chapter 9 for specific information about nutritional needs.

Vision aids. Most people older than 40 years of age require corrective lenses, so it is no surprise that most elderly will use eyeglasses. The visual capacity of the elderly can change frequently enough that regular evaluation of vision and the effectiveness of prescribed lenses is warranted. Annual eye examinations are helpful not only in ensuring the appropriateness of corrective lenses, but also in early detection of the many eye disorders that increase in prevalence with age.

Table 15-2 *Deaths by Injuries by Gender and Age (in thousands)*

AGE (Y)	BOTH SEXES	MEN	WOMEN
Total	95.3	65.5	29.7
< 15	8.1	5.2	2.9
15–24	20.0	15.5	4.5
25–34	16.9	13.3	3.4
35–44	10.3	7.9	2.4
45–54	7.0	5.2	1.8
55–64	7.7	5.3	2.4
65–74	8.5	5.1	3.4
75–84	9.6	4.9	4.7
85 and older	7.0	2.8	4.2

From US Department of Commerce. Statistical abstract of the US. 110th ed. Washington, DC: Bureau of the Census, 1990:49.

Hearing aids. The ability to hear directions and warnings is basic to safety. Audiometric evaluation should be obtained for persons with hearing impairments to determine possible corrective measures and the benefit of hearing aids. Older persons should be ad-

Table 15-3 Aging and Risks to Safety

AGE-RELATED FACTOR	POTENTIAL NURSING DIAGNOSIS
Decrease in intracellular fluid	Fluid volume deficit related to easier development of dehydration
Loss of subcutaneous tissue; less natural insulation; lower basal metabolic rate	High risk for injury and alterations in thought processes related to hypothermia
Decreased efficiency of heart	Activity intolerance related to alterations (decrease) in cardiac output
Reduced strength and elasticity of respiratory muscles; decreased lung expansion; inefficient cough response; less ciliary activity	High risk for infection related to reduced ability to expel accumulated or foreign matter from lungs
Reduced oxygen use under stress	Altered tissue perfusion related to changes in cardiovascular response to stress
Poor condition of teeth	High risk for infection related to dental disease or aspirated tooth particles
Weaker gag reflex	High risk for infection related to aspiration
Altered taste sensation	Altered nutrition: more than body requirements of salt or sweets related to taste deficit
Reduction in filtration of wastes by kidneys	High risk for injury related to ineffective elimination of wastes from blood stream
Higher prevalence of urinary retention	High risk for infection related to stasis of urine
More alkaline vaginal secretions	High risk for infection related to inadequate acid environment to inhibit bacterial growth
Decreased muscle strength	High risk for injury related to reduced muscle strength
Demineralization of bone	High risk for injury and impaired physical mobility related to increased tendency of bones to fracture
Delayed response and reaction time	High risk for injury related to inability to respond in timely manner
Poorer vision and hearing	High risk for injury, impaired home maintenance management, and sensory-perceptual alterations related to misperception of environment
Reduced lacrimal secretions	High risk for injury and infection related to decreased ability to protect cornea
Distorted depth perception	High risk for injury related to decreased ability to judge changes in level of walking surface
Increased threshold for pain and touch	High risk for injury, infection, sensory–perceptual alterations and impaired skin integrity related to less ability to sense problems such as pain and pressure
Less elasticity and more dryness and fragility of skin	Impaired skin integrity and high risk for infection related to easier skin breakdown
Poorer short-term memory	High risk for injury and noncompliance related to inability to recall medication administration, treatments
Higher prevalence of polypharmacy	Altered health maintenance and high risk for injury related to drug interactions and side effects
Different norms for vital signs, laboratory values	Altered health maintenance and high risk for injury related to unknowledgeable provider attempting to achieve middle-aged norms in the elderly
Reduced income	High risk for injury related to limited ability to afford protection of safe neighborhood, home repairs, adequate environmental temperature

vised not to purchase a hearing aid without an evaluation and prescription for their specific needs.

Stable body temperature. Temperature fluctuations can be hazardous to older individuals. The normal body temperature of many elderly persons is lower than that found in younger persons (*e.g.*, temperatures as low as 97°F [36°C] can be a normal finding in the elderly). Temperature elevation indicating a health problem can be missed if one is not aware of the person's baseline norm. For instance, a 99°F (37°C) temperature may not be alarming to the caregiver; however, if it is 2° above the individual's norm, an infection may be present and, if undiscovered, can lead to complications. In addition to having an undetected, untreated underlying problem, an unrecognized temperature elevation places an added burden on the heart. For every 1°F elevation, the heart rate increases approximately 10 beats per minute—a stress that older hearts do not tolerate well. At the other extreme, hypothermia develops more easily in older people and can cause serious complications and death.

Infection prevention. The risk of developing infections is considerably greater in the elderly person than the younger adult; thus, avoidance of situations that contribute to infection is necessary. Contact with persons who have known or suspected infections should be avoided, as should crowds (*e.g.*, in shopping malls, classrooms, movie theaters) during flu season. Vaccines (*e.g.*, pneumococcal, influenza, tetanus) should be kept up to date. In addition to care in avoiding external sources of infection, the elderly must be careful to ensure they do not create situations that predispose them to infection, such as immobility, malnutrition, and poor hygiene. Of course, good infection control practices are a must for preventing iatrogenic infections in elderly persons who receive services by health-care providers.

Sensible clothing. Shoes that are too large, offer poor support, or have high heels can lead to falls, as can loose hosiery and robes or slacks that drag on the floor. Garters and tight-fitting shoes or garments can obstruct circulation. Hats and scarves can decrease the visual field. Clothing that is practical, properly fitting, and conducive to activity is advisable.

Wise medication use. The high number of drugs consumed by the elderly and the differences in the pharmacokinetics in the aged can lead to serious adverse effects. Drugs should be prescribed only when necessary and after nonpharmacological measures of treatment have proven ineffective. The elderly and their caregivers should be taught the proper use, side-effects, and interactions of all drugs they are taking, and be advised in the discreet use of over-the-counter drugs. See Chapter 35 for more drug information.

Safe environment. Although it is fully discussed in Chapter 16, the importance of a safe environment must be mentioned here. Considerations should include lighting, noise, temperature, cleanliness, clutter, appliances, and plumbing and heating systems.

Crime avoidance. The elderly are a particularly vulnerable to criminals who view them as ready targets for an easy dollar. Older people should use caution in negotiating contracts and seek the advice of family members or professionals as needed. Likewise, discretion should be used in traveling alone or at night, and in opening their doors to strangers.

Early Detection

Identifying and correcting problems early aids in minimizing risks to safety. Regular assessment by professionals is important; however, self-evaluation by the elderly can be equally beneficial because they will recognize changes or abnormalities in themselves that signal problems. It could be useful for older people to be taught how to perform the following measures:

Take their temperature and pulse. Do not assume that everyone knows the right way to use and read a thermometer.

Listen to their lungs with a stethoscope. They may not be able to diagnose the sounds they hear, but they will be able to recognize a new or changed sound.

Observe changes in their sputum, urine, and feces that could indicate problems.

Identify the effectiveness, side effects, and adverse reactions of their medications.

Recognize symptoms that should warrant professional evaluation.

Confusion, disorientation, poor judgment, and decreased memory handicap the elderly's ability to protect themselves from hazards to their health and well-being. When these symptoms occur, they are not to be taken lightly or accepted as normal. Often, the root of the problem can be a reversible disorder such as hypotension, hypoglycemia, or infection. A competent evaluation is crucial to selecting the appropriate treatment modality and correcting the problem before complications occur.

A review of the individual's behaviors and function can pinpoint potential safety risks. Examples of situations to note include the following:

- a smoker who smokes in bed
- an incontinent individual
- an individual who uses a walker inappropriately
- a person who is dizzy from a new medication
- an automobile driver with poor vision
- a frail individual who cashes Social Security checks in a high-crime area
- an active pet that is constantly underfoot.

By observing and asking about routine activities, responsibilities, and typical tasks performed, these situations can be identified. Steps should be taken before an incident occurs to correct potential problems.

The Functionally Impaired

A particularly high risk to safety exists when persons are functionally impaired, as exemplified by victims of Alzheimer's disease, for instance. These individuals may not understand the significance of symptoms, may lack the capability to avoid hazards, and may be unable to communicate needs and problems to others. Examples of impairments that could heighten safety risks include the following:

- significant memory deficits
- disorientation
- dementia
- delirium
- depression
- deafness
- low vision
- aphasia
- paralysis.

When such conditions exist, an assessment should be made to determine how activities of daily living (*e.g.*, food preparation, telephone use, medication administration, laundry, and housekeeping) are affected. Interventions are then planned to address specific problems and could include the following:

Refer the individual to occupational therapists, audiologists, ophthalmologists, psychiatrists, and other specialists for evaluation of the existing condition and prescription of appropriate treatment

Provide assistive devices and mobility aids and instruct the elderly in their use.

Help the person to prepare and label drugs for unit dose administration; develop a triggering and recording system for drug administration.

Arrange for telephone reassurance, home health aid, home-delivered meals, housekeeper, emergency alarm system, or other community resources to assist the impaired person.

Instruct and support family caregivers as they supervise and care for the impaired individual.

Modify the individual's environment to reduce hazards and promote function.

Falls

One of the significant concerns about safety in later life relates to the incidence of falls. Various studies have indicated that approximately 30% of the elderly experience a fall each year, with a higher incidence of falls among persons who are experiencing episodes of illness.(Myers and Sharpe, 1990) The consequences of falls are serious; nearly one-fourth of fall victims sustain a serious injury from the fall and the likelihood of dying from the complications associated with falling increases with age.(Tinetti, Speechley, and Ginter, 1988) Even if no physical injury occurs, fall victims may develop a fear of falling again (*i.e.*, postfall syndrome) and reduce their activities as a result; this can lead to unnecessary dependency, loss of function, decreased socialization, and a poor quality of life.

Many factors contribute to the high incidence of falls in older adults, such as the following:

Age-related changes: reduced visual capacity; problems differentiating shades of the same color, particularly blues, greens, violets; cataracts; poor vision at night and in dimly lit

areas; less foot and toe lift during stepping; altered center of gravity leading to balance being lost more easily; slower responses; urinary frequency.

Improper use of mobility aids: using canes, walkers, wheelchairs without being prescribed, properly fitted, or instructed in safe use; not using brakes during transfers.

Medications: particularly those that can cause dizziness, drowsiness, orthostatic hypotension, and incontinence, such as antihypertensives, sedatives, antipsychotics, diuretics.

Unsafe clothing: poor-fitting shoes and socks, long robes or pants legs.

Disease-related symptoms: orthostatic hypotension, incontinence, reduced cerebral blood flow, edema, dizziness, weakness, fatigue, brittle bones, paralysis, ataxia, mood disturbances, confusion.

Environmental hazards: wet surfaces, waxed floors, objects on floor, poor lighting.

Caregiver-related factors: improper use of restraints, delays in responding to requests, unsafe practices, poor supervision of problem behaviors.

A history of falls can predict an individual's risk of future falls; therefore, persons who have experienced a fall or even a minor stumble should be carefully assessed to identify factors that may increase their risk of this problem (Display 15-1). Interventions should be planned accordingly.

Health-care facilities can find it beneficial to have an active falls-prevention program that incorporates some of the interventions described in the Nursing Diagnosis Highlight. Regular, careful inspection of the environment and prompt correction of environmental hazards (e.g., leaks, cracks in walkways, broken bed rails) are essential (Display 15-2). An evaluation of risk of falling should be incorporated into the assessment of each older client (see Nursing Diagnosis Highlight). Staff should orient older clients to new environments and reinforce safe practices such as using bed rails, braking wheelchairs and stretchers during transfers, and promptly cleaning spills.

Some falls will occur, despite the best preventive measures. The fall victim should be assessed and kept immobile until a full examination for injury is done. Skin breaks or discoloration, swelling, bleeding, asymmetry of extremities, lengthening of a limb, and pain are among the findings to note. Medical examination and x-rays are warranted for

DISPLAY 15-1   *Checklist of Risk Factors for Falls*

History of falls
Newly admitted to hospital
Impaired vision
Gait disturbance
Physical disability
Incontinence
Confusion
Mood disturbance
Dizziness
Weakness
Fatigue
Ataxia
Paralysis
Edema
Postural hypotension
Use of cane, walker, wheelchair, crutch, brace
Presence of IV, indwelling catheter
Unstable cardiac condition
Neurological disease
Parkinsonism
Cerebrovascular accident
Diabetes mellitus
Peripheral vascular disease
Orthopedic disease
Multiple diagnoses
Use of tranquilizers
Use of sedatives
Use of antihypertensives
Use of antipsychotics
Use of diuretics
Use of multiple medications

From Eliopoulos C. The older hospitalized patient. Glen Arm, MD: Health Education Network, 1991:66.

even the slightest suspicion of a fracture or other serious injury. Fractures often are not readily apparent immediately after the fall; it may be only when the person attempts to resume normal activity that the injured bone becomes misaligned. Also, areas other than the direct point of impact may be injured in the fall—for instance, a person may have fallen on the knee, but the force of the fall may have placed enough stress on the hip to fracture the femur. Careful examination and observation can aid in the prompt diagnosis of injury and introduction of appropriate treatment.

DISPLAY 15-2   Environmental Checklist

Smoke detector
Telephone
Fire extinguisher
Vented heating system
Minimal clutter
Functioning refrigerator
Proper food storage
Adequately lighted hallways and stairways
Handrails on stairs
Floor surface even, easy to clean, requiring no wax, free of loose scatter rugs and deep-pile carpets
Doorways unobstructed, painted a contrasting color from wall
Bathtub or shower with nonslip surface, safety rails, no electrical outlets nearby
Hot water temperature less than 110°F (43°C)
Windows screened, easy to reach and open
Ample number of safe electrical outlets, probably 3 feet higher than level of floor for easy reach, not overloaded
Safe stove with burner control on front
Shelves within easy reach, sturdy
Faucet handles easy to operate, clearly marked hot and cold
Proper storage of medications, absence of outdated prescriptions
Proper storage of cleaning solutions, paints, poisonous substances

For Wheelchair Use

Doorways and hallways clear and wide enough for passage
Ramps or elevator
Bathroom layout to provide maneuvering
Sinks, furniture low enough to reach

Safety Aids

When a fall, infection, or other problem occurs, the elderly take longer to recover and risk significantly more complications; thus, the key word in safety is prevention. A variety of practical methods, most of which are inexpensive, promote safety and should be considered in the care of the elderly.

To compensate for reduced peripheral vision, affected individuals should be approached from the front rather than from the back or side, and furniture and frequently used items should be arranged in full view. Altered depth perception may hamper the ability of the aged to detect changes in levels; this may be alleviated by providing good lighting, eliminating clutter on stairways, using contrasting colors on stairs, and providing signals to indicate when a change in level is being approached. The filtering of low-tone colors is an important consideration when decorating areas for the elderly; bright reds, oranges, and yellows and contrasting colors on doors and windows can be appealing and helpful. Difficulty in differentiating between low-tone colors should be considered if urine testing is being taught to older diabetics, because these tests often require color differentiation. Cleaning solutions, medications, and other materials should be labeled in large letters to prevent accidents or errors.

Directions and warnings can be missed because of poor hearing. Explanations and directions for diagnostic tests, medication administration, or other therapeutic measures should be explained in written as well as verbal form. These individuals should live close to someone with adequate hearing, who can alert them when fire alarms or other warnings are sounded. Specially trained dogs for the hearing impaired similar to Seeing Eye dogs may prove useful; local hearing and speech associations can provide information on this and other resources.

Other sensory deficits, although more subtle, can predispose the elderly to serious risks. A decreased sense of smell can cause warnings to be missed and scents of harmful versus harmless substances to be undifferentiated. Electric stoves can be helpful in preventing gas intoxication from the inability to detect a gas odor. The loss of taste receptors may cause the elderly to use excessive amounts of salt and sugar in their diets, which is a possible health hazard. Reduced tactile sensation to pressure from shoes, dentures, or an unchanged positions can cause skin breakdown, and the inability to differentiate between temperatures can cause burns. Careful observation, education, and environmental modifications to compensate for specific deficits should be planned.

Slower response and reaction times may be safety hazards. Older pedestrians may misjudge their ability to cross streets as traffic lights change, and older drivers may not be able to react quickly enough to avoid accidents; if family members are

not available to escort and transport these individuals, assistance may be obtained through local social service agencies. Slower movement and poor coordination subject the elderly to falls and other accidents; loose rugs, slippery floors, clutter, and poorly fitting slippers and shoes should be eliminated. Rubber mats and nonslip strips are essential in the bathtub, where fainting and falls often occur as a result of hypotension caused first from the warm temperature of the bath water, which dilates the peripheral vessels, and then again from the orthostatic effect of rising to a standing position.

NURSING DIAGNOSIS HIGHLIGHT
High Risk for Injury

Overview

Many older persons are limited in their ability to protect themselves from hazards to their health and well-being. Indications that this diagnosis exists can be manifested through a history of frequent falls or accidents, the presence of an unsafe environment, sensory deficits, multiple health problems, weak or immobile state, and altered mood or cognition.

Causative or contributing factors

Age-related changes, health problems, improperly fitted or used mobility aids, unsafe use of medications, unsafe environment, altered mood or cognitive function.

Goal

The patient is free from injury.

Interventions

- Assess risk of injury to patient (*e.g.,*) falls risk, activities of daily living and impaired activities of daily living function, mental status, gait, medication use, nutritional status, environment, knowledge of injury prevention practices).
- Identify patients at high risk for injury and plan measures to reduce their specific risks.
- Orient patients to new environments.
- Encourage patients to wear prescribed eyeglasses, hearing aids, and prosthetic devices.
- Ensure patients use canes, walkers, and wheelchairs properly and only when prescribed.
- Avoid the use of physical or chemical restraints unless assessed to be absolutely necessary; use proper procedures to ensure safety when they are used.
- Advise patients to change positions slowly, holding on to a stable object as they do.
- Keep floors free from litter and clutter.
- Provide good lighting in all areas used by patient.
- Store cleaning solutions and other noningestible substances in a safe area.
- Encourage patients to use handrails and grab bars.
- Assist patients as needed with transfers.
- Review medications used for continued need, effectiveness, appropriateness of dosage; instruct patients in safe medication use.
- Be sure patients wear well-fitted, low-heeled shoes and robes and pants of an appropriate length.
- Promptly detect and obtain treatment for changes in physical or mental health status.
- Review home environment for safety risks and assist patient in obtaining assistance in eliminating risks (*e.g.,* low-cost home improvements, housekeeping aid, senior housing).
- If safety risks are associated with insufficient finances (inability to purchase prescriptions, heating oil, home repairs) refer patient to social service agency to explore possibility of obtaining assistance.

Using a stool in the tub and resting before rising are useful measures. Because poor judgment, denial, or lack of awareness of their limitations may prevent them from protecting themselves, older people should be advised not to take risks such as washing windows or climbing ladders.

The environmental checklist (see Display 15-2) may also be useful in reviewing the safety of the elderly person's home.

References

Bush LM, Kaye D. Epidemiology and pathogenesis of infectious diseases. In: Abrams WB, Berkow R, eds. The Merck manual of geriatrics. Rahway, NJ: Merck Sharp & Dohme Research Laboratories, 1990:883.

Myers AH, Sharpe AC. Injuries in the elderly: risks and prevention. In: Eliopoulos C, ed. Caring for the elderly in diverse care settings. Philadelphia: JB Lippincott, 1989:110.

Tinetti ME, Speechley M, Ginter S. Risk factors for falls among elderly persons living in the community. N Engl J Med 1988;319(26): 1701.

Recommended Readings

Berryman E, Gaskin D, Jones A, Tolley F, MacMullen J: Point by point: predicting elders' falls. Geriatr Nurs 1989;10(4):199.

Janken JK, Reynolds BA, Swiech K. Patients falls in the acute care setting: identifying risk factors. Nurs Res 1986; 35:215.

Soderlind S. Weaving a safety net. Geriatr Nurs 1989; 10(4):187.

Whedon MB, Shedd P. Prediction and prevention of patient falls. Image: Journal of Nursing Scholarship 1989; 21:108.

16

Environmental Considerations

The environment is a statement by and to us, an expression of our unique selves. Whether it is cluttered with family heirlooms, accented by our handiwork, dramatic in design, or stark and simple, our environment expresses a great deal about our preferences, attitudes, life-styles, and personalities. In turn, we perceive messages from environments, such as the behavior expected, the degree of welcome, and the consideration for our needs. Although it is seldom given conscious thought, the communication between us and our surroundings is dynamic and significant.

The environment can be considered in two parts—the microenvironment and the macroenvironment. The microenvironment refers to our immediate surroundings with which we closely interact (e.g., furnishings, wall coverings, lighting, room temperature, and room sounds). The macroenvironment consists of the elements in the larger world that affect groups of people or even entire populations (e.g., the weather, pollution, traffic, and natural resources). Although nurses should be concerned with improving the macroenvironment to benefit public health, this chapter emphasizes the microenvironment, which can be more easily manipulated and from which more immediate benefits can be realized.

Purpose of the Environment

The environment should provide more than shelter; it should promote continued development, stimulation, and satisfaction to enhance our psychological well-being. This is particularly important for the elderly, many of whom spend considerable time in their homes or a bedroom of an institution and have reduced interaction with the larger environment of their communities. To achieve the fullest satisfaction from their microenvironments, the elderly must have other levels of needs met within their surroundings. This can be exemplified by comparing environmental needs with the basic human needs postulated by Maslow (Table 16-1). Similar to Maslow's theory, it can be hypothesized that higher level satisfaction from the environment cannot be achieved unless lower level needs are fulfilled. This may explain why some elderly have the following priorities and problems:

Do not care about installing a free smoke detector if they fear the rodents running around their apartment.

Refuse to have their house painted if it will make them look too affluent in a high-crime neighborhood and be a target for a burglary.

Table 16-1 *Environmental Needs Based on Maslow's Hierarchy*

BASIC HUMAN NEEDS	ENVIRONMENTAL NEEDS
Self-actualization	A space that promotes the realization of all potential, inspiring objects, beautiful grounds, relaxation aids
Self-esteem	A home one can feel pride in having, elegant decor, status symbols
Trust	A niche in which one can feel confident, control over life style, consistent layout/furnishings/temperature/lighting
Love	A place one derives pleasure from being, familiar and comfortable furniture, favorite objects, attractive
Security	A haven from external threats, ability to safeguard personal possessions, adequate lighting, locks, smoke detectors, alarms
Physiological needs	A shelter in which to live, adequate ventilation, room temperature about 70°F (21°C), functioning utilities and appliances, pest control

Data from Maslow AH. Toward a psychology of being. New York: Van Nostrand Reinhold, 1968.

Table 16-2 *Environmental Assessment*

STANDARD	YES	NO	COMMENTS
Room temperature 75°F (24°C)	____	____	_____
Low noise level	____	____	_____
Protected wandering area	____	____	_____
Filtered lighting via several sources	____	____	_____
No shadows or glare	____	____	_____
Contrasting colors at doorways, stairs	____	____	_____
Locked closets for medications, solutions	____	____	_____
Plexiglass in windows and doors of heavily used areas	____	____	_____
Permanently placed screens	____	____	_____
Signal alarm on exits	____	____	_____
Even floor surface	____	____	_____
Nonskid surface on tub, shower	____	____	_____
Nonslippery floor surface	____	____	_____
No jagged-edged surfaces	____	____	_____
Protective coverings on heaters, machinery, fans	____	____	_____
Covered electrical outlets	____	____	_____
Protected wires	____	____	_____
Routine checks of utility systems, equipment, paint	____	____	_____
Uncluttered, simple surroundings	____	____	_____
Furniture functional, easy to use	____	____	_____
Consistent identifier to mark personal belongings	____	____	_____
Familiar objects	____	____	_____
Designated spaces for items	____	____	_____
Orientation aids: clocks, picture cues	____	____	_____
Supervised smoking area	____	____	_____
Mechanism for regular environmental assessment	____	____	_____

Feel their home is no longer their own because a daughter-in-law has decided to redecorate it.

Remain socially isolated rather than invite guests to a house perceived to be shabby.

Are unwilling to engage in creative arts and crafts if they are adjusting to a new and unfamiliar residence.

Nurses must be realistic in their assessment of the environment to determine what levels of needs are being addressed and to plan measures to promote the fulfillment of higher-level needs (Table 16-2). The most common nursing diagnosis related to this assessment, Impaired home maintenance management, is presented in the Nursing Diagnosis Highlight.

Special Problems of the Elderly

Previous chapters have described some of the changes experienced with aging. These, along with limitations imposed by highly prevalent chronic diseases, create special environmental problems for elderly people, such as the following.

LIMITATION	POTENTIAL ENVIRONMENTAL IMPACT
Presbyopia	Decreased ability to focus and visualize near objects
Cornea less translucent, transmits less light	More external light needed to produce adequate image on retina
Decreased opacity of sclera, allows more light to enter eye	Colors more washed out, more contrast required
Yellowing of lens	Distorted color vision, particularly for browns, beiges, blues, greens, violets
Senile cataracts cloud lens	Glare more bothersome
Macular degeneration	Vision more difficult, more magnification needed
Senile miosis, pupil size decreased, less light reaches retina	Slower light-to-dark accommodation
Decreased visual field	Peripheral vision narrower
Presbycusis	Distortion of normal sounds
Dependency on hearing aid	Amplification of all environmental sounds
Reduced olfaction	Odors, smoke, gas leaks difficult to detect
Less discriminating touch sensation	Less stimulation from textures
Less body insulation, lower body temperature	More sensitivity to lower environmental temperatures
Slower nerve conduction	Slower response to stimuli, less ability to regain balance
Decreased muscle tone and strength	Increased difficulty rising from a seated position, fatigue easier, less elevation of toes during aubulation, shuffling gait.
Stiff joints	Difficulty climbing stairs, manipulating knobs and handles
Urinary frequency, nocturia	Frequent need for easily accessible bathroom
Shortness of breath, easily fatigued	Stairs, long hallways difficult to negotiate
Poor short-term memory	Forget to lock doors, turn off appliances
High use of medications, causing hypotension, dizziness	Increased risk of falls

Of course, specific handicaps accompany various diseases and create unique environmental problems, as is witnessed with a person who is cognitively impaired. Based on common limitations found among older people, most elderly need an environment that is:

- safe and functional, and compensates for their limitations
- comfortable, and that recognizes their special losses and changes
- personal and normalizing.

Lighting

Light has a more profound effect than simply illuminating an area for better visibility. For example, light affects the following:

Function. The individual may move around more and participate in more activities in a brightly lighted area, whereas the person may be more sedate in a dim room.

Orientation. The individual may lose his perspective of time if kept in a room that is constantly lighted or darkened for long periods, as witnessed with persons exposed to the bright lighting in intensive care units for several days, who cannot determine if it is day or night. A person who awakens in a pitch dark room may be disoriented for a few seconds.

Mood and behavior. Blinking psychedelic lights cause a different reaction than candlelight. In restaurants, customers are quieter and eat more slowly with soft, low illumination levels than with harsh high ones.

Several diffuse lighting sources rather than a few bright ones are best in areas used by the elderly. Fluorescent lights are the most bothersome because of eyestrain and glare. The use of fluorescent lighting for economic reasons actually may not be cost effective. Although less expensive to operate, they have higher maintenance costs. Sunlight can be filtered by sheer curtains. The environment should be assessed for glare, paying particular attention to light bouncing off shining floors and furniture. Observe the environment's lighting from a seated position because insufficient lighting, shadows, glare, and other problems can appear different at a chair or bed level than they do at standing height.

Night-lights are useful in facilitating orientation during the night and in providing enough visibility to locate light switches or lamps for nighttime mobility. A soft red light can be useful at night in the bedroom because it tends to improve night vision.

Temperature

Since Galen's time in 160 A.D., it has been realized that hot and cold temperatures affect human beings and their performance. Research has shown the following to be true.(Kobrick and Fine, 1983)

Tactile sensitivity is best at 85°F (29°C).

Visual vigilance performance is best at 90°F (32°C).

Vigilance performance in general is best between 85°F (29°C) and 90°F (32°C).

Psychomotor tasks become impaired below 55°F (13°C).

A direct correlation exists between body temperature and performance.

The normally lower body temperature and decreased amounts of natural insulation make the elderly especially sensitive to lower temperatures; thus, the maintenance of adequate environmental temperature becomes significant. The recommended room temperature for an older person should not be lower than 75°F (24°C). The older the person is, the narrower the range of temperature tolerated without adverse reactions. Room temperatures less than 70°F (21°C) can cause hypothermia in the elderly.(Hayter, 1980)

Although it is not as significant a problem as hypothermia, hyperthermia can create difficulty for older persons, who are more susceptible to its ill effects also. Brain damage can result from temperatures exceeding 106°F (41°C). Even in geographic areas that do not experience excessively high temperatures, consideration must be given to the temperature of rooms or homes in which doors and windows are not opened and no air conditioning is present. Persons with diabetes or cerebral atherosclerosis are high-risk groups for becoming hyperthermic.(Hayter, 1980)

Colors

Debates concerning the best color scheme to use in environments for older people can go on forever.

Warm colors such as reds, oranges, and yellows can be stimulating and increase pulse, blood pressure, and appetite, whereas cool-tone blues and greens can be excessively relaxing.(Newcomer and Gaggiano, 1976) Although certain colors are associated with certain effects, experiences with colors play a significant part in individual reactions to and meanings inferred from various colors. Because individual response can vary, it may be best to focus on the use of colors to enhance function and, whenever possible, personal preference of the room's resident. Contrasting colors are helpful in defining doors, stairs, and level changes within an area. When the desire is to not draw attention to an area, (e.g., a storage closet), walls should be of a similar color or within the same color family. Certain colors may be used to define different areas; bedrooms may be blue and green, eating and activity areas orange and red, lounge areas gray and beige. Although color coding to identify an individual's room and bed seem to promote memory and orientation, there is no evidence that this is any more helpful than labels or other factors.(Hiatt and West, 1980)

Patterned wall and floor coverings can add appeal to the environment; however, wavy patterns and diagonal lines can cause a sensation of dizziness and could worsen the confusion of persons with cognitive impairments. Using a simple pattern or a mural on one wall of the room can be more effective and pleasing.

Floor Coverings

Most people believe that carpeting represents warmth, comfort, and a homelike atmosphere and that it is an effective sound absorber. There even has been speculation that the use of carpeting in institutional settings can reduce the amount of fall-associated fractures. Carpeting does create problems, however, which include the following:

Static electricity and cling. Many older persons have a shuffling gait and incomplete toe lift during ambulation. Uncomfortable static electricity can be produced. The clinging of slippers and shoe soles to the carpeting could promote falls.

Difficult wheelchair mobility. The more plush the carpet, the more difficult it becomes to roll wheels on its surface.

Cleaning. Spills are more difficult to clean on a carpeted surface; even with washable surfaces, unattractive discoloration can result.

Odors. The smell of cigarette smoke and other odors can cling to carpeting, creating unpleasant odors. Urine, vomitus, and other substances can demand special deodorizing efforts that may not prove totally effective.

Pests. The undersurface of carpeting provides a wonderful environment in which roaches, moths, and other pests can reside.

To derive some of the benefits of carpeting, consideration may be given to carpeting some of the wall surface rather than the floor. This can provide a noise buffer, textural variation, and an attractive decor with fewer housekeeping and maintenance problems than floor carpeting.

Scattered and area rugs provide an ideal source for falls and should not be used. Tiled floor covering should be laid on a wood foundation rather than directly on a cement surface for better insulation and cushion. Bold designs can cause dizziness and confusion in ambulation; a single solid color is preferable. A nonglare surface is essential for the elderly. Floor treatments that create a nonslip surface are particularly useful in bathrooms, kitchens, and areas leading from outside doors.

Furniture

Furnishings should be appealing, functional, and comfortable. Firm chairs with armrests provide support and assistance in rising or lowering into the seat. Low, sinking cushions are difficult for older people to use. Love seats have the advantage over larger sofas in that no one risks being seated in the center without armrests for assistance. Rockers provide relaxation and some exercise. Chairs should be of an appropriate height to allow the individual's feet to rest flat on the floor with no pressure behind the knees.

Upholstery for all furniture must be easy to clean; thus, leather and vinyl coverings are more useful than cloth. Upholstery should be fire resistant with a firm surface without buttons or seams in areas that come in contact with the body. Rather than the back, seat, and armrest being one connecting unit, open space where these sections meet allows for ventilation and easier cleaning. Recliners can promote relaxation and provide a

means for leg elevation, but they should not require strenuous effort to change positions.

Tables, bookcases, and other furniture should be sturdy and able to withstand weight from persons leaning for support. If table lamps are used, consideration may be given to bolting them to the table surface so they are not knocked over in an attempt to locate them in the dark. Footstools, candlestick tables, plant stands, and other small pieces of furniture would be best placed in low-traveled areas if they must be present.

Drawers should be checked for ease in use. Sanding and waxing the corners and slides can facilitate their movement. In hanging mirrors, the height and function of the user must be taken into account; wheelchair-bound persons will need a lower level than their ambulatory counterparts.

Individuals with cognitive impairments need a particularly simple environment. Furniture should look like furniture and not pieces of sculpture. The use of furniture should be clear. Placement of a commode chair next to a sitting chair can be confusing and result in improper use of both.

Sensory Stimulation

By making thoughtful choices and capitalizing on the objects and activities of daily life, much can be done to create an environment pleasing and stimulating to the senses. Some suggestions are listed below:

- textured wall surfaces
- soft blankets and spreads
- differently shaped and textured objects to hold (*e.g.*, a round sheepskin-covered toss pillow and a square tweed-covered one)
- murals, pictures, sculptures, and wall hangings
- plants, freshly cut flowers
- coffee brewing, food cooking, perfumes
- birds to listen to, animals to pet
- soft music.

Different areas in the person's living space can be created for different sensory experiences. The appetite of nursing home residents could be much improved if within their own dining area they could smell the aroma of their coffee brewing or bread toasting rather than just having the finished product placed on a tray before them.

For bed-bound persons or those with limited opportunity for sensory stimulation, special efforts are necessary and could include the following:

Changing the wall hangings in their rooms. Many libraries and museums will loan artwork free of charge. Collaboration with a local school can yield unique art for the older person and meaningful art projects for the students.

Bringing in plants and fresh flowers.

Using a "sensory stimulation box" containing objects with different textures, shapes, colors, and fragrances for an activity.

Having a visiting or resident pet.

Noise Control

Many of the sounds we take for granted—television, traffic noise, conversation from an adjoining room, appliance motors, leaking faucets, paging systems—can create difficulties for the older person. Many elderly already experience some hearing limitation as a result of presbycusis and need to be especially attentive to compensate for this deficit. Environmental sounds compete with the sounds that the elderly want or need to hear, such as telephone conversation or the evening news, resulting in poor hearing and frustration. Unwanted or chronic noise can be a stressor and cause physical and emotional symptoms.

Ideally, noise control begins with the design of the building. Careful landscaping and walls can buffer outdoor noise. Acoustical ceilings, drapes, and carpeting—also useful on walls—are helpful, as is attention to appliance and equipment maintenance. Radios and televisions should not be playing when no one is listening; if one person needs a louder volume, earphones for that individual can prevent others from being exposed to high volumes. In institutional settings, individual pocket pagers are less disruptive than intercoms and paging systems.

Bathroom Hazards

Many accidental injuries occur in the bathroom and can be avoided with common sense and inexpensive measures. Particular attention should be paid to the following:

Lighting. A small light should be lit in the bathroom at all times. With urinary frequency and nocturia being the norm, the elderly will be using the bathroom often and can benefit from the increased visibility. This is especially helpful if the switch is located inside the bathroom so that the individual does not have to enter a dark area and then search for a switch.

Floor surface. Towels, hair dryers, and other items should not be left on the bathroom floor, and throw rugs should not be used. For older people, falls are dangerous under any circumstance, but with the high likelihood of falling and striking one's head on the hard surface of a tub or toilet, the potential seriousness of the fall increases. Leaks should be corrected to avoid creating slippery floors and another cause of falls.

Faucets. Lever-shaped faucet handles are easier to use than round ones or those that must have pressure exerted on them. Older people can risk falling as they struggle to turn a faucet handle or burning themselves by releasing too much hot water. This latter problem supports the need to control hot-water temperature centrally. Color-coding faucet handles makes differentiation of hot and cold easier than small letters alone.

Tubs and shower stalls. Nonslip surfaces are essential for tubs and shower floors. Grab bars on the wall and safety rails attached to the side of the tub offer support during transfers and a source of stabilization while bathing. A shower/bath seat offers a place to sit while showering and, for tub bathers, a resting point while lifting to transfer out of the tub. Because a drop in blood pressure may follow bathing, it may be beneficial to have a seat alongside the tub to enable the bather to rest while drying.

Toilets. Grab bars or support frames aid in the difficult task of sitting down and rising from a toilet seat. Because the low height of toilet seats makes it difficult for many elderly to use, a raised seat attachment could prove useful.

Electrical appliances. The use of electric heaters, hair dryers, and radios in the bathroom produces a considerable safety risk. Even healthy, agile persons can accidentally slip and pull an electric appliance into the tub with them.

Medical supply stores and health-care equipment suppliers offer a variety of devices that can make the bathroom and other living areas safer and more functional. Sometimes, less expensive replicas can be homemade and be equally effective. It is much wiser to invest in and use these assistive devices to prevent an injury than to wait until an injury occurs.

Psychosocial Considerations

Objects form only a partial picture of the environment. The human elements make the picture complete. Feelings and behavior influence and are influenced by the individual's surroundings.

From the bag lady who claims the same department store alcove to be her resting place each night to the nursing home resident who forbids anyone to open her bedside stand, most people want a space to define as their own. This territoriality is natural and common; many of us would become uncomfortable with a visitor to our office sifting through the papers on our desk, a house guest looking through our closets, or a stranger snuggling close to us on a subway when the rest of the seats are empty. The annoyance we feel at having someone looking into our window, peering over a privacy fence into our yard, playing music loudly enough to be heard in our home, or staring at us demonstrates that our personal space and privacy can be invaded without direct physical contact. To the dependent, ill elderly person, privacy and personal space are no less important, but they are more difficult to achieve. In an institutional setting, staff and other patients may make uninvited contact with a person's territory and self at any time, ranging from the confused resident who wanders into others' rooms to staff members who lift blankets to check if the bed is dry. Even in the home, well-intentioned relatives may not think twice about discarding or moving personal possessions in the name of housekeeping or entering a bathroom unannounced just to ensure that all is well. The more dependent and ill individuals are, the more personal space and privacy may be invaded. Unfortunately, for these individuals who have experienced multiple losses and a shrinking social

world, the regulation of privacy and personal space may be one of the few controls they can exercise. It is important that this be realized and respected by caregivers through basic measures such as the following:

Define a specific area and possessions that are the individual's (*e.g.*, this side of the room; this room in the house; this chair, bed, or closet).

Provide privacy areas for periods of solitude. If a private room is not available, arrange furniture to achieve maximum privacy (*e.g.*, beds on different sides of the room facing different directions, use of bookshelves and plants as room dividers).

Request permission to enter personal space. Imagine an invisible circle of about 5 to 10 feet around the person and ask before coming into it: "May I sit your new roommate next to you?" "Is it all right to come in?" "May I clean the inside of your closet?"

Allow maximum control over one's space.

Components of the environment can facilitate or discourage mental and social activity. Clocks,

---

NURSING DIAGNOSIS HIGHLIGHT
Impaired Home Maintenance Management

Overview

Impaired home maintenance exists when the patient is unable to maintain a safe, clean home environment. This condition can be caused by physical, mental, or social factors that limit the ability to care for the home and can be displayed through observations of a dirty, odorous environment; malfunction of electrical or plumbing systems; presence of vermin or rodents; accumulation of wastes; overgrown grass; unsafe home temperature; large amount of unwashed dishes or laundry; overdue utility, rent or mortgage bills; and the patient's verbalization of displeasure with or inability to care for home.

Causative or contributing factors

Injury or illness of patient or family member, loss of family member or caregiver, fatigue, pain, altered cognition or mood, substance abuse, medication side-effects, limited finances, added expenses, lack of knowledge or skills regarding home maintenance, lack of information regarding community resources.

Goal

The patient will reside in a clean, safe home environment.

Interventions

- Perform comprehensive assessment to identify all factors responsible for home maintenance management impairment.
- Assist patient in correcting or arranging for correction of home environment problems (*e.g.*, alleviate overloaded electrical outlets, discard wastes, call plumber, contact social service agency for financial aid for home improvements, screen windows, contracting for cleaning service).
- Instruct patient in techniques of home maintenance management, such as proper food storage, disinfection, insect control, avoidance of safety hazards.
- Identify assistive devices that can increase patient's independence in home maintenance management.
- If patient desires, enlist support and assistance of family or neighbors.
- Encourage patient to eat well, obtain adequate rest, and pace activities.
- Assist patient in realistically reviewing capabilities to remain in current housing situation; offer alternatives as necessary.
- Identify and refer patient to resources, such as alternate housing, homemaker assistance, shared housing program, home-delivered meals.

calendars, and newspapers promote orientation and knowledge of current events. Easily accessible books and magazines challenge the mind and expand horizons. Games and hobbies can offer stimulation and an alternative to watching television. The placement of chairs in clusters or in busy but not heavily trafficked areas is conducive to interaction and involvement with a larger world.

Although less than 5% of the elderly reside in nursing homes, slightly more than one in seven older persons will spend at least 6 months in such a facility during their last years of life.(Vincente, Wiley, and Carrington, 1979) Nursing homes are not reflections of normal homelike environments; adjustment to them can be difficult. Familiar surroundings are replaced with new and strange sights, sounds, odors, and people. Cues that triggered memory and function are gone, and new ones must be mastered at a time when reserves are low. Relatives and neighbors who possessed love and understanding are replaced with people who know only that person before them now and who have many tasks to be done. The individual experiencing this may experience a variety of reactions, such as the following:

Depression over the loss of health, personal possessions, independence.

Regression because of the inability to manage the stress at hand.

Humiliation by having to request basic necessities and minor desires such as toileting, a cup of tea, or a cigarette.

Anger at the loss of control and freedom.

Nursing homes cannot offer the same satisfaction as the person's own home, but the institutional environment can be enhanced through the following:

- an attractive decor
- inclusion of the individual's personal possessions
- respect for privacy and personal territory
- recognition of the individuality of the resident
- allowance of maximum control over activities and decision- making
- environmental modifications to compensate for deficits.

The human environment will be more important to the nursing home resident than the physical surroundings. Superior interior decoration and lovely color schemes mean little when respect, individuality, and sensitivity are not present.

References

Hayter J. Hypothermia-hyperthermia in older persons. J Gerontol Nurs 1980;6(2):65.

Hiatt L, West S. Orientation strategies of older hospital patients. Paper presented at the Eleventh Annual Conference of the Environmental Design Research Association, 1980.

Kobrick JL, Fine BJ. Climate and human performance. In: Osborne DJ, Gruneberg MM, eds. The physical environment at work. New York: John Wiley & Sons, 1983:69.

Newcomer RJ, Gaggiano MA. Environment and the aged person. In: Burnside IM, ed. Nursing and the aged. 2nd ed. New York: McGraw-Hill, 1980:568.

Vincente L, Wiley JA, Carrington RA. The risk of institutionalization before death. Gerontologist 1979;19:361.

Recommended Readings

Carp FM. Living environments of older adults. In: Murrow E, ed. Perspective on gerontological nursing. Newbury Park, CA: SAGE, 1991:185.

Kolanowski AM. Restlessness in the elderly: the effect of artificial lighting. Nurs Res 1990;39:181.

17

Nursing Assessment

Assessment pertains to the collection and analysis of data regarding the physical, emotional, and socioeconomic status of the individual. Not only are self-care capacities and limitations determined during this activity; nursing diagnoses and actions are identified as well. Although assessment is considered the first step of the nursing process, it is not an activity that is done once and forgotten. Instead, it is an ongoing process, whereby all observations and interactions are used to collect new data, recognize changes, and analyze needs. This dynamic nature of assessment is essential in gerontological nursing, where the status of patients changes often.

Sometimes assessment is viewed as an isolated nurse–patient activity solely for the purpose of gathering data. This can be observed during a clinic visit, when a patient is initially interviewed or completes a questionnaire pertaining to health status. In institutional settings, nurses may plan their first encounter with patients and their families to include an interview and examination for baseline data collection. It can be perfectly appropriate for assessment to be an isolated activity in some situations; however, it also is possible to integrate data collection into other activities, such as informal conversations at mealtime or during a back rub. As nurses gain experience and skill in assessment, they may be able to integrate data collection into their other care activities and later document their findings on a tool, rather than depend on a tool to

guide their assessment. Regardless of the approach, standard, comprehensive, baseline data must be collected, documented, and regularly reevaluated.

Interviewing for Data Collection

Among the various skills required in assessment, good communication is especially important if honest and thorough information is to be obtained. To facilitate communication, make patients comfortable and at ease during the interview. The room must be at a comfortable temperature although a comfortable environment for active staff may be too cool for older persons. Limit interruptions, and control noise and traffic flow. Be aware of the importance of privacy (e.g., do not conduct the interview in an open hallway or in a room shared by other patients). Provide seating with good support, and allow approximately 4 feet of distance between the patient and nurse—close enough to facilitate verbal exchange but far enough away to maintain a suitable social distance. Explain the type of questions that will be asked, how this information will be used, and with whom it will be shared. Many older persons have limited experience in being interviewed by service agencies and may be reluctant to share information about their innermost feelings, family conflicts, sexual dysfunction, voiding pattern, and financial status with "strangers." Rapport and trust must be established for complete and full information to be shared. Patients

should be reassured that the information they share will be handled discreetly and that they have a right to refuse to share information if they are uncomfortable doing so.

A variety of barriers can result in a poor exchange of information. An obvious barrier is some patients' limited use and understanding of the English language; special efforts to compensate for this through the use of interpreters and translation resources should be sought. English-speaking bilingual persons may resort to their native tongue when faced with a stressful situation such as a clinic visit or admission to a hospital or nursing home. The language level needs to be individualized so as not to overwhelm or insult patients. Jargon should be avoided; medical terminology can be accompanied by lay terms to facilitate understanding (e.g., "Do you use a diuretic or fluid pill?" "Do you ever faint or fall down?").

The manner in which questions are asked can influence the answer given. Sometimes brief, direct answers are needed, for which closed-ended questions are asked (e.g., "Where do you get your prescriptions filled?" "How many levels does your home have?" "How many aspirin tablets do you take each day?") Open-ended questions lend themselves to more lengthy responses and can be useful in obtaining more in-depth information or in evaluating mental status (e.g., "How do you manage when you run out of money and your check isn't due for another week?" "Please describe the pain you are having." "Could you tell me a little more about the thoughts you have when you're feeling depressed?") Nurses must be careful not to influence the response by the manner in which they ask the question (e.g., "You're not using laxatives, are you?" "You're eating well, aren't you?" "You understand that entering the nursing home is the best thing for you and your family, don't you?"). Not only the content of the answer but also the manner in which it is given can aid in uncovering problems. For instance, the patient may say she knows it is best that she be in the nursing home, but say it in a depressed, hopeless manner; responses in a loud tone of voice can be associated with hearing impairments, anxiety, or anger. During questioning, speech and thought disorders may be identified.

In addition to asking questions, nurses can obtain valuable data through a conscious use of their other senses. Problems can be identified by looking at the patient's general cleanliness, grooming, dress style, posture, skin color, body language, breathing pattern, facial expressions, mobility, and the normalcy of body structure and function. Sounds can be heard that will give clues to problems, such as wheezes, gurgling, clicking dentures, coughs, and an altered voice quality. Paying attention to breath and body odors can be useful in identifying problems ranging from poor hygienic practices to acidosis. Skin temperature and turgor, pain, and reactions to physical contact can be assessed by simple touching. Attentiveness to all data received by each of the sensory organs can enhance the interview process.

At the conclusion of the interview, it is helpful to summarize findings so that they can be validated or clarified. Patients should be given time to consider data that they have forgotten to share and to ask questions. It is helpful to describe how the collected data will be used and recommend that the patient feel free to share additional data perhaps remembered at a later time. If the patient tires or becomes uncomfortable during the interview, or if the time allotted proves insufficient, the interview may need to be conducted in several sessions; this time investment can yield high returns in the quality of data on which future care activities will be built.

Components of the Assessment

A wide range of data will be collected as part of the comprehensive nursing assessment. The nurse will work in collaboration with other health team members in the collection and analysis of this information. Some of the standard components of the assessment include profiles of the patient, his family, occupation, home, economic situation, health insurance, health and social service providers, social and leisure activities, health history, current health status, and medications.

Patient Profile

Identifying information includes full name, gender, race, religion and name and location of preferred church or synagogue, date of birth, address, telephone number, languages spoken, and name of spouse or nearest contact person.

Family Profile

If the spouse is living, information should be obtained pertaining to spouse's full name, date of birth, address, telephone number, occupation, and length of marriage. An assessment of the spouse's health status is also beneficial, not only to identify problems but also to evaluate the ability of this person to assist the patient should the need arise. If the spouse is deceased, it is useful to know the date and cause of death. Sometimes through exploring this information with the patient, unresolved grief, guilt, or other feelings surface.

Names and addresses of children add helpful information to the record, as do their ages and health status, which provide a realistic estimate of their ability to assist the patient. It is increasingly common to find such situations as an ill 85-year-old parent whose only source of assistance with daily home care is an ill 68-year-old daughter or son. One in five aged individuals has a child older than age 65 years! Deceased children and the date and cause of death should also be explored, and profiles of any other members of the household should be obtained. Just because the aged person may have no living family does not mean that friends or boarders in the household are not providing a strong support system.

The individual's relationship with family members is useful to know. Some elderly people would prefer living in a shabby room alone rather than in the new home of a child with whom they never got along. Likewise, if an elderly couple has had a satisfying marriage and have never been apart, the health team could make sure that when they are admitted to a nursing home, it is one in which they can share the same room and have their relationship respected.

Occupational Profile

If the individual is employed, information pertaining to the type of work, length of time at the present job, and working hours should be collected. The type of work can give clues to occupationally caused illnesses and indicate the type of diversionary activities the patient may prefer. It may be useful to explore the reason for working if the person is of retirement age. Continuing employment because of the satisfactions obtained from the job and a sincere desire to remain employed will have

different implications from disliking one's job but having to work from financial necessity. If the person is unemployed or retired, it is useful to evaluate the reason. Being unemployed because one desires to retire and travel has different implications from unwanted mandatory retirement or being unemployed because of poor health. The length of unemployment and the means of income are valuable to know and may help the nurse assess factors such as interests and financial concerns. Here again, the nurse should question the patient for occupational history.

Home Profile

The patient's home environment is essential to know, although this information is often overlooked by those who provide care for the aged in institutional settings. The home profile should include the type of dwelling, number of levels, locations of bathroom and patient's bedroom, number of stairs climbed in an average day, location of nearest neighbor, availability of a telephone, type of community, safety hazards, and whether the person owns or rents the home. The capacity of the individual to fulfill responsibilities in the home should also be explored.

The nursing history should reflect the presence of pets in the household. This may appear to be an insignificant consideration, but to the aged individual a pet may provide an important source of satisfaction and companionship. Some aged individuals may resist an emergency hospitalization or new housing because of their concern for the welfare of their pet. Knowledge pertaining to the cause of certain health problems (*e.g.*, allergies) may also be revealed by collecting information regarding pets.

Economic Profile

Various sources and amounts of income and whether the person is receiving all available benefits should be ascertained. Sometimes the elderly are not aware that they may qualify for certain benefits, or they are unable to understand the application process for these benefits. Monthly income should be balanced with the monthly expenses to evaluate the capacity of the individual to meet financial obligations. While obtaining these

data, the nurse may learn that the aged person is eating a poor quality diet due to budget constraints or that the patient is fearful of losing a home through inability to pay the annual property tax. Clues to specific financial concerns should be sought while questioning the person about financial status.

Health Insurance

The type of health insurance and policy number are basic information. If uninsured, measures can be taken to enroll the person in a program suited for individual needs. Lack of health insurance sometimes discourages people from seeking health care; it can be a source of stress if hospitalization is required. Multiple policies that may be duplicative or unnecessary should be identified.

Health and Social Services Providers

The names and locations of other physicians, social workers, visiting nurses, public health nurses, clinics, and hospitals involved with the individual should be recorded. They can provide additional insights about the patient and should be consulted to promote continuity of care. It is important to obtain information and avoid duplication regarding community resources used by the patient, such as home health aides or delivered meals.

Social and Leisure Activities

Knowing what organizations the person belongs to and preferred hobbies and interests helps guide the nurse in planning individual care and also indicates the person's health status, energy level, and opportunities for socialization. Sometimes organizations to which the individual has belonged will provide visits and continued communication if the individual is hospitalized or enters a nursing home.

Health History

The health history of an aged person need not explore every childhood disease or minor health problem that has ever existed, unless this information is significant to current health status. Information pertaining to a family tendency toward stroke, diabetes, heart disease, cancer, or hypertension may be more relevant. Health problems of current concern, or for which treatment is being obtained, should be recorded. A history of diabetes, hypertension, tuberculosis, and cancer should be indicated, even if the patient states that he or she is free of the disease at present. Previous major hospitalizations, surgeries, and fractures may give insight into current problems and should be explored. Women should be questioned as to the number and course of pregnancies. Allergies to foods and other items and drug sensitivities should be recorded.

Current Health Status

Current health problems should be recorded, and the patient's and family's knowledge and understanding of these problems should be ascertained. Perceptions regarding these problems should be indicated if significant (*e.g.,* the belief by an individual that his cancer was "caught" from his wife who recently died of the disease.) Any limitations in functions or inability to perform the activities of daily living should be assessed, as well as the methods in which these problems are managed. Any appliance or prosthesis used in the management of health problems should be listed. The main concerns and goals of the patient and family in relation to the patient's health status should be discussed and reflected in the assessment.

Medications

The high quantity and wide range of drugs used by older adults can lead to significant risks. A careful medication review can identify interactions, ineffectiveness, inappropriate dosages, and other problems associated with drug use. Ideally, the patient should have all medications, both prescription and over-the-counter, present during the assessment. For each of the medications, the nurse should review the following:

The reason for the drug. Review the record to determine the rationale for the drug's use. Question the patients about their understanding of the drug's purpose. Problems can arise from the patient's misunderstanding of the drug's intent (*e.g.,* if the patient believes that digoxin is a "fluid pill," he may feel he

can skip administration of the drug on days when he seems to be voiding excessively).

How the drug was obtained. Ask the patient who prescribed or recommended the drug's use and under what circumstances. It could be that a drug was prescribed by someone other than the patient's regular physician and the regular physician is unaware that the patient is using the drug.

The dosage of the drug. Check the dosage to ensure that it has been age adjusted.

Drug interactions. Note the impact the various drugs being used have on each other.

The patient's understanding and use of the drug. Review each medication with the patient and determine the patient's knowledge of the drug's purpose, route and schedule of administration, related precautions, and adverse effects.

The effectiveness of the drug. Determine if the drug is achieving its intended purpose; if the patient believes the drug is being as helpful now as it has been in the past.

Monitoring of the drugs. Review record for indications that serum levels and other factors have been evaluated, as appropriate.

Side-effects and adverse reactions of the drug.

Review signs and symptoms associated with side-effects and adverse reactions to each drug being used.

The continued need of the drug. Determine if changes in the patient's status have changed the need for the drug.

Physical Assessment

Physical examination of patients is part of the assessment process and, like other forms of data collection, can be a separately defined procedure or integrated into other care activities. The physical assessment conducted by the nurse serves a different purpose from the physical examination performed by the physician. For example, the physician may diagnose the type of arthritis present in the joint; the nurse recognizes this loss but may be more concerned with how the arthritis affects self-care capacity, providing effective pain relief measures, and devising required nursing actions to compensate for deficits. Thus, the focus of the nurse's physical assessment is to recognize self-care capacities, limitations, and pathology and their impact on the patient's ability to meet universal self-care and therapeutic (*e.g.*, illness-related)

PHYSICAL ASSESSMENT SKILLS

Auscultation

Purpose

To hear internal body sounds by use of a stethoscope

Procedure

Clean earpieces.
Select the portion of chestpiece that is appropriate for hearing specific sound:
    Diaphragm side for high-frequency sounds (*e.g.*, blood pressure, bowel sounds, respirations)
    Bell side for low-frequency sounds (*e.g.*, hear murmurs)
Apply minimal pressure when using the bell portion, or it will function as a diaphragm.
Auscultate desired areas.
Clean earpieces.

Percussion

Purpose

To determine location, size, and density of organs by tapping on body surface

Procedure (Fig. 17-1)

Position hands over area to be assessed (*e.g.*, lungs, liver, spleen, abdomen).
If right handed, place distal phalanx and joint of left middle finger firmly over surface to be percussed. (Do not place any other part of hand on surface.)
Partially flex middle finger of right hand and position above area of left middle finger. Quickly strike distal portion of left middle finger joint with tip of right middle finger. Striking motion should occur from wrist movement, not movement of entire arm.

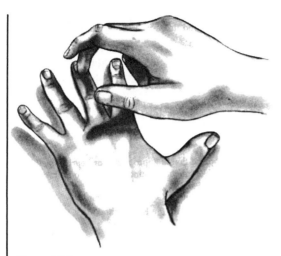

Figure 17-1.

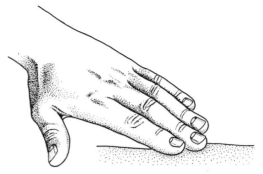

Figure 17-2. *The pads of the index and middle fingers lightly touch the skin surface (e.g., palpating the pulse).*

Withdraw finger immediately after striking.

If left handed, reverse hands in above directions.

Note sound produced:

Flat sound: soft, high-pitched, short duration; heard over solid organs

Dull sound: lower pitch and longer duration than flat sound; heard over hollow areas that contain fluid or tissue

Resonance: low pitch, loud, long duration; heard over hollow areas

Hyperresonance: louder, lower pitched, and of longer duration than resonance; usually associated with emphysematous lung

Tympany: loud, clear, hollow sound; indicates presence of air

Palpation

Purpose

To determine the size, temperature, texture, and mobility of various body parts by touching and direct manipulation

Procedure

Position hands over surface to be palpated.

Begin with light then progress to deeper palpation.

Light palpation (Fig. 17-2):

Useful in detecting tenderness, muscular resistance, spasm, masses, and superficial organs.

Use pads of fingertips to lightly press surface.

Move fingertips in wavelike motion.

Do not poke or jab.

Deep palpation:

Useful in delineating abdominal organs and masses.

Use same procedure as light palpation, but with more pressure.

If patient is obese, use one hand to palpate and the other to apply pressure on the palpating hand (Fig. 17-3).

Describe abnormal findings (*e.g.,* slippery 1 × 2 painful mass in left upper quadrant of abdomen)

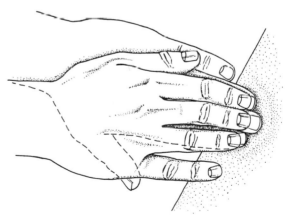

Figure 17-3. *The pads of the left hand touch the skin surface. The pads of the fingers of the right hand press down on the nail-bed areas of the fingers of the left hand. The skin surface is indented approximately 3 to 5 cm.*

demands, and resulting nursing diagnoses that will guide nursing actions.

There are some standard components of the physical assessment. The first basic step is a head-to-toe inspection of the body for normalcy of struc-ture and function, followed by auscultation, per-cussion, and palpation of selected body parts (see Physical Assessment Skills). Specific components of the physical examination include the following.

(Text continues on page 153)

ASSESSMENT ACTIONS	NORMAL FINDINGS	ABNORMAL FINDINGS
Head and Neck		
Inspect hair and scalp. Note consistency, texture, amount, distribution and care of hair. Ask about hair loss, itching or soreness of scalp. Note lesions, redness, sensitivity of scalp; describe exact location and measurement.	Gray, dry, thinning hair Men: baldness	Coarse, dry, brittle hair (hypothyroidism)
		Excessively oily hair (poor grooming practices, parkinsonism)
		Irregular patches of hair loss (fungal infection)
		Smooth, round nodules (sebaceous cysts)
		Nodular, ulcerative, raised, glossy, painless growth (melanoma, basal cell carcinoma)
		Red patches of dry skin with silver-white, light gray, or brown scale, less than 1 cm (solar [actinic] kerotoses)
		Redness and tenderness near hairline, over temporal artery (giant cell arteritis)
Note active and passive range of motion of head and neck.	Neck extension 55°, flexion 45°, lateral bending 40°, rotation 70°	Limited range of motion (arthritis, meningitis)
Ask patient to tilt head back and swallow.	No protrusion of thyroid gland	Prominence of thyroid gland (enlarged gland)
Ask patient to lie down, gently place hand on side of head and ask patient to resist your efforts to turn head; repeat for other side.	Ability to resist force to move head	Inability to resist force to move head (weakness or damage of sternocleidomastoid muscle, disorder of spinal accessory nerve)
Inspect and palpate carotid pulse.	Regular, strong carotid pulse	Weak carotid pulse with diminished stroke volume (left ventricular failure)
		Double carotid pulsation (aortic stenosis with insufficiency)
Inspect jugular veins.	No distention of jugular vein when patient erect or with head elevated 45°	Distended jugular veins when patient erect or with head elevated 45° (congestive heart failure, pericarditis)
		Unilateral jugular vein distention (kinking of innominate vein)
Inspect face. Note symmetry, scars, rashes, lesions.	Symmetrical features Freckles	Asymmetry, paralysis, numbness (CVA, Bell palsy)

ASSESSMENT ACTIONS	NORMAL FINDINGS	ABNORMAL FINDINGS
Ask about facial pain and numbness.	Lines, wrinkles, decreased skin elasticity	Raised, yellow, shiny growth, 1–5 mm in diameter (senile sebaceous adenoma)
Test function of trigeminal nerve: ask patient to close eyes while you gently touch forehead, cheek, and chin with cotton wisp and then a pin; repeat on other side of face.	Patient able to differentiate sharp from soft sensations at each site	Raised, well-marginated nodular lesion, waxy looking skin, ranging from few mm to over 1 cm (basal cell epithelioma)
Ask patient to hold mouth open while you gently attempt to close it by pushing on head and chin.	Patient able to resist efforts to close mouth.	Raised, circumscribed pigmentation with papules within lesion (malignant melanoma)
Inspect eyes. Note drooping eyelids, moisture of eyes, discharge, unusual movements, discoloration of sclera.	Loss of tissue elasticity around eyes, "baggy" eyelids	Ptosis (impairment of oculomotor nerve, edema)
	White sclera; black-skinned persons can have slight yellow discoloration	Edematous eyelids (allergy, infection, nephrosis, heart failure)
		Yellow sclera (liver disease)
		Protruding eyes (hyperthyroidism)
		Excessively dry eyes (Shogren syndrome)
Ask patient to close eyes and gently palpate eyeballs.		Soft, spongy-feeling eyes (dehydration)
Ask about visual capacity and changes, symptoms.		Extremely hard-feeling eyes (increased introcular pressure)
		Eye pain, dilated pupils, perception of halos around lights (acute glaucoma)
		Tearing, headaches, complaint of "smeared" or unclear vision (chronic glaucoma)
		Blind spot in visual field: scotoma (macular degeneration)
		Blindness in same half of both eyes: homonymous hemianopsia (CVA)
Test visual acuity by having patient read a Snellen chart or various sized print on a newspaper.		Inability to see small print (farsightedness)
Test extraocular movement by having patient follow your finger as you move it to various horizontal and vertical points.		Irregular, jerking movements of eyes (disturbance of cranial nerves III, IV, VI)
Ask about date of last ophthalmologic exam; refer for exam if one has not been done within past year.		

(Continued)

ASSESSMENT ACTIONS	NORMAL FINDINGS	ABNORMAL FINDINGS
Inspect ears. Ask about pain, itching, discharge, care of ears.	Increased cerumen accumulation	Itching (cerumen, chronic external otitis)
Note hearing capacity, patient's ability to hear watch tick.	Larger lobes, greater protrusion of ears	Small, crusted ulcerated lesion on pinna (basal or squamous cell carcinoma)
	Increased hair growth in ear	
	Atrophy of tympanic membrane (appears white or gray)	Tinnitus (hypertension, adverse drug reaction)
	Increased difficulty hearing high-pitched sounds	Hearing deficit (sensorineural or conductive hearing loss, cerumen impaction, upper respiratory or ear infection, ototoxic drugs, diabetes)
Inspect nares. Note lesions, masses, perforated septum.	Drier nasal cavity	Obstructed nasal breathing (mass, polyp, dried crusts)
Test patency of each naris by obstructing one at a time and asking the patient to inhale with mouth closed.		
Ask about nosebleeds, feeling of obstruction, pain, other symptoms.		Nosebleeds (hypertension, vitamin C deficiency, irritation from picking)
Determine ability to differentiate common scents (*e.g.,* orange peel, coffee grounds, rose)	Some decreased olfaction	Inability to smell (impairment of olfactory nerve, local irritation or bleeding)
Inspect oral cavity with tongue depressor and light. Examine tongue. Note lesions, discoloration, moisture.	Vertical wrinkling of skin surrounding mouth	Blue lips (anoxia, anemia)
	Drier, thinner, less vascular buccal mucosa	Dryness of lips and oral cavity (dehydration)
		Sore, lesion (infection, cancer)
	Varicosities on ventral surface of tongue	Fissure at corner of mouth (vitamin B complex deficiency, infection, overclosure of mouth due to missing teeth or poorly fitting dentures)
	Decreased secretion of salivary ptyalin	
	Dark-skinned persons may have bluish hue to lips and brownish markings on gum as normal findings	Bluish, black line along gumline (lead, arsenic, or mercury poisoning)
		Smooth, red tongue (iron, vitamin B_{12}, or niacin deficiency)
		White patches on tongue (moniliasis, leukoplakia)
Note voice tone and quality, articulation, speech pattern.	Interpret and use language appropriately	Aphasia (neurological disease, altered cognition)
		Monotonous, slurred speech (parkinsonism)
		Slurred speech (hypoglycemia, intoxication, neurological disease)

ASSESSMENT ACTIONS	NORMAL FINDINGS	ABNORMAL FINDINGS
Test gag reflex, rise of soft palate when patient says "ah."	Gag reflex present, although may be weaker Rise of soft palate	Failure of soft palate to rise (vagus nerve paralysis)
Note breath odor.		Sweet, fruity smelling breath (ketoacidosis)
Inspect the number and condition of teeth. Ask about last dental exam. If dentures are present, examine fit and condition; remove dentures and inspect and palpate gums (with gloved hand).		Breath odor of urine (uremic acidosis) Breath odor of clover (liver failure) Foul breath odor (halitosis, decaying teeth, lung abscess)

Respiratory System

ASSESSMENT ACTIONS	NORMAL FINDINGS	ABNORMAL FINDINGS
Ask patient about ease of breathing, symptoms, coughing, sputum production.	Reduced efficiency of cough response	Orthopnea, dyspnea, shortness of breath (respiratory infection or disease)
Ask about dates of last influenza and pneumoccal vaccines, tuberculin test or chest x-ray.		Ruddy, pink coloring of face, trunk, limbs (COPD)
Inspect bare chest. Note coloring, symmetrical expansion during respiration, scars, structural abnormalities. Evaluate respiratory rate, rhythm, depth, and length.		Bluish, gray hue to face and neck (chronic bronchitis) Asymmetrical lung expansion (acute pleurisy, pleural fibrosis, pleural effusion, pain, fractured rib)
Inspect and palpate for spinal curvatures.		
Note anteroposterior and lateral chest diameter.	Slight increase in anteroposterior chest diameter	Significant increase anteroposterior diameter or anteroposterior diameter that is greater than lateral diameter (COPD)
Palpate posterior chest by placing both hands on the patient's back (thumbs alongside the spine and fingers fanned over intercostal spaces). Feel depth of respirations and chest movement; be alert to areas of sensitivity, masses.	Bilateral movement during respirations Lack of basilar inflation	Crepitus (crunchy feeling to skin resulting from air getting trapped under epidermis)
Evaluate tactile fremitus (vibratory tremors felt during palpation of chest wall) by placing palmar bases of fingers or ulnar surface of hands along different areas of lung fields and feeling for vibrations as the patient says "99."	Fremitus best in upper lobes	Increased fremitus in lower lobe (pneumonia, mass) Lack of fremitus in upper lobe (COPD, pneumothorax)

(continued)

ASSESSMENT ACTIONS	*NORMAL FINDINGS*	*ABNORMAL FINDINGS*
Percuss lungs, starting at the upper lobe and percussing downward; alternate from one side to the other to compare sounds.	Resonance (clear, low-pitched sounds)	Diminished breath sounds (emphysema, shallow respirations, pleural thickening)
Auscultate to assess pitch, intensity, quality, and duration of breath sounds.	Bronchial breath sounds over trachea (short inspirations; long expirations)	Increased breath sounds (extensive lung damage)
	Vesicular breath sounds over entire lung field (long inspirations; short expirations)	Crackles, rales (extrainterstitial fluid due to CHF, pulmonary edema, bronchitis, pneumonia)
	Bronchovesicular breath sounds over sternum and scapula (equal inspiratory and expiratory phase)	Rhonchi, rattling (increased mucus production and partial airway obstruction due to bronchitis, bronchiectasis)
		Wheezes (presence of large amounts of thick mucus or narrowing of airway due to asthma, pulmonary stenosis)

Cardiovascular System

Note generalized coloring, energy level, breathing pattern, mental status.	No distress, symptoms or discoloration	Pallor, confusion, fatigue, dyspnea (cardiac disease)
Inspect veins; note varicosities.		Confusion, blackouts, fatigue, dizziness (decreased carotid blood flow, aortic stenosis, reduced cardiac output, digitalis toxicity)
Note condition of nails, presence of hair on extremities, color and temperature of extremities.	Extremities warm, hair present	Coughs, wheezes (left-sided heart failure)
Ask about symptoms such as dizziness, lightheadedness, edema, cold extremities, palpitations, chest pain, blackouts.		Hemoptysis (pulmonary embolus, heart failure)
		Chest pain, pressure (MI, angina)
Assess blood pressure using a two-step palpatory-auscultatory method: Palpate the radial pulse, inflate the cuff and note the level where the pulse disappears; deflate the cuff, wait 30 s, palpate the brachial pulse and place the stethoscope over the artery; inflate the cuff 30 mm Hg above palpated systolic; deflate at a rate of 2–3 mmHg/s and listen.	BP levels must be elevated individually and in relationship to physical and mental status at various BP levels.	Repeated BP >160/95 (hypertension)
Assess the blood pressure in lying, sitting, and standing positions.	Positional drops <20 mm Hg	
Assess rate, rhythm and volume of pulse.	Pulse rate can range 60–100 beats.	Arrhythmias (digitalis toxicity, hypokalemia, infection, hemorrhage, cardiac disease)
	Some tachycardia may be present, related to stress of being examined; reevaluate in several hours.	

ASSESSMENT ACTIONS	*NORMAL FINDINGS*	*ABNORMAL FINDINGS*
Palpate PMI in the apical or left ventricular areas (5th left intercostal space or slightly medial to the midclavicular line).		Displaced PMI (marked kyphoscoliosis, left ventricular hypertrophy)
Palpate the right ventricular area at the lower left sternal border, the pulmonary area at the second left intercostal space, the aortic area at the second right intercostal space, and the epigastric area at the fifth intercostal space near the sternum. Note thrills (palpable vibrations similar to the feeling of a cat purring).		Thrills in apical area (mitral valve disease) Thrills in right ventricular area (ventricular septal defect) Thrills in pulmonary area (pulmonic stenosis) Thrills in aortic area (aortic stenosis)
Auscultate the entire heart: use the bell portion of the stethoscope to hear low-frequency sounds (*e.g.,* diastolic murmur of mitral stenosis) and diaphragm portion to hear high-frequency sounds (*e.g.,* murmurs associated with aortic and mitral regurgitrelated to problems such as local obstruction)		
Measure jugular venous pressure: Expose neck and chest. If pressure is significantly elevated, have patient sit erect; if pressure is moderately elevated, elevate patient to 45° angle; if pressure is slightly elevated or normal, have patient lie flat. Support head and neck to relax sternocleidomastoid muscle. Turn patient's head slightly away and shine light tangentially across sternocleidomastoid muscle. Observe pulsations. Repeat for other side. Inspect carotid arteries for abnormally large, bounding pulses.	Full neck veins disappear when patient is supine; pulsations are < 2 cm above clavicle when in 45° elevation.	Bilateral jugular neck distension (CHF, pericarditis, superior vena cava obstruction) Unilateral jugular vein distension (kinking of left innominate vein)
Palpate pulse at medial edge of sternocleidomastoid muscle. To avoid carotid massage, palpate only one side at a time. Listen for bruits by asking the patient to hold his breath while you auscultate the arteries with the bell portion of the stethoscope.	Palpable carotid pulse	

(continued)

ASSESSMENT ACTIONS	NORMAL FINDINGS	ABNORMAL FINDINGS
Gastrointestinal System		
Ask about appetite, diet, swallowing problems, indigestion, regurgitation, pain, nausea, vomiting, flatus, constipation.		Bleeding, irritation of esophagus (esophageal varicosities)
		Excessive salivation, hiccups, dysphagia, anemia, thirst, chronic bleeding (esophageal cancer)
		Heartburn, dysphagia, belching, vomiting, regurgitation, pain, symptoms worse in recumbent position (hiatal hernia)
Obtain weight. Ask patient about recent changes in weight.	See Table 9-1 for age-adjusted weight norms.	Weight loss >5% in last 30 days; >10% in last 6 mo
Obtain triceps and biceps skinfold measurements; review biochemical data (see Chap. 9).		
Inspect abdomen. Note discoloration, asymmetry, dilated vessels, bulges, distention, rashes, scars, strong contractions. Ask the patient to raise head and note herniations that may become evident.	Symmetrical sides, rounded, adipose tissue	Pink or blue striae (recent stretching due to tumors, ascites, obesity)
	Silver-white striae secondary to pregnancy, weight changes	Jaundice (cirrhosis, gallstones, pancreatitis)
		Rashes (irritation, drug reaction)
		Small painless nodules (skin cancer)
		Symmetrical distention of abdomen (tumor, obesity, hernia, ascites)
		Central lower quadrant distention (distended bladder, ovarian or uterine tumor)
		Central upper quadrant distention (gastric dilatation, pancreatic cysts or tumor)
Auscultate abdomen prior to touching it for percussion or palpation to avoid stimulating bowel activity. Listen for bowel sounds over intestines using diaphragm portion of stethoscope. If sounds are not heard, listen for 5 min and then flick finger against abdominal wall to stimulate intestinal motility.	Peristaltic sounds every 5–15 s	Absent or reduced bowel sounds (late bowel obstruction, peritonitis, electrolyte imbalances, handling of bowel during surgery)
	Continuous bowel sounds if food has been ingested within past several hours	Increased bowel sounds (early bowel obstruction, gastroenteritis, diarrhea)
Auscultate vascular sounds by placing bell portion of stethoscope over major arteries.	Heartbeat can be heard	Murmurs over abdominal aorta (aneurysm)

ASSESSMENT ACTIONS	NORMAL FINDINGS	ABNORMAL FINDINGS
Auscultate over the liver and spleen for friction rubs (grating sound similar to shoes rubbing on cement) indicating enlarged organ coming in contact with peritoneum.		Friction rub (enlarged organ)
Percuss all quadrants of abdomen.	Tympany (drumlike sound) over air-filled areas Dullness over organs	Dullness over air-filled spaces (ascites, masses)
Palpate in all quadrants, beginning with light palpation and progressing to deep palpation.		Bulge (hernia) Lumps, masses (nodules, cancer)
Inspect the rectum; perform digital exam unless contraindicated.		Palpable spleen (enlarged spleen) Rectal mass (fecal impaction, tumor)
Note masses, blood, hemorrhoids, fissures.		Bright red blood (lower GI bleeding, hemorrhoids, diverticulitis)
Ask about pattern of bowel elimination.	Regular passage of moist, formed stool without straining	Infrequent passage of stool, abdominal fullness and discomfort, lethargy, poor appetite (constipation) Diarrhea or seepage of stool, palpable mass in rectum (fecal impaction)
Obtain a stool specimen.		Dark, tarry stools (hemorrhoids, lower GI cancer, diverticulitis) Gray, tan, unpigmented stool (obstructive jaundice) Pale, fatty stool (malabsorption) Mucus in stool (inflammation) Small worms in stool or rectal area (pinworms)

Reproductive System

For women:

Ask about history of pregnancies menstrual pattern, gynecological problems, sexual function, and date of last gynecological exam, including Pap smear and mammogram.		Postmenopausal bleeding (estrogen therapy, cancer) Dyspareunia (age-related changes to vagina, prolapsed uterus, mass) Vaginal discharge, odor, irritation, soreness, itching (vaginitis, moniliasis, trichomoniasis)
Inspect genitalia. Note inflammation, irritation, discharge, lesions, prolapse. Palpate genitalia for masses and tenderness.	Loss of pubic hair; flattening of labia; dry vaginal canal; smaller-sized uterus (may not be palpable) Atrophy of breast tissue	Protrusion of vaginal wall outside vulva, pelvic pressure or heaviness, urinary tract symptoms (prolapsed uterus, cystocele, rectocele)

(continued)

ASSESSMENT ACTIONS	NORMAL FINDINGS	ABNORMAL FINDINGS
Ask about breast changes, pain, tenderness, nipple discharge. Inquire about patient's knowledge and practice of self-examination of breasts. Inspect and palpate breasts for discharge, masses, abnormalities.		Palpable mass (cancer) Dimpling and retraction of nipple; nontender, nonmovable hard mass in breast (carcinoma)
Refer to GYN exam and mammogram as necessary.		
For men: Ask about sexual function, symptoms, date of last prostate exam.	Decreased frequency of sexual activity	Impotency (stress, depression, drug side-effects, fatigue, overeating, neuropathy, long period of sexual inactivity)
Inspect genitalia for lesions, edema, discharge, masses, deformity.	Potency	Penile discharge (urethritis, prostatitis, venereal disease)
		Crooked, painful erection (Peyronie's disease)
Palpate scrotum for symmetry of testicles, tenderness, masses.	Reduced size and firmness of testes	Mass (carcinoma)
Obtain rectal examination of prostate.	Some degree of prostatic enlargement present in most older men	Scrotal pain, swelling (epididymitis, orchitis, carcinoma)
Inspect breast tissue and nipples; ask about pain, changes.		Prostatic enlargement (benign prostatic hypertrophy, cancer)
		Painful, edematous, reddened breasts (irritation from suspenders, restraints)
		Disk-shaped, firm, movable, tender mass under areola (fibroadenosis, carcinoma)
		Noninflammatory breast enlargement (obesity, drug side-effect [*e.g.,* digitalis, phenothiazines], liver dysfunction, testicular tumor, bronchogenic cancer)
Ask about pattern, frequency, and characteristics of bladder elimination; history of incontinence.	Urinary frequency, nocturia Continence	Incontinence (urinary tract infection, prostatic enlargement, neurogenic bladder, tumor, cerebral cortex lesion, calculi, medications, altered cognition)
		Increased urinary frequency (urinary tract infection, diuretic therapy, increased fluid intake, diabetes, hypocalcemia, anxiety)
Obtain urine specimen for evaluation.		Cloudy, alkaline, odorous urine; temperature elevation; frequency (urinary tract infection)
		Hematuria, pain, signs of urinary tract infection (renal calculi)

ASSESSMENT ACTIONS	*NORMAL FINDINGS*	*ABNORMAL FINDINGS*
		Painless hematuria, signs of urinary tract infection (bladder cancer)
		Yellow-brown or green-brown urine (jaundice, obstructive bile duct)
		Pink, red, or rust-colored urine (presence of blood)
		Dark brown or black urine (hematuria, carcinoma)
		Orange urine (presence of bile, ingestion of phenazopyridine [Pyridium])
Musculoskeletal System		
Ask about joint pain, restricted movement, tremors, spasms; inquire as to how the patient manages these problems.	Reduction in muscle mass and strength	Back pain (degenerative arthritis, muscle strain, osteoporosis)
	Range of motion adequate to perform ADL	Joint pain, stiffness, crepitus, bony nodules/Heberden's nodes (osteoarthritis)
Place all joints through active and passive range of motion.		Joint pain, stiffness, redness, warmth, subcutaneous nodules over bony prominences, atrophy of surrounding muscle, flexion contractures (rheumatoid arthritis)
Palpate all muscles for tenderness, contractions, masses.		Calf cramps during exercise, relieved by rest (intermittent claudication)
Test muscle strength.		Red, dry, thickened piece of skin over bony prominence (corn)
		Medial allocation of first metatarsophalangeal joint (digiti flexus [hammer toe])

ADL, activities of daily living; BP, blood pressure; CHF, congestive heart failure; COPD, chronic obstructive pulmonary disease; CVA, cerebrovascular accident; GI, gastrointestinal; GYN, gynecological; MI, myocardial infarction; PMI, point of maximal impulse.
Adapted from Eliopoulos C. Assessing normal from abnormal. In: Eliopoulos C. Nursing the elderly in diverse care settings. Philadelphia: JB Lippincott, 1990:26.

Cognitive and Emotional Status

Considerable insight into cognitive and emotional status can be gained throughout the general assessment process by observing how alert and lucid the patient is and how appropriately and rapidly he responds to stimuli. Observations and information derived from the patient and the family can indicate specific emotional problems. Attention should be paid to the presence of anxiety, depression, suspiciousness, fearfulness, emotional lability, nervous mannerisms, disinterest in self or life in general, and hyperactive or hypoactive behavior. Current stress factors in the individual's life should be explored along with coping mechanisms used. It is also revealing to learn the older person's attitude and concerns about death. Specific assessment actions for assessing mental health are as follows.

ASSESSMENT ACTIONS	NORMAL FINDINGS	ABNORMAL FINDINGS
Ask if patient has ever had a problem with mental health, been treated for depression, anxiety, "bad nerves," "nervous breakdown," mood problems; if medications have ever been or are currently being used for emotional problems; if patient has noticed any change in mental function, mood; if appetite, sleep pattern, or activity level has changed; if patient sees or hears things that others do not; how patient feels about self. Inquire if patient has ever considered suicide; if patient has, ask if he has planned how he would commit suicide.	Positive self-concept Interest in life	Recent changes in cognitive or emotional status (depression, delirium, adverse drug reaction, physical illness)
State three, unrelated words and ask the patient to remember them. Ask for immediate recall and for recall after 15 min.	Ability to retain and recall items immediately and 15 min after being instructed to do so	Inability to retain and recall (delirium, dementia, lack of interest in participating in exam due to depression, limited intellectual ability)
Ask patient to state name of self, president, knowledge of location, day, season, time (ensure patient has reason to know this information).	Orientation to person, place, time	Disorientation (delirium, dementia, lack of interest in participating in exam due to depression, limited intellectual ability)
Test judgment by presenting a situation and asking the patient how he would respond to it, such as "What would you do if the trashcan had a fire in it?"	Appropriate, reasonable response	Inappropriate response (delirium, dementia, lack of interest in participating in exam due to depression, limited intellectual ability)
Ask the patient to follow a simple direction consisting of three parts, such as "Pick up that piece of paper, fold it in half, and give it to me."	Ability to follow three-stage command	Inability to follow three-stage command (delirium, dementia, lack of interest in participating in exam due to depression, limited intellectual ability)
Ask the patient to count backwards from 100 by sevens or to spell the word *world* backward.	Ability to subtract 7 from answer five times (*i.e.*, to 65) or to spell the word world backward	Inability to count backwards from 100 by 7s, perform simple calculations, or spell the word world backward (delirium, dementia, lack of interest in participating in exam due to depression, limited intellectual ability)
Observe the appropriateness of the patient's use of language. Ask patient to give name of simple objects that you point to, to read a simple sentence, and write a simple dictated sentence (ensure patient has educational ability to read and write).	Proper use and understanding of language	Aphasia, paraphasia (delirium, dementia, neurological disease, lack of interest in participating in exam due to depression, limited intellectual ability)

ASSESSMENT ACTIONS	*NORMAL FINDINGS*	*ABNORMAL FINDINGS*
Note general mood and behavior.	Appropriate actions Stable mood	Suspiciousness, insecurity (paranoid disorder, sensory deficit, history of being abused) Hyperactivity, euphoria, hostility, paranoia, feelings of grandiosity (mania) Feelings of hopelessness, helplessness, sighing, crying, low activity level, sleep or appetite changes (depression)

Organizing and Documenting Data

More likely than not, a thorough assessment will yield a rich abundance of data, valuable to care planning and delivery. Whether these data are stored in the chart as an academic exercise or regulatory requirement fulfillment or are used to guide individualized, effective care can be determined by how understandable, retrievable, and user-friendly it is. A consistent format should be used to organize data; it can be in the form of a standard outline/narrative approach or a fill-in-the-blank assessment tool. The needs of the agency may cause the format to vary.

If the information obtained is compiled on a nursing history form, it will provide guidance and organization in data collection and ease in data retrieval. A sample of such a form is provided in Table 17-1. The type of format will vary, depending on the type of information and the function it is to fulfill.

The Minimum Data Set for Nursing-Home Resident Assessment and Care Screening

In 1991, as a result of the nursing home reform law known as the Omnibus Budget Reconciliation Act, (OBRA), a new requirement for assessment of long-term care facility residents has been implemented. The law mandates that long-term care facilities conduct a standardized, comprehensive, accurate, and reproducible assessment of all residents. The assessments must be done on admission and whenever the resident's status changes; the ongoing ap-

propriateness of the assessment is to be evaluated every 3 months.

The federal government has specified the basic, minimum data that should be included in the assessment and described it as the Minimum Data Set for Nursing Home Resident Assessment and Care Screening (MDS). A suggested format for documenting this data has been provided by the Health Care Financing Administration and is shown in the Appendix. It is anticipated that this form will change as experience with the use of the MDS is gained; in addition, individual states have the option to develop their own tools for data collection that include more than the minimum data required by the federal government. As can be noted on the MDS tool, the major categories of areas assessed include the following:

- cognitive patterns
- communication/hearing problems
- vision patterns
- physical function and structural problems
- continence
- psychosocial well-being
- mood and behavior patterns
- activity pursuit patterns
- disease diagnoses
- health conditions
- oral and nutritional status
- skin condition
- medication use
- special treatment and procedures.

When certain problems are identified during the assessment, the need to follow Resident Assessment Protocols (RAPs) is triggered. RAPs give

(Text continues on page 161)

Table 17-1 *Nursing History for Older Adults*

Profile of Patient
Name _____ Sex _____ Race _____ Religion _____ Date of birth _____
Address _____Telephone _____
Language spoken _____ Nearest contact person _____

Profile of Family

Spouse

_____ Living
    Health status:
    Age:
    Occupation:
_____ Deceased
    Year deceased:
    Cause of death:
Others in household:

Children

_____ Living
    Names and addresses:
_____ Deceased
    Year deceased:
    Cause of death:
Quality of relationships:

Occupational Profile

_____ Employed
    Type of Work:
    Length of employment:
    Working hours:
    Sources of income:

_____ Unemployed
    Reason:
    Length of unemployment:
    Previous occupations:

Home Profile

_____ Single dwelling
_____ Multiple dwelling
_____ Own
_____ Rent
_____ Telephone
_____ Pets (describe)

Number of levels:
Location of bathroom:
Location of bedroom:
Nearest neighbor:
Household responsibilities:
Safety:

Economic Profile
Sources in income:
Monthly income:
Monthly expenses:
Financial concerns:

Health Insurance
_____ Medicaid
_____ Medicare
_____ Blue Cross/Blue Shield
_____ Other:
Policy number:

Health and Social Resources Currently Used

_____ Private MD
_____ Hospital
_____ Clinic

_____ HMO
_____ Adult day care
_____ Home health nurse

_____ Social worker
_____ Meals-on-Wheels
Other:

Social/Leisure Activities
Organization membership:
Hobbies/interests:

_____ Allergies
    Food:
    Drug:
    Other:
_____ Diabetes
_____ Hypertension
_____ Cancer

_____ Hospitalizations:
_____ Surgery:
_____ Fractures:
_____ Major health problems:

Table 17-1 *(Continued)*

Current Health Status
Knowledge and understanding of health problems:
Limitations of function or performance of ADL: Management of limitations:

Health goals:

Medications

Name	Dosage	How and When Taken	How Obtained	Knowledge and Understanding of Medication

Physical Status
T _____ (A,O,R)   Height _____   Urine:
P _____   Weight _____ (recent changes:)   S/A: _____
R _____   BP _____ (sitting, standing, lying)   Specific gravity:
                                                            How obtained:
                                                            Characteristics:

Skin condition
_____ Intact   _____ Rash (describe)   _____ Wounds
_____ Dry   _____ Discoloration (describe)   (describe)
_____ Pruritus   _____ Abnormal finding (describe)

Hair condition _____ | Nail condition _____
_____ | _____
_____ | _____

Mobility
_____ Ambulatory   _____ Able to rise from chair or toilet
_____ Nonambulatory   _____ Able to climb stairs
_____ Ambulatory with assistance (specify)   _____ Able to transfer

(Continued)

Table 17-1 (Continued)

Extremity function

	Location	Degree of Limitation	Assistive/Relief Measures
Contracture			
Arthritis			
Painful movement			
Paralysis			
Spasm			
Amputation			
Dominant hand			

Respiration

	Precipitating Factors	Degree of Limitation	Assistive/Relief Measures
Orthopnea			
Dyspnea			
Shortness of breath			
Wheezing			
Asthma			
Coughing			

Sputum characteristics
_____ Smoking history   _____ Tracheostomy

Circulation

	Precipitating Factors	Degree of Limitation	Assistive/Relief Measures
Chest Pain			
Tachycardia			
Edema			
Cramping in extremities			

Equality of pulse, temperature, and color in extremities:

Table 17-1 *(Continued)*

Nutrition

Teeth: Dentures: Chewing problems:
   Number: _____ Partial/Complete   Swallowing problems:
   Status: Fit: Feeding tube:
Date last dental exam:

	Precipitating Factors	Assistive/Relief Measures
Indigestion		
Constipation		
Diarrhea		

Usual meal pattern:	Fluid intake: Alcohol use:
Food preferences and restrictions:	Appetite:

Bladder
_____ Nocturia   _____ Burning   _____ Incontinence   _____ Catheter
_____ Frequency   _____ Urgency   _____ Stress incontinence _____ Ostomy
   Voiding pattern:
   Urine characteristics:

Bowel

_____ Hemorrhoids	_____ Pain during movement	_____ Chronic constipation	Incontinence
_____ Straining	_____ Recent change in pattern	_____ Chronic diarrhea	_____ Ostomy

Stool
   Bowel movement pattern:
   Characteristics:

	Frequency of Use	Results Obtained
Laxatives		
Suppositories		
Enemas		

(Continued)

Table 17-1 *(Continued)*

Sensory status

	Degree of Limitation	Assistive/Relief measures

Hearing
  All sounds
  High frequency		

Vision
  Full vision
  Night vision
  Peripheral vision
  Reading
  Color discrimination
  Depth perception		

Taste		
Smell		

Touch
  Feels pressure and pain
  Differentiates temperature
  Pain
  Speech		

Other sensory data:

_____ Hearing aid   _____ Contact lenses   Date last hearing exam:
_____ Eyeglasses   Date last vision exam:

Rest and sleep
_____ Insomnia (describe)   Medicines and alcohol used to induce sleep:
_____ Night restlessness   Factors interfering with rest:
_____ Night confusion   Usual sleep and rest pattern:

Female reproductive factors		Male reproductive factors

Female reproductive factors

_____ Vaginal discharge   _____ Nipple discharge   _____ Scrotal swelling
_____ Itching   _____ Breast pain   _____ Lesions
_____ Lesions   _____ Mastectomy   _____ Discharge
_____ Breast mass   (indicate right or left)   _____ Impotency
                           _____ Prosthesis

Date last GYN exam:
Date last mammogram:

Male reproductive factors

Sexual profile

_____ Interest   _____ Dyspareunia   _____ Attitude:
_____ Sexually active   _____ Limitations: _____ Frequency:

Table 17-1 (Continued)

Mental Status

_____ Alert

_____ Rapid response to verbal stimuli

_____ Slow response to verbal stimuli

_____ Confused

_____ Stuporous

_____ Comatose

Memory of recent events:

Orientation

_____ Person

_____ Place

_____ Time

Attention span:

Ability to follow three-stage command:

Memory of past events:

Emotional Status

_____ Anxious

_____ Fearful

_____ Depressed

_____ Hostile

_____ Hyperactive

_____ Hypoactive

_____ Suspicious

_____ Euphoric

_____ Disinterest in life

_____ Emotionally labile

_____ Suicidal

_____ Other (describe)

Self concept _____

Current stress factors _____

Attitude and concerns about death _____

Other data _____

Informant

_____ Patient

_____ Other (specify)

Signature of Nurse	Date

guidelines for additional factors to assess and imply that further evaluation of the problem is necessary. For example, if the assessment has revealed that the resident shows decline in cognitive function, the RAP for "Delirium" is indicated; that protocol lists factors that may be associated with the problem, clarifying information to be considered in establishing a diagnosis, and the environment conducive to reducing symptoms. The nurse will be expected to document the nature of the problem, complications, risk factors, referrals needed, and rationale for deciding for or against including the problem on the care plan. The problems identified through the resident assessment process should be reflected on the care plan unless rationale is given for omitting them.

Although the MDS is mandated for long-term care facilities, the data available from this process can be significantly helpful to nurses in other settings who care for residents transferred from nursing homes. If the MDS form does not accompany residents to hospitals, home health agencies, or other care settings, the nurses in those settings should request the form from the long-term care facility. Continuity of care is enhanced with the communication of this information.

Recommended Readings

Abbey JC. Physiological illness in aging. In: Murrow E, ed. Perspective on gerontological nursing. Newbury Park, CA: SAGE, 1991:275.

Duffy ME, MacDonald E. Determinants of functional health of older persons. Gerontologist 1990;30:503.

Eliopoulos C, ed. Health assessment of the older adult. 2nd ed. Redwood City, CA: Addison-Wesley, 1990.

Eliopoulos C. Resident assessment handbook. Glen Arm, MD: Health Education Network, 1991.

Fields SD. History-taking in the elderly: obtaining useful information. Geriatrics 1991;46(8):36.

Foreman MD. Reliability and validity of mental status questionnaires in elderly hospitalized patients. Nurs Res 1987;36: 216.

Haight BK. Psychological illness in aging. In: Murrow E, ed. Perspectives on gerontological nursing. Newbury Park, CA: SAGE, 1991:296.

Morris JN, Hawes C, Fries BE, et al. Designing the national resident assessment instrument for nursing homes. Gerontologist 1990;30:293.

Teng EL, Chui HC. The modified mini-mental state (3MS) examination. J Clin Psychiatry 1987;48(8):314.

18

Planning and Providing Care

Chapter 17 discussed data collection for nursing assessment. This first phase of the nursing process sets the foundation for care; however, analysis of the data is essential to developing the blueprint for care, or the care plan. In analyzing data, a variety of questions should be considered, including the following:

What deficits exist in the patient's ability to fulfill the universal self-care requirements?

What potential risks to self-care ability exist?

What health problems are present, and how capable is the patient to meet the demands imposed by them?

What measures could enhance the health, independence, and satisfaction of the patient and family unit?

This should yield a list of actual and potential problems for the nurse to consider.

Nursing Diagnosis

When analyzing and deriving the patient's problem list, nurses need to focus on nursing problems that nurses can legally diagnose and treat. For example, nurses cannot diagnose or prescribe treatment for the medical problem of diabetes; however, various problems emerge from this disease that nurses can diagnose and independently manage, such as anxiety, potential for infection, knowledge deficit, noncompliance, and disturbance in self-concept.

The diagnostic categories accepted by the North American Nursing Diagnosis Association are listed in Chapter 1; these can serve as guidelines as data are analyzed for nursing problems.

Ideally, a nursing diagnosis statement consists of two parts: the nursing diagnosis and the related cause or contributing factor. Examples include the following:

Anxiety related to reduced income

Fluid volume excess related to excessive sodium intake

Noncompliance related to cognitive impairments

Altered oral mucous membrane related to dehydration

Powerlessness related to nursing home admission

Disturbance in self-concept related to retirement

Sexual dysfunction related to reduced vaginal lubrication

Social isolation related to incontinence.

Obviously, a nursing diagnosis can be related to a variety of factors; thus, defining the specific causative or contributing factor helps to identify the specific interventions needed. For instance, interventions for a patient with sexual dysfunction would be different if the cause were a medication side-effect than if it were separation from one's partner. To assist the reader, each of the chapters on universal self-care demands (see Chaps. 8–15)

and those on pathologies of aging (see Chaps. 19–33) include a list of nursing diagnoses and potential causes or contributing factors; these can be consulted for specific nursing diagnoses.

Planning Care

Prioritization

Most older adults possess multiple problems. Because some of these problems require more immediate action than others and because human and material resources are limited, priorities must be set in planning care. Nurses must consider not only those problems requiring the most urgent attention but also the risks involved with placing a problem low on the priority list. For example, monitoring vital signs and administering medications are important to the patient who has experienced a myocardial infarction, but not addressing the potential for skin breakdown can be detrimental.

Active Participation of Patient

If possible, patients and significant others should participate actively in the development of the care plan so that interventions are understood and conflicts in priorities or approaches can be avoided. Consider the following example:

A visiting nurse was concerned about the housing situation of the 72-year-old woman for whom she was caring. The house was too large for the woman to clean adequately and consequently was dirty and cluttered. Leaking faucets, peeling wallpaper, and roaches added to the nurse's impression that it was necessary to seek new housing for the woman.

The nurse worked diligently with the local housing authorities and social service agencies to locate an affordable apartment in a modern high-rise apartment building. She felt positive about her efforts to arrange improved housing that would maintain the independence of the elderly woman in a safe community setting.

With excitement, the nurse shared her accomplishment with the woman, anticipating that the woman would be delighted at the prospect of improved housing. The nurse was shocked at the woman's anger and refusal to relocate. Didn't this woman understand? Was she confused? How could she deny an opportunity to leave her shabby old house and move into a modern apartment?

If the participation of the elderly woman had been elicited initially in establishing plans for her housing problem, perhaps the nurse could have saved herself and others much time and energy and delivered more efficient, effective care. To this 72-year-old woman, maintaining the family house in which she had spent most of her lifetime was of utmost importance. The familiar furnishings, the memories, the yard in which her dog could romp and she could garden, and her friendly neighbor of many years were all part of that old house. Of course, she did not like the dirt, disrepair, and roaches either, but they were worth the price of maintaining her own home. If the nurse had explored these factors and jointly established priorities with the patient, perhaps other acceptable solutions could have been found, such as arranging a homemaker's service, obtaining a community handyman to make repairs, or sharing with someone who could assist with household responsibilities. Nurses must be careful not to develop ideal plans that will not be supported by the patient; a compromise plan that works is much more effective.

Multidisciplinary Collaboration

It is wise to enlist the cooperation of other professionals who will be involved in the patient's care, such as the physician, social worker, nutritionist, and paraprofessionals. A multidisciplinary approach is beneficial to addressing the many interwoven problems that older adults frequently possess. Without such coordination, various caregivers might work toward different and sometimes conflicting goals, which is a waste of time, energy, and resources. The most effective and efficient care is achieved through multidisciplinary interdependence, cooperation, and respect.

Prevention Considerations

Nurses should consider not only the care or management of existing problems but also the prevention of problems. A basic approach to this is a review of each of the universal self-care requirements, using data from the nursing assess-

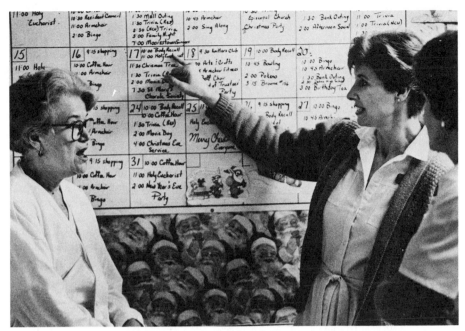

Care planning is a multidisciplinary process. (Photography by Eric Schenk.)

ment. For example, from the assessment it may be learned that the patient has occasional periods of depression that can lead to eating problems. Although no current nutritional problem exists, planning could include arranging for the patient to attend a senior citizen lunch program to provide an opportunity for socialization and food intake in an effort to prevent poor eating habits from developing. Likewise, an older person's skin may be in fine condition when the person is admitted to the hospital and placed on complete bed rest. To maintain skin integrity, the nurse would plan to turn the patient frequently, offer massages, and use bath oil when bathing the patient.

Specific Direction

In addition to knowing precisely what actions are intended, staff can more objectively and accurately evaluate the effectiveness of nursing plans when they are specific. For example, if the nursing care plan stated "reduce fluid at bedtime," one caregiver could interpret this as meaning only 100 ml after 9 P.M., another could interpret it as 500 ml after dinner, and the third could allow no fluids after midnight. It would be difficult to evaluate the effective-

ness of reducing fluid intake to control nocturnal incontinence because the daily approach is inconsistent. On the other hand, with a nursing order of "reduce fluid intake to 300 ml between 8 P.M. and 6 A.M.," the nurse can judge the effectiveness of the particular plan and identify exactly the type of change needed to result in the desired outcome.

Developing Goals

Nursing actions are driven by nursing diagnoses and the patient's unique needs and desires as identified through the assessment process. To achieve optimal effectiveness, these actions must be consistent and work toward a specific outcome. The formation of goals provides general direction to care and a realistic understanding of the outcome of care activities.

A goal is an objective or desired outcome that specifically describes what the patient will achieve through care activities.(Eliopoulos, 1990) For example, for the diagnosis "Impaired physical mobility related to amputation" could lead to the need for the patient to learn to ambulate with a prosthetic device. The goal is not to instruct the patient in the use of the prosthesis—that is an action re-

lated to the goal—but rather, that the patient ambulates independently a distance of at least 20 feet three times daily within the next month.

Another characteristic of a goal is that it be measurable. If the goal example in the previous paragraph is phrased "the patient will ambulate," the success of the patient in meeting the goal could be evaluated differently by various nurses. One nurse may believe the goal has been met because the patient ambulates 10 feet daily with the assistance of one staff member; another nurse may judge that the patient has not achieved the goal although he walks approximately 40 feet four times daily independently. By describing the exact conditions by which the goal is achieved and the target date, no individual interpretation is imposed and all staff can evaluate the patient's progress accurately.

Goals can reflect a variety of aims, including the following:

Maintenance: to stabilize blood glucose within normal range
Improvement: to heal pressure ulcer
Prevention: to be free from skin breakdown
Palliation: to control arthritic pain.

Both short- and long-term goals provide insight into the direction of care activities. A long-term goal gives a general statement of major anticipated outcomes, such as the following:

The patient will return to community living in 6 months.
The patient will resolve grief by the end of the year.
The patient will verbalize acceptance of her new housing situation within the next 3 months.

Short-term goals describe the small steps along the way to achieving larger outcomes, such as the following:

The patient will learn to use assistive devices for cooking within the next 2 weeks.
The patient will attend at least one meeting of the widowhood support group within the next month.
The patient will meet at least one neighbor in her new housing development within the next 2 weeks.

Similar to planning for a trip, a long-term goal gives the ultimate destination of care, whereas the short-term goals describe the landmarks during the process of getting to the endpoint.

As with all components of the care plan, goals should be developed in collaboration with the patient, and as appropriate, significant others. By understanding and agreeing to goals, compliance can be promoted, and the patient can understand the rationale for and outcomes of care activities.

Implementing Actions

Implementation is the phase of the nursing process in which care planning is made operational. A proficient blend of intellectual, interpersonal, and technical skill is necessary for care implementation. As stated earlier in the book, nursing actions fall within the spheres of the following:

Strengthen the patient's self-care capacity.
Eliminate or minimize self-care limitations.
Provide direct care services by acting for, doing for, or partially assisting the patient when universal or illness-imposed demands cannot be fulfilled independently.

Frequently, nursing actions must be delegated to family caregivers or other nursing personnel; nurses must still ensure that care is provided appropriately and safely.

It is a nursing responsibility to recognize when changes in the patient's capacities and limitations require a different level of care. Perhaps the patient has recovered from an illness and has restored energy; a nursing assistant may no longer be required to bathe the patient as the patient may now be able to perform this act independently. On the other hand, if the patient becomes more limited in the ability to self-inject insulin because of arthritic fingers, a visiting nurse may have to administer the insulin to compensate for this deficit. Both the need for different care actions and different care providers must be considered.

With all care activities, it must be remembered that older patients may require more nursing time than younger patients because of slower responses and the multitude of problems that often exist. Rather than trying to rush through care or frustrating themselves and their patients, nurses should allocate more time for care activities with older patients. It is useful to keep this in mind when planning assignments and case loads.

Evaluating Care

An often overlooked although important step of the nursing process is evaluation, that is, a judgment of the degree to which plans and actions were effective in achieving desired outcomes. If plans and actions continue to be effective and no change in status exists, no change is necessary. However, some actions may have been ineffective in achieving desired results, and specific alterations of the care plan may be required. Oversights and omissions may be detected, and additions may have to be made to the care plan. Thus, the evaluation process can result in no change, an alteration of the original plan, or the addition of new plans.

The individual for whom care is being provided, the patient's family, and all caregivers should be included in the evaluation process. It may be learned that although the action is bringing the desired result, the action itself is not satisfactory to the patient or caregivers; perhaps a different action that achieves the same result is necessary. For example, a goal of increasing socialization opportunities for an elderly widow who lives alone may have been established, and specific plans may have included daily attendance at the senior citizen center. If the woman has attended daily and developed friendships, the nurse could evaluate this action as effective in reaching the desired outcome. However, if the widow feels that visiting the center fatigues her to the extent she is unable to perform her household responsibilities and is requiring that she use part of her food budget for transportation costs, different plans to achieve the same goal may be warranted. The nurse can alter the plan to provide a different means of transportation, to arrange for visits to the center every other day with friendly visitors to her home in between, and to obtain assistance for household chores. It cannot be assumed that a desired outcome has been achieved in the most preferable, beneficial, and effective manner.

Through evaluation, it is learned whether or not accurate, effective, and efficient planning and actions have occurred. Nursing audits are becoming increasingly common as a means to evaluate nursing care in a more formal manner. When problems or needs to alter care are determined, revised care plans and actions should follow. Ideally, nursing care is a dynamic process through the cycle of assessing → diagnosing → planning → implementing → evaluating → reassessing → diagnosing → and so forth.

Reference

Eliopoulos C. Effective care plans. Long-Term Care Educator 1990;1(6):2.

Recommended Readings

Burggraf V, Mickey S. Nursing and the elderly: a care plan approach. Philadelphia: JB Lippincott, 1989.

Eliopoulos C. Nursing care planning guides for long-term care. Baltimore: Williams & Wilkins, 1990.

Maas M, Buckwalter K, Hardy M. Nursing diagnoses and new interventions for the elderly. Redwood City, CA: Addison Wesley, 1991.

Naylor MD. Comprehensive discharge planning for hospitalized elderly: a pilot study. Nurs Res 1990;39:156.

Wilson EB, Clancy C, Deeves ME, Schmitt A. Take a fresh look at discharge planning. Geriatr Nurs 1991;12(1):23.

unit III

Pathologies of Aging

19

Cardiovascular Problems

Improved technology for early diagnosis and treatment and increased public awareness of the importance of proper nutrition, exercise, and smoking cessation have resulted in a decline in heart disease in the population as a whole. Future generations will experience fewer deaths and disabilities associated with cardiovascular diseases. Unfortunately, today's older population carries the insults of many years of inadequate preventive, diagnostic, and treatment practices and faces cardiovascular problems as the major cause of disability and death.

Aging and the Cardiovascular System

Significant anatomical changes to the heart do not normally occur with age. The heart size remains unchanged unless factors such as inactivity or obesity exist. Increased amounts of lipofuscin granules and subpericardial fat accumulate in the heart. The heart muscle possesses increased collagen and scarring and is less elastic. The valves get thick and rigid, secondary to fibrosis and sclerosis, particularly in the mitral valve and the base or aortic cusps. The aorta and arteries are less elastic, and the carotid artery may kink to the extent that it is mistaken for an aneurysm.

The heart manifests its reduced efficiency in a variety of ways. Heart contractions may be weaker and cardiac output reduced about 1% each year beginning at approximately 25 years of age. Maximum coronary blood flow at 60 years of age is estimated to be 35% less than that of younger persons. The lessened elasticity of the aorta and the presence of atrial atrophy produce problems in filling and emptying the heart. Oxygen use, the cardiac reserve, and the capacity for cardiac work are decreased. Systolic blood pressure rises to compensate for the inelasticity and increased resistance of peripheral vessels. Increased vasopressor lability may raise both systolic and diastolic blood pressure. Vasomotor tone decreases and vagal tone increases. The heart is more sensitive to carotid sinus stimulation and less sensitive to the effects of atropine.

Stress is managed less well by older hearts. The heart rate elevation to stress is not as high in the elderly as in younger persons; therefore, stroke volume may increase, which can elevate the blood pressure. An elevated heart rate in the elderly takes longer to return to normal.

The electrocardiogram of the older adult may reflect differences secondary to these aging changes. There may be a slight prolongation of the PR, QRS, and QT intervals, left axis deviation, and, possibly, decreased voltage of all waves.

Display 19-1 summarizes the various changes affecting the cardiovascular system with age.

Assessment

The early detection of cardiac problems can be difficult because of the atypical presentation of symptoms, the subtle nature of the progression of cardiac disease, and the ease with which cardiac symptoms can be mistakenly attributed to other

DISPLAY 19-1   Age-Related Changes to the Cardiovascular System

Thickening and rigidity of heart valves

Dilation and elongation of aorta

Reduced elasticity and narrower lumen of vessels

Greater prominence of vessels in head, neck, and extremities

Decreased efficiency and contractile strength of heart muscle

Reduced cardiac output

Reduced stroke volume

Prolongation of isometric contraction phase and relaxation time of left ventricle

Decreased efficiency of cardiovascular stress response

Increased vagal tone

Increased blood pressure

Decreased baroreceptor sensitivity; increased incidence of orthostatic hypotension

health conditions (*e.g.,* indigestion, arthritis). Careful questioning and observation can yield valuable insight into problems that have recently developed or escaped recognition.

General Observation

Assessment of the cardiovascular system can begin at the moment the nurse sees the patient by observing indicators of cardiovascular status. Such observations would note the following:

Generalized coloring: pallor can accompany cardiovascular disorders.

Energy level: fatigue and the amount of activity that can be tolerated should be noted.

Breathing pattern: respirations can be observed while the patient ambulates, changes position, and speaks. Acute dyspnea warrants prompt medical attention because it can be a symptom of myocardial infarction in older adults.

Condition of nails: inspection of the color, shape, thickness, curvature, and markings in nail beds can give insight into problems. Blanching should be checked; circulatory insufficiency can delay the nails' return to pink after blanching. Advanced cardiac disease can cause clubbing of the nails.

Status of vessels: the vessels on the extremities, head, and neck should be inspected. Varicosities should be noted, as well as redness on the skin above a vessel.

Hair on extremities: hair loss can accompany poor circulation.

Edema: swelling of the ankles and fingers is often indicative of cardiovascular disorders.

Mental status: inadequate cerebral circulation often manifests itself through confusion. Cognitive function and level of consciousness should be evaluated.

Interview

The interview should include a review of function, signs, and symptoms. Questions should be asked pertaining to the following:

Symptoms: inquiry should be made into the presence of dizziness, lightheadedness, edema, cold extremities, palpitations, blackouts, breathing difficulties, coughing, hemoptysis, chest pain or unusual sensations in chest, neck, back or jaws. It is helpful to use specific examples in questions: "Do you ever feel as though there is a vise pressing against your chest?" "Have you ever become sweaty and had trouble breathing while you felt that unusual sensation in your chest?" "Do you find that rings and shoes become tighter on you as the day goes on?" "Do you ever get the sensation of the room spinning when you rise from lying down?" When symptoms are reported, explore their frequency, duration, and management.

Family history of cardiac problems.

Changes in function: the patient can be asked if changes in physical or mental function have been noticed using questions such as: "Do you have difficulty or have you noticed any changes in your ability to walk, work, or take care of yourself?" "Do you ever have periods in which your thinking doesn't seem clear?" "Have you had to restrict activities or change your life-style recently?"

Physical Examination

There should be an inspection of the patient from head to toe, noting areas of irritation or redness over a vessel, distended vessels, edema, and pallor.

Blanching of the nail beds gives information about circulation. An examination of the extremities should include palpation of the pulses and temperature of the extremities and observation of hair distribution on the legs. Assessment of apical and radial pulses is done and should normally reveal a pulse that ranges between 60 and 100 beats per minute. Remember that older hearts take longer to recover from stress; thus, tachycardia may be detected as a result of a stress that occurred several hours earlier. If tachycardia is discovered in an elderly person, reassess in several hours. Blood pressure assessment in three positions is important to determine the presence of postural hypotension; positional drops greater than 20 mmHg are significant. Auscultation of the heart is done to detect thrills and bruits. Palpation of the point of maximal impulse can identify displacement, which can occur with problems such as left ventricular hypertrophy. Jugular venous pressure should be measured. Refer to Chapter 17 for specific guidance on assessment of the cardiovascular system.

Review of Selected Disorders

Congestive Heart Failure

The incidence of congestive heart failure increases with age and is particularly a potential complication in older patients with arteriosclerotic heart disease. The conditions that can precipitate congestive heart failure in older adults include coronary artery disease, hypertensive heart disease, cor pulmonale, mitral stenosis, subacute bacterial endocarditis, bronchitis, pneumonia, congenital heart disease, and myxedema. This problem is common in older adults because of age-related changes such as reduced elasticity and lumen size of vessels and rises in blood pressure that interfere with the blood supply to the heart muscle. The decreased cardiac reserves limit the heart's ability to withstand effects of disease or injury. Symptoms of this problem in older patients include confusion, insomnia, wandering during the night, agitation, depression, anorexia, nausea, weakness, dyspnea, shortness of breath, orthopnea, weight gain, and bilateral ankle edema. The detection of any of these symptoms should be promptly communicated to the physician.

The management of congestive heart failure in the elderly is basically the same as in middle-aged adults, commonly consisting of bed rest, digitalis, diuretics, and a reduction in sodium intake. The patient may be allowed to sit in a chair next to the bed; usually, complete bed rest is discouraged to avoid the potential development of thrombosis and pulmonary congestion. The patient should be assisted into the chair, be adequately supported, and, while sitting, observed for signs of fatigue, dyspnea, and changes in skin color and pulse.

The nurse should be aware that the presence of edema and the poor nutrition of the tissues associated with this disease, along with the more fragile skin of the aged, predisposes the patient to a greater risk of skin breakdown. Regular skin care and frequent changes of positioning are essential. It must be recognized that this is a frightening, and often recurring, condition requiring a great deal of reassurance and emotional support.

Pulmonary Heart Disease

Changes in the respiratory system associated with normal aging and certain disease processes in the elderly can reduce pulmonary function, contributing to pulmonary heart disease. Factors that reduce pulmonary function include decreased elasticity of the lungs, alveolar dilation, fibrosis, kyphosis, emphysema, chronic bronchitis, tuberculosis, and mitral valve disease. The forms of pulmonary heart disease discussed below, pulmonary emboli and cor pulmonale, primarily affect the older person.

Pulmonary Emboli

The incidence of pulmonary emboli is high in the elderly, but the detection and diagnosis of it in this age group are rare. Patients who are in particular danger when they develop this problem are those with a fractured hip, congestive heart failure, arrhythmias, and a history of thrombosis. Immobilization and malnourishment, frequent problems in the aged population, can contribute to pulmonary emboli. Symptoms that should be observed include confusion, apprehension, increasing dyspnea, slight temperature elevation, pneumonitis, and an elevated sedimentation rate. Older patients may not experience chest pain because of altered pain sensations, or their pain may be attributed to other existing problems. A lung scan or angiography may be done to confirm the diagnosis and establish the location, size, and extent of the prob-

lem. Treatment of pulmonary emboli in the elderly does not significantly differ from that used for the young.

Cor Pulmonale

Acute cor pulmonale is usually a result of a massive pulmonary embolus, respiratory infection, atrial fibrillation, or chronic failure. This is often a problem experienced by older hemiplegics. With the exception of the use of morphine or barbiturates, treatment is the same as for younger adults. Chronic cor pulmonale is primarily a result of emphysema. This disease can develop into acute cor pulmonale, and nursing measures should focus on preventing this occurrence. Treatment does not differ from that for the young, including antismoking education.

Coronary Artery Disease

Coronary artery disease is the popularly used phrase for ischemic heart disease. The prevalence of coronary artery disease increases with advanced age, so that some form of this disease exists in most persons 70 years of age or older.

Anginal Syndrome

A symptom of myocardial ischemia, the anginal syndrome presents in an atypical pattern, creating difficulty in detection. Pain may be diffuse and of a less severe nature than described by younger adults. The first indication of this problem may be a vague discomfort under the sternum, frequently following a large meal. The type of pain described and the relationship of the onset of pain to a meal may cause the patient, and the health professional, to attribute this discomfort to indigestion. As this condition progresses, the patient may experience precardial pain radiating down the left arm. The recurrence of anginal syndromes over many years can result in the formation of small areas of myocardial necrosis and fibrosis. Eventually, diffuse myocardial fibrosis occurs, leading to myocardial weakness and the potential risk of congestive heart failure.

Nitroglycerin has been effective in the prevention and treatment of anginal attacks. Because this drug may cause a drop in blood pressure, the patient should be cautioned to sit or lie down after taking the tablet to prevent fainting episodes and falls. To prevent swallowing the tablet and thus blocking its absorption, patients should be re-

minded not to swallow their saliva for several minutes after sublingual administration. Specific information on nitroglycerin is presented in Chapter 35. Long-acting nitrates are usually not prescribed for older adults. To prevent anginal syndromes, the patient should be taught and helped to avoid those factors that may aggravate this problem, such as cold wind, emotional stress, strenuous activity, anemia, tachycardia, arrhythmias, and hyperthyroidism. Because the pain associated with a myocardial infarction may be similar to that of angina, patients should be instructed to notify the physician or nurse if pain is not relieved by nitroglycerin. Patients' charts should include factors that precipitate attacks, as well as the nature of the pain and its description by the patient, the method of management, and the usual number of nitroglycerin tablets used to alleviate the attack.

Myocardial Infarction

Myocardial infarction is frequently seen in older persons, especially in men with a history of hypertension and arteriosclerosis. Myocardial infarction diagnosis can be delayed or missed in the aged because of an atypical set of symptoms and the frequent absence of pain. Symptoms include pain radiating to the left arm, the entire chest, the neck, and abdomen; moist, pale skin; decreased blood pressure; low-grade fever; and an elevated sedimentation rate. Output should be observed because partial or complete anuria may develop as this problem continues. Arrhythmias may occur, progressing to fibrillation and death, if untreated. Cardiac rupture may also occur, especially in older women.

The trend in treating myocardial infarction has been to reduce the amount of time in which the patient is limited to bed rest and to replace complete bed rest with allowing the patient to sit in an armchair next to the bed. The patient should be assisted into the chair with minimal exertion by the patient. Arms should be supported to avoid strain on the heart. Not only does this armchair treatment help to prevent many of the complications associated with immobility, but also it prevents pooling of the blood in the pulmonary vessels, thereby decreasing the work of the heart.

Because older persons are more susceptible to cerebral and intestinal bleeding, close nursing observation for signs of bleeding is essential if anticoagulants are used in the patient's treatment.

Nurses should be alert to signs of developing pulmonary edema and congestive heart failure, potential complications for the geriatric patient with a myocardial infarction. These and other observations, such as persistent dyspnea, cyanosis, decreasing blood pressure, rising temperature, and arrhythmias, reflect a problem in the patient's recovery and should be brought to the physician's attention promptly.

Acute Coronary Insufficiency

Arterial narrowing and myocardial damage and increased cardiac stress can result in acute coronary insufficiency. Symptoms of this problem that the nurse can recognize include a low-grade fever and prolonged chest pain. Treatment includes the use of oxygen and analgesics as well as rest. Areas of necrosis can develop after repeated episodes of this problem, leading to diffuse fibrosis.

Hypertension

The incidence of hypertension increases with advancing age and is a problem the gerontological nurse commonly encounters. Many aged people have high blood pressure arising from the vasoconstriction associated with aging, which produces peripheral resistance. Hyperthyroidism, parkinsonism, Paget disease, anemia, and a thiamine deficiency can also be responsible for hypertension. Usually, if the older person's blood pressure is equal to or greater than 200 mmHg systolic and 100 mmHg diastolic and if the person is symptomatic, treatment is initiated. The nurse should carefully assess the patient's blood pressure by checking it several times with the person in standing, sitting, and prone positions. Anxiety, stress, or activity before the blood pressure check should be noted, because these factors may be responsible for a temporary elevation. The anxiety of being examined by a physician or of preparing for and experiencing a visit to a clinic frequently causes elevated blood pressure in a usually normotensive individual.

Awakening with a dull headache, impaired memory, disorientation, confusion, epistaxis, and a slow tremor may be symptoms of hypertension. The presence of these symptoms with an elevated blood pressure reading usually warrants treatment. Hypertensive older patients are advised to rest, reduce their sodium intake, and, if necessary, reduce their weight. Aggressive antihypertensive therapy is discouraged for older persons because of the risk of a sudden dangerous decrease in blood pressure. Nurses should observe for signs indicating blood pressure that is too low to meet the patient's demands, such as dizziness, confusion, syncope, restlessness, and drowsiness. An elevated blood urea nitrogen level may be present also. These signs should be observed for and communicated to the physician if they appear. In the management of the older hypertensive person, it is a challenge to achieve a blood pressure level high enough to provide optimum circulation yet low enough to prevent serious related complications.

Arrhythmias

Digitalis toxicity, hypokalemia, acute infections, hemorrhage, anginal syndrome, and coronary insufficiency are some of the many factors that cause an increasing incidence of arrhythmias with age. Of the causes mentioned, digitalis toxicity is the most common.

The basic principles of treatment of arrhythmias do not vary much for older adults. Tranquilizers, digitalis, and potassium supplements are part of the therapy prescribed. Patient education may be warranted to help the individual modify diet, smoking, drinking, and activity patterns. The nurse should be aware that digitalis toxicity can progress in the absence of clinical signs and that the effects can be evident even 2 weeks after the drug has been discontinued. The aged have a higher mortality rate from cardiac arrest than other segments of the population, which emphasizes the necessity for close nursing observations and early problem detection to prevent this serious complication.

Tachycardia

Tachycardia is one form of conduction disturbance seen in older persons. The most common types are paroxysmal atrial tachycardia and ventricular tachycardia. With the exception of acute myocardial infarction, ventricular tachycardia—a serious problem for both the young and the old—does not occur frequently. However, ventricular tachycardia has been noted at the time of a person's death and for minutes following clinical death. Decreased blood pressure, impaired cerebral circulation, and congestive heart failure may develop if tachycardia is not corrected.

Premature Contractions

Atrial and ventricular premature contractions are cardiac arrhythmias experienced by the aged. Premature contractions can be caused by gastrointestinal disturbances, stress, and agents such as coffee, tea, alcohol, and tobacco. If not corrected, this problem can lead to a serious ventricular arrhythmia.

Atrial Fibrillation

As a result of severe cardiovascular disease, hyperthyroidism, high fevers, digitalis intoxication, and pulmonary emboli, atrial fibrillation can occur. If prolonged, it encourages the development of an atrial thrombus; thus, prompt treatment is important. The patient should be observed for signs of a possible embolus. Dyspnea and chest pain may indicate a pulmonary embolus; an embolus lodged in the mesenteric arteries will cause abdominal pain. Discolored urine may result from a renal embolus, and changes in cerebral function may indicate an embolus in the brain.

Some research has indicated that atrial fibrillation makes it hard to identify the onset and disappearance of Korotkoff sounds (*i.e.*, the arterial vibrations heard during auscultation). This may account for the distortion of blood pressure assessment in persons with this condition. Repeated assessments can compensate for this distortion.(Sykes et al, 1990)

Heart Block

Arteriosclerosis, digitalis overdose, quinidine, certain poisons, and changes in the heart structure can cause heart block. Older persons experiencing heart block have a greater risk of suffering cardiac standstill and Stokes–Adams attack, whereby unconsciousness and possible seizures occur as a result of hypoxia from interrupted cerebral circulation.

Bacterial Endocarditis

Subacute Bacterial Endocarditis

This may be a potential complication experienced by aged patients with staphylococcal, fungal, and other infections and those with collagen disorders, diabetes, and a history of recent surgery; patients who have been receiving steroids, cancer chemotherapy, and antibiotics for a long time also may develop this condition. Diagnosis can be compli-

cated in the elderly because of nonspecific symptoms such as anorexia, fatigue, weight loss, anemia, confusion, weakness, pallor, tachycardia, and an elevated sedimentation rate. The difficulty in relating these symptoms to subacute bacterial endocarditis in the aged contributes to the high mortality rate associated with this problem. As this disease progresses, atrial fibrillation and heart failure may occur. The treatment for this problem in the elderly is similar to that for younger persons.

Acute Bacterial Endocarditis

This occurs in older adults to a significantly lesser degree than the subacute form, but with similar difficulty in diagnosis because its symptoms are much like those of many other geriatric problems.

Rheumatic Heart Disease

Rheumatic heart disease may occur in aged people who either have had rheumatic fever earlier in life or have had acute episodes during old age. Older individuals who have rheumatic fever suffer moderate joint discomfort, sudden soreness and diffuse redness of the throat, enlarged lymph nodes, and temperature elevation. Any joint lesions are more disabling to the elderly than to the young. It is not unusual for repeated episodes to occur, and the nurse needs to be alert to symptoms in patients with a history of this disease. With proper therapy, the prognosis for an older person with acute rheumatic fever is favorable, and rheumatic heart disease, which is of higher incidence in elderly women, can be prevented. Residual valvular deformities from acute rheumatic fever progress differently in each individual. Usually, the mitral and aortic valves are most affected. Some persons have minimal limitations because of adequate compensation by the myocardium; some develop murmurs, hypertension, atrial fibrillation, and congestive heart failure. Aggressive therapy for the disease itself usually is not warranted, and the emphasis is on managing the symptoms and any complications that develop.

Syphilitic Heart Disease

Ten percent of the heart disease in persons aged 50 years or older is a result of syphilis. Aged persons with syphilitic heart disease may have contracted the disease at a time when a definite stigma was attached to venereal diseases and open dis-

cussion and education regarding these diseases were nonexistent or minimal. The individual may have been fearful, felt guilty, or may not have noticed or been aware of the significance of the associated symptoms and therefore may not have sought treatment. Treatment before the 1940s, when penicillin was developed, may not have eliminated the disease. Older persons who have had recent exposure to syphilis may be reluctant to seek treatment because they are concerned about what others might think of sexual activity in old age.

The first sign of syphilitic heart disease may occur years after the initial infection. The valvular defect most frequently associated with this disease is aortic insufficiency, whereby a leak in the aortic valve during diastole causes blood to be forced back into the left ventricle. The systolic blood pressure is increased, the diastolic blood pressure is reduced, and the pulse pressure is significantly greater than normal. When the heart is no longer able to compensate for these changes, cardiac failure can occur. The most effective treatment may be the replacement of the damaged valve with a ball-valve prosthesis, a procedure viewed with increasing optimism for the aged.

Congenital Heart Disease

Because of the limited medical and surgical correctives for congenital defects available when today's aged population was young, people born with serious heart problems most likely did not survive to adulthood. Thus, congenital heart disease is not common among the elderly and is sometimes unrecognized as such. It is believed that some of the arrhythmias, murmurs, and other cardiac diseases found in the geriatric patient are caused by congenital lesions.

Atrial and Ventricular Septal Defects

These are the most common congenital heart defects discovered in the aged. Symptoms of atrial septal defect are similar for all ages, except that older people may have a higher pulse rate, increased blood pressure, dyspnea, recurrent bronchopneumonia, and a greater incidence of coronary artery disease. Most patients with ventricular septal defects are asymptomatic, although they may experience fatigue and episodes of heart failure. Surgery is sometimes effective in improving both of these defects in older persons.

General Nursing Interventions Related to Cardiovascular Problems

Facilitating Cardiovascular Health

The prevention of cardiovascular problems in all age groups is an important goal for all nurses to consider. By teaching the young and old to identify and lower risk factors related to cardiovascular disease, nurses promote optimum health and function. Important practices to reinforce include the following:

Proper nutrition. A diet that provides all daily requirements, maintains weight within an ideal range for height and age, and controls cholesterol intake is beneficial.

Adequate exercise. Automobiles, elevators, modern appliances, and less physically exerting jobs lead to a more sedentary life-style than may be optimally healthy. Related to this may be the practice of being physically inactive during the week and then filling weekends with housecleaning, yard work, and sports activities. A sensible distribution of exercise throughout the week is advisable and is more beneficial to cardiovascular function than periodic spurts of activity. Persons who dislike scheduled exercise programs should be encouraged to maximize opportunities for exercise during their routine activities (e.g., using stairs instead of an elevator, parking their car on the far end of the lot, or walking to the corner to buy a newspaper instead of having it delivered).

Avoiding cigarette smoking. Nearly everyone is aware of the ill effects of smoking. The difficulty is breaking the habit and, for this, people need more than to be told to stop. They need considerable support and assistance, which are often obtainable through smoking cessation programs. Even if the patient has had repeated failures in attempting to quit, the next try could be successful and should be encouraged. In addition to avoiding cigarette smoking themselves, people should be instructed to limit their exposure to the cigarette smoke produced by others, which also can be detrimental.

Managing stress. Stress is a normal part of all our lives. People should be taught to identify the stressors in their lives, their unique reactions to stress, and how they can more effectively manage stress. Relaxation exer-

Table 19-1 *Nursing Diagnoses Related to Cardiovascular Problems*

NURSING DIAGNOSIS	CAUSES OR CONTRIBUTING FACTORS
Activity intolerance	Insufficient oxygen transport, poor circulation, electrolyte imbalance, bedrest, pain, fatigue, effects of medications, fear of harming self
Anxiety	Change in self-concept, fear of unknown procedures or diagnosis, hospitalization
Constipation	Bedrest, medications, diet, stress, inactivity, insufficient fluids, pain, hospital environment
Altered cardiac output: decreased	Bradycardia, tachycardia, congestive heart failure, myocardial infarction, hypertension, cor pulmonale, stress, medications
Pain	Vasospasm, occlusion, phlebitis, spasms, diagnostic tests, surgery, poor positioning, exertion
Ineffective individual coping	Hospitalization, altered self-concept, helplessness
Ineffective family coping	Separation of patient from family, lack of knowledge
Diversional activity deficit	Hospitalization, forfeiture of activities, fear of impact
Altered family processes	Patient's illness; financial, physical, and psychological burdens of illness; hospitalization; role changes
Fear	Change in function, disability, procedures, pain, lack of knowledge
Fluid volume deficit	Ascites, hypovolemia, anorexia
Fluid volume excess	Decreased cardiac output, excess fluid intake, dependent venous pooling/stasis
Grieving	Change in body function or life style, pain
Altered health maintenance	Lack of knowledge, loss of independence
Impaired home maintenance management	Disability, pain, fatigue
High risk for infection	Impaired oxygen transport, invasive procedures, medications, immobility
High risk for injury	Poor circulation, fatigue, immobility, pain, medications
Knowledge deficit	Unfamiliar diagnostic tests, diagnosis, treatments, diet, ineffective coping, denial
Impaired physical mobility	Pain, fatigue, bedrest, edema, medications
Noncompliance	Lack of knowledge or skill, prescribed plan in conflict with beliefs and practices, insufficient funds
Altered nutrition; less than body requirements	Anorexia, depression, stress, medications, nonacceptance of prescribed diet, anxiety
Powerlessness	Inability to participate in usual activities, lack of knowledge, hospitalization
Self-care deficit	Immobility, pain, edema, fatigue
Disturbance in self-concept	Change in body function, new diagnosis, hospitalization, immobility, pain
Sensory–perceptual alterations	Metabolic changes, impaired oxygen transport, medications, immobility, pain, stress, hospital environment

Table 19-1 Nursing Diagnoses Related to Cardiovascular Problems (Continued)

NURSING DIAGNOSIS	CAUSES OR CONTRIBUTING FACTORS
Sexual dysfunction	Pain, fatigue, fear, anxiety, depression, medications, hospitalization, lack of knowledge
Impaired skin integrity	Edema, immobility, impaired oxygen transport
Sleep pattern disturbance	Impaired oxygen transport, immobility, hospitalization, pain, anxiety, inactivity, medications, depression
Altered thought processes	Metabolic or electrolyte imbalances, medications, anxiety, depression
Altered tissue perfusion	Decreased cardiac output, myocardial infarction, angina, congestive heart failure, hypertension, vasoconstriction, hypotension, immobility, medications
Altered patterns of urinary elimination	Diuretics, bed rest, hospital environment, anxiety

cises, yoga, meditation, and a variety of other stress-reducing activities can prove beneficial to nearly all persons.

Gerontological nurses understand that it is much easier and more useful to establish good health practices early in life than to change them or deal with their outcomes in old age.

Care Planning

Actual or potential problems can be discovered during the assessment of the cardiovascular system. Assessment data should be reviewed for those problems that fall within the realm of nursing to diagnose and manage, and related nursing diagnoses developed accordingly. Table 19-1 lists some of the major nursing diagnoses related to cardiovascular disorders.

The development of realistic goals guides care and provides a yardstick by which the patient's progress can be measured. Although the goals developed for individual patients will be specific to their unique needs, some potential goals in the care of cardiovascular problems for older patients are listed in the Sample Care Plan. Patients and their significant others should be active participants in the development of goals and establish-

ment of priorities. See Chapter 18 for more information on planning and providing care.

Keeping the Patient Informed

Basic diagnostic and treatment measures for cardiovascular problems of the elderly will not differ greatly from those used with younger patients, and the same nursing measures can be applied. Because of sensory deficits, anxiety, poor memory, or illness, the older patient may not fully comprehend or remember the explanations given for diagnostic and treatment measures. Full explanations with reinforcement are essential. Patients and their families should have the opportunity to ask questions and to discuss their concerns openly. Often procedures that seem relatively minor to the nurse, such as frequent checks of vital signs, may be alarming to the unprepared patient and family.

Preventing Complications

The edema associated with many cardiovascular diseases may promote skin breakdown, especially in older people who typically have more fragile skin. Frequent changes of position are essential. The body should be supported in proper alignment, and dangling arms and legs off the side of a

bed or chair should be avoided. A frequent check of clothing and protective devices can aid in detecting constriction due to increased edema. Protection, padding, and massage of pressure points are beneficial. If the patient is to be on a stretcher, an examining table, or an operating room table for a long time, protective padding can be placed on pressure points beforehand to provide comfort and prevent skin breakdown. When much edema is present, excessive activity should be avoided because it will increase the circulation of the fluid, with the toxic wastes it contains, and can subject the patient to profound intoxication. Weight and circumferences of extremities and the abdomen should be monitored to provide quantitative data regarding changes in the edematous state.

Accurate observation and documentation of fluid balance are especially important. Within any prescribed fluid restrictions, fluid intake should be encouraged to prevent dehydration and facilitate diuresis—water is effective for this. Fluid loss through any means should be measured; volume, color, odor, and specific gravity of urine should be noted. Intravenous fluids must be monitored carefully, particularly because excessive fluid infusion results in hypervolemia and can subject the elderly to the risk of congestive heart failure. Intravenous administration of glucose solution could stimulate the increased production of insulin, resulting in a hypoglycemic reaction if this solution is abruptly discontinued without an adequate substitute.

Vital signs must be checked regularly, with close attention to changes. A temperature elevation can reflect an infection or a myocardial infarction. The body temperature for the elderly may be normally lower than for younger adults; it is important to record the patient's normal temperature when well to have a baseline for comparison. It is advisable to detect and correct temperature elevations promptly, because a temperature elevation increases metabolism, thereby increasing the body's requirements for oxygen, and causes the heart to work harder. A decrease in temperature slows metabolism, causing less oxygen consumption and less carbon dioxide production and fewer respirations. A rise in blood pressure is associated with a reduced cardiac output, vasodilation, and lower blood volume. Hypotension can result in insufficient circulation to meet the body's needs; symptoms of confusion and dizziness could indicate insufficient cerebral circulation resulting from a reduced blood pressure. Pulse changes are significant. In addition to cardiac problems, tachycardia could indicate hypoxia caused by an obstructed airway. Bradycardia may be associated with digitalis toxicity.

Oxygen is frequently administered in the treatment of cardiovascular diseases, and in elderly patients it requires most careful use. The patient should be observed closely for hypoxia. Patients using a nasal catheter may breathe primarily by mouth and reduce oxygen intake. Although a face mask may remedy this problem, it does not guarantee sufficient oxygen inspiration. Older patients may not demonstrate cyanosis as the initial sign of hypoxia; instead, they may be restless, irritable, and dyspneic. These signs also can indicate high oxygen concentrations and consequent carbon dioxide narcosis, a particular risk to elderly patients receiving oxygen therapy. Although blood gas levels will provide data to reveal these problems, early correction is facilitated by keen nursing observation.

Anorexia may accompany cardiovascular disease, and special nursing assistance may be necessary to help patients meet their nutritional needs. Several smaller meals throughout the entire day rather than a few large ones may compensate for poor appetite and reduce the work of the heart. Favorite foods, served attractively, can be effective. Patients should be encouraged to maintain a regular intake of glucose, the primary source of cardiac energy. Education may be necessary regarding low-sodium, low-cholesterol, and low-calorie diets. Therapeutic dietary modifications should attempt to incorporate ethnic food enjoyed by patients; patients may reject a prescribed special diet if they believe they must forfeit the foods that have been an important component of their lives for decades. It may be necessary to negotiate compromises; a realistic, although imperfect, diet with which patients are satisfied is more likely to be followed than an ideal one that patients cannot accept. The foods included in the diets should be reviewed, and patients should be informed of the sodium, cholesterol, and caloric contents of these items. These foods can then be categorized as those that should be eaten "never," "only on special occasions," "occasionally or not more than once monthly," and "as desired." Patients should be taught to read labels of food, beverages, and drugs for sodium content; they must understand that

carbonated drinks, certain analgesic preparations, commercial alkalizers, and homemade baking soda mixtures contain sodium.

Straining from constipation, enemas, and removal of fecal impactions can cause vagal stimulation, a particularly dangerous situation for patients with cardiovascular disease. Measures to prevent constipation must be an integral part of the care plan for these patients; a stool softener may be prescribed. If bed rest is prescribed, range-of-motion exercises should be performed, because they will cause muscle contractions that compress peripheral veins and thereby facilitate the return of venous blood.

Patients who are weak or who fall asleep while sitting need to have their heads and necks supported to prevent hyperextension or hyperflexion of the neck. All elderly persons, not only those with cardiovascular disease, can suffer a reduction in cerebral blood flow from the compression of vessels during this hyperextension or hyperflexion. Those with congestive heart failure need good positioning and support. A semirecumbent position with pillows supporting the entire back maintains good body alignment, promotes comfort, and assists in reducing pulmonary congestion. Cardiac strain is reduced by supporting the arms with pillows or armrests. Footboards help prevent footdrop contracture; patients should be instructed in how to use them for exercising.

If hepatic congestion develops, drugs may detoxify more slowly. Because the elderly may already have a slower rate of drug detoxification, nurses must be acutely aware of signs indicating adverse reactions to drugs. Digitalis toxicity particularly should be monitored and could present with a change in mental status, nausea, vomiting, arrhythmias, and a slow pulse. Because hypokalemia sensitizes the heart to the effects of digitalis, prevention through proper diet and the possible use of potassium supplements is advisable. Chapter 35 reviews some of the drug groups that may be used in the treatment of cardiovascular disorders.

Promoting Normality

An often unasked question of elderly patients relates to the impact of their cardiovascular condition on sexual activity. They may be reluctant to inquire because they fear being ridiculed or causing shock that "someone their age would still be interested in sex." They may resign themselves to forfeiting sexual activity under the misconception that they will further harm their hearts. Nurses should encourage discussion of this subject and introduce the topic if patients seem unable to do so themselves. Realistic explanations should be provided, including when sex can be resumed, how medications can affect sexual function, how to schedule medications for beneficial impact during sexual activity, and sexual positions that produce the least cardiac strain.

Relaxation and rest are both important in the treatment of cardiovascular disease, and it is wise to remember that a patient who is at rest is not necessarily relaxed. The stresses from hospitalization, pain, ignorance, and fear regarding disability; alterations in life-style; and potential death can

---

Sample Care Plan Goals for the Patient With a Cardiovascular Problem

To have cause of cardiac symptoms and signs diagnosed

To verbalize an understanding of the cardiovascular problem and its management

To tolerate increased activity without symptoms of cardiac distress

To maintain vital signs within predetermined range

To be free from arrhythmias or to have arrhythmias controlled

To demonstrate knowledge of and compliance with prescribed dietary restrictions

To be free from edema

To possess fluid and electrolyte balance

To describe the purpose, administration, side-effects, adverse reactions, interactions, and special precautions associated with prescribed cardiovascular medications

To correctly self-administer cardiovascular medications

To participate in a regular exercise program as prescribed

To demonstrate positive measures to manage stress

To describe signs and symptoms that indicate changes in cardiovascular status

Resources to Assist Patients With Cardiovascular Problems

The following organizations provide educational materials on cardiovascular health and specific cardiovascular diseases:

American Heart Association
7320 Greenville Ave.
Dallas, TX 75231
(214)750-5551

High Blood Pressure Information Center
120/80 National Institutes of Health
Bethesda, MD 20205
(301)496-1809

National Heart, Lung, and Blood Institute
Office of Information
Bethesda, MD 20205

The following organizations provide support services through local chapters:

International Association of Pacemaker Patients
P.O. Box 54305
Atlanta, GA 30308
(800)241-6993

Mended Hearts (heart surgery patients)
7320 Greenville Ave.
Dallas, TX 75231
(214)750-5442

cause the patient to become anxious, confused, and irrational. Reassurance and support are needed, including full explanations of diagnostic tests, hospital or institutional routines, and other activities. Opportunities for patients and their families to discuss questions, concerns, and fears must be provided. Realistic explanations of any required restrictions and life-style changes should emphasize that patients need not become "cardiac cripples" just because they have a cardiac disease. Most patients can live a normal life and need to be reassured of this. Refer to the Resource List for names of organizations with resources to help patients live with cardiovascular disorders.

Reference

Sykes D, et al. Measuring blood pressure in the elderly: does atrial fibrillation increase observer variability? Br Med J 1990;300:162.

Recommended Readings

Gantz NM. Geriatric endocarditis: avoiding the trend toward mismanagement. Geriatrics 1991;46(4):66.

Horowitz LN, Lynch RA. Managing geriatric arrhythmias. Geriatrics 1991;46(3):31.

Leibovitch ER. Congestive heart failure: a current overview. Geriatrics 1991;46(1):43.

Miller M, Gottleib SO. Preventive maintenance of the aging heart. Geriatrics 1991;46(7):22.

Moser M. Physical changes in the elderly: are they clinically important in the management of hypertension? Geriatrics 1989;44(10):4.

Rosenthal J. Aging and cardiovascular system. Gerontology 1987;33 (suppl 1):3.

Schron EB, Friedman LM. Cardiovascular options for the 1990s. Geriatr Nurs 1990;11(4):187.

Souter S. After the bypass. Geriatr Nurs 1990;11(6):271.

Taylor JL. Overcoming barriers to blood pressure control in the elderly. Geriatrics 1990;45(2):35.

20

Peripheral Vascular Disease

Complaints of leg pain and poor circulation among the elderly, as well as the greater prominence of tortuous vessels, make it obvious that peripheral vascular problems increase with advancing years. These problems can significantly impair mobility and function and lead to life-threatening complications. Effective recognition and management of these problems are important.

Aging and the Vessels

With age, greater amounts of calcium, cholesterol, and other lipids are found in arteries, and increased amounts of connective tissue and mucopolysaccharides are present in the intima. A loss of elasticity causes the vessels to dilate and elongate, and the tortuous nature of the vessels can be detected by the naked eye. Valves become less efficient. Vessels occlude and rupture more frequently in old age, resulting in compromised circulation to the tissues dependent on those vessels. Display 20-1 summarizes the age-related changes in the vessels.

Assessment
General Observations

Clues to peripheral vascular disorders often can be detected through general contact with patients, who may comment that their feet always feel cold and numb, that they experience burning sensations in the calf, or that they become dizzy on rising. They may ambulate slowly, rub their legs, or kick off their shoes. Varicosities may be noted on the legs. Such observations can be used to introduce discussions of peripheral vascular problems.

Interview

Some patients may be able to relate symptoms to vascular problems; however, others may be unaware that signs such as lightheadedness, scaling skin, edema, or discoloration can be associated with peripheral vascular disorders; they must be asked specific questions. Information can be elicited through questions such as the following:

> "Do your arms or legs ever become cold or numb?"
> "Do dark spots or sores ever develop on your legs?"
> "Do your legs get painful or swollen when you walk or stand?"
> "Do you ever have periods of feeling dizzy, lightheaded, or confused?"
> "Does one leg ever look larger than the other?"

Physical Examination

Pulses are palpated bilaterally for condition of the vessel wall, rate, rhythm, quality, contour, and equality at the following sites.

Temporal pulse the only palpable artery of the head, located anterior to the ear, overlying the temporal bone; normally appears tortuous

Brachial pulse   located in the groove between the biceps and triceps; usually palpated if arterial insufficiency is suspected

Radial pulse   branching from the brachial artery, the radial artery extends from the forearm to the wrist on the radial side and is palpated on the flexor surface of the wrist laterally

Ulnar pulse   also branching from the brachial artery, the ulnar artery extends from the forearm to the wrist on the ulnar side and is palpated on the flexor surface of the wrist medially; usually palpated if arterial insufficiency is suspected

Femoral pulse   the femoral artery is palpated at the inguinal ligament midway between the anterosuperior iliac spine and the pubic tubercle

Popliteal pulse   located behind the knee, the popliteal artery is the continuation of the femoral artery; having the patient flex the knee during palpation can aid in locating this pulse

Posterior tibial pulse   palpable behind and below the medial malleolus

Dorsalis pedis pulse   palpated at the groove between the first two tendons on the medial side of the dorsum of the foot; this and the posterior tibial pulse can be congenitally absent

Pulses are rated on a scale from 0 to 4:

0 = no pulse
1 = thready, easily obliterated pulse
2 = pulse difficult to palpate and easily obliterated
3 = normal pulse
4 = strong, bounding pulse, not obliterated with pressure.

Often, a stick figure is used to show the quality of pulses at different locations (Fig. 20-1).

While the nurse assesses pulses, the vessels can be inspected for signs of phlebitis. This signs could include redness, tenderness, and edema over a vein. Sometimes, visible signs of inflammation may not be present, and the primary indication that phlebitis exists can be tenderness of the vessel detected through palpation. A positive Homan sign (*i.e.,* pain when the affected leg is dorsiflexed) can accompany deep phlebitis of the leg.

The legs should be inspected for discoloration, hair loss, edema, scaling skin, pallor, lesions, and tortuous-looking veins. Inspection of the nails can reveal thickness and dryness in the presence of cardiovascular disease. Skin temperature can be assessed by touching the skin surface in various areas.

Examination of the jugular and carotid vessels is described in Chapter 17. Alterations in cerebral circulation can cause disruptions to cognitive function; therefore, a mental status evaluation can provide useful information about circulatory problems.

Review of Selected Disorders
Arteriosclerosis

Arteriosclerosis is a common problem among the aged, especially among diabetic patients. Unlike atherosclerosis, which generally affects the large vessels coming from the heart, arteriosclerosis most often affects the smaller vessels farthest from the heart. Arteriography and radiography can be used to diagnose arteriosclerosis, and oscillometric testing can assess the arterial pulse at different levels. If surface temperature is evaluated as a diagnostic measure, the nurse should keep the patient in a warm, stable room temperature for at least 1 hour before testing. Treatment of arteriosclerosis includes bed rest, warmth, Buerger–Allen exercises (Fig. 20-2), and vasodilators. Occasionally, a permanent vasodilation effect is achieved by performing a sympathetic ganglionectomy.

Arteriosclerosis Obliterans

Most of the occlusions that result in the development of ischemic lesions are due to arteriosclerosis. Aortoiliac occlusion, occurring in the terminal abdominal aorta and common iliac arteries, may not produce any difficulty for years. Resting pain and gangrene may be eventual effects as this problem progresses. In the lower extremities, the most

common site of occlusion is the superficial femoral artery, with the involvement of the popliteal artery tree or the tibial artery tree. Intermittent claudication is the most frequent problem associated with lower extremity occlusions, although some patients do develop ischemic rest pain, neuropathy, and, less frequently, ulcers and gangrene. Treatment of arteriosclerosis obliterans depends on the location of the occlusion.

Arterial Embolism

Aneurysms, atrial fibrillation, myocardial infarction, atherosclerosis, and arteriosclerosis are among the problems that give rise to arterial emboli, which lodge primarily in the lower extremity and brachial arteries. The elderly are seriously threatened by gangrene and death from an undetected or untreated embolism; therefore, the nurse should be alert to indicative symptoms and signs. Coldness and numbness below the location of the embolism may prevent the patient from feeling pain until the condition progresses. Any pressure or constriction to the affected part should be avoided. Anticoagulation therapy, which requires close nursing super-

vision (see Chap. 35), and embolectomies have proven beneficial.

Special Problems of the Diabetic Patient

Diabetic patients, who have a high risk of developing peripheral vascular problems and associated complications, commonly display the diabetes-associated neuropathies and infections that affect vessels throughout the entire body. Arterial insufficiency can present in several ways. Resting pain may occur as a result of intermittent claudication; arterial pulses may be difficult to find or totally absent; and skin discoloration, ulcerations, and gangrene may a be present. Diagnostic measures, similar to those used to determine the degree of arterial insufficiency with other problems, include oscillometry, elevation–dependency tests, and palpation of pulses and skin temperatures at different sites. When surgery is possible, arteriography may be done to establish the exact size and location of the arterial lesion. The treatment selected will depend on the extent of the disease. Walking can promote collateral circulation and may constitute sufficient management if intermittent claudication is

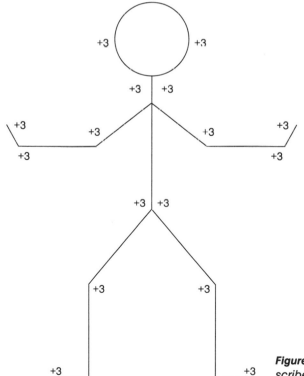

Figure 20-1. *A stick figure may be used to describe the quality of the various pulses.*

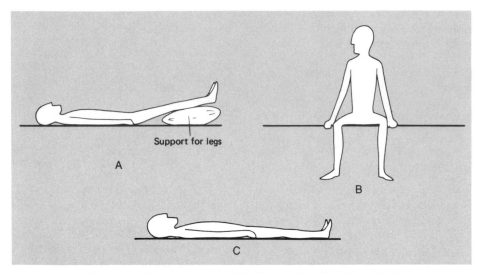

Figure 20-2. *Buerger–Allen exercises. (**A**) The patient lies flat with legs elevated above the level of the heart until blanching occurs (about 2 minutes). (**B**) The patient lowers legs to fill the vessels and exercises feet until the legs are pink (about 5 minutes. (**C**) The patient lies flat for about 5 minutes before repeating the exercises. The entire procedure is done five times, or as tolerated by the patient, at three different times during the day. The nurse should assist the patient with position changes, since postural hypotension can occur. The patient's tolerance and effectiveness of the procedure should be noted.*

the sole problem. Analgesics can provide relief from resting pain.

Because many of today's older diabetic patients may have witnessed severe disability and death among others with the disease they have known throughout their lives, they need to be assured that improved methods of medical and surgical management—perhaps not even developed at the time their parents and grandparents had diabetes—increase their chances for a full, independent life.

Aneurysms

In older adults, advanced arteriosclerosis is usually responsible for the development of aneurysms, although they may also result from infection, trauma, syphilis, and other factors. Sometimes they can be seen by the naked eye and are able to be palpated as a pulsating mass; sometimes they can only be detected by radiography. A thrombosis can develop in the aneurysm, leading to an arterial occlusion or rupture of the aneurysm—the most serious complications associated with this problem.

Aneurysms of the abdominal aorta most fre-

quently occur in older people. Patients with a history of arteriosclerotic lesions, angina pectoris, myocardial infarction, and congestive heart failure more commonly develop aneurysms in this area. A pulsating mass, sometimes painful, in the umbilical region is an indication of an abdominal aorta aneurysm. Prompt correction is essential because, if not corrected, rupture can occur. Fewer complications and deaths result from surgical intervention before rupture. Among the complications that the elderly can develop after surgery for this problem are hemorrhage, myocardial infarction, cerebral vascular accident, and acute renal insufficiency. The nurse should observe closely for signs of postoperative complications.

Aneurysms can develop in peripheral arteries, the most common sites being the femoral and popliteal arteries. Peripheral aneurysms can usually be palpated, thus establishing the diagnosis. The most serious complication associated with peripheral aneurysms is the formation of a thrombus, which can occlude the vessel and cause loss of the limb. As with abdominal aortic aneurysms, early treatment reduces the risk of complications and death. The lesion may be resected and the portion of the

vessel removed replaced, commonly with a prosthetic material. For certain patients, a lumbar sympathectomy can be performed. The nurse should be aware that these patients can develop a thrombus postoperatively and should assist the patient in preventing this complication.

Varicose Veins

Varicosities, a common problem in old age, can be caused by lack of exercise, jobs entailing a great deal of standing, and loss of vessel elasticity and strength associated with the aging process. Varicosities in all ages can be detected by the dilated, tortuous nature of the vein, especially the veins of the lower extremities. The person may experience dull pain and cramping of the legs, sometimes severe enough to interfere with sleep. Dizziness may occur as the patient rises from a lying position because blood is localized in the lower extremities and cerebral circulation is reduced. The effects of the varicosities make the skin more susceptible to trauma and infection, promoting the development of ulcerative lesions, especially in the obese or diabetic patient.

Treatment of varicose veins is aimed toward reducing venous stasis. The affected limb is elevated and rested to promote venous return. Exercise, particularly walking, also will enhance circulation. The nurse should make sure that elastic stockings and bandages are properly used and not constricting and that the patient is informed of the causes of venous status (e.g., prolonged standing, crossing the legs, wearing constricting clothing) to prevent the development of complications and additional varicosities. Ligation and stripping of the veins require the same principles of nursing care used for other age groups undergoing this surgery.

Venous Thromboembolism

An increasing incidence of venous thromboembolism is found among the aged. Patients who have been restricted to bed rest or have had recent surgery or fractures of a lower extremity are high-risk candidates. Although the veins in the calf muscles are the most frequently seen sites of this problem, it also occurs in the inferior vena cava, iliofemoral segment, and various superficial veins. The symptoms and signs of venous thromboembolism depend on the vessel involved. The nurse should be alert for edema, warmth over the affected area, and pain in the sole of the foot. Edema may be the primary indication of thromboembolism in the veins of the calf muscle, because discoloration and pain are often absent in aged persons with this problem. If the inferior vena cava is involved, bilateral swelling, aching and cyanosis of the lower extremities, engorgement of the superficial veins, and tenderness along the femoral veins will be present. Similar signs will appear with involvement of the iliofemoral segment but only on the affected extremity.

The location of the thromboembolism will dictate the treatment used. Elastic stockings or bandages, rest, and elevation of the affected limb may promote venous return. Analgesics may be given to relieve any associated pain. Anticoagulants may be administered, and surgery may be performed as well. The nurse should help the patient to avoid situations that cause straining and to remain comfortable and well hydrated.

General Nursing Interventions Related to Peripheral Vascular Diseases
Facilitating Peripheral Circulation

Nurses can play a significant role in preventing peripheral vascular problems. Health education for persons of all ages should reinforce the importance of exercise in promoting circulation; factors that can interfere with optimal circulation, such as crossing legs and wearing garters, should be reviewed. Weight control can be encouraged because obesity can interfere with venous return. Tobacco use should be discouraged because it may cause arterial spasms. Immobility and hypotension should be prevented to avoid thrombus formation. Buerger–Allen exercises (see Fig. 20-2) may be prescribed, and the patient and family members or caregivers will need to learn how they are done correctly and comfortably. Instruction in the correct use of support hose or special elastic stockings is important.

Care Planning

Actual or potential problems can be discovered during the assessment of peripheral vessels. Assessment data should be reviewed for those problems that fall within the realm of nursing to diagnose and manage, and related nursing diagnoses

Table 20-1 *Nursing Diagnoses Related to Peripheral Vascular Disease*

NURSING DIAGNOSIS	CAUSES OR CONTRIBUTING FACTORS
Activity intolerance	Pain, numbness of extremities, dizziness, confusion
Anxiety	Pain, limited mobility
Pain	Insufficient circulation
Altered family processes	Pain, limitations in functional ability
Fear	Pain, loss of function or limb
Impaired home maintenance management	Impaired mobility, pain
High risk for infection	Impaired circulation, stasis ulcers, high risk for injury
High risk for injury	Altered mobility, pain, altered cerebral circulation, altered sensory function
Knowledge deficit	Diagnostic tests, treatments, medications, precautions
Impaired physical mobility	Pain, spasms, amputation
Noncompliance	Lack of knowledge, skill, competency, or motivation
Altered nutrition: more than body requirements	Decreased activity, anxiety, depression
Powerlessness	Decreased ability to perform activities of daily living, lack of knowledge, hospitalization
Self-care deficit	Altered functional ability, lack of knowledge, decreased mobility, amputation
Disturbance in self-concept	Change or loss of body part or function, hospitalization
Sensory–perceptual alterations	Impaired oxygen transport to tissues, amputation, pain, immobility
Sexual dysfunction	Pain, altered self-concept
Impaired skin integrity	Impaired oxygen transport, infection, immobility, fragile skin
Sleep pattern disturbance	Impaired oxygen transport, pain, immobility, inactivity, drugs, anxiety, depression
Impaired social interactions	Change or loss of body part or function, anxiety, pain, altered self-concept
Social isolation	Impaired function, amputation, altered self-concept
Altered thought processes	Impaired cerebral circulation, anxiety, depression, fear
Altered tissue perfusion	Varicosities, arteriosclerosis, thrombus, edema, immobility

should be developed accordingly. Table 20-1 lists some of the major nursing diagnoses that can be related to peripheral vascular disease.

The development of realistic goals guides care and provides a yardstick by which the patient's progress can be measured. Although the goals developed for individual patients will be specific to their unique needs, some possible goals in the care of peripheral vascular diseases for older patients are listed in the Sample Care Plan. Patients and their significant others should be active participants in the development of goals and establishment of priorities. See Chapter 18 for more information on planning and providing care.

Foot Care

Persons with peripheral vascular disease must pay special attention to the care of their feet, which should be bathed and inspected daily. To avoid in-

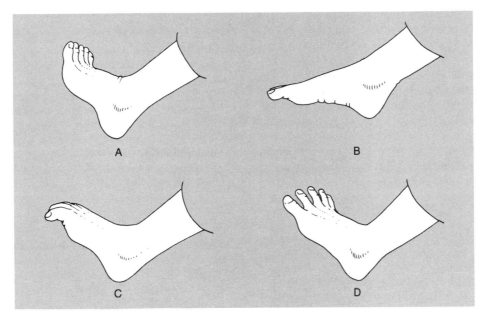

Figure 20-3. *Foot and toe exercises.* (**A**) *Foot flexion.* (**B**) *Foot extension.* (**C**) *Curling toes.* (**D**) *Moving toes apart.*

jury, patients should not walk in bare feet. Any foot lesion or discoloration should be brought promptly to the attention of the physician or nurse. These patients are at high risk of developing fungal infections from the moisture produced by normal foot perspiration; it is not unusual for the elderly to develop fungal infections under their nails, emphasizing the importance of regular, careful nail inspection. If untreated, a simple fungal infection can lead to gangrene and other serious complications. Placing cotton between the toes and removing shoes several times during the day will help keep the feet dry. Shoes should be large enough to avoid any pressure and safe enough to prevent any injuries to the feet; they should be aired after wearing. Laces should not be tied tightly because they can exert pressure on the feet. Colored socks may contain irritating dyes and would be best to avoid; socks should be changed regularly. Although the feet should be kept warm, the direct application of heat to the feet, as with heating pads, hot water bottles, and soaks, can increase the metabolism and circulatory demand, thereby compounding the existing problem. Exercises that may benefit patients with peripheral vascular disease are shown in Figure 20-3.

Caring for Special Problems

Ischemic foot lesions may be present in patients with peripheral vascular disease. If eschars are present, they should be loosened to allow drainage. Careful debridement is necessary to avoid bleeding and trauma; chemical debriding agents may be useful. Systemic antibiotic agents can be helpful in controlling cellulitis. Topical antibiotics usually are not used because epithelization must occur before bacterial flora can be destroyed. Analgesics may be administered to relieve associated pain. Good nutrition, particularly an adequate protein intake, and the maintenance of muscle strength and joint motion are essential. Various surgical procedures may be used in treating ischemic foot lesions, including bypass grafts, sympathectomies, and amputations.

Loss of a limb may represent a significant loss of independence to the elderly, regardless of the reality of the situation. With an altered body image, new roles may be assumed as other roles are forfeited. Patients and their families need opportunities to discuss their fears and concerns. Making them aware of the likelihood of a normal life and the availability of appliances that make ambulation,

driving, and other activities possible may help reduce anxieties and promote a smoother adjustment to the amputation. The rehabilitation period can be long for the elderly and may necessitate frequent motivation and encouragement by nursing staff. The Resource List indicates groups that may be of benefit to patients with peripheral vascular disorders.

Sample Care Plan Goals for the Patient With Periperal Vascular Disease

To participate in a regular exercise program as prescribed

To verbalize an understanding of the peripheral vascular disease and its management

To demonstrate proper procedures related to the care of the peripheral vascular disease

To describe factors that promote good circulation

To identify signs and symptoms of circulatory problems

To be free from complications associated with poor circulation

To demonstrate good foot care techniques

To adjust to the use of a prosthesis

To increase or maintain activity level

To be free from pain and dysfunction associated with circulatory problems

---

Resources to Assist Patients With Peripheral Vascular Disease

American Heart Association
7320 Greenville Ave.
Dallas, TX 75231
(214)750-5551

(Provides literature on cardiovascular health)

National Amputation Foundation
12-45 150th St.
Whitestone, NY 11357
(212)767-0596

(Offers a prosthetic center, rehabilitation services, and educational literature)

Recommended Readings

Levine JM. Leg ulcers: differential diagnosis in the elderly. Geriatrics 1990;45(6):32.

Spilane M. Peripheral vascular disease. In: Cassel CK, Walsh JR, eds. Geriatric medicine. vol. 1. New York: Springer-Verlag, 1984:197.

Spittell JA. Diagnosis and management of leg ulcer. Geriatrics 1984;38(6):57.

Thompson MK. The care of the elderly in general practice. New York: Churchill-Livingston, 1984:157.

Young JR. Peripheral vascular disease. In: Steinberg FU, ed. Care of the geriatric patient. 6th ed. St. Louis: CV Mosby, 1983:373.

21

Respiratory Problems

Respiratory health is vital to the elderly person's ability to maintain a physically, mentally, and socially active life-style. It can make the difference between whether or not a person will maximize opportunities to live life to the fullest or be too fatigued and uncomfortable to leave the confines of home. A lifetime of insults to the respiratory system from smoking, pollution, and infection takes its toll in old age, making respiratory disease a leading cause of disability and the fourth leading cause of death in persons over 70 years of age. However, positive health practices can benefit respiratory health at any age and minimize limitations imposed by problems.

Aging and the Respiratory System

The effects of aging create a situation in which respiratory problems can develop more easily and be more difficult to manage. Various connective tissues responsible for respiration and ventilation are weaker. The elastic recoil of the lungs during expiration is decreased due to less elastic collagen and elastin, and expiration requires the active use of accessory muscles. Alveoli are less elastic, develop fibrous tissue, and contain fewer functional capillaries. Arterial oxyhemoglobin saturation is reduced to 93% to 94%; PaO_2 becomes 75 to 80 mmHg; $PaCO_2$ remains at 35 to 46 mmHg; and blood pH remains at 7.40 to 7.45. The loss of skeletal muscle strength

in the thorax and diaphragm, combined with the resilient force that holds the thorax in a slightly contracted position, contribute to the slight kyphosis and barrel chest seen in many older adults. The net effect of these changes is a reduction in vital capacity and an increase in residual volume—in other words, less air exchange and more air and secretions remaining in the lungs.

Age-related changes external to the respiratory system can affect respiratory health in significant ways. A reduction in body fluid and reduced fluid intake can cause drier mucous membranes, impeding the removal of mucus and leading to the development of mucous plugs and infection. Altered pain sensations can cause signals of respiratory problems to be unnoticed or mistaken for nonrespiratory disorders. Different norms for body temperature can cause fever to present at an atypical level, potentially being missed and allowing respiratory infections to progress. Tooth brittleness can result in the aspiration of tooth fragments; relaxed sphincters and slower gastric motility further contribute to the risk of aspiration. Impaired mobility, inactivity, and numerous medications associated with the highly prevalent diseases in the older population can decrease respiratory function, promote infection, interfere with early detection, and complicate treatment of respiratory problems. Display 21-1 lists some of the age-related changes affecting the respiratory system.

DISPLAY 21-1   Age-Related Changes of the Respiratory System

Increased rigidity of rib cage
Increase in anteroposterior chest diameter
Weaker thoracic muscles
Decreased elastic recoil, increased rigidity of lungs
Decreased number, stretching of alveoli
Increase in residual capacity, decrease in vital capacity and maximum breathing capacity
Lack of basilar inflation

Assessment

Early detection and diagnosis of respiratory problems often are complicated by the elderly's acceptance or lack of awareness of symptoms and altered presentation of the disorder. Nurses must aggressively examine the elderly for even the most subtle clues of respiratory problems.

General Observation

Much can be determined regarding the status of the respiratory system through careful observation of the following:

Color: coloring of the face, neck, limbs, and nail beds can be indicative of respiratory status. Ruddy, pink complexions often occur with chronic obstructive pulmonary disease (COPD) and are associated with hypoxia, which is caused by a high carbon dioxide level in the blood that inhibits involuntary neurotransmission from the pons to the diaphragm for inspiration. In the presence of chronic bronchitis, patients can have a blue or gray discoloration caused by the lack of oxygen binding to the hemoglobin.

Chest structure and posture: the anteroposterior chest diameter increases with age—significantly so in the presence of COPD. Abnormal spinal curvatures (*e.g.,* kyphosis, scoliosis, lordosis) should be noted.

Breathing pattern: the chest should be observed for symmetrical expansion during respirations, as well as the depth, rate, rhythm, and length of respirations. Decreased expansion of the chest can be caused by pain, fractured ribs, pulmonary emboli, pleural effusion, or pleurisy. The patient should be asked to change positions, walk, and cough to see if these activities result in any changes.

Interview

Some older persons can give unreliable accounts of their past respiratory symptoms or have grown so accustomed to living with their symptoms that they do not consider them unusual. Specific questions can assist in revealing disorders, such as the following:

"Do you ever have wheezing, chest pain, or a heavy feeling in your chest?"
"How often do you get colds? Do you get colds that keep returning? How do you treat them?"
"How far can you walk? How many steps can you climb before getting short of breath?"
"Do you have any breathing problems when the weather gets cold or hot?"
"How many pillows do you sleep on? Do breathing problems (*e.g.,* coughing, shortness of breath) ever awaken you from sleep?"
"How much do you cough during the day? During each hour? Can you control it?"
"Do you bring up sputum, phlegm, or mucus when you cough? How much? What color? Is it the consistency of water, egg white, or jelly?"
"How do you manage respiratory problems? How often do you use cough syrups, cold capsules, inhalers, vapors, rubs, or ointments?"
"Did you ever smoke? If so, for how long and when and why did you stop? How many cigarettes or cigars do you smoke daily? Do people you live with or spend a lot of time with smoke?"
"What kind of jobs have you had over your lifetime? Any in factories or chemical plants?"
"Do you live or have you lived near factories, fields, or high-traffic areas?"

More specific questions increase the likelihood of obtaining a full and accurate history of factors related to respiratory health. The dates of influenza and pneumonia vaccines should be ascertained and documented.

Physical Examination

The posterior chest is palpated to evaluate the depth of respirations, degree of chest movement, and presence of masses or pain. Normally there is bilateral movement during respirations and reduced expansion of the base of the lungs. Tactile fremitus is usually best felt in the upper lobes; increased fremitus in the lower lobes occurs with pneumonia and masses. COPD and pneumothorax can cause a lack of fremitus in the upper lobes. Percussion of the lungs should produce a resonant sound. Auscultation of the lungs should reflect normal bronchial, vesicular, and bronchovesicular breath sounds; crackles, rhonchi, and wheezes are abnormal findings. Refer to Chapter 17 for specific guidelines on palpation, percussion, and auscultation of the lungs.

Review of Selected Disorders

Pneumonia

Pneumonia, especially bronchopneumonia, is common in the elderly and, as mentioned, it is one of the leading causes of death in this age group. At one time, pneumonia in an aged person meant death, but the discovery of antibiotics has significantly reduced the mortality and morbidity associated with this disease. Several factors contribute to its high incidence. Changes to the respiratory system with age may cause poor chest expansion and more shallow breathing. The elderly may have other respiratory diseases that promote mucus formation and bronchial obstruction. Upper respiratory infection is more frequent in the aged, especially because they have a lowered resistance to infection. The reduced sensitivity of pharyngeal reflexes in many older persons may promote aspiration of foreign material. They are more likely to be debilitated and immobile.

The signs and symptoms of pneumonia may be altered in older persons, and serious pneumonia may exist without symptoms being evident. Pleuritic pain, for instance, may not be as severe as that described by younger patients. Differences in body temperature may cause little or no fever. Symptoms may include a slight cough, fatigue, and rapid respiration. Confusion, restlessness, and behavioral changes may occur as a result of cerebral hypoxia. Nursing care for the geriatric patient with pneumonia is similar to that used for the younger patient. Close observation for subtle changes is especially important. The aged patient can also develop the complication of paralytic ileus, which can be prevented by mobility.

Asthma

Some older persons have been affected with asthma throughout their lives; some develop it during old age. The symptoms and management do not differ much from those of other age groups. Because of the added stress that asthma places on the heart, older asthmatics have a high risk of developing complications such as bronchiectasis and cardiac problems. The nurse should assist in detecting causative factors and educate the patient regarding early recognition and prompt attention to an asthma attack when it does occur. Careful assessment of the aged asthmatic patient's use of aerosol nebulizers is advisable. Cardiac arrhythmias leading to sudden death may be risked by the overuse of sympathomimetic bronchodilating nebulizers. Cromolyn sodium is one of the least toxic respiratory drugs that can be used, although several weeks of therapy may be necessary for benefits to be realized. Some of the new steroid inhalants are effective and carry a lower risk of systemic absorption and adverse reactions than older steroids.

Chronic Bronchitis

Many elderly persons demonstrate the persistent, productive cough, wheezing, recurrent respiratory infections, and shortness of breath caused by chronic bronchitis. These symptoms may develop gradually, sometimes taking years for the full impact of the disease to be realized, when, because of bronchospasm, the patient notices increased difficulty breathing in cold and damp weather. They experience more frequent respiratory infections and greater difficulty managing them. Episodes of hypoxia begin to occur because mucus obstructs the bronchial tree and causes carbon dioxide retention. As the disease progresses, emphysema may develop and death may occur from obstruction. The management of this problem, aimed at removing bronchial secretions and preventing obstruction of the airway, is similar for all age groups. Older patients may need special encouragement to maintain a good fluid intake and expectorate se-

cretions. The nurse can be most effective in preventing the development of chronic bronchitis by discouraging chronic respiratory irritation, such as from smoking, and by helping older adults prevent respiratory infections.

Emphysema

Of increasing incidence in the aged population is emphysema, a progressive COPD. Factors causing this destructive disease include chronic bronchitis and chronic irritation from dusts or certain air pollutants and morphologic changes in the lungs, which include distention of the alveolar sacs, rupture of the alveolar walls, and destruction of the alveolar capillary bed. Cigarette smoking also plays a major role in the development of emphysema. The symptoms are slow in onset and initially may resemble age-related changes in the respiratory system, causing many patients to experience delayed identification and treatment of this disease. Gradually, increased dyspnea is experienced, which is not relieved by sitting upright as it may have been in the past. A chronic cough develops. As more effort is required for breathing and hypoxia occurs, fatigue, anorexia, weight loss, and weakness are demonstrated. Recurrent respiratory infections, malnutrition, congestive heart failure, and cardiac arrhythmias are among the more life-threatening complications the elderly can experience from emphysema.

Treatment usually includes postural drainage, intermittent positive-pressure breathing, bronchodilators, the avoidance of stressful situations, and breathing exercises, which are an important part of patient education. Cigarette smoking definitely should be stopped. The older patient may have a problem with adequate food and fluid intake, requiring special nursing attention. If oxygen is used, it must be done with extreme caution and close supervision. It must be remembered that for these patients, a low oxygen level rather than a high carbon dioxide level stimulates respiration. The older patient with emphysema is a high-risk candidate for the development of carbon dioxide narcosis. Respiratory infections should be prevented, and any that do occur, regardless of how minor they may seem, should be promptly reported to the physician. Sedatives, hypnotics, and narcotics may be contraindicated because the patient will be more sensitive to these drugs. Patients with emphysema

need a great deal of education and support to be able to manage this disease. It is difficult for the patient to adjust to the presence of a serious chronic disease requiring special care or even a change in life-style. The patient must learn to pace activities, avoid extremely cold weather, administer medications correctly, and recognize symptoms of infection.

Tuberculosis

The incidence of tuberculosis is increasing among the older population, and a high incidence is found in institutional settings. A reactivation of an earlier asymptomatic or improperly treated infection is more common than new infection in the elderly. Diagnosis may be delayed, either because the classic symptoms are not demonstrated or because symptoms resemble changes associated with the aging process. For instance, anorexia and weakness may be the primary symptoms. Night sweats may not occur because of reduced diaphoresis with advanced age. Likewise, fever may not be detected due to alterations in the aged's body temperature. These factors emphasize the importance of periodic evaluation for this disease. Screening for tuberculosis should be performed for all patients entering a hospital or facility for geriatric care, and groups of aged persons, such as senior citizen organizations, should be checked periodically. A two-step Mantoux test is recommended for the elderly because of the high prevalence of false-negative results (*i.e.*, if the result is negative after the first test, the test should be repeated in 1 week, which could cause a conversion if the infection is present due to a waned response).

Treatment follows the same principles as for any age group, basically consisting of rest, good nutrition, and medications. Some of the side-effects of medications commonly prescribed for tuberculosis have special implications for older persons. Streptomycin can cause damage to the peripheral and central nervous systems, demonstrated through hearing limitations and disequilibrium. The safety hazards created by these adverse reactions are significant to the aged. Para-aminosalicylic acid can cause irritation to the gastrointestinal tract, anorexia, nausea, vomiting, and diarrhea, which can predispose the elderly to the risk of malnutrition. Changes in gastric secretions can cause these tablets to pass through the gastrointestinal sys-

tem without being dissolved, thereby preventing a therapeutic benefit. Stools should be examined for undissolved tablets. Isoniazid, although not as toxic as the other drugs mentioned, can have toxic effects on the peripheral and central nervous systems. The nurse must assess the patient continuously for the appearance of adverse reactions to such medications.

A diagnosis of tuberculosis can be extremely difficult for older persons to accept. Having lived through an era when people with tuberculosis were sent away to sanitariums for long periods of time, they may be unaware of new approaches to treatment and fear institutionalization. Believing they could infect family and friends, they may avoid contact with others, promoting social isolation. It is possible that other people will fear contracting the disease and be reluctant to maintain social contact. Education of patients, their families, and friends is essential to clarify these misconceptions and promote a normal life-style. Patients should be taught their responsibilities in managing this disease. Medication is essential for the treatment of tuberculosis, and because the older person may have a problem remembering to take it, nurses should devise a system for helping the patient remember how to administer the medication. For example, medications and denture cream could be placed in the same box so that during daily denture care medications would be remembered; the patient, a family member, or a visiting nurse could fill seven envelopes with medications, labeling them for each day of the week, and devise a chart for recording when medication is taken; a family member or friend could call the patient daily to ask whether medication was taken. With prompt and proper therapy, the older person can recover from tuberculosis with minimal residual effects.

Lung Cancer

It is uncertain whether the increased incidence of lung cancer in the aged population is due to more cases of lung cancer actually occurring or improved diagnostic tools and greater availability of medical care. Lung cancer occurs more frequently in men although the rate among women is rising. The mortality rate from lung cancer is higher among Caucasians. Cigarette smokers have twice the incidence as nonsmokers. A high incidence oc-

curs among individuals who are chronically exposed to agents such as asbestos, coal gas, radioactive dusts, and chromates. This emphasizes the significance of obtaining thorough information regarding a patient's occupational history as part of the nursing assessment. Although conclusive evidence is unavailable, some association has been reported between the presence of lung scars, such as those resulting from tuberculosis and pneumonitis, and lung cancer.

The individual may have lung cancer long before any symptoms develop. This suggests that individuals at high risk should be screened regularly and periodic roentgenograms obtained to detect this disease in an early stage. Dyspnea, coughing, chest pain, fatigue, anorexia, wheezing, and recurrent upper respiratory infections are part of the symptomatology seen as the disease progresses. Diagnosis is confirmed through chest roentgenogram, sputum cytology, bronchoscopy, and biopsy. Treatment may consist of surgery, chemotherapy, or radiotherapy, requiring the same type of nursing care as that for patients of any age with this diagnosis.

Lung Abscess

A lung abscess may result from pneumonia, tuberculosis, a malignancy, or trauma to the lung. Aspiration of foreign material can also cause a lung abscess, and this may be a particular risk to aged persons who have decreased pharyngeal reflexes. Symptoms, which resemble those of many other respiratory problems, include anorexia, weight loss, fatigue, temperature elevation, and a chronic cough. Sputum production may occur, but this is not always demonstrated in older persons. Diagnosis and management are the same as that for other age groups. Modifications for postural drainage, an important component of the treatment, have been discussed earlier in this chapter. Because protein can be lost through the sputum, a high-protein, high-calorie diet should be encouraged to maintain and improve the nutritional status of the elderly patient.

Bronchiectasis

Bronchiectasis does not occur as frequently in older age groups as it does in the young. Aged persons can develop this problem from chronic

bronchitis, asthma, recurrent upper respiratory infections, or aspiration of foreign material. The weakening of the bronchioles with increased age may cause a breakdown of the alveolar and bronchiolar walls. The most outstanding symptoms that older persons demonstrate are temperature elevation and a chronic cough that produces large amounts of foul-smelling sputum. Diagnostic measures and treatment are similar to those for other age groups. Postural drainage and a high-protein, high-calorie diet are essential components of the treatment plan.

General Nursing Interventions Related to Respiratory Problems

Facilitating Respiratory Health

The high risk that every older person faces in developing respiratory disorders warrants that preventive measures be incorporated into all care plans. In addition to basic health practices, special attention to promoting respiratory activity is important. All older adults should be encouraged to do deep-breathing exercises several times daily. Keeping in mind that full expiration is more difficult than inspiration, these exercises should emphasize an inspiration ratio of 1:3. See Chapter 8 for a full description of breathing exercises. Even healthy, active people can benefit from including these exercises in their daily activities.

Smoking is the most important factor contributing to respiratory disease. Many elderly smokers started their habit at a time when the full effects of smoking were not realized, and smoking was considered fashionable, sociable, and sophisticated. Although smokers may be aware of the health hazards associated with smoking, it is an extremely difficult habit to break. The effects on respiratory health initially may be so subtle and gradual that they are not realized. Unfortunately, by the time signs and symptoms become apparent, considerable damage to the respiratory system may have occurred. Smokers have twice the incidence of lung cancer; a higher incidence of all respiratory disease; more complications with respiratory problems; and commonly suffer from productive coughs, shortness of breath, and reduced breathing capacity. Although maximum benefit is obtained by not starting to smoke in the first place or quitting early in life, smoking cessation can be beneficial at any age.

Local chapters of the American Lung Association, health departments, clinics, and commercial agencies offer a wide range of smoking cessation approaches that may be useful.

Immobility is a major threat to pulmonary health, and the elderly frequently experience problems that decrease their mobility. Preventing fractures, pain, weakness, depression, and other problems that could decrease mobility is an essential goal. The elderly, family members, and caregivers all need to be educated about the multiple problems associated with immobility. It may be tempting for the older person to rest or for caring family to encourage that person to rest on days when arthritis or other discomforts are bothersome, unless it is understood that by doing so, more discomfort and disability can result. When immobility is unavoidable, hourly turning, coughing, and deep breathing will promote respiratory activity; blow bottles and similar equipment can be beneficial also. Persons who are chair-bound may need the same attention to respiratory activity as the bed-bound.

Older persons should be advised against self-treating respiratory problems. Many over-the-counter cold and cough remedies can have serious effects in older adults, and can interact with other medications being taken. These drugs also can mask symptoms of serious problems, thereby delaying diagnosis and treatment. The elderly should know that a cold lasting more than 1 week may not be a cold at all, but something more serious that needs medical attention.

All medications used with the elderly should be evaluated for their impact on respirations. Decreased respirations or rapid, shallow breathing can be caused by many of the drugs commonly prescribed for this group; these drugs include analgesics, antidepressants, antihistamines, antiparkinson agents, synthetic antispasmodics, sedatives, and tranquilizers. As always, alternatives to drugs should be used whenever possible.

Care Planning

Actual or potential problems can be discovered during the assessment of the respiratory system. Assessment data should be reviewed for those problems that fall within the realm of nursing to diagnose and manage, and related nursing diagnoses should be developed accordingly. Table 21-1

Table 21-1 *Nursing Diagnoses Related to Respiratory Problems*

NURSING DIAGNOSIS	CAUSES OR CONTRIBUTING FACTORS
Activity intolerance	Altered oxygen transport, fatigue, dyspnea
Anxiety	Breathing problems, potential disability or dependency
Altered cardiac output: decreased	Altered oxygen transport
Pain	Dyspnea, inflammation, overactivity, procedures
Impaired verbal communication	Shortness of breath, pain
Ineffective individual coping	Stress from disease or its management
Diversional activity deficit	Inability to tolerate activities, disability, pain, demands of disease
Altered family processes	Illness or disability of patient, care needs
Fear	Disability, altered function or body image, treatments, lack of knowledge
Fluid volume deficit	Infection, fever, reduced motivation to drink or eat, hyperpnea, diaphoresis
Grieving	Loss of function, pain, change in life style
Altered health maintenance	Disability, dependency, lack of knowledge
Impaired home maintenance management	Disability, anxiety, pain, lack of knowledge
High risk for infection	Impaired oxygen transport, immobility, procedures (*e.g.*, suctioning), medications
High risk for injury	Altered cerebral circulation, pain, fatigue, lack of knowledge (*e.g.*, safe use of O_2)
Knowledge deficit	Diagnostic tests, new diagnosis, treatments, drugs
Impaired physical mobility	Fatigue, weakness, pain, dyspnea
Noncompliance	Lack of knowledge, denial, self-care deficit
Altered nutrition: less than body requirements	Infection, anorexia, stress, fatigue, pain
Altered oral mucous membrane	Mouth breathing, inadequate oral hygiene, endotrachial tube
Powerlessness	Inability to fulfill role or participate in activities of daily living, lack of knowledge
Altered respiratory function: ineffective airway clearance; ineffective breathing patterns; impaired gas exchange	Infection, excessive or thick secretions, inelasticity of lungs, edema of airway structures, medications, pain, anxiety, fatigue, obstruction, aspiration, smoking, chronic cough or ineffective cough, mouth breathing
Self-care deficit	Fatigue, pain, immobility
Disturbance in self-concept	Altered body function or image, pain, immobility
Sexual dysfunction	Shortness of breath, anxiety, fear, pain, fatigue, drugs
Impaired skin integrity	Impaired oxygen transport; irritation from mucous contract; friction from nasal cannulas, masks, tubes
Sleep pattern disturbance	Impaired oxygen transport, orthopnea, dyspnea, fear, anxiety, medications
Impaired social interactions	Altered body function or image, pain, fatigue

lists some of the major nursing diagnoses that can be related to respiratory disorders.

The development of realistic goals guides care and provides a yardstick by which the patient's progress can be measured. Although the goals developed for individual patients will be specific to their unique needs, some potential goals in the care of respiratory problems for older patients are listed in the Sample Care Plan. Patients and their significant others should be active participants in the development of goals and establishment of priorities. See Chapter 18 for more information on planning and providing care.

Preventing Complications

Often overlooked in the prevention of respiratory problems is the significance of a healthy oral cavity. Infections of the oral cavity can lead to respiratory infections or can decrease appetite and facilitate a general poor health status. Loose, brittle teeth can dislodge or break, leading to lung abscesses and infections. Respiratory infections may decline when loose or diseased teeth are removed.

Once respiratory diseases have developed, close monitoring of the patient's status is required to minimize disability and prevent mortality. Close nursing observation can prevent and detect respiratory complications and should include the following:

- respiratory rate and volume
- pulse (e.g., a sudden increase can indicate hypoxia)
- blood pressure (e.g., elevations can occur with chronic hypoxia)
- temperature (e.g., not only to detect infection but also to prevent stress on the cardiovascular and respiratory systems as they attempt to meet the body's increased oxygen demands imposed by an elevated temperature)
- neck veins (e.g., for distention)
- patency of airway
- coughing (e.g., frequency, depth, productive)
- quality of secretions
- mental status.

Oxygen administration can have serious, even fatal, consequences for older persons and must be used with extreme caution (Fig. 21-1). The gauge should be checked frequently to ensure that it is set at the prescribed level; the oxygen flow should be checked for any interruption or blockage from an empty tank, kinked tubing, or other problem. Nurses should evaluate and recommend the method of administration that will be most effective for the individual patient. Older patients who breathe by mouth or have poor control in keeping their lips sealed most of the time may not receive the full benefit of a nasal cannula. An emaciated person whose facial structure does not allow for a tight seal of a face mask may lose a significant portion of oxygen through leakage. A patient who is insecure and anxious inside an oxygen tent may spend oxygen for emotional stress and not gain full therapeutic benefit. The patient's nasal passages should be regularly cleaned to maintain patency. Indications of insufficient oxygenation must be closely monitored; some older persons will not become cyanotic when hypoxic, so other signs must be evaluated. With increasing numbers of patients being discharged from hospitals on oxygen for home use, and with the realization that many elderly lack capabilities, knowledge, and caregiver support, realistic appraisals of the patient's ability to safely use home oxygen are crucial. Information must be reinforced and supervision through home health agencies or other community resources used until the patient or caregiver is comfortable and competent with this treatment. The home environment must be evaluated for safety. Consideration must be given to the impact of oxygen on the patient's and family's total life-style; whether home oxygen results in the family having a new lease on life or becoming prisoners in their home can be influenced by the assistance and support they are given.

Postural drainage often is prescribed for removing bronchial secretions in certain respiratory conditions. The basic steps for this procedure are the same as those for other adults, with some slight modifications. If aerosol medications are prescribed, they should be administered preceding the postural drainage. The position for postural drainage depends on the individual patient and on the portion of the lung involved. The older patient needs to change positions slowly and be allowed a few minutes to rest between position changes to adjust to the new position. The usual last position for postural drainage—lying face down across the bed with the head at floor level—may be stressful for the older person and have adverse effects. The nurse can consult with the physician as to the ad-

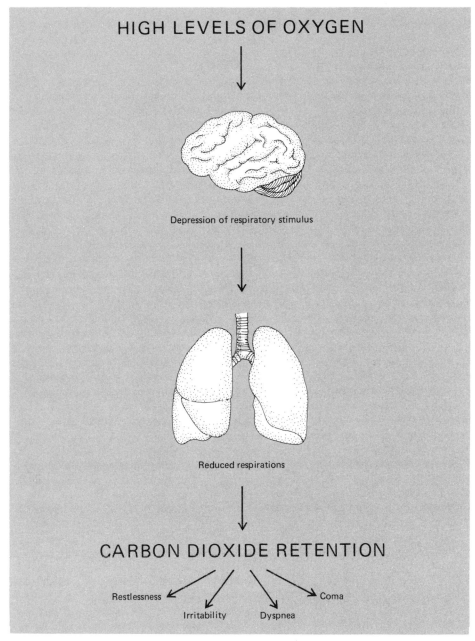

HIGH LEVELS OF OXYGEN

Depression of respiratory stimulus

Reduced respirations

CARBON DIOXIDE RETENTION

Restlessness   Coma

Irritability   Dyspnea

Figure 21-1. *Oxygen must be administered with caution to the aged. High levels of oxygen can depress the respiratory stiumlus in the brain, thereby reducing respiration and promoting carbon dioxide retention.*

visability of this position and possible alterations to meet the needs of the individual patient. Cupping and vibration facilitate drainage of secretions; it must be emphasized that old tissues and bones are more fragile and may be injured more easily. The procedure should be discontinued immediately if dyspnea, palpitation, chest pain, diaphoresis, apprehension, or any other sign of distress occurs. Thorough oral hygiene and a period of rest should follow postural drainage. Documentation of the tolerance of the procedure and the amount and characteristic of the mucus drained is essential.

Coughing to remove secretions is important in the management of respiratory problems; however, nonproductive coughing may be a useless expenditure of energy and stressful to the older patient. Various measures can be used to promote productive coughing. Hard candy and other sweets increase secretions, thereby helping to make the cough productive. The breathing exercises discussed earlier can be beneficial. An intermittent positive-pressure breathing machine may be prescribed, proving especially beneficial to a weak patient or one who will not comply with breathing exercises; bronchodilators may or may not be used with this machine. A variety of humidifiers can be obtained without prescription for home use; the patient needs to be taught the correct, safe use of such apparatus. Expectorants also may be prescribed to loosen secretions and make coughing more productive. A basic, although extremely significant, measure to reinforce is good fluid intake. Patients should be advised to use paper tissues, not cloth handkerchiefs, for sputum expectoration. Frequent hand washing and oral hygiene are essential and have many physical and psychological benefits.

Promoting Self-Care

Bronchodilators may be prescribed in pocket nebulizer form for treatment of bronchial asthma and other conditions causing bronchospasm, such as chronic bronchitis or emphysema. Effective use of these devices depends on the ability of the individual to manipulate the apparatus and coordinate the spray with inhalation—areas that can be problematic for older persons with slower responses, poorer coordination, arthritic joints, or general weakness. Before an inhaler is prescribed, the ability of the patient to use it correctly must be assessed. If the patient is able to manage the skills required for use, instructions and precautions should be reviewed in depth. The patient and caregivers must understand the serious cardiac effects of excessive use. Normally, one or two inhalations are sufficient to relieve symptoms for 4 hours. To ensure that the inhaler does not become empty unexpectedly and leave the person without medication when needed, the fullness of the inhaler should be evaluated periodically by placing it in a bowl of water. When full, the inhaler will sink, and, empty, it will float, with varying levels in between indicating partial levels of fullness.

Not long ago, patients on ventilator support were found in intensive care units of acute hospitals. Today, growing numbers of ventilator-dependent persons are being managed at home or in long-term care facilities. Each ventilator has unique features, and nurses should seek the guidance of a respiratory-care specialist to ensure a thorough understanding and correct use of the equipment. Whether in their own homes or an institutional setting, these patients need strong multidisciplinary support to assist with the complex web of physical, emotional, and social care needs they may present. Nurses can play a significant role in providing a realistic assessment of the abilities of patients and family caregivers to manage ventilator-related care. It makes little sense to use a ventilator to save a patient's life and then threaten that life by sending the person home with a family who cannot meet care needs. Special attention also must be paid to the quality of life of the ventilator-dependent patient; counseling, sensory stimulation, expressive therapies, and other resources should be used.

Polyvalent influenza and pneumococcal vaccines can benefit most elderly persons and are particularly advisable for those with respiratory disease. Patients should be encouraged to discuss these vaccines with their physicians.

Respiratory problems are frightening and produce anxiety. Patients with these conditions require psychological support and reassurance, especially during periods of dyspnea. Patients need a complete understanding of their disease and its management to help reduce their anxiety. Repeated encouragement may be required to assist the patient in meeting the demands of a chronic disease. Some patients may find it necessary to spend most of their time indoors to avoid the ex-

tremes of hot and cold weather; some may have to learn to transport oxygen with them as they travel outside their homes; some may need to move to a different climate for relief. These changes in lifestyle may have a significant impact on their total lives. Groups with information available for respiratory patients are presented in the Resources List. As with any persons having chronic diseases, patients with respiratory problems can benefit from being assisted to live the fullest life possible with their conditions, rather than become prisoners to them.

Sample Care Plan Goals for the Patient With a Respiratory Problem

To have cause of respiratory symptoms and signs diagnosed

To breathe deeply and regularly without distress

To verbalize an understanding of the respiratory problem and its management

To prevent respiratory infection

To increase breathing capacity

To tolerate increased activity without respiratory distress

To possess blood gas levels within a normal range

To correctly self-administer medications prescribed for the treatment and prevention of respiratory problems

To describe the purpose, administration, side-effects, adverse reactions, interactions, and special precautions associated with prescribed respiratory care medications

To describe changes in sputum characteristics that should be reported

To reduce or cease smoking tobacco products

To demonstrate the correct use of oxygen

To identify and promptly report signs and symptoms of a worsening or complication of the respiratory condition

To perform deep breathing exercises at least three times daily

---

Resources to Assist Patients With Respiratory Problems

American Lung Association
1740 Broadway
New York, NY 10019
(212)245-8000

Asthma and Allergy Foundation of America
19 W. 44th St.
New York, NY 10036
(212)921-9100

Emphysema Anonymous
P.O. Box 66
Fort Myers, FL 33902
(813)334-4226

Recommended Readings

Cunha BA, Gingrich D, Rosenbaum GS. Pneumonia syndromes: a clinical approach in the elderly. Geriatrics 1990;45(10):49.

Gleckman RA. Pneumonia: update on diagnosis and treatment. Geriatrics 1991;46(2):49.

Kinzel T. Managing lung disease in late life: a new approach. Geriatrics 1991;46(1):54.

Kovach CR, Shore B. Managing a tuberculosis outbreak. Geriatr Nurs 1991;12(1):29.

Poe RH, Utell MJ. Theophylline in asthma and COPD: changing perspectives and controversies. Geriatrics 1991;46(4):55.

Webster JR, Kadah H. Unique aspects of respiratory disease in the aged. Geriatrics 1991;46(7):31.

22

Gastrointestinal Problems

Significantly fewer older people die from gastrointestinal problems than from diseases of other major body systems; however, these problems often are the source of many complaints and discomforts in this age group. Indigestion, belching, diarrhea, constipation, nausea, vomiting, anorexia, weight gain or loss, and flatulence are among the bothersome problems that increasingly occur, even in the absence of organic cause. Gallbladder disease and various cancers of the gastrointestinal tract increase in incidence in later life. In addition, poor nutrition, medications, emotions, inactivity, and a variety of other factors influence the status of gastrointestinal health.

Aging and the Gastrointestinal System

Every component of the gastrointestinal system is affected by the aging process. At the entrance of this system, age-related changes begin with a drier mucous membrane of the oral cavity. Salivary gland activity is lessened, and the number of taste buds is reduced—particularly those for sweet and salty flavors. Although tooth loss is not a normal consequence of growing old, teeth often are missing; if teeth are present, they frequently are in poor condition, having thinner enamel and being more brittle.

Aspiration poses a greater risk in old age than in younger people. The gag reflex is weaker and food remains in the esophagus for a longer time.

A slight relaxation of the cardiac sphincter may allow food to reenter the esophagus more easily.

Reduced secretion of gastric acids contributes to the high incidence of indigestion. Stomach discomfort is further increased by food remaining in the stomach for an extended time. Although significant changes in the small intestine are not apparent with advanced age, the same cannot be said for the large intestine. Weakened intestinal musculature, decreased peristalsis, and a tendency for incomplete emptying of the bowel at one voiding make elimination-related complaints prevalent.

With advanced age, the liver decreases in size and consequently has reduced storage capacity and protein synthesis, but normally its functional capacity remains within an acceptable range. The gallbladder experiences difficulty with emptying, and bile is of thicker consistency and lesser quantity. The pancreas decreases its production of digestive enzymes and may release insulin in an altered manner that may not be correlated to the level of glucose present. Display 22-1 lists some of the changes that occur in the gastrointestinal system with age.

Assessment

Usually, older adults are aware of their gastrointestinal discomforts and use various measures to manage symptoms of these problems. In some situations, misinformation can interfere with good

DISPLAY 22-1 Age-Related Changes of the Gastrointestinal System

Decreased dentin production

Retraction of gingiva

Shrinkage and fibrosis of root pulp

Loss of bone density in alveolar ridge

Atrophy of taste buds (particularly affecting sweet and salty flavors)

Decrease in amount of saliva and salivary ptyalin produced

Loss of papillae on tongue

Decreased esophageal motility

Weaker gag reflex

Reduced stomach motility and emptying time

Reduced hunger contractions

Atrophy of gastric mucosa

Decreased secretion of hydrochloric acid, pepsin, lipase, pancreatic enzymes

Slower fat absorption

Increased difficulty in absorption of dextrose, xylose, calcium, iron, vitamins B_1 and B_{12}

Atrophy in small and large intestines

Fewer cells on absorbing surface of intestines

Slower peristalsis

Loss of tone of internal anal sphincter

Decreased size of liver

Increased incidence of gallstones

Dilation and distention of pancreatic ducts

gastrointestinal health (*e.g.,* assuming that tooth loss is normal, believing a daily laxative is essential); in other circumstances, self-treatment can delay the diagnosis of pathologies (*e.g.,* using antacids to mask symptoms of stomach cancer). Astute assessment can reveal problems that patients may have omitted sharing with their physicians and identify practices that can interfere with good health.

General Observations

General appearance: pallor can be associated with blood loss from gastrointestinal bleeding. Weakness and fatigue can be due to malnutrition, fluid and electrolyte imbalances, or bleeding. Obesity or unusual thinness should be noted.

Odors: unusual breath odors can be associated with disorders. Halitosis can indicate poor oral hygiene practices, disease of the oral cavity or esophagus, lung abscess or infection, liver disease, or uremia.

Skin: dry, poorly turgored skin can indicate dehydration; scaling, itching, discolored skin, or skin eruptions can result from a variety of nutritional deficiencies.

Interview

Carefully structured questions can reveal hidden problems, particularly in older adults who accept some gastrointestinal symptoms as normal or who have lived with these symptoms for so long that they no longer consider them abnormalities. Questions should review topics such as the following:

Status of teeth or dentures. "When was your last dental exam? How do you care for your teeth/dentures? When did you get your dentures; how do they fit? Do you have any pain, bleeding or other symptoms?"

Taste, appetite. "Does food taste differently to you than it did in the past? What do you do to make food taste better? How is your appetite; how does it compare to earlier years?"

Symptoms. "Do you ever have a sore mouth, difficulty swallowing, choking, a sense that something has 'gone down the wrong hole,' nausea, vomiting, bleeding from your mouth, blood in your vomitus or stool, pain or burning in your stomach or intestines, diarrhea, constipation, bleeding from your rectum?" Specific questions should be asked to explore each positive response.

Weight. "Have you noticed any recent changes in your weight? Have you been trying to gain or lose weight?"

Digestion. "How often do you have indigestion? What seems to cause it and how is it managed? Is there a sense of fullness or discomfort in the chest after meals? Does regurgitation or belching ever occur?"

Elimination. "How often do you have a bowel movement? Do you have to take special measures to move your bowels? If so, what are they? Do you strain to have a bowel movement? Is there ever blood in your stools or on

the toilet tissue? What are the color and consistency of your bowel movements?"

Diet. "Describe what and when you eat in a typical day. Do foods have a different taste to you? Can you shop for and cook meals on your own? Has your eating pattern changed?"

Further questions may be necessary in response to certain problems that emerge through the interview.

Physical Examination

Inspection, auscultation, percussion, and palpation aid in validating problems identified through the interview and detecting undisclosed disorders. A systematic examination of the gastrointestinal system would review the following:

Lips: note symmetry, color, moisture, and general condition. Because capillaries are abundant in the lips, a bluish discoloration could reflect poor oxygenation. Cracks and fissures can be associated with riboflavin deficiencies; jagged teeth or poorly fitting dentures also can be responsible for cuts and cracks on the lips.

Oral cavity: with a tongue depressor and flashlight, inspect the mouth. The mucous membrane should be moist and pink. Black persons may have a pigmented mucosa. Excessive dryness of the mucosa or tongue can indicate dehydration. Note lesions or areas of irritation, which could be caused by teeth, dentures, or pathological conditions. White beads in the oral cavity can be a sign of moniliasis infections and should be cultured. Bleeding, swollen gums are most commonly associated with periodontal disease. Swollen gums also can result from phenytoin therapy or leukemia. Lead poisoning causes a bluish black line along the edge of the gums, but only if teeth are present. Older persons can develop lead poisoning due to occupational exposure or contact within their home environment.

Tongue: examine the top and bottom surface of the tongue. A coating on the tongue can be associated with poor hygiene or dehydration. A smooth, red tongue occurs with iron, vitamin B_{12}, or niacin deficiencies. Thick, white patches can indicate leukoplakia, which could be precancerous. Attention should be given to lesions on the tongue that have been present for several weeks because they can be cancerous; they more frequently occur on the bottom surface than on the top of the tongue. Varicosities on the undersurface of the tongue are not unusual findings.

Pharynx: during normal swallowing, the vagus nerve causes the soft palate to rise and block the nasopharynx so that aspiration is prevented. To test this function, press a tongue depressor on the middle of the tongue, but not so far back that gagging results, and ask the patient to say "ah." The soft palate should rise when "ah" is said. If soreness, redness, or white patches are present in the throat, a culture is warranted.

Abdomen: have the patient lie supine on a firm surface and inspect the abdomen. Have the patient void first. Ask about any scars that are present; the patient may have forgotten to mention an appendectomy that occurred 50 years ago. Striae, or stretch marks, are pink or blue if newly developed and silvery white if old; they can result from obesity, ascites, pregnancy, or tumors. Rashes, indentations, and other findings should be noted. Both sides of the abdomen should be symmetrical with no bulging areas. A symmetrical distention most commonly is due to obesity, although it also can be associated with ascites or tumors. Central, lower-abdominal (*i.e.,* below the umbilicus) distention occurs with bladder distention or tumors of the uterus or ovaries. Central, upper-abdominal distention may result from gastric dilation or pancreatic tumors. The abdomen should rise and fall in conjunction with respirations. Peristaltic activity may be observed; sometimes, gently flicking a finger on the abdomen will stimulate peristalsis. With the diaphragm of the stethoscope, bowel sounds can be heard about once every 5 to 15 seconds; they usually are irregular. If no bowel sounds are heard, try stimulating them by flicking a finger on the abdomen. No sounds for at least 5 minutes can indicate the absence of bowel sounds, and medical evaluation would be warranted. Loud, gurgling sounds indicate increased peristaltic activity.

Palpation of the abdomen should normally reveal no masses.

Rectum: a rectal examination can be performed with the patient in a standing position, bent over the examination table, or in a left lateral position with the right hip and knee flexed. Inspect the perianal area first. Flaccid skin sacs around the anus are hemorrhoids. Fissures, tumors, inflammation, and poor hygienic practices may be noted. Ask the patient to bear down, which could make additional hemorrhoids or rectal prolapse visible. Ask the patient to bear down again and insert a lubricated gloved finger into the anal canal. Assure the patient that it is normal to feel as if a bowel movement is imminent. The sphincter should tighten around the finger. Masses or other abnormalities along the rectal wall should be noted. A hard mass that prevents full palpation of the rectum may be a fecal impaction. Impactions may or may not be movable. If it is a fecal impaction, fecal material will be found on the glove or a discharge will occur when the examining finger is withdrawn.

Stool: a stool specimen should be obtained; fecal material withdrawn during the rectal examination can give clues to problems. Black, tarry stools can be associated with the ingestion of iron preparations or iron-rich foods or can indicate upper gastrointestinal bleeding; bright-red blood accompanies bleeding from the lower bowel or hemorrhoids; pale, fatty stool can occur with absorption problems; gray or tan stool is caused by obstructive jaundice; and mucus in the stool may result from inflammation.

Review of Selected Disorders

Anorexia

Anorexia can be related to a variety of conditions, including medication side-effects, anxiety, depression, inactivity, or physical illness. The initial step in managing this problem is to identify its cause. Treatment could consist of a high-calorie diet, tube feeding, hyperalimentation, psychiatric therapy, or medications, depending on the cause. Intake, output, and weight should be monitored.

Dental Problems

Continued dental care is important throughout an individual's lifetime. Dental examination can be instrumental in the early detection and prevention of many problems that affect other body systems. Poor teeth can restrict food intake, which can cause constipation and malnourishment; they also detract from appearance, which can affect socialization, and this can result in a poor appetite, which also can lead to malnourishment. Periodontal disease can predispose the aged to systemic infection. Although dental care is important in preventing these problems, financial limitations prevent many older persons from seeking dental attention. Some have the misconception that dentures eliminate the need for regular visits to the dentist; others, like many younger persons, fear the dentist. The nurse should encourage regular dental examination and promote dental care, explaining that serious diseases can be detected by the dentist and helping patients find free or inexpensive dental clinics. Understanding how modern dental techniques minimize pain can alleviate fears. Although older persons may not have had the benefit of fluoridated water or fluoride treatments when younger, topical fluoride treatments are as beneficial to the teeth of the aged as they are to younger teeth. Patients should be instructed to inform their dentists about health problems and medications they are taking to help them determine how procedures need to be modified, what healing rate to expect, and which medications cannot be administered.

Dental problems can be caused by altered taste sensation, a poor diet, or a low-budget carbohydrate diet with excessive intake of sweets, which can cause tooth decay. Deficiencies of the vitamin-B complex, hormonal imbalances, hyperparathyroidism, diabetes, osteomalacia, Cushing disease, and syphilis can be underlying causes of dental problems, and certain drugs such as aspirin and phenytoin can play a part. The aging process itself takes its toll on teeth. Surfaces are commonly worn down from many years of use, varying degrees of root absorption occur, and loss of tooth enamel increases the risk of irritation to deeper dental tissue. Although benign neoplastic lesions develop more frequently than malignant ones, cancer of the oral cavity, especially in men, increases in incidence

with age, as does moniliasis, which is often associated with more serious problems such as diabetes or leukemia. It should not be assumed that all white lesions found in the mouth are moniliasis—biopsy is important to make sure they are not cancerous. Periodontal disease, which damages the soft tissue surrounding teeth and supporting bones, is of high incidence among the elderly. Dental caries occur less frequently in older people, but they remain a problem.

Good oral hygiene is especially important to the aged, who already may be having problems with anorexia or food distaste. Teeth, gums, and tongue should be regularly brushed using a soft toothbrush, which also can be used in gentle gum massage for people with dentures. Daily flossing of natural teeth should be performed, and brushing is superior to using swabs, even for the teeth of unconscious patients. Because the buccal mucosa is thinner and less vascular with age, trauma to the oral cavity should be avoided. The nurse should notify the dentist and physician of an atonic or atrophic tongue, lesions, mucosa discoloration, loose teeth, soreness, bleeding, or any other problem identified during inspection and care of the oral cavity.

Esophageal Diverticulum

Dysphagia, gagging, and the regurgitation of undigested food are among symptoms indicating esophageal diverticulum. The accumulation and decomposition of food in the diverticulum may cause the breath to have an extremely foul odor. Difficulty or pain with swallowing can be present, as can coughing caused by irritation and compression of the trachea and a gurgling sound high in the chest. A particularly dangerous complication of this disorder for older people is aspiration, which leads to many serious respiratory problems. A barium swallow confirms the diagnosis. For mild symptoms, treatment consists of a bland diet, small-portioned meals eaten four to six times a day, antacids, and cholinergic-blocking agents. Surgical repair may be performed using a thoracic approach. Close nursing observation is important postoperatively to detect leakage from the esophagus, which could cause the formation of a fistula. Nasogastric feedings are used until the patient can progress to oral feedings.

Hiatal Hernia

The incidence of hiatal hernia increases with age and is of greater incidence in older women. The two types of hiatal hernia are paraesophageal and sliding. In the paraesophageal type, the fundus and greater curvatures of the stomach roll up through the diaphragm; in the sliding type, a part of the stomach and the junction of the stomach and esophagus slide through the diaphragm. Heartburn, dysphagia, belching, vomiting, and regurgitation are common symptoms associated with hiatal hernia. These symptoms are especially problematic when the patient is recumbent. Pain, sometimes mistaken for a coronary attack, and bleeding may occur also. Diagnosis is confirmed by a barium swallow and esophagoscopy. A majority of patients are managed medically. If the patient is obese, weight reduction can minimize the problem. A bland diet may be recommended, as may the use of milk and antacids for symptomatic relief. Several small meals each day rather than three large ones are beneficial in bringing about improvement and may be advantageous to the aged in coping with other age-related gastrointestinal problems. Eating before bedtime should be discouraged. Some patients may find it helpful to sleep in a partly recumbent position.

Cancer of the Esophagus

Most persons affected by cancer of the esophagus are aged. This disease commonly strikes between the ages of 60 and 65 years and is of higher incidence in men, blacks, and alcoholics. Poor oral hygiene and chronic irritation from tobacco, alcohol, and other agents contribute to the development of this problem. Dysphagia, excessive salivation, thirst, hiccups, anemia, and chronic bleeding are symptoms of this disease. Barium swallow, esophagoscopy, and biopsy are performed as diagnostic measures. Treatment consists of an esophagectomy, and a poor prognosis is common among aged patients. Benign tumors of the esophagus are rare in the elderly.

Peptic Ulcer

Although peptic ulcers occur most frequently at younger ages, the incidence of this problem is on the rise for the aged. In addition to stress, diet, and

genetic predisposition as causes, particular factors are believed to account for the increased incidence of ulcers in the aged, including longevity, more precise diagnostic evaluation, and the fact that ulcers can be a complication of chronic obstructive pulmonary disease, which is increasingly prevalent. Drugs commonly prescribed for the elderly that can increase gastric secretions and reduce the resistance of the mucosa include aspirin, reserpine, tolbutamide, phenylbutazone, colchicine, and adrenal corticosteroids.

Early symptoms commonly associated with peptic ulcer may not occur in the older patient. Pain, bleeding, and perforation may be the only indications of this problem. Diagnostic and therapeutic measures resemble those used for younger adults. The nurse should be alert to complications associated with peptic ulcer, which may be especially threatening to the geriatric patient, such as constipation or diarrhea caused by antacid therapy and pyloric obstruction resulting in dehydration, peritonitis, hemorrhage, and shock.

Cancer of the Stomach

Although stomach cancer is of lower incidence in the aged, it is not uncommon. The incidence is greater among men, in patients with pernicious anemia or atrophy of the gastric mucosa, and in persons between the ages of 75 and 85 years. Anorexia, epigastric pain, weight loss, and anemia are symptoms of gastric cancer. Bleeding and enlargement of the liver may occur. Symptoms related to pelvic metastasis may develop also. Diagnosis is confirmed by barium swallow and gastroscopy with biopsy. Surgical treatment consisting of a partial or total gastrectomy is preferred. Unfortunately, the elderly with gastric cancer have a poor prognosis.

Superior Mesenteric Vascular Occlusion

The aged, especially older men, experience superior mesenteric vascular occlusion more frequently than do younger adults. This occlusion usually involves the jejunum and ileum. Congestion, obstruction, peritonitis, and ischemic necrosis can result from this problem and seriously threaten the aged person's life. Pain, vomiting, abdominal distention, and bloody diarrhea are symptoms associated with superior mesenteric vascular occlusion. Surgical intervention, possibly a bowel resection, is used, and the prognosis is not favorable for older adults with this disorder.

Abdominal Angina

Arterial insufficiency may cause the older patient to experience abdominal angina. Upper abdominal pain after meals and while walking, which can be relieved by a recumbent position, are manifestations of this problem. Back pain also may be a symptom. Aortography is used to diagnose abdominal angina. Medical management is preferred and includes a feeding schedule of several small meals instead of three large ones. Sometimes surgical intervention is used to replace the involved artery.

Diverticulosis and Diverticulitis

Multiple pouches of intestinal mucosa in the weakened muscular wall of the large bowel, known as diverticulosis, are common among the elderly. Chronic constipation, obesity, hiatal hernia, and atrophy of the intestinal wall muscles with aging contribute to this problem. Slight bleeding may occur with diverticulosis, and usually a barium enema identifies the problem. Surgery is not performed unless severe bleeding develops. Medical management is most common and includes a bland diet, weight reduction, and avoidance of constipation. Bowel contents can accumulate in the diverticuli and decompose, causing inflammation and infection; this is known as diverticulitis. Although fewer than half the patients with diverticulosis develop diverticulitis, most patients who do are elderly. Older men tend to experience this problem more than any other group.

Overeating, straining during a bowel movement, alcohol, and irritating foods may contribute to diverticulitis in the patient with diverticulosis. Pain in the left lower quadrant, similar to that of appendicitis but over the sigmoid area, is a symptom of this problem. Nausea, vomiting, constipation, diarrhea, low-grade fever, and blood or mucus in the stool may also occur. These attacks can be severely acute or slowly progressing; although the acute attacks can cause peritonitis, the slower forms can also be serious because of the possibility of

lower bowel obstruction resulting from scarring and abscess formation. In addition to the mentioned complications, fistulas to the bladder, vagina, colon, and intestines can develop. During the acute phase, efforts are focused on reducing infection, providing nutrition, relieving discomfort, and promoting rest. Usually nothing is ingested by mouth, and intravenous therapy is used. When the acute episode subsides, the patient is taught to consume a low-residue diet. Surgery, performed if medical management is unsuccessful or if serious complications occur, may consist of a resection or temporary colostomy. Continued follow-up should be encouraged.

Cancer of the Colon

Cancer at any site along the large intestine is common in the elderly and affects both sexes equally. The sigmoid colon and rectum tend to be frequent sites for carcinoma. Bloody stools, a change in bowel function, epigastric pain, jaundice, anorexia, and nausea may be symptoms of this problem, although the pattern of symptoms frequently varies for each person. Some older patients ignore bowel symptoms, believing them to be from constipation, poor diet, or hemorrhoids. The patient's description of bowel problems is less reliable than a digital rectal examination, which detects half of all carcinomas of the large bowel and rectum. The standard diagnostic tests, including barium enema and sigmoidoscopy with biopsy, are used to confirm the diagnosis. Surgical resection with anastomosis or the formation of a colostomy is usually performed. Medical–surgical nursing textbooks can provide information on this surgery, and nurses should consult them for specific guidance on caring for patients with this condition.

It is important to realize that a colostomy can present many problems for the aged. In addition to having to adjust to many bodily changes with age, a colostomy presents a major adjustment and a threat to a good self-concept. The elderly may feel that a colostomy further separates them from society's view of normal. Socialization may be impaired by the patient's concern over the reactions of others or by fear of embarrassing episodes. Reduced energy reserves, arthritic fingers, slower movement, and poorer eyesight are among the problems that may hamper the ability to care for a colostomy, thus causing dependency on others to assist with this procedure. This need for assistance may be perceived as a significant loss of independence for the aged. Tactful, skilled nursing intervention can promote a psychological as well as physical adjustment to a colostomy. Continued follow-up is beneficial to assess the patient's changing ability to engage in this self-care activity, identify problems, and provide ongoing support and reassurance.

Acute Appendicitis

Although acute appendicitis does not occur frequently in aged persons, it is important to note that it can occur and that it may present with altered signs and symptoms. The severe pain that occurs in younger persons may be absent in aged persons, whose pain may be minimal and referred. Fever may be minimal, and leukocytosis may be absent. These differences often cause a delayed diagnosis. Prompt surgery will improve the patient's prognosis. Unfortunately, delayed or missed diagnosis and the inability to improve the general status of the patient before this emergency surgery can lead to greater complications and mortality in older persons with appendicitis.

Chronic Constipation

It is not uncommon for the elderly to be bothered by and concerned about constipation. An inactive life-style, less bulk and fewer fluids in the diet, depression, and laxative abuse contribute to this problem. Certain medications, such as opiates, sedatives, and aluminum hydroxide gels, will promote constipation. Dulled sensations may cause the signal for bowel elimination to be unnoticed, leading to constipation. Not allowing sufficient time for complete emptying of the bowel can also cause constipation. The aged may not fully empty the bowel at one voiding, and it is not unusual for a second bowel movement to be required one-half hour after the initial bowel movement. A diet high in bulk and fluid and regular activity can promote bowel elimination, and particular foods that patients find effective (*e.g.,* prunes, chocolate pudding) can be incorporated into the regular diet. Providing a regular time for bowel elimination is often helpful; mornings tend to be the best time for the elderly to empty their bowels. Sometimes rocking the trunk from side to side and back and forth

while sitting on the toilet will stimulate a bowel movement. Only after these measures have failed should medications be considered.

Older persons may need education concerning bowel elimination. The misconception that daily bowel movements are necessary must be corrected with realistic explanations. Safe use of laxatives should be emphasized to prevent laxative abuse. The patient should be aware that diarrhea resulting from laxative abuse may cause dehydration and be a serious threat to life. The aged in a hospital or nursing home may benefit from a stool chart that reflects the time, amount, and characteristics of bowel movements. This chart can help the nurse prevent constipation and impaction by providing easily accessible data regarding bowel function. Even aged persons in the community can benefit from the use of a stool chart that they can maintain themselves.

Chronic constipation that does not improve with the usual measures may require medical evaluation, including anal, rectal, and sigmoid examinations, to determine the presence of any underlying cause.

Fecal Impaction

Constipation frequently leads to fecal impaction in older adults. The absence or insufficient amount of stool should create suspicion of an impaction. What may appear to be diarrhea may occur as a result of the oozing of liquid feces around the impaction. While taking a rectal temperature, the nurse may detect resistance to the thermometer and find feces on the thermometer when it is withdrawn. A movable mass may be palpated by digital examination. The best approach to fecal impactions is to prevent them from developing; the preventive measures discussed with constipation should be exercised. Once the impaction has developed, it must be softened, broken, and removed.

Because policies may vary, nurses are advised to review the permissive procedures of their employing agency to ensure that removal of a fecal impaction is an acceptable nursing action. An enema, usually oil retention, may be prescribed to assist in the softening and elimination process. Manual breaking and removal of feces with a lubricated gloved finger will promote removal of the impaction. Sometimes, injecting 50 ml hydrogen peroxide through a rectal tube will cause breakage of the impaction as the hydrogen peroxide foams. Care should be taken not to traumatize or overexert the patient during these procedures.

Cancer of the Pancreas

Pancreatic cancer is a difficult disease to detect until it has reached an advanced stage. Anorexia, weakness, weight loss, and wasting are generalized symptoms easily attributed to other causes. Dyspepsia, belching, nausea, vomiting, diarrhea, constipation, and obstructive jaundice may occur as well. Fever may or may not be present. Epigastric pain radiating to the back may be experienced. This pain is relieved when the patient leans forward and is worsened when a recumbent position is assumed. Surgery is performed to treat this problem. Unfortunately, the disease is generally so advanced by the time diagnosis is made that the prognosis is usually poor.

Biliary Tract Disease

The incidence of gallstones increases with age and affects women more frequently than men. Pain is the primary symptom associated with this problem. Treatment measures include nonsurgical therapies, such as rotary lithotrite treatment and extracorporeal shock wave lithotripsy, and the standard surgical procedures. Obstruction, inflammation, and infection are potential outcomes of gallstones and should be monitored. Cancer of the gallbladder primarily affects older persons, especially women. Fortunately, this disease does not occur frequently. Pain in the right upper quadrant, anorexia, nausea, vomiting, weight loss, jaundice, weakness, and constipation are the usual symptoms. Although surgery may be performed, the prognosis for the patient with cancer of the gallbladder is poor.

General Nursing Interventions Related to Gastrointestinal Problems
Facilitating Gastrointestinal Health

A variety of gastrointestinal problems can be avoided by good health practices. Good dental hygiene and regular visits to the dentist can prevent

disorders that can threaten nutritional intake, general health, comfort, and self-image. The proper quantity and quality of foods can enhance general health and minimize the risks of indigestion and constipation. Refer to Chapter 9 for more specific information on ways to promote nutritional health. Knowledge of the relationship of medications to gastrointestinal health is important.

Care Planning

Actual or potential problems can be revealed during the assessment of the gastrointestinal system. Assessment data should be reviewed for those problems that fall within the realm of nursing to diagnose and manage, and related nursing diagnoses should be developed accordingly. Table 22-1 lists some of the major nursing diagnoses that can be related to gastrointestinal disorders.

The development of realistic goals guides care and provides a yardstick by which the patient's progress can be measured. Although the goals developed for individual patients will be specific to their unique needs, some potential goals in the care of gastrointestinal problems in older adults

are listed in the Sample Care Plan. Patients and their significant others should be active participants in the development of goals and establishment of priorities. See Chapter 18 for more information on planning and providing care.

Gavage Feeding

Gavage feedings may be required to supply nutrition for some older persons. When feeding the patient in this manner and instructing other caregivers how to gavage feed, the following points must be remembered:

Place the patient in a high Fowler position and have the patient remain in this position for at least 20 minutes after the feeding.

Check that the tube is in the stomach. This is accomplished by aspirating some of the gastric contents with a syringe, placing a stethoscope over the stomach and listening for a swishing sound as 5 ml to 10 ml of air is injected into the tube, and placing the end of the tube in a glass of water and noting air bubbles that correspond to respirations, indicating that the tube is in the lungs.

Table 22-1 *Nursing Diagnoses Related to Gastrointestinal Problems*

NURSING DIAGNOSIS	CAUSE OR CONTRIBUTING FACTOR
Activity intolerance	Anemia, constipation, obesity, vitamin and mineral deficiencies, dehydration
Altered bowel elimination: constipation	Anorexia, obesity, hemorrhoids, lack of roughage in diet, dehydration, habitual laxative use
Altered bowel elimination: diarrhea	Medications, peptic ulcer, gastritis, ulcerative colitis, diverticulitis, diabetes, fecal impaction, tube feedings, stress
Pain	Indigestion, constipation, hemorrhoids, flatus
Fluid volume deficit	Uncontrolled diabetes, infection, peritonitis, diarrhea, vomiting, blood loss, insufficient fluid intake, high-solute tube feedings
High risk for infection	Diabetes, malnutrition, hemorrhoids
Altered nutrition: less than body requirements	Intestinal obstruction, anorexia, nausea, vomiting, poor dental status, altered taste sensations, constipation
Altered nutrition: more than body requirements	Altered taste sensations, ethnic preferences, inactivity, lack of motivation to eat well
Altered oral mucous membrane	Diabetes, cancer, gingivitis, periodontal disease, jagged teeth, poorly fitting dentures, dehydration, malnutrition

Administer the feeding with a slow, steady flow, keeping the reservoir at the level of the patient's nose.

Stay with the patient through the entire feeding. Allowing the feeding to flow in unattended could lead to serious complications and death.

Discontinue the feeding immediately if dyspnea, coughing, cyanosis, or other unusual signs develop.

Clamp the tube immediately after the feeding to prevent the entry of air into the stomach.

Figure 22-1 demonstrates the proper way to anchor the nasogastric tube to the patient's face. The tube is not to be pulled and taped to the side of the nose; this causes the tube within the nasal passage to place pressure on the nasal mucosa, predisposing the elderly's fragile skin to break down in that area. Sometimes, applying a small amount of lubricant in the nostril will prevent irritation. The nostrils are to be cleansed and kept patent. Gentle manipulation with a cotton-tipped applicator can be effective in removing dried crusts and preventing any interference with breathing. Frequent oral hygiene also is essential.

In some chronic care settings, the older patient may be receiving gastric feedings over a long period of time. Special attention must be paid to the development of complications associated with prolonged use of a nasogastric tube, including respiratory infection, ulceration anywhere along the area in which the tube is located—especially the nasal and gastric mucosa, sinusitis, and esophagitis. Regular assessment of the continued need for feeding in this fashion is an important nursing measure. At no time should tube feeding be used as a faster, easier way to feed an older patient.

Gastrointestinal symptoms, although common, can indicate serious medical problems and need to be taken seriously. The diagnosis of these problems can be difficult because of atypical symptomatology and easy confusion with disorders of other systems. Therefore, the nurse can add as much information as possible to the patient's history to increase the likelihood of prompt, appropriate treatment.

Some of the available resources to assist patients with gastrointestinal problems are presented in the Resource List.

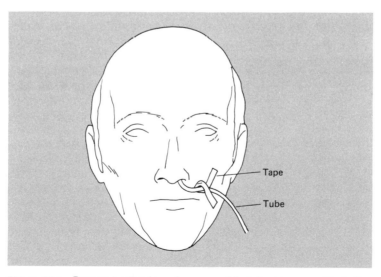

Figure 22-1. *Proper anchoring of nasogastric tube to prevent irritation and breakdown of the nasal mucosa.*

Sample Care Plan Goals for the Patient With a Gastrointestinal Problem

To ingest a well balanced diet that meets daily nutritional requirements

To maintain weight within predetermined range

To increase or decrease weight to specified level

To identify and avoid foods that cause gastrointestinal discomfort

To demonstrate good oral hygiene practices

To be evaluated by a dentist annually

To be free from symptoms of indigestion

To regularly eliminate normal consistent stool without straining or discomfort

To substitute laxative or enema with natural measures to facilitate bowel movement

To have cause of gastrointestinal symptoms and signs diagnosed

To verbalize understanding of the gastrointestinal problem and its management

To possess fluid and electrolyte balance

To describe the purpose, administration, side-effects, adverse reactions, interactions and special precautions associated with prescribed gastrointestinal medications

To correctly self-administer gastrointestinal medications

To describe and identify signs and symptoms that indicate changes in gastrointestinal status

Resources to Assist Patients With Gastrointestinal Problems

National Foundation for Ileitis and Colitis
295 Madison Avenue
New York, NY 10017
(212)685-3440

United Ostomy Association
2001 W. Beverly Blvd.
Los Angeles, CA 90057
(213)413-5510

Recommended Readings

Freston MS, Freston JW. Peptic ulcer in the elderly: unique features and management. Geriatrics 1990;45(1):39.

Henderson CT. Safe and effective tube feeding of bedridden elderly. Geriatrics 1991;46(8):56.

Kayser-Jones J. The use of nasogastric feeding tubes in nursing homes: patient, family and health care provider perspectives. Gerontologist 1990;30:469.

Morley JE. Anorexia in older patients: its meaning and management. Geriatrics 1990;45(12):59.

Yen PK. The picture of malnutrition. Geriatr Nurs 1989; 10(3):159.

23

Diabetes

A proficient blend of various kinds of knowledge and skills is required in caring for diabetic patients; older ones, with their unique set of problems, present an even greater challenge. Diabetes, the seventh leading cause of death among the aged, has a particularly high prevalence among blacks and people 65 to 74 years of age. Consequently, nurses must be adequately informed of how the detection and management of diabetes in aged persons differs from that in other age groups. The increasing number of individuals attaining old age and the expanding health-care services for the aged further emphasize the necessity for nurses to be prepared to meet the needs of older diabetic individuals.

Assessment

Approximately 50% of the elderly have a problem with glucose intolerance. Several explanations are offered for the high prevalence of hyperglycemia among the aged. Research has shown that a physiological deterioration of glucose tolerance occurs with increasing age. Diagnostic techniques are improved. Also, some believe that the high prevalence of glucose intolerance is a result of an increase in the incidence of diabetes throughout the general population. Regardless of the reason, it is agreed that different standards must be applied in evaluating glucose tolerance in the elderly.

Early diagnosis of diabetes in older persons is often difficult. The classic symptoms of diabetes may be absent, leaving nonspecific symptoms as the only clues. Some indications of diabetes in the elderly include orthostatic hypotension, stroke, gastric hypotony, impotence, neuropathy, confusion glaucoma, Dupuytren contracture, and infection. Laboratory tests, as well as symptoms, may be misleading. Because the renal threshold for glucose increases with age, older individuals can be hyperglycemic without evidence of glycosuria, thus limiting the validity of urine testing for glucose.

Among all the diagnostic measures, the glucose tolerance test is the most effective. To avoid a false-positive diagnosis, more than one test should be performed. The American Diabetes Association recommends that a minimum of 150 g carbohydrate be ingested daily for several days before the test; older malnourished individuals may be prescribed 300 g. Recent periods of inactivity, stressful illness, and inadequate dietary intake should be communicated to the physician, because these situations can contribute to glucose intolerance. In such circumstances, more accurate results can be obtained if the test is postponed for a month after the episode. Nicotinic acid, ethacrynic acid, estrogen, furosemide, and diuretics can decrease glucose tolerance and should not be administered before testing. Monoamine oxidase inhibitors (MAOIs), propranolol, and high dosages of salicylates may lower blood sugar levels and also interfere with testing.

Usual nursing measures are applied during glucose tolerance testing of the aged. If unusual symptoms, such as confusion, develop during the test, it is important to tell the physician. Those interpreting the glucose tolerance test may find it beneficial

to use age-related gradients. For each decade after age 55 years, 10 mg/dl is added to the standard values at the first, second, and third hours. Thus, a glucose level that would be significantly elevated for a 35-year-old may be within normal limits for an 85-year-old.

The diagnosis of diabetes usually is established if one of three criteria exist:(Davidson, 1990)

1. Random plasma glucose concentrations are ≥200 mg/dl
2. Fasting blood glucose concentrations are ≥140 mg/dl
3. Plasma glucose concentrations after oral glucose intake are ≥ 200 mg/dl.

General Nursing Interventions for the Patient With Diabetes

Care Planning

Although the basic principles of diabetic management are applicable to all age groups, special considerations and adjustments must be made for the older diabetic patient. It is impractical and unrealistic to expect that individuals who have established specific practices over the past six or seven decades will drastically alter their life-styles when diagnosed with diabetes. Many compromises may be required by the diabetic individual and the professionals managing the patient's care.

While assessing and caring for diabetic patients, problems that fall within the realm of nursing to diagnose and manage should be identified, and nursing diagnoses developed accordingly (Table 23-1). Goals are then developed to assist the patient in the management of the illness, prevention of complications, and achievement of a satisfactory lifestyle. The development of realistic goals guides care and provides a yardstick by which progress can be measured. Although the goals developed for individual patients will be specific to their unique needs, some possible goals for the diabetic patient are listed in the Sample Care Plan. Patients and significant others should be active participants in the development of goals and establishment of priorities. See Chapter 18 for more information on planning and providing care.

Table 23-1 *Nursing Diagnoses Related to Diabetes Mellitus*

NURSING DIAGNOSIS	CAUSES OR CONTRIBUTING FACTORS
Anxiety	Fear of disease's impact
Fear	High risk loss of body part or function
High risk for infection	Hyperglycemia
High risk for injury	Decreased sensations, confusion, or dizziness from hypoglycemia
Knowledge deficit	Diagnostic tests, care demands, denial
Noncompliance	Lack of knowledge, self-care limitation
Altered nutrition: less than body requirements	Insufficient calories to meet energy, insulin demands
Altered nutrition: more than body requirements	Caloric intake in excess of energy, insulin coverage
Powerlessness	Inability to meet therapeutic demands
Sensory–perceptual alterations	Peripheral neuropathies, retinopathy
Sexual dysfunction	Peripheral neuropathy, vaginitis
Impaired skin integrity	Susceptibility to fungal infections, pruritus from hyperglycemia
Sleep pattern disturbance	Urinary frequency
Altered tissue perfusion	Altered neurovascular function secondary to neuropathies

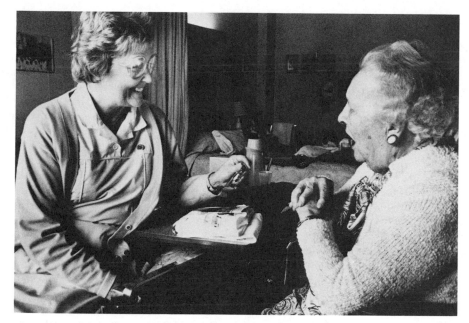

Figure 23-1. *The teaching–learning process is highly individualized. (Photograph by Eric Schenk.)*

Educating the Older Diabetic Patient

Once the diagnosis has been confirmed, a teaching plan should be established by the nurse (Fig. 23-1). Diabetes is known as a serious and chronic problem to most lay individuals, and it is frightening to have it diagnosed. Fear and anxiety can interfere with the learning process for newly diagnosed older diabetic patients, who may have witnessed the crippling or fatal effects of diabetes in others and anticipate such occurrences in themselves. Having lived through a period in which diabetes was not successfully managed and was always severely disabling or fatal, the older individual may not be aware of the advances in diabetic management. Insulin was isolated in 1921, when many of today's elderly were children and young adults.

Elderly people may be depressed or angry that this disease further threatens to decrease the remaining period of their lives; they may question the trade-off value in exchanging an unrestricted life-style for a potentially longer but restricted one. Concerns may arise as to how a special diet and medications will be afforded on an already limited budget. Social isolation may develop from fear of becoming ill in public or facing restrictions that make them different from their peers. They may question their ability to manage their diabetes independently and worry that institutionalization will be necessary. These and a multitude of other concerns that the older diabetic patient may have must be recognized and dealt with by the nurse to reduce the risk of other limitations and promote the individual's self-care capacities. Reassurance, support, and information can reduce barriers to learning about and managing diabetes. The steps described in Display 23-1, helpful in any patient education situation, may offer guidance in teaching the older diabetic patient.

Monitoring Health Status

One factor that must be considered in the management of the older diabetic person is the ability of the patient to handle a syringe and vial of insulin. Several return demonstrations of this skill should be performed during the hospitalization, especially on days in which arthritis discomfort is present. Because most elderly persons have some degree of visual impairment, the ability to read the calibrations on an insulin syringe must be evaluated. The yellowing of the lens with age tends to

DISPLAY 23-1   *Patient Education Guidelines*

Assess Readiness to Learn. Discomfort, anxiety and depression may block learning and the retention of knowledge. Relieving these symptoms and allowing time for patients to develop to the point where they desire and can hope with information may be necessary.

Assess Learning Capacities and Limitations. This includes consideration of educational level, language problems, literacy, present knowledge, willingness to learn, cultural background, previous experience with the illness, memory, vision, hearing, speech, and mental status.

Outline Content of Presentation. Your outline should not only be specific and clear but should also consider learning priorities. Nurses sometimes feel obligated to teach every detail about an illness, condensing a multitude of new facts and procedures into a short time frame. Most people need time to receive, absorb, sort, and translate new information into behavioral changes; the elderly are no different. Altered cerebral function or slower responses may further interfere with learning in the aged. Patients and their families should have a role in setting teaching priorities; the most vital information should be given first, followed by other relevant material. Visiting nurses and other resources should be used after hospital discharge to continue the teaching plan if the proposed outline is not completed during the hospitalization.

Alter the Teaching Plan in View of Capacities and Limitations. The nurse may feel that an explanation of the physiological effects of diabetes is significant for new diabetics. However, the older person who tends to be confused or has a poor memory may not have long-range benefit from this type of information. It may be better to use that time to reinforce diet information or to make sure the most significant information required for self-care is retained.

Prepare the Patient for the Teaching–Learning Session. Patients should understand that education is an integral part of care. Whenever possible, a specific time should be arranged in advance to avoid conflict with other activities and to allow the family to be present if desired.

Provide Environment Conducive to Learning. An area that is quiet, clean, relaxing, and free from odors and interference will help to create a good atmosphere for learning. Distraction should be minimal, especially in view of the aged's reduced capacity to manage multiple stimuli.

Use the Most Effective Individualized Educational Material. The nurse must recognize the limitations of standard teaching aids and the importance of individualized methods. An aid that was successful for one person may not be effective for another. The variety of sophisticated audiovisual aids that are commercially prepared and available in many agencies as resources for nurses are impressive, but they may not necessarily be effective for the given patient. The quality of an audio cassette may be excellent, but it is of little benefit to the older person with a hearing problem. A slide presentation, even slowly paced, may present facts more rapidly than can be absorbed by an older person with delayed response time. The print on a commercial pamphlet may appear minute to older eyes. The language used in many commercial materials may not be one to which the person is accustomed. Original handmade aids suited for the individual's unique needs may have a value equal to or greater than commercially prepared ones. Selectivity in methodology is essential.

Use Several Approaches to the Same Body of Knowledge. The greater the number of different exposures to new material, the higher the probability that the material will be learned. Combine verbal explanation with flipcharts, diagrams, pamphlets, demonstrations, discussions with other patients, and audiovisual resources.

Leave Material With the Patient for Later Review. Often, it is helpful to summarize the teaching session in writing, using language familiar to the patient. This provides concrete material that the patient can review independently later and share with the family.

Reinforce Key Points. Reinforcement should be regular and consistent, with all staff members supporting the teaching plan. For example, if the objective of the nurse caring for the patient has been to increase competency in self-injection of insulin, then the person substituting on the nurse's day off should comply with the established objectives rather than administering the

insulin for the individual. Informal reinforcement of information during other daily activities should also be planned.

Obtain Feedback. Evaluate whether the patient and family have accurately received and understood the information communicated. This can be done by observing return demonstrations, asking questions, and listening to discussions among patients.

Reevaluate Periodically. To ascertain retention and effectiveness of the teaching sessions, informally reevaluate at a later time. Remember that retention of information may be especially difficult for the older individual.

Document. Describe specifically what was taught, when, who was involved, what methodology was used, the patient's reaction and understanding, and future plans for remaining learning needs. This assists the staff caring for patients during their hospitalization and serves as a guide for those providing continued care after discharge.

filter out low-tone colors such as blues and greens; because these colors are frequently used to identify various levels of glycosuria in urine testing kits, it is important to assess the older individual's ability to discriminate between these shades. Older people may also be limited in their ability to purchase and prepare adequate meals because of financial, energy, or social limitations. This can interfere with management of the illness. Meals on Wheels, food stamps, the assistance of a neighbor, and other appropriate resources should be used to assist the individual.

Altered tubule reabsorption of glucose may lead to inaccurate results from urine testing. As mentioned, the older individual can be hyperglycemic without being glycosuric. On the other hand, higher blood glucose levels are common in the aged, and minimal or mild glycosuria usually is not treated with insulin. Although nurses are not responsible for prescribing insulin coverage, they need to be aware that the insulin requirements of the older diabetic patients are individualized. Responses to various insulin levels are to be carefully observed and communicated to the physician. Table 23-2 reviews the various insulins that may be prescribed. Because insulins are selected not only for their timing but for their specific tolerance by the patient, the nurse must be careful to administer the correct type of insulin prescribed. Patients must understand that they cannot borrow a vial

Table 23-2 *Insulins Used in the Management of Diabetes Mellitus*

TYPES OF INSULIN	ONSET OF ACTION	PEAK	DURATION
Fast-acting			
Injection: Regular, unmodified	20–30 min	1–2 h	5–8 h
Zinc suspension: prompt, crystalline (semilente)	50–60 min	2–3 h	6–8 h
Medium-acting			
Globin, with zinc	1–2 h	8–16 h	18–24 h
Isophane suspension (NPH)	1–2 h	10–20 h	28–30 h
Zinc suspension (lente)	1–2 h	10–20 h	20–32 h
Long-acting			
Zinc suspension, extended (ultralente)	4–6 h	16–24 h	24–36 h
Protamine zinc suspension (protamine zinc)	4–6 h	16–24 h	24–36 h

of insulin from a friend if their own supply is exhausted.

Many diabetic patients must perform blood glucose level testing using a finger-prick method. Patients must be instructed in this technique and successfully demonstrate competency in performing this procedure. The finger-prick technique will most likely be replaced in the near future by an infrared device that determines blood glucose level by measuring how light is absorbed by the body. The patient sticks a finger into a small meter that shines an infrared light through the skin. The infrared method of glucose testing should make glucose testing more convenient and pain-free for diabetic persons.

Regular exercise is important for older diabetic patients and provides multiple health benefits. Physical activity can improve the patient's response to insulin during the period in which the exercise regimen is done if the exercise is sufficient to lower the resting heart rate. In the diabetic individual, however, a vigorous exercise program or changes in an exercise program must be reviewed with the physician to prevent adverse consequences. For example, moderate to vigorous exercise increases the absorption of insulin and heightens the use of glucose by the exercising muscles, potentially leading to hypoglycemia.

Attempts should be made to maintain a consistent daily food intake because the insulin dosage is prescribed to cover a specific amount of food. This may be a problem if the elderly person has a minimal food intake during the week when alone but an increased intake when visiting with family on weekends, or if the patient skimps on meals when financial resources are low. Sociological and psychological factors can influence consistent food intake as much as physical factors. The nurse and physician must carefully assess, plan, and manage insulin needs in view of the individual's unique problems and life-style. Special attention must also be paid to the aged in a hospital or nursing home setting to ensure that food intake is regular and adequate.

At times, oral agents are prescribed for the elderly diabetic patient. Chlorpropamide is an oral hypoglycemic agent with approximately six times the potency of tolbutamide. It is readily absorbed in the gastrointestinal tract, reaching its maximum level in 2 to 4 hours, and is slowly excreted in the urine. The biological half-life of chlorpropamide is normally 36 hours, with most of the dose excreted within 96 hours. Chlorpropamide is contraindicated in individuals with severe impairment of hepatic, renal, or thyroid function. This drug can prolong the action of barbiturates, a consideration for gerontological nurses because elderly patients may be receiving both medications. Close nursing observation is essential when patients receiving oral hypoglycemic agents are prescribed antibacterial sulfonamides, phenylbutazone, salicylates, probenecid, dicumarol, or MAOIs, because these drugs can potentiate a hypoglycemic reaction. Chlorpropamide may cause an exaggerated hypoglycemic effect in individuals with Addison disease.

If hypoglycemia occurs in the patient receiving chlorpropamide, it could be prolonged. A slightly higher blood glucose level is considered acceptable for adequate functioning in the aged; therefore, the nurse should note and communicate to the physician observations indicating dysfunction from a reduced blood sugar level. A higher than normal glucose level may promote optimum function in a given individual. Adverse reactions to chlorpropamide include pruritus, rash, jaundice, dark-colored urine, light-colored stools, diarrhea, low-grade fever, and sore throat. Tolbutamide, acetohexamide, tolazamide, and phenformin are among the other oral hypoglycemic agents that may be prescribed. Suggestions, special precautions, and adverse reactions for these drugs resemble those mentioned with chlorpropamide.

Some individuals only need oral hypoglycemic agents to control their diabetes. Those on insulin therapy who have lost weight or have not been ketoacidotic may have their insulin substituted by oral hypoglycemic agents. Still others will need periodic changes in their insulin dosages to meet changing demands. These factors, combined with other management difficulties in the older diabetic person, necessitate frequent reevaluation of the patient's status. The continuation of health supervision is an essential part of diabetic management.

Preventing Complications

The elderly are subject to a long list of complications from diabetes and have a greater risk of developing these complications than younger adults. Hypoglycemia seems to be a greater threat to older diabetic patients than ketoacidosis, and this is especially problematic because of the possible presentation of a different set of symptoms. Classic symptoms such as tachycardia, restlessness, per-

spiration, and anxiety may be totally absent in the older individual with hypoglycemia. Instead, any of the following may be the first indication of the problem: behavior disorders, convulsions, somnolence, confusion, disorientation, poor sleep patterns, nocturnal headache, slurred speech, and unconsciousness. Uncorrected hypoglycemia can cause tachycardia, arrhythmias, myocardial infarctions, cerebrovascular accident, and death.

Peripheral vascular disease is a common complication in the older diabetic individual, and is influenced by the poorer circulation and atherosclerosis often associated with increased age. Symptoms may range from numbness and weak pulses to infection and gangrene. The nurse should identify and promptly communicate to the physician symptoms of peripheral vascular disease. Educating the patient in proper foot care can help reduce the risk of this problem; referral to a podiatrist also can prove beneficial.

Another significant vascular problem of older diabetic patients is retinopathy with consequent blindness. More than 25% of diabetic persons older than age 75 years are likely to have some degree of retinopathy.(Sherman, 1991) Individuals who are hypertensive or who have had diabetes for a long time have a greater risk of developing this complication. Hemorrhage, pigment disturbances, edema, and visual disorders are manifested with this problem.

Drug interactions can be a major source of complications for older diabetic patients. Some research has revealed that in a given month more than 50% of diabetic patients had taken between one to five drugs that had the potential to interact with their antidiabetic therapy.(Sherman, 1991) Nurses should review all medications the patient is taking to identify those drugs that may interact with antidiabetic medications. See Chapter 35 for a full discussion of antidiabetic drugs and those medications that interact with them.

A variety of additional complications can affect older diabetic individuals. Cognitive impairment is greater among elderly people with type II diabetes mellitus than in nondiabetic persons.(U'Ren et al, 1990) Older persons may develop neuropathies, demonstrated through tingling sensations progressing to stinging or stabbing pain; carpal tunnel syndrome; paresthesias; nocturnal diarrhea; tachycardia; and postural hypotension. They have twice the mortality rate from coronary artery disease and cerebral arteriosclerosis, and a higher incidence of urinary tract infections. There is a higher risk of problems developing with virtually every body system. Early detection of complications is essential and can be facilitated by nursing intervention and patient education. Competent management of the older diabetic patient is a vital activity that requires great skill and poses a great challenge and responsibility to the practice of nursing. The recognition of differences in symptomatology, diagnosis, management, and complications is crucial. Resources of benefit to patients with diabetes are presented in the Resource List.

Sample Care Plan Goals for the Patient With Diabetes

To verbalize understanding of diabetes and its management

To demonstrate proper technique for administration of antidiabetic medication

To demonstrate correct method of blood glucose testing

To be free from signs of hypoglycemia and hyperglycemia

To describe signs and symptoms of hypoglycemia and insulin shock

To adapt management of diabetes to life style

To maintain weight at appropriate level or to lose specified amount

To engage in a regular exercise program

To be free from injury

To be free from infection

To be free from impairments in skin integrity

To be free from complications associated with diabetes

Resources to Assist Patients With Diabetes

American Diabetes Association
2 Park Avenue
New York, NY 10016
(212)683-7444

Diabetes Education Center
4959 Excelsior Blvd.
Minneapolis, MN 55416
(612)927-3393

References

Davidson MB. Carbohydrate metabolism and diabetes mellitus. In: Abrams WB, Berkow R, eds. The Merck manual of geriatrics. Rahway, NJ: Merck Sharp & Dohme Research Laboratories, 1990:793.

Sherman D. Diabetes mellitus: complications in treatment. Contemporary Long-Term Care 1991;14(7):79.

U'Ren RC, et al. The mental efficiency of the elderly person with type II diabetes mellitus. J Am Geriatr Soc 1990;38:505.

Recommended Readings

Cohen JA, Gross KF. Autonomic neuropathy: clinical presentation and differential diagnosis. Geriatrics 1990; 45(7):33.

Dere WH, Groggel GC. Update on diabetic nephropathy in NIDDM. Geriatrics 1990;45(7):48.

Fukagawa NK, Minaker KL, Rowe JW, Matthews DE, Bier DM, Young VR. Glucose and amino acid metabolism in aging man: differential effects of insulin. Metabolism 1988; 37:371.

Jackson RA, Hawa MI, Roshania RD, Sim BM, DiSilvio L, Jaspan JB. Influence of aging on hepatic and peripheral glucose metabolism in humans. Diabetes 1988;37:119.

Kane RL, Ouslander JG, Abrass IB. Essentials of clinical geriatrics. 2nd ed. New York: McGraw-Hill, 1989:271.

Leichter SB, Schaffer JC, O'Brien JT. New concepts in managing diabetic foot infections. Geriatrics 1991;46(5):24.

Riddle MD. Diabetic neuropathies in the elderly: management update. Geriatrics 1990;45(9):32.

Walter RM. Hypoglycemia: still a risk in the elderly. Geriatrics 1990;45(3):69.

Yen PK. Following the diabetic diet. Geriatr Nurs 1990; 11(6):303.

24

Musculoskeletal Problems

It is the rare older individual who does not experience some degree of discomfort, disability, or deformity from musculoskeletal disorders. Stiff and aching joints, muscle cramps, reduced range of motion, and greater ease of fracturing bones are challenges that must be confronted in the elderly. Because activity and mobility are vital to the total health of older adults, musculoskeletal problems that limit functional capacity can have devastating effects. Prevention of these problems and aggressive intervention to minimize their impact if they are present should be integral parts of gerontological nursing care.

Aging and the Musculoskeletal System

Loss of bone minerals and mass occurs throughout life, causing the skeletal structure to become brittle and weak. The vertebrae are less firm and the vertebral column may compress or bow. Shortening of the vertebral column contributes to the general reduction in height. The cartilage deteriorates, most notably at the weight-bearing joints, and bone formation at the joint surface declines. Some decrease in the range of joint motion may be evident.

Muscle fibers progressively decrease in number and bulk with age, which is evident in the flabby, thin muscles of the arms and legs of many older people. Muscle strength, endurance, and agility decline. Muscle movements and tendon jerks are reduced. Muscles may take longer to contract because of a slowing of impulse conduction along the motor units, especially at the distal regions of the axon. A decrease in oxidate activity results from a reduction in glycolytic enzymes, causing the muscles to fatigue more easily and to require more rest. Muscle tremors may occur, even during resting states. Display 24-1 lists some of the changes to the musculoskeletal system that occur with age.

Assessment

In assessing the musculoskeletal system, function and pain are the major areas to consider. A head-to-toe review is essential to identify problems.

General Observation

Assessment of the musculoskeletal system can begin even before the formal examination by noting the patient's actions, such as transfer activities, ambulation, and use of hands. Observations that should be noted include the following:

- abnormal gait (Table 24-1)
- abnormality of structure
- dysfunction of a limb
- favoring of one side
- paralysis
- weakness
- atrophy of a limb
- redness, swelling of a joint
- use of cane, walker, wheelchair.

Interview

Although it may seem tedious, it is best to go from head to toe and question the patient about limited function or discomfort in specific parts of the body. Examples of questions could include the following:

"Does your jaw ever get stiff or hurt when you chew?"

"Do you get a stiff neck?"

"Does your shoulder ever tighten?"

"Do your hips hurt after you have walked for a while?"

"Are your joints stiff in the morning?"

"Do you have muscle cramps?"

"How far are you able to walk?"

"Are you able to take care of your home, get in and out of a bathtub, and climb stairs?"

Specific inquiry should be made into how the patient manages musculoskeletal pain, particularly in reference to the use of analgesics, heat, and topical preparations.

Physical Examination

The active and passive range of motion of all joints should be examined. Note the degree of movement with and without assistance. Specific areas to review include the following:

Shoulder: the patient should be able to lift both arms straight above the head. With arms straight at the sides, the patient should be able to lift them laterally above the head (*i.e.,* 180°) with hands supine and 110° with hands prone. The patient should be able to extend the arms 30° behind the body from the sides.

Neck: the patient should be able to turn the head laterally and to flex and extend the head approximately 30° in all directions.

Elbow: the patient should be able to open the arms fully and flex the joint enough to allow the hand to touch the shoulder.

DISPLAY 24-1   Age-Related Changes of the Musculoskeletal System

Decrease and atrophy of muscle fibers
Fibrous tissue replaces muscle tissue
Decrease in muscle mass, strength, movements
Reduction in bone mass and mineral content
Thinning of vertebral disks

Table 24-1 *Gait Disturbances*

GAIT PATTERN	ASSOCIATED DISORDER
Ataxic Unsteady, uncoordinated, feet raised high while stepping and then dropped flat on floor Intoxication	Cerebellum disease
Foot-slapping Wide based, feet raised high while stepping and then slapped down against floor, no staggering or weaving	Lower motor neuron disease Paralysis of pretibial and peroneal muscles
Hemiplegic Unilateral footdrop and foot dragging, leg circumducted, arm flexed and held close to side	Unilateral upper motor neuron disease
Parkinsonian Trunk leans forward, slight flexion of hip and knees, no arm swing while stepping, short and shuffling steps, starts slowly and then increases in speed	Parkinsonism
Scissors Slow, short steps; legs cross while stepping	Spastic paraplegia Dementia Cerebral palsy
Spastic Uncoordinated, jerking gait; legs stiff; toes drag	Spastic paraplegia Spinal cord tumor Multiple sclerosis

Wrist: the patient should be able to bend the wrist 80° in the palmar direction and 70° in the dorsal direction. With a hand-waving motion, the patient should be able to bend the wrist laterally 10° toward the radial or thumb side and 60° in the direction of the ulnar side. The patient should be able to move the hand to 90° in the prone and supine positions.

Finger: the patient should be able to bend the distal joint of the finger approximately 45° and the proximal joint 90°. Hyperextension of 30° should be possible.

Hip: while lying down, the patient should be able to abduct and adduct the leg 45°. With the patient lying on his back, the leg should be able to be lifted 90° with the knee straight and 125° with the knee bent.

Knee: while lying on the stomach, the patient should be able to flex the knee approximately 100°.

Ankle: the patient should be able to point the toes 10° toward the head and 40° toward the foot of the bed or examining table. There should be a 35° inversion and a 25° eversion.

Toe: the patient should be able to flex and hyperextend the toes approximately 30°.

The patient's active and passive range of motion should be noted, as well as any weakness, tightness, spasm, tremor, or contracture that may be evident.

Some muscle weakness can be anticipated, although the exact degree will vary among individuals. The upper extremity usually shows greater strength on the side of the dominant hand; there should be equal strength in the lower extremities. To test muscle strength in holding its shortest position, have the patient hold the muscle in its shortest position and apply force to cause the muscle to extend. Normally, a muscle will be able to hold its shortest position under moderate resistance. Palpate all muscles for tenderness, contractures, and masses.

Review of Selected Disorders

Fractures

Trauma, cancer metastasis to the bone, osteoporosis, and other skeletal diseases contribute to fractures in aged persons. The neck of the femur is a common site for fractures in the aged, especially in older women. Not only do the more brittle bones of older persons fracture more easily, but their rate of healing is slower than in younger persons, potentially predisposing the aged to the many complications associated with immobility. Knowing that the risk of fracture and its multiple complications is high among the elderly, the gerontological nurse must aim toward prevention, drawing on the effectiveness of basic common sense measures. Because their coordination and equilibrium are poorer, the aged should be advised to avoid risky activities (e.g., climbing on ladders or chairs to reach high places). To prevent dizziness and falls resulting from postural hypotension, older individuals should rise from a kneeling or sitting position slowly. Safe, properly fitting shoes with a low, broad heel can prevent stumbling and loss of balance, and handrails for climbing stairs or rising from the bathtub provide support and balance.

Placing both feet near the edge of a curb or bus before stepping up or down is safer than a poorly balanced stretch of the legs (Fig. 24-1). Older persons should be reminded to carefully notice where they are walking to avoid tripping in holes and on damaged sidewalks or slipping on pieces of ice. Older eyes are more sensitive to glare, so sunglasses may be helpful for improving vision outdoors. A night-light is extremely valuable in preventing falls during night visits to the bathroom. Loose rugs and clutter on floors and stairs should be removed. Because even the most healthy aged person can experience some confusion when waking during the night, bed rails can be used to prevent falls from bed and attempts at sleepwalking, whether at home or away. Putting the bed against a wall with a straight chair at the other side is an effective substitute.

The high prevalence and ease of fractures in the elderly warrant that this injury be suspected whenever an older adult falls or otherwise subjects their bones to trauma. Symptoms to look for include pain, change in the shape or length of a limb, abnormal or restricted motion of a limb, edema, spasm of surrounding tissue, discoloration of tissue, and bone protruding through the tissue. The absence of these symptoms does not negate the possibility of a fracture. Overt signs and symptoms can be absent; in addition, the position of the fracture can prevent it from being apparent on the initial roentgenogram. As the patient is transported

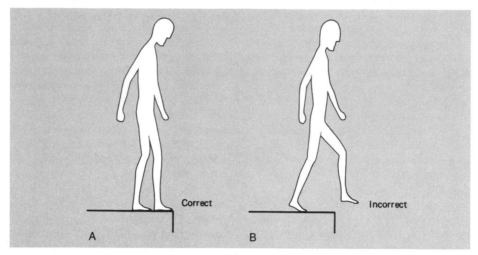

Figure 24-1. (A) *The correct method for stepping to or from a curb is to place both feet near the edge of the curb before stepping up or down.* **(B)** *The incorrect method is to stretch the legs apart before stepping.*

for evaluation, immobility of the injured site and control of bleeding are essential.

As mentioned, fractures heal more slowly in older adults, and the risk of complications is greater. Pneumonia, thrombus formation, pressure ulcers, renal calculi, fecal impaction, and contractures are among the complications that special nursing attention can help prevent. Activity, within the limits determined by the physician, should be promoted, including deep-breathing and coughing exercises, isometric and range-of-motion exercises, and frequent turning and position changes. Fluids should be encouraged, and the characteristics of urine output noted. Good nutrition will facilitate healing, increase resistance to infection, and decrease the likelihood of other complications. Joint exercise and proper positioning can prevent contractures. Correct body alignment can be maintained with the use of footboards, trochanter rolls, and sandbags. Keeping the skin dry and clean, preventing pressure, stimulating circulation through massage, and frequent turning may reduce the risk of decubiti. Sheepskin, water beds, and alternating-pressure mattresses are beneficial, but they are not substitutes for good skin care and frequent position changes.

The patient should be mobilized as early as possible. The patient may fear using the fractured limb and avoid doing so. Explanations and reassurance are required to help the patient understand that the healed limb is safe to use. Progress in small steps may be easier for the patient to tolerate physically and psychologically; the first attempt at ambulation may be to stand at the bedside, the next to walk to a nearby chair, and the next to walk to the bathroom. Initially, it may be helpful for two people to assist the patient with ambulation, especially because weakness and dizziness are common. The principles of nursing management for specific types of fractures are available in medical–surgical nursing textbooks, and the nurse is advised to explore that literature for more detailed information.

Osteoarthritis

Osteoarthritis is the deterioration and abrasion of joint cartilage, with the formation of new bone at the joint surfaces. This problem is increasingly seen with advanced age and affects women more than men. Unlike rheumatoid arthritis, osteoarthritis does not cause inflammation, deformity, and crippling—a fact that is reassuring to the affected individual who fears the severe disability often seen in persons with rheumatoid arthritis. The wear and tear of the joints as an individual ages is thought to have a major role in the development of

osteoarthritis. Excessive use of the joint, trauma, obesity, and genetic factors may also predispose an individual to this problem. Patients with acromegaly have a high incidence of osteoarthritis. Usually osteoarthritis affects several joints rather than a single one. Weight-bearing joints are most affected, the common sites being the knees, hips, vertebrae, and fingers, and the classic symptoms associated with arthritis are present—aching, stiffness, and limited motion of the joint.

Systemic symptoms do not accompany osteoarthritis. Crepitation on joint motion may be noted, and the distal joints may develop bony nodules (*i.e.*, Heberden nodes). The patient may notice that the joints are more uncomfortable during damp weather and periods of extended use. Rest, heat, and gentle massage will help relieve joint aches. Although isometrics and mild exercises are beneficial, excessive exercise will cause more pain and degeneration. Analgesics may be prescribed to control pain; splints, braces, and canes provide support and rest to the joints. The importance of maintaining proper body alignment and using good body mechanics should be emphasized in educating the patient. Weight reduction may improve the obese patient's status and should be encouraged. It is beneficial if a homemaker's service or other household assistance relieves the patient of strenuous activities that cause the joints to bear weight. Occupational and physical therapists can be consulted for assistive devices to promote independence in self-care activities.

Rheumatoid Arthritis

Rheumatoid arthritis affects many persons, particularly in the 20- to 40-year-old age group, and is a major cause of arthritic disability in later life. The deformities and disability associated with this disease primarily begin during early adulthood and peak during middle age; in old age, greater systemic involvement occurs. This disease occurs more frequently in women and in persons with a family history of this problem. The joints affected by rheumatoid arthritis are extremely painful, stiff, swollen, red, and warm to the touch. Joint pain is present during rest and activity. Subcutaneous nodules over bony prominences and bursae may be present, as may deforming flexion contractures. Systemic symptoms include fatigue, malaise, weakness, weight loss, wasting, fever, and anemia.

Encouraging patients to rest and providing support to the affected limbs are helpful measures. Limb support should be such that decubiti and contractures are prevented. Splints are commonly made for the patient in an effort to prevent deformities. Range-of-motion exercises are vital to maintain musculoskeletal function; the nurse may have to assist the patient with active exercises. Physical and occupational therapists can provide assistive devices to promote independence in self-care activities, and heat, gentle massage, and analgesics can help to control pain. Patients with rheumatoid arthritis may be prescribed anti-inflammatory agents, corticosteroids, antimalarial agents, gold salts, and immunosuppressive drugs. The nurse should be familiar with the many toxic effects of these drugs and detect them early if they occur.

The patient with rheumatoid arthritis and his family need considerable education to be able to manage this condition. Patient education should include a knowledge of the disease, treatments, administration of medications, identification of side effects, exercise regimens, use of assistive devices, methods to avoid and reduce pain, and an understanding of the need for continued medical supervision. Accepting this chronic disease is not an easy task for either the patient or his family. The patient may be a prime target for salespeople offering a quick cure or relief for arthritis and should be advised to consult a nurse or physician before investing many dollars on useless fads.

Osteoporosis

Osteoporosis is the most prevalent metabolic disease of the bone; it primarily affects adults in middle to later life. Demineralization of the bone occurs, evidenced by a decrease in the mass and density of the skeleton. Any health problem associated with inadequate calcium intake, excessive calcium loss, or poor calcium absorption can cause osteoporosis. Many of the following potential causes are problems commonly found among aged persons:

Inactivity or immobility. A lack of muscle pull on the bone can lead to a loss of minerals, especially calcium and phosphorus. This particularly may be a problem for limbs in a cast.
Cushing syndrome. An excessive production of glucocorticosteroids by the adrenal gland is

thought to inhibit the formation of bone matrix.

Reduction in anabolic sex hormones. Decreased production or loss of estrogens and androgens may be responsible for insufficient bone calcium; therefore, postmenopausal women may be at high risk of developing this problem.

Diverticulitis. Excessive diverticulitis can interfere with the absorption of sufficient amounts of calcium.

Hyperthyroidism. This increased metabolic activity causes more rapid bone turnover. Bone resorption occurs at a rate faster than bone formation, causing osteoporosis.

Poor diet. An insufficient amount of calcium, protein, and other nutrients in the diet can cause osteoporosis.

Heparin. Prolonged use of heparin can increase bone resorption and inhibit bone formation.

Diabetes mellitus. Although the direct relationship is uncertain at this time, diabetes can contribute to the development of osteoporosis.

Osteoporosis may cause kyphosis and a reduction in height. Spinal pain can be experienced, especially in the lumbar region. The bones may tend to fracture more easily. Some patients may be asymptomatic, however, and unaware of the problem until it is detected by radiography. Treatment depends on the underlying cause of the disease and may include calcium supplements, vitamin D supplements, hormones, anabolic agents, fluoride, or phosphate. A diet rich in protein and calcium is encouraged. Braces may be used to provide support and reduce spasms. A bed board is also beneficial and should be recommended. The patient must be advised to avoid heavy lifting, jumping, and other activities that could result in a fracture. Persons providing care for these patients must remember to be gentle when moving, exercising, or lifting them because fractures can occur easily. Compression fractures of the vertebrae are a potential complication of osteoporosis. Range-of-motion exercises and ambulation are important to maintain function and prevent greater damage.

Gout

Gout is a metabolic disorder in which excess uric acid accumulates in the blood. As a result, uric acid crystals are deposited in and around the joints, causing severe pain and tenderness of the joint and warmth, redness, and swelling of the surrounding tissue. Attacks can last from weeks to months, with long remissions between attacks possible. Treatment is aimed at reducing sodium urate through a low-purine diet (*e.g.*, avoidance of bacon, turkey, veal, liver, kidney, brain, anchovies, sardines, herring, smelt, mackerel, salmon, and legumes) and the administration of drugs. Colchicine or phenylbutazone can be used to manage acute attacks; long-term management could include colchicine, allopurinol, probenecid, or indomethacin. Gout attacks can be precipitated by the administration of thiazide diuretics, which raise the uric acid level of the blood.

General Nursing Interventions Related to Musculoskeletal Problems
Facilitating Musculoskeletal Function

A good diet is important in preventing and managing musculoskeletal problems. A well-balanced diet rich in proteins and minerals will help maintain the structure of the bones and muscles. A minimum of 800 mg calcium should be included in the diet daily. Good sources of calcium include the following:

SOURCE	PORTION	CALCIUM (mg)
Plain lowfat yogurt	1 cup	415
Skim milk	1 cup	302
Buttermilk	1 cup	300
Instant, enriched cooked farina	1 cup	200
Swiss cheese	1 ounce	272
Lowfat (2%) cottage cheese	1 cup	154
Cooked turnip greens	½ cup	150

In addition to the quality of the diet, attention also must be paid to its quantity. Obesity places strain on the joints, which aggravates conditions such as arthritis. Weight reduction frequently will ease musculoskeletal discomforts and reduce limitations and should be promoted as a sound health practice for persons of all ages.

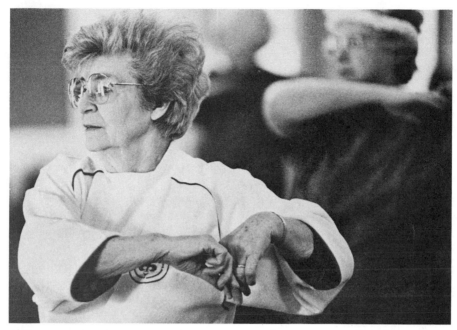

Individually planned exercises are essential to the musculoskeletal health of aging persons. (Photograph by Eric Schenk.)

Activity promotes optimal musculoskeletal function and reduces the many complications associated with immobility. Fear of reinjuring a healing bone or causing pain could cause an unnecessary limitation of activities. Realistic explanations describing the healing process or the benefit of exercise to aching joints are most important. Patients and their families can benefit from an understanding of the hazards arising from immobility; sympathetic family members who believe they are helping their elderly relatives by allowing them to be inactive may be more willing to encourage activity if they are aware of the harm that immobility can cause. Continued support, encouragement, and positive reinforcement by nurses can help patients considerably.

Care Planning

Actual or potential problems can be revealed during the assessment of the musculoskeletal system. Assessment data should be reviewed for those problems that fall within the realm of nursing to diagnose and manage, and related nursing diagnoses developed accordingly. Table 24-2 lists some of the major nursing diagnoses that can be related to musculoskeletal disorders.

The development of realistic goals guides care and provides a yardstick by which the patient's progress can be measured. Although the goals developed for individual patients will be specific to their unique needs, some potential goals in the care of musculoskeletal problems in older adults are listed in the Sample Care Plan. Patients and their significant others should be active participants in the development of goals and establishment of priorities. See Chapter 18 for more information on planning and providing care.

Managing Pain

Pain often accompanies musculoskeletal problems. Degenerative changes in the tendons and arthritis often are responsible for painful shoulders,

Table 24-2 *Nursing Diagnoses Related to Musculoskeletal Problems*

NURSING DIAGNOSIS	CAUSE OR CONTRIBUTING FACTOR
Activity intolerance	Muscle fatigue, pain, deformity
Anxiety	Pain, fear of injury
Altered bowel elimination: constipation	Inactivity or immobility from pain or disability
Pain	Fracture, contracture, spasms, arthritis
Fear	Change or loss of function or appearance
Impaired home maintenance management	Arthritis, contracture, pain, impaired range of motion
High risk for injury	Unsteady gait, pain, improper use of heat
Impaired physical mobility	Spasms, atrophy, pain, deformity
Powerlessness	Impaired self-care capacity
Self-care deficit	Immobility, pain, deformity
Disturbance in self-concept	Change in body structure or function, pain, immobility, increased dependency
Sexual dysfunction	Pain, fatigue, positioning difficulties, altered body image
Sleep pattern disturbance	Pain, spasms, cramps
Impaired social interactions	Change in body structure or function, altered self-concept, pain
Social isolation	Immobility, pain, disfigurement

elbows, hands, hips, knees, and spines; cramps, especially during the night, commonly are experienced in calves, feet, hands, hips, and thighs; joint strain and damp weather more frequently cause musculoskeletal pain in the elderly than in the young. Pain relief is essential in promoting optimal physical, mental, and social function. Unrelieved pain can interfere with elderly people's abilities to engage in self-care, manage their households, and maintain social contact. To enrich the quality of life, every effort should be made to minimize or eliminate pain. Often, heat will relieve muscle spasms, and a warm bath at bedtime accompanied by blankets and clothing to keep the extremities warm can reduce spasms and cramps throughout the night and promote uninterrupted sleep. The elderly are at high risk for burns; care must be taken to avoid injury if heat applications or soaks are used. Passive stretching of the extremity can be helpful in controlling muscle cramps. Excessive exercise and musculoskeletal stress should be avoided, as well as situations known to cause pain,

such as heavy lifting or damp weather. Pain in the weight-bearing joints can be alleviated by resting those joints, supporting painful joints during transfers, and using a walker or cane (Fig. 24-2). Correct positioning, whereby all body parts are in proper alignment, can help prevent and manage pain. Accidental bumping against the patient's bed or chair and rough handling of the patient during care activities must be prevented. Nurses may need to emphasize to other caregivers the need for extra gentleness in turning and lifting older patients. Diversional activities are useful in preventing the patient's preoccupation with pain. The goal is to aid the patient in achieving the maximum level of activity with the least degree of pain.

Preventing Injury

Safety considerations are essential for all elderly persons because of their high incidence of accidents and musculoskeletal injuries and their pro-

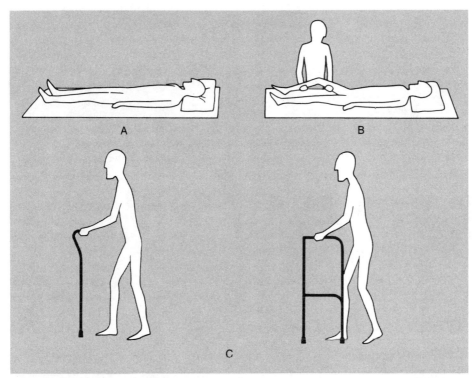

Figure 24-2 *Methods for reducing musculoskeletal pain.* (**A**) *Good body alignment.* (**B**) *Support of parts of the limb adjacent to the painful joint when moving or lifting.* (**C**) *Use of a walker or cane.*

longed time required for healing. Prevention includes paying attention to the area where one is walking; climbing stairs and curbs slowly; using both feet for support as much as possible; using railings and canes for added balance; wearing properly fitting, safe shoes for good support; and avoiding long trousers, nightgowns, or robes. The importance of the safe use of heat has already been mentioned; it is useful for patients to learn how to measure water temperature and use hot water bottles and heating pads safely. Patients with peripheral vascular disease must be warned that the local application of heat can cause circulatory demands that their body will be unable to meet; they should be informed that other means of pain relief may be more beneficial to them. Warm baths can reduce muscle spasm and provide pain relief, but they also can cause hypotensive episodes leading to dizziness, fainting, and serious injury.

Carelessly turning patients so that legs hit the

bed rail, dropping them into a chair during a transfer, restraining them in an unaligned position, roughly handling a limb, or attempting to use force to straighten a contracture can lead to muscle strain and fractures. Gentle handling will prevent unnecessary musculoskeletal discomfort and injury.

Promoting Independence

Any loss of independence associated with the limitations imposed by musculoskeletal problems has a serious impact on physical, emotional, and social well-being; therefore, nurses must explore all avenues to help patients minimize limitations and strengthen capacities, thereby promoting the highest possible level of independence. Canes, walkers, and other assistive devices can often provide significant aid in compensating for handicaps and should be used when feasible (Fig. 24-3); physical

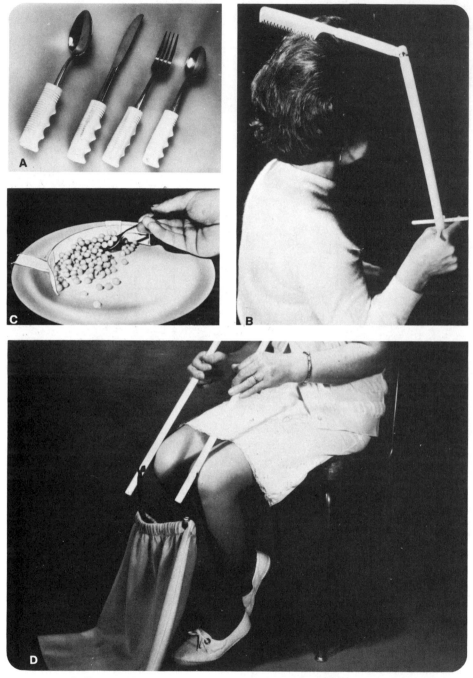

Figure 24-3. *Self-care devices can help the patient achieve the maximum indepen-dence possible. (**A**) Set of four built-up hand utensils. (**B**) Long-handled comb. (**C**) Food-bumper. (**D**) Dressing sticks with carter clips. (**E**) Universal ADL cuff. (**F**) Dor-sal wrist splint. (**G**) Tall-Ette with safety bars. (Courtesy of Maddak, Inc., subsidary of Bel-Air Products, Pequannock, NJ.)*

(continued)

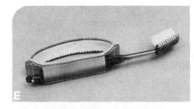

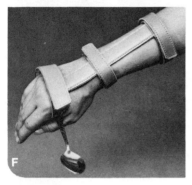

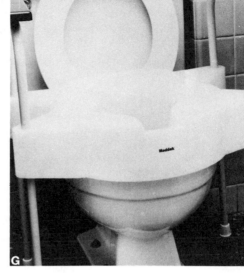

Figure 24-3. (continued)

Sample Care Plan Goals for the Patient With Musculoskeletal Problems

To possess maximum possible range of motion for all joints

To be free from musculoskeletal injury

To safely manage musculoskeletal pain

To have cause of musculoskeletal symptoms and signs diagnosed

To describe the purpose, administration, side-effects, adverse reactions, interactions, and special precautions associated with drugs prescribed to manage musculoskeletal problems

To correctly self-administer medications prescribed to treat musculoskeletal problems

To participate in a regular exercise program according to individual capability

To demonstrate the proper and safe use of adaptive equipment and self-care devices

To learn proper transfer techniques

To demonstrate safe techniques for ambulation

To regain ability to ambulate

To be maximally independent in self-care

---

and occupational therapists can be valuable resources in determining appropriate assistive devices for use with specific deficits. Resources to assist patients with musculoskeletal problems are presented in the Resource List.

Resources to Assist Patients With Musculoskeletal Problems

Arthritis Foundation
3400 Peachtree Road
Suite 1101
Atlanta, GA 30326
(404)266-0795

Arthritis Information Clearinghouse
P.O. Box 34427
Bethesda, MD 20034
(301)881-9411

Recommended Readings

Ettinger WH. Joint and soft tissue disorders. In: Abrams WB, Berkow R, eds. The Merck manual of geriatrics. Rahway, NJ: Merck Sharp & Dohme Research Laboratories, 1990:686.

Gerhart TN. Fractures. In: Abrams WB, Berkow R, eds. The Merck manual of geriatrics. Rahway, NJ: Merck Sharp & Dohme Research Laboratories, 1990:69.

Holm K, Walker J. Osteoporosis: treatment and prevention update. Geriatr Nurs 1990;11(3):140.

Mazanec DJ. Conservative treatment of rheumatic disorders in the elderly. Geriatrics 1991;46(5):41.

Present D, Shaffer B. Disease associated with fracture: detection and management in the elderly. Geriatrics 1990;45(3):48.

Riggs BL, Melton LJ, eds. Osteoporosis: etiology, diagnosis and management. New York: Raven, 1988.

Rosenbaum JT. Toward a new understanding of rheumatoid arthritis. Geriatrics 1990;45(4):76.

25

Genitourinary Problems

Genitourinary problems, although bothersome, frequent, and potentially life-threatening, are disorders not easily discussed by older adults. Some feel embarrassment or distaste at making others aware of these problems; others fear societal reactions to an older person's concern about sexual function; still others may associate genitourinary problems with sexual "wrongdoing" and feel guilty over the development of these disorders; and some individuals accept symptoms of genitourinary disorders as a normal part of aging. These factors, along with reluctance to obtain gynecological and urological examinations, often delay early detection and treatment. Untreated, these problems can jeopardize total body health and profoundly affect psychological well-being. Nurses are in ideal positions to develop close relationships with geriatric patients, which can help them to more comfortably discuss problems of the urinary tract and reproductive system. By demonstrating sensitivity, acceptance, and understanding of patients' problems, nurses can facilitate prompt, appropriate intervention.

Aging and the Genitourinary System

The urinary tract undergoes many changes with age. Muscles lose their elasticity, and supportive structures lose some of their tone. Arteriosclerotic changes reduce this system's resistance to injury and infection. Nephrons are lost, and kidney size decreases because renal tissue growth declines. The glomerular filtration rate begins to decline in midlife: by 90 years of age, filtration is half what it was at 20 years of age. Renal blood flow decreases, and by 70 years of age, the blood urea nitrogen level nearly doubles to become 21.2 mg/dl. The kidney's ability to concentrate urine is decreased as a result of reduced tubular function, and an increase in the renal threshold for glucose can cause the elderly to be hyperglycemic without evidence of glycosuria. Bladder capacity decreases, as evidenced by urinary frequency and nocturia. Weaker bladder muscles cause difficulty in bladder elimination and increase the risk of retention.

The female reproductive system experiences a variety of evident changes. Pubic hair is lost and the labia flatten. The vulva has a reduction in elasticity, subcutaneous fat, and blood flow, causing it to gain an atrophic appearance. The vagina has a thinner, less vascular epithelium and is drier and more alkaline; vaginal infections and dyspareunia often result. The cervix and uterus shrink, and the fallopian tubes and ovaries atrophy. Menopause brings an end to ovulation and estrogen production. Breast tissue loses its firmness, causing breasts to sag.

The aging man will discover that more time and direct physical stimulation are required to achieve an erection. He will still ejaculate and have satisfying orgasms, but his ejaculations will be less rapid and forceful. His testes will be smaller and less firm although testosterone production will continue. Display 25-1 lists some of the changes to the genitourinary system with age.

DISPLAY 25-1   *Age-Related Changes of the Genitourinary System*

Urinary Tract

Loss of nephrons

Decrease in renal mass (primarily on cortex); decline in kidney weight from 250 to 270 g in young adulthood to 180 to 200 g in eighth decade*

Reduction in number of glomeruli

Decline in glomerular filtration rate

Appearance of sclerotic changes in renal blood vessels

Decrease in renal blood flow from 1200 ml/min to 600 ml/min by age 80 years*

Increase in blood urea nitrogen level by age 70 years to 21.2 mg/dl

Decrease in creatinine clearance after fourth decade by approximately 8 ml/min per 1.73 m² per decade

Increased renal threshold for glucose

Decrease in plasma renin and plasma aldosterone levels

Replacement of smooth muscle and elastic tissue with fibrous connective tissue in bladder

Weaker bladder muscles; incomplete emptying of the bladder; tendency for urinary retention

Decreased bladder capacity; urinary frequency

Reduction in muscle elasticity and tone of supportive structures

Lower resistance to infections and injury

Female Reproductive System

Loss of pubic hair

Flattening, atrophy, and shrinkage of labia associated with loss of estrogen and progesterone stimulation

Reduced elasticity, subcutaneous fat, and blood flow of vulva

Atrophy and thinning of vaginal tissue secondary to loss of estrogen

Decreased secretions and vascularity of vagina

Increase in vaginal pH

Shrinkage of cervix and uterus

Atrophy of fallopian tubes and ovaries

Replacement of breast glandular tissue by fat tissue after midlife; atrophy of fat and glandular tissue after age 60 years; sagging and loss of firmness of breasts

Male Reproductive System

Decrease in size and firmness of testes

Decline in testosterone production

More direct physical stimulation required to achieve erection

Ejaculations slower, less forceful

Hypertrophy of prostate gland

---

*Data from Rowe JW. Renal system. In: Abrams WB, Berkow R, eds. The Merck manual of geriatrics. Rahway, NJ: Merck Sharpe & Dohme Research Laboratories, 1990:598.

Assessment

A complete history and examination are essential in pinpointing specific areas that require further investigation; however, obtaining data about genitourinary function and problems can be difficult. Older persons may feel embarrassment, distaste, or guilt about discussing these problems. A comfortable tone should be set and sensitivity displayed during the assessment to facilitate good data collection.

Interview

The interview should include a review of function, signs, and symptoms. Questions should be asked pertaining to the following:

Frequency of voiding. "How often do you need to urinate during the day and during the night? Has there been any recent change in that pattern?"

Continence. "Do you ever lose control of your urine? Do you experience a steady stream of urine dribbling at all times or at certain times? Is urine released when you cough or sneeze? How soon do you need to toilet after getting the urge to void before you lose control?"

Retention. "Do you ever feel that you have not fully emptied your bladder after you have voided? Do you have a sense of fullness in your bladder after voiding?"

Pain. "Does it burn when you void? Do you experience pain in your lower abdomen or anywhere else? Is there any tenderness, discomfort, itching, or pain anywhere along your genital area?"

Discharge. "Do you ever have secretions, blood, or other discharge from your genitals?"

Urine. "Have you ever seen crystals or particles in your urine? Is your urine ever pink, bloody, or discolored? Is it as clear as tap water or as dark as rusty water? Does your urine ever have a strong odor? If so, what is that odor like?"

Sexual dysfunction. "Can you obtain an erection and hold it through intercourse? What are your ejaculations like? Is your vagina sensitive or overly dry during intercourse? Do you feel extra pressure or that your partner's penis is hitting a blockage during intercourse? Can you have satisfying orgasms? Has there been any change in your sexual pattern?"

Urine Sample

A urinalysis can provide basic information about this system. The specific gravity should range from 1.005 to 1.025, and the *p*H from 4.6 to 8. Although alkaline urine is most often associated with infections, it can be present if the specimen has been sitting for a few hours. Normally the urine should be free of glucose and protein, but renal changes in the older adult cause proteinuria and glycosuria to be less reliable findings. It is beneficial to note characteristics of the urine sample such as the following:

Color: examination of the urine's color can yield insight into the presence of health problems.

Dark colors can indicate increased urine concentration.

Red or rust color usually is associated with the presence of blood.

Yellow-brown or green-brown color can be caused by an obstructed bile duct or jaundice.

Orange urine results from the presence of bile or the ingestion of phenazopyridine.

Very dark brown urine is associated with hematuria or carcinoma.

Odor: a faint aromatic odor of the urine is normal.

Strong odor, which can indicate concentrated urine associated with dehydration, should be noted.

Ammonialike odor can accompany infections.

Physical Examination

Inspect, percuss, and palpate the abdomen for bladder fullness, pain, or abnormalities. Test women for stress incontinence by doing the following:

Have the patient drink at least one full glass of fluid and wait until she senses fullness of the bladder.

Instruct the patient to stand. If this is not possible, have her sit as upright as possible.

Ask the patient to hold a 4 × 4 gauze at her perineum.

Instruct the patient to cough vigorously.

The test is negative if no leakage or leakage of only a few drops occurs. If residual urine is a problem, a postvoid residual may be ordered in which the patient is catheterized within 15 minutes of voiding to determine the volume of urine remaining in the bladder. If incontinence is present, the patient should be referred for a comprehensive evaluation; it can prove useful to maintain a record or have the patient maintain a diary of each occurrence of incontinence and factors associated with these incidents.

The genitalia should be inspected for lesions, sores, breaks, or masses. Note bleeding, discharges, odors, and other abnormalities. If the patient has not had a gynecological examination or mammogram within the past year, she should be referred accordingly. Likewise, the male patient should receive a prostate examination if one has not been done within the past year.

The breasts should be palpated for masses. The procedure for self-examination of the breasts should be reviewed (see Chap. 30) and instruction provided if the patient is unskilled in this technique.

Review of Selected Disorders
Urinary Incontinence

A common and bothersome disorder of the aged that requires skillful nursing attention is the involuntary loss of urine, or urinary incontinence. Stud-

ies have shown that urinary incontinence is present in 30% of the community-based elderly, 50% of the institutionalized aged, and 30% of hospitalized older adults; this problem is twice as prevalent in women as compared to men.(Diokno, 1990) The following are various types of incontinence:(Eliopoulos, 1991)

> *Stress:* caused by weak supporting pelvic muscles. When pressure is placed on the pelvic floor (*e.g.*, from laughing, sneezing, coughing), urine is involuntarily lost.
>
> *Urgency:* caused by urinary tract infection, enlargement of the prostate, diverticulitis, or pelvic or bladder tumors. Irritation or spasms of the bladder wall cause a sudden elimination of urine.
>
> *Overflow:* associated with bladder neck obstructions and medications. Bladder muscles fail to contract or periurethral muscles do not relax, leading to an excessive accumulation of urine in the bladder.
>
> *Neurogenic:* arising from cerebral cortex lesions, multiple sclerosis, and other disturbances along the neural pathway. There is an inability to sense the urge to void or control urine flow.
>
> *Functional:* caused by dementia, disabilities that prevent independent toileting, sedation, inaccessible bathroom, or any other factor interfering with the ability to reach a commode.
>
> *Mixed incontinence:* incontinence can be due to a combination of these factors.

Nurses should not assume that individuals with incontinence, even long-term incontinence, have necessarily had this problem identified and evaluated. Embarrassment at discussing this disorder or the belief that incontinence is a normal outcome of aging can cause incontinence to be unreported. This reinforces the importance of questioning about incontinence during every routine assessment. In addition to referring the patient for a comprehensive medical evaluation, nurses can aid in the identification of the cause and determination of appropriate treatment measures through the process of nursing assessment. Display 25-2 lists some of the factors to consider in assessing the incontinent individual.

The initial goal for incontinent individuals is to have the cause of the incontinence identified; thereafter, treatment goals are developed based on the underlying cause. Kegel exercises, biofeedback, and medications (*e.g.*, estrogen, anticholinergics) may be useful for the improvement of stress incontinence; in some circumstances, surgery may be warranted. Urge incontinence can be aided by adherence to a toileting schedule, biofeedback, and medications (*e.g.*, anticholinergics, adrenergic antagonists); overflow incontinence may benefit from adherence to a toileting schedule, the use of the Credé maneuver, intermittent catheterization, and medications (*e.g.*, parasympathomimetics). Interventions to assist with functional incontinence could range from improvement of mobility to provision of a bedside commode. General nursing measures should include the following:

> *Promote good fluid intake.* Some incontinent persons may restrict their fluid intake to reduce their episodes of incontinence. Incontinent patients need to understand that concentrated urine can irritate the bladder and worsen their incontinence.
>
> *Protect skin integrity.* Urine can be irritating to the skin and facilitate breakdown. Urine-soaked clothing, briefs, or linens should be changed promptly, and the skin should be cleansed after having contact with urine.
>
> *Prevent falls.* Urine spills can be a cause of falls and lead to serious injury for incontinent persons. Until control can be established, patients should use products such as incontinence briefs or condom catheters to contain their urine. Of course, spills should be cleaned from floors immediately.
>
> *Maintain or establish positive self-concept.* Incontinence can be extremely embarrassing and alter the self-perception and perception by others of incontinent persons. Socialization and the general quality of life can be jeopardized. Correcting the underlying cause, when possible, is essential to avoiding these consequences, as are the use of effective containment measures and the sensitive treatment of this problem by caregivers.

The nurse can assist patients in the development of a program for bladder training. The success of this program depends on each patient's physical capacity to regain bladder control, their comprehension of the program, and their motivation. Therefore, a complete assessment of capacities and limitations and joint planning with the patient are

DISPLAY 25-2 *Factors to Review When Assessing the Incontinent Patient*

Medical History

Note diagnoses that could contribute to incontinence, such as delirium, dementia, cerebrovascular accident, diabetes mellitus, congestive heart failure, urinary tract infection.

Medications

Review all prescription and nonprescription drugs used for those that can affect continence, such as diuretics, antianxieties, antipsychotics, antidepressants, sedatives, narcotics, antiparkinsonism agents, antispasmotics, antihistamines, calcium channel blockers, and α-blockers and α-stimulants.

Functional Status

Assess activities of daily living and impaired activities of daily living capacities; ask about recent changes in function; determine degree of dependency on others for mobility, transfers, toileting.

Mental Status

Test cognitive function; review symptoms such as depression, hallucinations; ask about recent changes in mood or intellectual function.

Neuromuscular Function in Lower Extremity

Test patient's ability to keep leg lifted against your efforts to gently push it down; touch various areas along both legs with pin point and smooth side of safety pin to determine patient's ability to detect and differentiate sensations.

Control and Retention

Test for stress incontinence in women; determine postvoid residual.

Bladder Fullness and Pain

Inspect, percuss, and palpate the bladder for distention, discomfort, and abnormalities.

Elimination Pattern

Record bladder and bowel elimination patterns and associated factors for several days; inquire about changes to elimination pattern; note frequency, pattern, amount, and relationship to other factors.

Fecal Impaction

Palpate the rectum for the presence of fecal impaction (unless contraindicated).

Symptoms

Ask about urgency, burning, vaginal itching, pain, pressure in bladder area, fever.

Reactions to Incontinence

Explore how incontinence has affected activities, life-style, self-concept; determine patient's appraisal of problem.

---

prerequisites to the initiation of this regimen. When the patient is fully prepared to begin the program, a schedule is developed indicating the times for voiding. Usually, 2-hour intervals are planned first, with increased intervals as the patient's progress indicates, and intervals are reduced during the night. Approximately one-half hour before the time scheduled, the patient should drink a full glass of fluid and make a conscious effort to retain urine. At the scheduled time, the patient should attempt to void; if difficult, massaging the bladder area or rocking forward and backward may facilitate voiding (Fig. 25-1). It is important to keep an accurate record of intake and output and of the patient's responses to the training program and its effectiveness. The essential role for the nursing staff in this procedure is to make sure the schedule is strictly adhered to by all. Inconsistency on the part of the nursing staff will be destructive to the progress of patients and denigrating to their efforts. Conversely, positive reinforcement and encouragement are most beneficial to the patient during this difficult program. Indwelling catheters should be used only in special circumstances, and

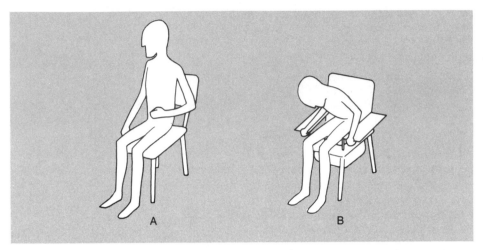

Figure 25-1. *Measures to facilitate voiding.* (**A**) *Massaging bladder area.* (**B**) *Rocking back and forth.*

certainly never for the convenience of staff. Half of patients will develop bacteriuria within the first 24 hours of being catheterized; 35% to 40% of all nosocomial infections are catheter-associated urinary tract infections.(Bush and Kaye, 1990) In addition, the risk of developing urinary calculi is high when indwelling catheters are present.

Urinary Tract Infections

Infections of the urinary tract are the most common infection in the aged and increase in prevalence with age. Primarily responsible for urinary tract infections are *Escherichia coli* in women and *Proteus* species in men. The presence of any foreign body in the urinary tract or anything that slows or obstructs the flow of urine (*e.g.,* immobilization, urethral strictures, neoplasms, or a clogged indwelling catheter) predisposes the individual to these infections. They can result from poor hygienic practices, improper cleansing after bowel elimination, a predisposition created by low fluid intake and excessive fluid loss, and hormonal changes, which reduce the body's resistance. Persons in a debilitated state or who have neurogenic bladders, arteriosclerosis, or diabetes also have a high risk of developing infections.

The gerontological nurse should be alert to the signs and symptoms of this problem. Early indicators include burning, urgency, and fever. Awareness of the patient's normal body temperature helps the nurse recognize the presence of fever, for

instance, 99°F (37°C) in a patient whose normal temperature is 96.8°F (35°C). Some urologists believe that many urinary tract infections in the aged seem asymptomatic because of unawareness of elevations in normal temperature. The gerontological nurse can significantly facilitate diagnosis by informing the physician of temperature increases. Bacteriuria greater than 10^5 CFU/ml confirms the diagnosis of a urinary tract infection.

As a urinary tract infection progresses, retention, incontinence, and hematuria may occur. Treatment is aimed at establishing adequate urinary drainage and controlling the infection through antibiotic therapy. The nurse should carefully note the patient's fluid intake and output. Forcing fluids is advisable, provided that the patient's cardiac status does not contraindicate this action. Observation for new symptoms, bladder distention, skin irritation, and other unusual signs should continue as the patient recovers.

Bladder Cancer

The incidence of bladder cancer increases with age; older men have twice the rate of older women. Chronic irritation of the bladder and cigarette smoking, both avoidable factors, are among the risk factors associated with bladder tumors. Some of the symptoms resemble those of a bladder infection, such as frequency, urgency, and dysuria. A painless hematuria is the primary sign and characterizes cancer of the bladder. Standard diagnos-

tic measures for this disease are used with the aged patient, including cystoscopic examination. Treatment can include surgery or radiation, depending on the extent and location of the lesion. The nurse should use the nursing measures described in medical–surgical nursing literature. Observation for signs indicating metastasis, such as pelvic or back pain, is part of the nursing care for these patients.

Renal Calculi

Renal calculi occur most frequently in middle-aged adults. In the aged, the formation of stones can be caused by immobilization, infection, changes in the *p*H or concentration of urine, chronic diarrhea, dehydration, excessive elimination of uric acid, and hypercalcemia. Pain, hematuria, and symptoms of urinary tract infection are associated with this problem, and gastrointestinal upset may occur also. Standard diagnostic and treatment measures are used for the aged, and the nurse can assist by preventing urinary stasis, providing ample fluids, and facilitating prompt treatment of urinary tract infections.

Glomerulonephritis

Most frequently, chronic glomerulonephritis already exists in aged persons who develop an acute condition. The symptoms of this disease may be so subtle and nonspecific that they are initially unnoticed. Clinical manifestations include fever, fatigue, nausea, vomiting, anorexia, abdominal pain, anemia, edema, arthralgias, elevated blood pressure, and an increased sedimentation rate. Oliguria may occur, as can moderate proteinuria and hematuria. Headache, convulsions, paralysis, aphasia, coma, and an altered mental status may be consequences of cerebral edema associated with this disease. Diagnostic and treatment measures do not differ significantly from those used with the young. The use of antibiotics, a restricted sodium and protein diet, and close attention to fluid intake and output are basic parts of the treatment plan. If the aged person is receiving digitalis, diuretics, or antihypertensive drugs, close observation for cumulative toxic effects resulting from compromised kidney function must be maintained. The patient should be evaluated periodically after the acute illness is resolved for exacerbations of chronic glomerulonephritis and signs of renal failure.

Pyelonephritis

Although urinary obstruction is the primary cause of pyelonephritis in older persons, autoimmune reactions may have some relationship as well. Symptoms of this problem vary from mild to severe. Dull back pain, fever, gastrointestinal upset, frequency, dysuria, burning, bacteriuria, and pyuria are usually present with acute pyelonephritis. As the chronic form develops, progressive kidney damage leads to polyuria, anorexia, weight loss, fatigue, and the classic symptoms associated with uremia. Aged patients have been found to have no fever and no voiding difficulty, even when high bacterial counts have been present. The treatment depends on the causative factor and usually includes antibiotic therapy to eliminate the causative organism, correcting the obstruction, and strengthening the patient's resistance. As with glomerulonephritis, periodic evaluation for the recurrence of infection and close follow-up are essential.

Infections and Tumors of the Vulva

The vulva loses hair and subcutaneous fat with age, and this is accompanied by a flattening and folding of the labia. General atrophy occurs as well. These changes cause the vulva to be more fragile and more easily susceptible to irritation and infection. Senile vulvitis is the term used to describe vulvar infection associated with hypertrophy or atrophy. Vulvar problems in the aged may reflect serious disease processes such as diabetes, hepatitis, leukemia, and pernicious anemia. Incontinence and poor hygienic practices can also be underlying causes of vulvitis. Pruritus is the primary symptom associated with vulvitis. Patients who are confused and noncommunicative may display restlessness, and the nurse may discover that they are suffering from irritation and thickening of the vulvar tissue as a result of scratching. Initially, treatment is aimed at finding and managing any underlying cause. Good nutritional status assists in improving the condition, as does special attention to cleanliness. Sitz baths and local applications of saline compresses or steroid creams may be included in the treatment plan. Special attention is required to keep the incontinent patient clean and dry as much as possible.

Although pruritus is commonly associated with vulvitis, it may be a symptom of a vulvar tumor. Pain and irritation also may be associated with this

problem. Any mass or lesion in this area should receive prompt attention and be biopsied. The clitoris is commonly the site of a vulvar malignancy. Cancer of the vulva, the fourth most common gynecological malignancy in later life, may be manifested by large, painful, and foul-smelling fungating or ulcerating tumors. The adjacent tissues may also be affected. A radical vulvectomy is usually the treatment of choice and tends to be well tolerated by the aged woman. Less commonly used is radiation therapy, which is not tolerated as well as surgery. Counseling regarding self-care practices, body image, and sexual activity should be provided. Early treatment, before metastasis to inguinal lymph nodes, promotes a good prognosis.

Problems of the Vagina

Vaginitis

With advancing age, the vaginal epithelium thins, which is accompanied by a loss of tissue elasticity. Secretions become alkaline and of lesser quantity. The flora changes, affecting the natural protection the vagina normally provides. These changes predispose the older female to the common infection, senile vaginitis. Soreness, pruritus, burning, and a reddened vagina are symptoms, and the accompanying vaginal discharge is clear, brown, or white. As it progresses, this vaginitis can cause bleeding and adhesions.

Local estrogens in suppository or cream form are usually effective in treating senile vaginitis. Nurses should make sure that patients understand the proper use of these topical medications and do not attempt to administer them orally. Acid douches may be prescribed also; if the patient is to administer a douche at home, it is important to emphasize the need to measure the solution's temperature with a dairy thermometer. Altered receptors for hot and cold temperatures and reduced pain sensation predispose the patient to burns from solutions excessively hot for fragile vaginal tissue. Good hygienic practices are beneficial for the treatment and the prevention of vaginitis.

Cancer of the Vagina

Cancer of the vagina is rare in older women; it results more frequently from metastasis than from the vaginal area as a primary site. All vaginal ulcers and masses detected in aged women should be viewed with suspicion of malignancy and be biop-

sied. Because chronic irritation can predispose women to vaginal cancer, those who have chronic vaginitis or who wear a pessary should obtain frequent Papanicolaou smears, commonly known as Pap smears. Treatment is similar to that used for younger women and may consist of irradiation, topical chemotherapeutic agents, or surgery, depending on the extent of the carcinoma.

Problems of the Cervix

With age, the cervix becomes smaller, and this is accompanied by an atrophy of the endocervical epithelium. Occasionally the endocervical glands can seal over, causing the formation of nabothian cysts. As secretions associated with these cysts accumulate, fever and a palpable tender mass may be evident. It is important, therefore, for the aged woman to receive regular gynecological examinations in which the patency of the cervix can be checked.

Cancer of the Cervix

The incidence of cervical cancer peaks in the fifth and sixth decades of life and thereafter declines. Although most endocervical polyps are benign in older women, they should be viewed with suspicion until biopsy confirms a benign diagnosis. Vaginal bleeding and leukorrhea are signs of cervical cancer in aged women. Pain does not usually occur. As the disease progresses, the patient can develop urinary retention or incontinence, fecal incontinence, and uremia. Treatment of cervical cancer can include radium or surgery. An annual Pap smear is recommended to aid in detecting this problem.

Problems of the Uterus

The uterus decreases in size with age, becoming so small in some older women that it cannot be palpated on examination. The endometrium continues to respond to hormonal stimulation.

Cancer of the Endometrium

Cancer of the endometrium is not uncommon in the aged and is of higher incidence in obese, diabetic, and hypertensive women. Any postmenopausal bleeding should give rise immediately to suspicion of this disease. Dilation and curettage usually are done to confirm the diagnosis because

not all cases can be detected by Pap smears alone. Treatment consists of surgery, irradiation, or a combination of both. Early treatment can prevent metastasis to the vagina and cervix. Endometrial polyps can also cause bleeding and should receive serious attention because they could be indicative of early cancer.

Problems of the Fallopian Tubes and Ovaries

Although masses are occasionally detected in the fallopian tubes, they rarely present any significant problem to the aged woman. The primary changes the fallopian tubes undergo with age are shortening, straightening, and atrophy. The ovaries also atrophy with age, becoming smaller and thicker. They may not be palpable during the gynecological examination because of their decreased size. Ovarian cancer is responsible for only 5% of malignant disease in older women although it is the leading cause of death from gynecological malignancies. Early symptoms are nonspecific and can be confused with gastrointestinal discomfort. As it progresses, the clinical manifestations of this disease include bleeding, ascites, and the presence of multiple masses. Treatment may consist of surgery or irradiation. Benign ovarian tumors commonly occur in the aged, and surgery is usually required to differentiate them from malignant ones.

Perineal Herniation

As a result of the stretching and tearing of muscles during childbirth and of the muscle weakness associated with advanced age, perineal herniation is a common problem among older women. Cystocele, rectocele, and prolapse of the uterus are the types most likely to occur. Associated with this problem are lower back pain, pelvic heaviness, and a pulling sensation. Urinary and fecal incontinence, retention, and constipation may also occur. Sometimes the woman is able to feel pressure or palpate a mass in her vagina. These herniations can make intercourse difficult and uncomfortable. Although rectoceles do not tend to worsen with age, the opposite is true for cystoceles, which will cause increased problems with time. Surgical repair is the treatment of choice and can be successful in relieving these problems. If surgery cannot be performed, the patient is usually fitted for a pes-

sary, although this method is discouraged because the pessary often is cumbersome to use and can cause ulceration and infection.

Dyspareunia

Dyspareunia is a common problem among older women but is not necessarily a normal consequence of aging. Nulliparous women experience this problem more frequently than women who have had children. Because vulvitis, vaginitis, and other gynecological problems can contribute to dyspareunia, a thorough gynecological examination is important, and any lesions or infections should be corrected to alleviate the problem. All efforts should be made to help the older woman achieve a satisfactory sexual life. A more detailed discussion of sexual problems is presented in Chapter 14.

Breast Problems

The breasts atrophy with age, sagging more and hanging at a lower level. Some retraction of the nipples may occur as a result of shrinkage and fibrotic changes. Firm linear strands may develop on the breasts from fibrosis and calcification of the terminal ducts.

Cancer of the Breast

Because of the visual manifestations of decreased fat tissue and atrophy in aged women's breasts, it is not unusual for tumors, possibly present for many years, to become more evident. Because breast cancer is a leading cause of cancer deaths in aged as well as younger women, regular breast examinations should be encouraged. A more detailed explanation of breast examination is presented in Chapter 30. Diagnostic and treatment measures for women with breast cancer are the same at any age.

Benign Prostatic Hypertrophy

A majority of older men have some degree of benign prostatic hypertrophy. Symptoms of this problem progress slowly but continuously; they include hesitancy, decreased force of urinary stream, frequency, and nocturia. As the condition progresses, dribbling, poor control, overflow incontinence, and bleeding may occur. Unfortunately, some men are

reluctant or embarrassed to seek prompt medical attention and may develop kidney damage by the time symptoms are severe enough to motivate them to be evaluated. Treatment can include prostatic massage, the use of urinary antiseptics and, if possible, the avoidance of diuretics, anticholinergics, and antiarrhythmic agents. The most common prostatectomy approach used for aged men with prostatism is transurethral surgery. The patient should be reassured that this surgery will not cause impotence. On the other hand, realistic explanations are needed so the patient understands that this surgery will not guarantee a sudden rejuvenation of sexual performance.

Cancer of the Prostate

Prostatic cancer increases in incidence with age and is the second most common cause of cancer death in men older than 75 years of age. Although this disease can be asymptomatic, a majority of prostatic cancers can be detected by rectal examination, which emphasizes the importance of regular physical examinations. Benign hypertrophy should be followed closely because it is thought to be associated with prostatic cancer, the symptoms of which can be similar. Symptoms such as back pain, anemia, weakness, and weight loss can develop as a result of metastasis. If metastasis has not occurred, treatment may consist of irradiation or a radical prostatectomy; the latter procedure will result in impotency. Estrogens may be used to prevent tumor dissemination. Palliative treatment, used if the cancer has metastasized, includes irradiation, transurethral surgery, orchiectomy, and estrogens. General principles associated with these therapeutic measures are applicable to the aged patient. Many men are able to continue sexual performance after orchiectomy and during estrogen therapy; the physician should be consulted for specific advice concerning the expected outcomes for individual patients.

Tumors of the Penis, Testes, and Scrotum

Cancer of the penis is rare and appears as a painless lesion or wartlike growth on the prepuce or glans. The resemblance of this growth to a chancre can cause a misdiagnosis or a reluctance on the part of the patient to seek treatment. A biopsy should be done of any penile lesion. Treatment may consist of irradiation and local excision for small lesions and partial or total penile amputation for extensive lesions. Testicular tumors are uncommon in the aged but are usually malignant when they do occur; testicular enlargement and pain and enlargement of the breasts are suspicious symptoms. Chemotherapy, irradiation, and orchiectomy are among the treatment measures. Scrotal masses, usually benign, can be caused by conditions such as hydrocele, spermatocele, varicocele, and hernia. Symptoms and treatment depend on the underlying cause and are the same as for younger men. As with any genitourinary problem, counseling regarding self-care practices, body image, and sexual activity is important.

General Nursing Interventions Related to Genitourinary Problems

Care Planning

Actual or potential problems can be revealed during the assessment of the genitourinary system. Assessment data should be reviewed for those problems that fall within the realm of nursing to diagnose and manage, and related nursing diagnoses developed accordingly. Table 25-1 lists some of the major nursing diagnoses that can be related to genitourinary disorders.

The development of realistic goals guides care and provides a yardstick by which the patient's progress can be measured. Although the goals developed for individual patients will be specific to their unique needs, some potential goals in the care of genitourinary problems in older adults are listed in Sample Care Plan. Patients and their significant others should be active participants in the development of goals and establishment of priorities. See Chapter 18 for more information on planning and providing care.

Preventing Problems

Basic health practices, which are easily incorporated into the daily schedule, can prevent a variety of urinary tract problems. A good fluid intake can reduce the amount of bacteria in the bladder. An acidic urine, beneficial in preventing infection, can be enhanced by the intake of vitamin C and foods such as cranberries, prunes, plums, eggs, cheese, fish, and grains. Activity can eliminate urinary stasis, and frequent toileting can avoid urinary reten-

Table 25-1 *Nursing Diagnoses Associated With Genitourinary Problems*

NURSING DIAGNOSIS	CAUSE OR CONTRIBUTING FACTOR
Anxiety	Sexual dysfunction, pain, embarrassment over symptoms or treatments
Pain	Infection, cancer, retention
High risk for infection	Concentrated urine, immobility, more alkaline urine, more alkaline and fragile vaginal canal, prostatic hypertrophy, catheterization
High risk for injury	Falls on urine puddles, fragile vaginal tissue
Self-care deficit, toileting	Immobility, dementia, weakness
Disturbance in self-concept	Incontinence, sexual dysfunction
Sexual dysfunction	Infection, pain, altered structures, embarrassment
Impaired skin integrity	Incontinence, vaginitis
Sleep pattern disturbance	Nocturia, retention, dysuria
Impaired social interactions	Embarrassment over symptoms, odor, frequency, discomfort
Altered patterns of urinary elimination	Infection, retention, calculi, prostatic enlargement, vaginitis, strictures, incontinence

tion. Catheterization significantly increases the risk of infection and should be avoided.

The value of regular examinations of the reproductive system needs to be reinforced. Nursing considerations in fostering sexual function in older adults are discussed in Chapter 14. An annual gynecological examination, including a Pap smear, is essential for the older woman; she should be knowledgeable about self-examination of the breasts (see Chap. 30). Men with prostatic hypertrophy should be examined at least every 6 months to ensure that a malignancy has not developed.

Promoting a Positive Self-Concept

Nurses need sensitivity in dealing with patients' genitourinary problems. In addition to being areas that are considered taboo for discussion, these disorders may raise fears and anxieties that tales of becoming incontinent and sexless in old age perhaps are valid. Realistic explanations and a committed effort to correcting these disorders are vital. All levels of staff need to be reminded of the importance of discretion and dignity in managing these problems. Staff members should not check to see if a patient's pants are wet in front of others, allow someone to sit on a bedside commode in a hallway, bring in a group of students without the patient's permission to show them his orchitis, or scold the patient for having an accident in bed last night. Every effort should be made to minimize embarrassment and promote a positive self-concept. Resources available to assist patients with genitourinary problems are presented in the Resource List.

Sample Care Plan Goals for the Patient With a Genitourinary Problem

To have genitourinary problem diagnosed and treated

To verbalize accurate knowledge of the normal structure and function of the genitourinary system

To have a balanced fluid intake and output

To void without difficulty or discomfort

To be free from infection

To be free from skin irritation and breakdown

To be free from discomfort and pain related to genitourinary problem

To restore continence

To maintain or restore sexual function

To be free from discomfort associated with sexual function

To obtain annual gynecological or prostate examination

Resources to Assist Patients With Genitourinary Problems

Help for Incontinent People
Box 544
Union, SC 29389
(803)585-8789

Kimberly Clark Corporation
2001 Marathon Avenue
Neenah, WI 54946
(414)721-2000

Procter and Gamble
Procter and Gamble Plaza
Cincinnati, OH 45202
(800)428-8363

References

Bush LM, Kaye D. Epidemiology and pathogenesis of infectious diseases. In: Abrams WB, Berkow R, eds. The Merck manual of geriatrics. Rahway, NJ: Merck Sharpe & Dohme Research Laboratories, 1990:887.

Diokno AC. Urinary incontinence. In: Abrams WB, Berkow R, eds. The Merck manual of geriatrics. Rahway, NJ: Merck Sharpe & Dohme Research Laboratories, 1990:89.

Eliopoulos C. Resident assessment handbook. Glen Arm, MD: Health Education Network, 1990:46.

Recommended Readings

Brink CA, Sampselle CM, Wells TJ, Diokno AC, Gillis GL. A digital test for pelvic muscle strength in older women with urinary incontinence. Nurs Res 1989;38:196.

Cunha BA, Marx J, Gingrich D. Managing prostatitis in the elderly. Geriatrics 1991;46(1):60.

Lonergan ET. Aging and the kidney: adjusting treatment to physiologic change. Geriatrics 1988;43(3):27.

Loughlin KR. Medical and nonmedical therapies for benign prostatic hypertrophy. Geriatrics 1991;46(6):26.

Morishita L. Nursing evaluation and treatment of geriatric outpatients with urinary incontinence: geriatric day hospital model: a case study. Nurs Clin North Am 1988;23(1):189.

National Institutes of Health Consensus Development Conference. Urinary incontinence in adults. J Am Geriatr Soc 1990;38(3):265.

Norton C. Nursing for continence. Bucks, England: Beaconsfield, 1986.

Palmer MH, McCormick KA. Alterations in elimination: urinary incontinence. In: Murrow E, ed. Perspectives on gerontological nursing. Newbury Park, CA: SAGE, 1991:339.

Pieper B, Cleland V, Johnson DE, O'Reilly JL. Inventing urine incontinence devices for women. Image: Journal of Nursing Scholarship 1989;21:203.

Wells T. Conquering incontinence. Geriatr Nurs 1990;11(3):133.

Wisby M, Denny MS, Kissane K. For men only. Geriatr Nurs 1991;12(1):26.

26

Neurological Problems

The nervous system has a profound influence on our interaction with the world. A healthy system enables us to sense the pleasures around us; protect ourselves from harm; solve problems; derive intellectual stimulation; and communicate our needs, thoughts, and desires. Every aspect of our basic activities of daily living depends on a good neurological status. Dysfunction of this system has a ripple effect on other systems and can profoundly affect health, safety, normalcy, and general well-being.

Aging and the Nervous System

With age, neurons are lost and overall brain weight is reduced 5% to 17%. No evidence demonstrates that any functional changes relate to these structural alterations. It takes more time for impulses to travel along the neural pathways; thus, response and reaction time are slower. Profound changes occur in the sensory organs; these are discussed in detail in Chapter 27. Display 26-1 summarizes the changes to the nervous system that occur with age.

Assessment

General Observations

Keen observation while interviewing the patient can aid in detecting a variety of neurological problems. On initial inspection of the patient, asymmetry, deformity, weakness, paralysis, and other ab-

normalities can be seen. If such problems are noted, inquire into their origin, length of time present, and resulting limitations or problems. Explore the presence of symptoms of neurological disorders, such as pain, tingling sensations, numbness, blackouts, headaches, twitching, seizures, dizziness, distortions of reality, weakness, and changes in mental status.

Speech

During something as basic as simple introductions, speech disorders can become evident. If speech problems exist, it is important to differentiate problems with articulation (*i.e.*, dysarthria) and problems with the use of symbols (*i.e.*, dysphagia). With dysarthria, the symbols, in this case, words, are used correctly, but speech may be slurred or distorted as a result of poor motor control. Subtle dysarthrias can be disclosed by asking the patient to pronounce the following syllables:

- me, me, me (to test the lips)
- la, la, la (to test the tongue)
- ga, ga, ga (to test the pharynx).

Dysphasias can be receptive, expressive, or a combination of both. To test for a receptive aphasia, ask the patient to follow a command (*e.g.*, pick up the pencil); the patient's inability to understand what these symbols mean will prevent the command from being followed. The patient with expressive aphasia will be able to understand com-

Decrease in number of nerve cells
Reduction in cerebral blood flow and metabolism
Lower nerve conduction velocity
Slower reflexes
Delayed response to multiple stimuli
Decreased kinetic sense
Alteration in sleep cycle: less prominent stages III and IV
Decrease in efficiency of sensory organs

mands but will not be able to put symbols together into an intelligent speech form. Point to several objects and ask the patient to name them; mild dysphasias (*i.e.*, paraphasia) may be noted if the patient substitutes a close, although inaccurate, word for the right one, such as calling a shoe a boot or a watch a clock. The ability to understand and express oneself through the written word is important to evaluate also. Ask the patient to write a short sentence that you dictate and to read a sentence from a newspaper. Ensure that the patient has the educational and visual abilities to fulfill these demands.

Physical Examination

One component of the physical assessment of the nervous system involves the test of sensations. To help document areas where problems are identified, a figure drawing may prove useful. Ask the patient to close his or her eyes and to describe the sensations felt. Touch various parts of the body (*e.g.*, forehead, cheeks, arms, hands, legs, feet) lightly with your finger or a cotton wisp and note if the patient is able to feel the sensation. Compare analogous areas on both sides of the body and distal and proximal areas on the same extremity. If these primary sensations are intact, test the patient's ability to identify two simultaneous stimuli (*e.g.*, touch the right cheek and the left forearm). To test cortical sensation (*i.e.*, stereognosis), have the patient, again with closed eyes, identify various objects placed in each hand (*e.g.*, key, marble, coin). The inability to sense these objects is known as astereognosis.

Several simple measures are used for coordination and cerebellar testing. Hold up your finger and ask the patient to touch it and then touch his nose;

have the patient continue this action as you move your fingers to different areas. Do this point-to-point testing with both of the patient's arms, and note uneven, jerking movements and the inability to touch your finger or his nose. To test coordination in the lower extremity, have the patient lie down and run the heel of one foot against the shin of the other leg. The ability to make rapid alternating movements can be tested by having the patient rapidly tap his index finger on the thigh or a table surface. Tandem walking, in which the patient walks heel to toe as though walking a tightrope, also tests coordination; patients with arthritic deformities may not be able to perform this test. Have weak or poorly coordinated patients hold your hand during the tandem walking test.

Nurses can perform some tests of reflexes. To test the corneal reflex, gently touch the cornea with a wisp of clean cotton. Tissue and gauze are too rough and can cause corneal abrasions. Normally, the eye should blink. The Babinski reflex (*i.e.*, plantar response) is tested by stroking the sole of the patient's foot. Normally the toes should flex; an abnormal response is extension and fanning of the toes.

Each of the cranial nerves can be tested to identify further problems in the following ways.

Olfactory nerve. To test the sense of smell, obstruct one nostril by gently pressing on the side of the nose and see if the patient can detect the smell of strong substances such as coffee or tobacco. It is more important that the patient be able to detect the odor than to differentiate exactly what it is.

Optic nerve. Although complete assessment of this nerve requires ophthalmoscopic and funduscopic examination, nurses can test basic vision. The use of the Snellen chart is beneficial in determining visual acuity; if the chart is not available, use a newspaper to see what size print can be read (*e.g.*, small print or headlines only). If the patient's vision is so impaired that large print cannot be seen, have the patient give the count of fingers held in front of him. Some degree of presbyopia (*i.e.*, farsightedness) is common among most older adults. Be sure that the patient's eyeglasses, if worn, are used during visual testing.

Another test of the optic nerve involves visual fields. Ophthalmologists will use a target

screen during their examination to test visual fields; nurses can perform a basic test during their examination. Sit 3 feet away from the patient, at eye level, and ask the patient to look at your eyes. Extend your arm laterally until you no longer see your pointed index finger. Gradually bring your finger into your visual field, while you and the patient stare at each another, and ask the patient to tell you when he first sees your finger. Test the visual field at all points in a 360° area. Deficits can be determined based on the differences between when you and the patient first see your finger entering the visual field.

Oculomotor nerve. Cranial nerves III, IV, and VI control extraocular movements and are usually tested together by having the patient follow your finger as you move it to different points, horizontally and vertically. Normally, the eyes should move smoothly together.

Pupillary response to light is another test of the oculomotor nerve. First look at the size of the patient's pupil; then bring a lighted flashlight from the side of the patient's face outside of the visual field and observe what happens to the pupil. Normally, the pupil will constrict.

The oculomotor nerve also controls the eyelid. Look at the relationship of the eyelid to the pupil. Normally, the lids should be equal and not cover the pupil.

Trochlear nerve. The function of this nerve is to control downward and inward movement of the eye and is determined during the test of cranial nerve III, in which the patient's eyes follow your moving finger.

Trigeminal nerve. This three-branch nerve is responsible for sensations in the face and motor control of mastication. Have the patient close his eyes. Using a wisp of cotton and a toothpick or pin, touch the forehead, cheek, and chin on both sides of the face. Normally, the patient should be able to feel the sensations similarly on both sides of the face and differentiate between the soft and sharp objects. To test the nerve supply to the muscles of mastication, ask the patient to open his mouth and hold it open as you exert gentle pressure to try to close it; normally, the patient should be able to resist your force.

Abducens nerve. This nerve controls lateral movement of the eye and is included in the test of cranial nerve III, in which the patient's eyes follow your moving finger.

Facial nerve. This nerve supplies the muscles of facial expression. Examine the patient's face for symmetry and the absence of drooping. Ask the patient to smile, pull the mouth to each side, and lift the lips to show the teeth. The patient should be able to perform these movements without displaying asymmetry. Taste sensations on the anterior two-thirds of the tongue are supplied by this nerve. This can be tested by having the patient differentiate various flavors.

Acoustic nerve. Throughout the entire examination, pay attention to the patient's hearing ability: Does the patient ask to have things repeated? Does the patient appear to lip read? Can the patient hear you when you speak from behind talk in a low voice? These types of problems should be noted. A gross test of high-frequency hearing can be done by determining the ability of the patient to hear a wristwatch. Weber and Rinne tests are used to assess conductive losses and involve vibrating tuning forks. Thorough audiometric evaluation is essential when hearing loss is suspected.

Glossopharyngeal nerve. Along with the vagus nerve, this nerve supplies the pharynx and palate. Look in the patient's mouth and have him say "ah." The uvula should rise, as should both sides of the palate. The gag reflex should be tested also.

Vagus nerve. This nerve's function is determined as part of the evaluation of the glossopharyngeal nerve, in which the gag reflex and rise of the uvula are tested.

Spinal accessory nerve. To test the nerve supply to the sternomastoid and trapezius muscles, ask the patient to shrug the shoulders. Normally, they should lift symmetrically.

Hypoglossal nerve. As the name implies, this nerve supplies the tongue. Have the patient stick out the tongue and move it to both sides. It should move symmetrically.

Lumbar puncture, cerebral angiography, pneumoencephalography, and computed tomography scans are among other screening devices used to evaluate neurological problems. A review of mental

status is included in the assessment of the nervous system. For information on mental status examination, refer to Chapter 33.

Review of Selected Disorders

Herpes Zoster

Herpes zoster, or shingles, is an acute viral infection usually caused in the elderly by a reactivation of the latent varicella virus in the dorsal root ganglia. The varicella virus is the same one that causes chickenpox. The weakening of immunity associated with aging is believed to contribute to the increased incidence of this problem with age; radiation, chemotherapy, or other factors that disturb immune mechanisms also can cause shingles. The disease begins with pain and itching of the skin, followed in several days by the formation of vesicles. The eruption follows the path of a sensory nerve and can occur anywhere on the body, although the thoracic and abdominal areas are the most common sites. Treatment is symptomatic, consisting of analgesics, corticosteroids, and topical preparations to dry the lesions. Older adults are more likely than other age groups to experience post-herpetic neuralgia. If herpes zoster is recurrent or if dissemination is widespread, the patient should be evaluated for the possibility of an underlying lymphoma or other immune deficiency.

Parkinson Disease

Parkinson disease affects the central nervous system's ability to control body movements. It is most common in men and occurs most frequently in the fifth decade of life. Although the exact cause is unknown, this disease is thought to be associated with a history of metallic poisoning, encephalitis, and cerebrovascular disease—especially arteriosclerosis. A faint tremor that progresses over a long time may be the first clue. The tremor is reduced when the patient attempts a purposeful movement. Muscle rigidity and weakness develop, evidenced by drooling, difficulty in swallowing, slow speech, and a monotone voice. The face of the patient assumes a masklike appearance, and the skin is moist. Appetite frequently increases, and emotional instability may be demonstrated. A characteristic sign is a shuffling gait while leaning forward at the trunk. The rate of movement increases

as the patient walks, and the patient may not be able to voluntarily quit walking. As the disease progresses, the patient may become entirely unable to ambulate.

A variety of measures are used to control the tremors and maintain the highest possible level of independence. Levodopa or anticholinergics may be prescribed to decrease the patient's symptoms. Joint mobility is maintained and improved by active and passive range-of-motion exercises; warm baths and massage may facilitate these exercises and relieve muscle spasms caused by rigidity. Contractures are a particular risk of the aged parkinsonian patient. Physical and occupational therapists should be actively involved in the exercise program to help the patient find devices that increase self-care ability. Surgical intervention is rare for aged patients because they do not tend to respond well.

Tension and frustration will aggravate the patient's symptoms; therefore, the nurse should offer psychological support and minimize emotional upsets. Teaching helps patients and their families gain realistic insight into the disease. The nurse should emphasize that the disease progresses slowly and that therapy can minimize disability. Although intellectual functioning is not impaired by this disease, the speech problems and helpless appearance of patients may cause others to underestimate their mental ability; this can be extremely frustrating and degrading to the patient, who may react by becoming depressed or irritable. Continuing support by the nurse can help the family maximize the patient's mental capacity and understand personality changes that may occur. Communication and mental stimulation should be encouraged on a level that the patient always enjoyed. As the disease progresses, increased assistance is required by the patient. Skillful nursing assessment is essential to ensure that the demands for assistance are met while the maximum level of patient independence is preserved.

Transient Ischemic Attacks

Transient ischemic attacks, or temporary episodes of central nervous system dysfunction, can be caused by any situation that reduces cerebral circulation. Hyperextension and flexion of the head, such as when an individual falls asleep in a chair, can impair cerebral blood flow. Reduced blood

pressure resulting from anemia and certain drugs (*e.g.*, diuretics and antihypertensives) and cigarette smoking, due to its vasoconstrictive effect, will also decrease cerebral circulation. Hemiparesis, hemianesthesia, aphasia, unilateral loss of vision, diplopia, vertigo, nausea, vomiting, and dysphagia are among the manifestations of a transient ischemic attack, depending on the location of the ischemic area. These signs can last from minutes to hours, and complete recovery is usual within a day. Treatment may consist of correction of the underlying cause, anticoagulant therapy, or vascular reconstruction. A significant concern regarding transient ischemic attacks is that they increase the patient's risk of cerebrovascular accident.

Cerebrovascular Accidents

Older persons with hypertension, severe arteriosclerosis, diabetes, gout, anemia, hypothyroidism, silent myocardial infarction, transient ischemic attacks, and dehydration, and those who are smokers are among the high-risk candidates for a cerebrovascular accident, the third leading cause of death in this age group. Although a ruptured cerebral blood vessel could be responsible for this problem, most cerebrovascular accidents in the aged are caused by partial or complete cerebral thrombosis. Lightheadedness, dizziness, headache, drop attack, and memory and behavioral changes are some of the warning signs of a cerebrovascular accident. A drop attack is a fall caused by a complete muscular flaccidity in the legs but with no alteration in consciousness. Patients describing or demonstrating these symptoms should be referred for prompt medical evaluation. Because nurses are in a key position to first learn of these signs, they can be instrumental in helping the patient avoid disability or death from a stroke. Cerebrovascular accidents can occur without warning, however, and show highly variable signs and symptoms, depending on the area of the brain affected. Major signs tend to include hemiplegia, aphasia, and hemianopia.

Although the aged have a higher mortality rate from cerebrovascular accident than the young, those who do survive have a good chance of recovery. Good nursing care can improve the patient's chance of survival and minimize the limitations that impair a full recovery. In the acute phase, nursing efforts have the following several aims:

Maintain a patent airway.
Provide adequate nutrition and hydration.
Monitor neurological and vital signs.
Prevent complications associated with immobility.

In addition, unconscious patients need good skin care and frequent turning because they are more susceptible to decubiti formation. If an indwelling catheter is not being used, it is important for the nurse to examine the patient for indications of an overdistended bladder and promptly remedy the situation if it occurs. The eyes of the unconscious patient may remain open for a long time, risking drying, irritation, and ulceration of the cornea. Corneal damage can be prevented by eye irrigations with a sterile saline solution followed by the use of sterile, mineral-oil eye drops. Eye pads may be used to aid in keeping the eyelids closed; these are changed daily and frequently checked to make sure the lids are actually closed. Regular mouth care and range-of-motion exercises are also standard measures.

When consciousness is regained and the patient's condition stabilizes, more active efforts can focus on rehabilitation. It may be extremely difficult for patients to understand and participate in their rehabilitation because of speech, behavior, and memory problems. Although these problems vary depending on the side of the brain affected, some general observations can be noted. Attention span is reduced, and long, complicated directions may be confusing. Memory for old events may be intact, whereas recent events or explanations are forgotten, a characteristic demonstrated by many aged persons without a history of cerebrovascular accident. Patients may have difficulty transferring information from one situation to another. For example, they may be able to remember the steps in lifting from the bed to the wheelchair but be unable to apply the same principles in moving from the wheelchair to an armchair. Confusion, restlessness, and irritability may arise from sensory deprivation. Emotional lability may be a problem also. To minimize the limitations imposed by these problems, the nurse may find the following actions helpful:

Talk to the patient during routine activities.
Explain in brief form the basics of what has occurred, the procedures being performed, and the activities to expect.

Speak distinctly but do not shout.

Devise an easy means of communication, such as a picture chart to which one can point.

Minimize environmental confusion, noise, traffic, and clutter.

Aim for consistency—of those providing care and of care activities.

Use objects familiar to patients—their own clothing, clock, and so forth.

Keep a calendar or sign in the room showing the day and date.

Supply sensory stimulation through conversation, radio, television, wall decorations, and objects for patients to handle.

Provide frequent positive feedback; even a minor task may be a major achievement for the patient.

Expect and accept errors and failures.

The reader is advised to consult general medical–surgical textbooks for more detailed guidance in the care of patients who have suffered a stroke. Local chapters of the American Heart Association also provide much useful material for the nurse, the patient, and the family on the topic of stroke.

Nurses should promote activities that reduce patients' risks of stroke. Management of hypertension is important in decreasing fatal and nonfatal stroke in the elderly. Likewise, smoking cessation is helpful. Elderly persons who quit smoking experience higher cerebral perfusion levels than persons who never smoked.(Aronow, 1990)

Brain Tumors

Although brain tumors are not of high incidence in the aged, the resemblance of their symptoms to those mistakenly attributed to Alzheimer disease often results in delayed diagnoses. For instance, poor memory, confusion, personality change, headache, visual difficulties, poor coordination, and sensory–motor changes may be associated with arteriosclerosis or a multitude of other age-related problems. If these signs are not evaluated thoroughly in an early stage, valuable and potentially successful treatment time may be lost. The nurse must be aware of the general course of the patient's symptoms and facilitate their prompt evaluation.

General Nursing Interventions Related to Neurological Problems

Promoting Independence

Older patients with neurological problems must deal with the limitations imposed both by the disease and those resulting from the aging process. Skillful and creative nursing assistance can help the patient achieve a maximum level of independence. Some of the self-help devices previously mentioned—rails in the hallways, grab bars in bathrooms, and numerous other household modifications—can extend the time that patients can live independently in the community. Periodic home visits by the nurse, regular contact with a family member or friend, and a daily call from a local telephone reassurance program can help the patient feel confident and protected, which promotes independence. Although these patients may perform tasks awkwardly and slowly, family members need to understand that allowing independent function is physically and psychologically more beneficial than doing tasks for them. Continuing patience, reassurance, and encouragement are essential to maximize patients' capacities for independence.

Personality changes may often accompany neurological problems. Patients may become depressed as they realize their limitations or become frustrated by their need to be dependent on others. Their reactions may be displaced and evidenced by irritability toward others, often their loved ones or immediate caregivers. Family members and caregivers may need help in understanding the reasons for this behavior and in learning effective ways of dealing with it. Getting offended or angry at such patients may only serve to anger or frustrate them further. Understanding, patience, and tolerance are needed.

Care Planning

Actual or potential problems can be revealed during the assessment of neurological function. Assessment data should be reviewed for those problems that fall within the realm of nursing to diagnose and manage, and related nursing diagnoses developed accordingly. Table 26-1 lists some of the major nursing diagnoses that can be related to neurological problems.

Table 26-1 *Nursing Diagnoses Related to Neurological Problems*

NURSING DIAGNOSIS	CAUSE OR CONTRIBUTING FACTOR
Activity intolerance	Impaired sensory or motor function, fatigue, pain, depression, need for equipment or aids that use energy
Anxiety	Altered self-concept, inability to communicate, dependency
Altered bowel elimination: constipation	Inability to sense signal, lack of motor control, immobility
Pain	Poor positioning, pressure on brain, neuritis
Impaired verbal communication	Dysphasia, dysarthria, altered mental status
Ineffective individual coping	Altered body structure or function, dependency
Ineffective family coping	Dependency, demands of patient
Diversional activity deficit	Barriers from disabilities
Altered family processes	Demands, dependency, and role changes due to patient's illness
Fear	Altered body structure and function, dependency
Grieving	Loss of function, life style change
Altered health maintenance	Dependency, disability, altered self-concept
Impaired home maintenance management	Disability, dependency, pain, impaired mental status
High risk for infection	Immobility, lack of sensation
High risk for injury	Impaired sensory function, fatigue, altered mental status, improper use of aids, altered mobility or coordination
Impaired physical mobility	Paralysis, weakness, vertigo, poor coordination
Altered nutrition: less than body requirements	Swallowing disorder, inability to feed self or express desires, depression, altered taste, anorexia
Altered oral mucous membrane	Inability to provide adequate oral hygiene
Powerlessness	Dependency, disability, impaired communication, role change
Self-care deficit	Weakness, paralysis, poor coordination, visual disorders
Disturbance in self-concept	Altered body structure or function, dependency, role change
Sensory–perceptual alterations	Decreased or lost sensory function, cerebral vascular accident, sensory deprivation
Sexual dysfunction	Impaired nerve supply, disability, altered self-image, depression
Impaired skin integrity	Altered ability to feel pressure or pain, immobility
Impaired social interactions	Altered body structure or function, dysphasia, dysarthria, visual or hearing deficits, depression, altered self-concept
Social isolation	Inability to communicate, disability, impaired mobility
Altered thought processes	Cerebral vascular accident, depression, anxiety, fear, altered cerebral function
Altered patterns of urinary elimination	Lack of sensory awareness to void or ability to control bladder emptying, inability to communicate needs or toilet self

The development of realistic goals guides care and provides a yardstick by which the patient's progress can be measured. Although the goals developed for individual patients will be specific to their unique needs, some possible goals in the care of neurological problems for older patients are listed in the Sample Care Plan. Patients and their significant others should be active participants in the development of goals and establishment of priorities. See Chapter 18 for more information on planning and providing care.

Preventing Injury

Protecting the patient from hazards is particularly important in caring for the person with a neurological disorder. Uncoordinated movements, weakness, and dizziness are among the problems that cause these patients to be at high risk for accidents. Whether in an institutional setting or the patient's own home, the environment should be scrutinized for potential sources of mishaps, such as

---

Sample Care Plan Goals for the Patient With a Neurological Problem

To regain motor skills
To verbalize an understanding of the neurological problem and its management
To demonstrate proper procedures related to the care of the neurological problem
To learn effective mechanism for communication
To be oriented to person, place, and time
To appropriately use adaptive equipment
To be free from injury
To regain continence
To be free from pain or verbalize reduction in pain experienced
To increase independent function
To verbalize a positive self-concept
To develop means to derive sexual satisfaction
To be free from infection
To be free from pressure ulcers
To be free from complications associated with neurological problems

---

Resources to Assist Patients With Neurological Problems

American Parkinson's Disease Association
116 John St.
New York, NY 10038
(212)732-9550

Epilepsy Concern
1282 Wynnewood Dr.
West Palm Beach, FL 33409
(305)967-7616

Epilepsy Foundation of America
4351 Garden City Dr.
Landover, MD 20785
(301)459-3700

National Institute of Neurological
   and Communicative Disorders
National Institutes of Health
Information Office
Bethesda, MD 20205

National Multiple Sclerosis Society
205 E. 42nd St.
New York, NY 10017
(212)986-3240

National Parkinson Foundation
1501 N.W. 9th Ave.
Miami, FL 33136
(305)547-6666

Paralyzed Veterans of America
4350 East-West Hwy.
Suite 900
Washington, DC 20014
(301)652-2135

Parkinson's Disease Foundation
William Black Medical Research Bldg.
640-650 W. 168th St.
New York, NY 10032
(212)923-4700

United Parkinson Foundation
220 S. State St.
Chicago, IL 60604
(312)922-9734

loose carpeting; poorly lit stairwells; clutter; ill-functioning appliances; and the lack of fire warning systems, fire escapes, tub rails, nonslip tub surfaces, and other safeguards. Safety considerations also include the prevention of contractures, decubiti, and other risks to health and well-being. It is an injustice to the patient to allow preventable complications to hamper progress and compound disability. Resources that can assist patients with neurological problems are presented in the Resources List.

Reference

Aronow WS. Risk factors for geriatric stroke: identification and follow-up. Geriatrics 1990;45(9):37.

Recommended Readings

Corman LC. Strokes and the carotid: myths and realities. Geriatrics 1990;45(7):28.

Morris JC, McManus DQ. The neurology of aging: normal vs. pathologic change. Geriatrics 1991;46(8):47.

27

Sensory Deficits

Good sensory function is an extremely valuable asset that is often taken for granted. Intact senses facilitate accurate perception of the environment. People are better able to protect themselves from harm when they can see, hear, smell, touch, and verbalize danger. The beauties of the earth are more fully appreciated when the senses are functioning at their optimum level. Communication, the sharing of experiences, and the exchange of feelings are more complete when all the senses can participate. The environment is perceived with distortion when sensory function is impaired (e.g., people might suspect they are being talked about if they are unable to hear the conversation of those around them). Everyday experiences, such as reading the newspaper and recognizing a familiar face on the street, can be hampered by poor eyesight. Food tastes bland without properly functioning taste buds. Freshly cut flowers lose their fragrances when olfactory functioning is poor.

The reduced ability to protect oneself from hazards due to sensory deficits can result in serious falls from unseen obstacles, missed alarms and warnings, ingestion of hazardous substances from not recognizing their taste, an inability to detect the odor of smoke or gas, and burns and skin breakdown because of decreased cutaneous sensation of excessive temperature and pressure. Alterations during the aging process, excessive use and abuse, and the disease processes that affect all age groups contribute to the problems of the elderly. Sensory deficits compound the other problems that threaten the health and well-being of the

aged—their increased vulnerability to accidents, their social isolation and declining physical function, and many other limitations regarding self-care activities. Because it is the rare older individual who does not suffer from some sensory deficit, it behooves the nurse working with the aged to have a sound knowledge of the sensory problems that may affect them and of the associated assistive techniques. Some of the nursing diagnoses associated with sensory deficits are listed in Table 27-1, and potential care plan goals can be found in the Sample Care Plan.

Aging and the Senses
Vision

As the eye undergoes a variety of structural and functional changes with age, the lids become thinner and wrinkled, displaying skin folds commonly known as bags (Fig. 27-1). Ptosis, inversion, and eversion of the lid are common. The conjunctiva, easily irritated by dust particles and air pollutants, is thinner and more fragile. The cornea gains a cloudy appearance, being less translucent and more spherical. Deposits of fat over the cornea and grayish plaques on the sclera may be detected. The pupil decreases in size and becomes less responsive to light, and the pupil sphincter undergoes sclerosis. Peripheral vision is more difficult as the visual field narrows, and vision at night and in dimly lit areas is a greater problem which results from the increase in the threshold of light percep-

Table 27-1 *Nursing Diagnoses Associated With Sensory Deficits*

NURSING DIAGNOSIS	CAUSE OR CONTRIBUTING FACTOR
Activity intolerance	Sensory deprivation or overload, impaired communication
Anxiety	Impaired communication, altered self-concept, reduced ability to protect self
Pain	Acute glaucoma, corneal ulcer, detached retina
Impaired verbal communication	Hearing deficit
Diversional activity deficit	Impaired vision or hearing
Impaired home maintenance management	Visual deficits, inability to protect self
High risk for infection	Reduced tactile sensations
High risk for injury	Inability to see, hear, smell, or feel hazards
Powerlessness	Inability to protect self, care for self, communicate
Self-care deficit	Visual disorders
Disturbance in self-concept	Dependency, impaired interactions, altered self-concept
Sensory–perceptual alterations	Impairment of any of the sensory organs
Impaired skin integrity	Reduced tactile sensations
Sleep pattern disturbance	Misperception of environment
Impaired social interactions	Visual or hearing deficits
Social isolation	Visual or hearing deficits, frustration of patient or others in attempting to communicate
Altered thought processes	Misperceptions or sensory deprivation due to altered sensory function

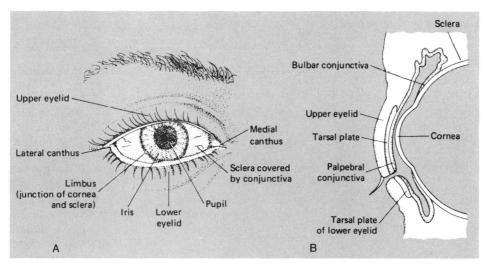

Figure 27-1. *Gross anatomy of the eye.* (**A**) *Anterior view.* (**B**) *Cross-sectional view.*

tion. Yellowing of the lens makes accurate perception of low-tone colors (*e.g.*, blues and greens) more difficult. Visual acuity is reduced, and adaptation to dark is slowed. Defective accommodation from loss of elasticity in the lens of the eye (*i.e.*, presbyopia) is common. The eyes have slower responses, fewer secretions, and a lower tissue resistance, predisposing the aged person to eye irritation and trauma. There may be a liquefaction of vitreous humor, accompanied by the release of supporting tissue, and cholesterol crystals may develop, causing bothersome but harmless spots before the aged individual's eyes.

Despite these changes, a majority of older persons have sufficient visual capacity to meet normal self-care demands with the assistance of corrective lenses. Serious visual problems can develop, however, and should be recognized early to prevent significant visual damage. Routine eye examinations by an ophthalmologist are important in detecting and treating eye problems early in the aged. Frequently, people postpone eye examinations because their present corrective lenses are still functional, because the need is not apparent, or because they have limited finances. The gerontological nurse can be instrumental in ensuring appropriate visual care by emphasizing that eye examinations are necessary to detect problems,

despite apparent need. It is important to inform people that although an optician prepares lenses and an optometrist fits the lenses to the visual deficit, only the ophthalmologist diagnoses and treats the full range of eye diseases.

In addition to annual eye examinations, prompt evaluation is required for any symptom that could indicate a visual problem, including burning or pain in the eye, blurred or double vision, redness of the conjunctiva, spots, headaches, and any other change in vision. A variety of disorders can threaten the aged person's vision. For instance, arteriosclerosis and diabetes can cause damage to the retina, and nutritional deficiencies and hypertension can result in visual impairment. The reader is advised to refer to the sections of this book that describe these diseases to gain an understanding of the pathophysiology involved.

Hearing

Hearing deficits can result from changes to the ear that occur with aging (Fig. 27-2). The external ear does not undergo significant change, although cerumen secretion is somewhat altered. Cerumen, secreted in lesser amounts, contains a greater amount of keratin in the aged, which makes it harder and easily impacted. The middle ear may experience

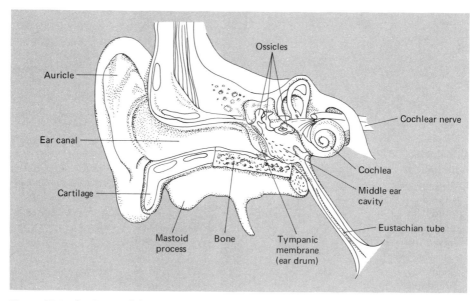

Figure 27-2. *Anatomy of the ear.*

atrophy or sclerosis of the tympanic membrane. The inner ear and retrocochlear lose their efficiency, and the cells at the base of the cochlea degenerate. The changes affecting the inner ear are demonstrated first by a loss in the ability to hear high-frequency sounds; this is followed by a loss of middle and then low frequencies as well. Presbycusis is the commonly used term to describe this progressive hearing loss associated with aging.

Assessment

General Observations

During interactions with the patient, signs of hearing deficits can be noted such as missed communication, requests to have words repeated, reliance on lip reading, and cocking of the head to one side in an effort to hear better. Eye problems can be identified by noticing if the patient uses eyeglasses, demonstrates difficulty seeing (*e.g.*, bumping into objects, unable to see small print), or possesses eye abnormalities such as drooping eyelids, discolored sclera, excess tearing, discharge, and unusual movements of the eyes. Foul odors (*e.g.*, associated with incontinence or vaginitis) that do not seem to bother the patient could reflect diminished olfactory function; cigarette burns on fingers or unrecognized pressure ulcers may indicate that the patient has reduced ability to sense pressure and pain. Display 27-1 lists common sensory problems in gerontological patients.

Interview

The patient should be asked about the date and type of the last ophthalmic and audiometric examinations (*e.g.*, where was the examination done; was an ophthalmologist or optometrist seen; did the eye examination include tonometry; was a full audiometric evaluation done or basic hearing screening). If eyeglasses or hearing aids are used, questions should be asked about where, when, and how these appliances were obtained (*e.g.*, reading glasses purchased from the local pharmacy versus prescription glasses; hearing aid obtained via television advertisement). Questions can be asked to disclose the presence of sensory problems, such as the following:

DISPLAY 27-1   Age-Related Changes of Sensory Function

Presbyopia
Narrowing of visual field
Decreased pupil responsiveness to light; decrease in pupil size
Increased light perception threshold
Yellowing of lens; altered perception of green, blue, and violet colors
Slower dark–light adaptation
Diminished corneal sensitivity
Increased incidence of "floaters"
Presbycusis
Harder consistency of cerumen
Degeneration of vestibular structures
Atrophy of cochlea, organ of Corti, and stria vascularis
Decreased number of taste buds; inefficiency in relaying flavors
Decreased number of sensory cells in nasal lining; fewer cells in olfactory bulb of brain
Reduced ability to feel pressure and pain
Decreased ability to differentiate temperatures

"Has there been any change in your vision? Please describe."
"Are your glasses as useful to you as they were when you first obtained them?"
"Do you experience pain, burning, or itching in the eyes?"
"Do you ever see spots floating across your eyes? How often does this happen and how large and numerous are the spots?"
"Do you ever see flashes of light or halos?"
"Are your eyes ever unusually dry or watery?"
"Do you have difficulty with vision at night, in dimly lit areas, or in bright areas?"
"Does any one in your family have glaucoma or other eye problems?"
"Have you noticed any change in your ability to hear? Please describe."
"Are certain sounds more difficult for you to hear than others?"
"Do you ever experience pain, itching, ringing, or a sense of fullness in your ears?"
"Do your ears accumulate alot of wax? How do you manage this?"
"Is there ever drainage from your ears?"

"Is your sense of smell as keen as it was in earlier years? Describe any differences."

"Do you have any problem or have you noticed changes in your ability to feel pain, pressure, or different temperatures?"

Physical Examination

The eyes should be inspected for unusual structure, drooping eyelids, discoloration, and abnormal movement. Loss of elasticity around the eyes, indicated by bags, is a common finding. Black-skinned persons may normally have a slight yellow discoloration of the sclera. Palpation of the eyeballs with the eyelids closed can reveal hard-feeling eyes with extremely elevated intraocular pressure and spongy-feeling eyes with fluid volume deficits. Lesions on the lids should be noted.

A gross evaluation of visual acuity can be done by having the patient read a Snellen chart or various-sized lettering on a newspaper. If the patient is unable to see letters on the chart or newspaper, an estimation of the extent of the visual limitation can be obtained by determining if the patient is able to see fingers held up before him or can merely make out figures.

If the patient has restrictions in seeing all portions of the visual field, the exact nature of this problem should be reviewed. A blind spot in the visual field (*i.e.*, scotoma) can occur with macular degeneration, a narrowing of the peripheral field may be associated with glaucoma, and blindness in the same half of both eyes (*i.e.*, homonymous hemianopia) can be present in persons who have experienced a cerebrovascular accident.

Extraocular movements are tested by having the patient follow the nurse's finger as it is moved to various points, horizontally and vertically. Irregular, jerking movements can result from disturbances in cranial nerves III, IV, or VI.

Inspection of the ears usually shows cerumen accumulation, increased hair growth, and atrophy of the tympanic membrane, which causes it to appear white or gray. Cerumen impactions should be noted and removed. A small, crusted, ulcerated lesion on the pinna can be a sign of basal or squamous cell carcinoma.

A gross evaluation of hearing can be made by determining the patient's ability to hear a watch ticking. Both ears should be checked. In addition to presbycusis and conductive hearing losses, ear or upper respiratory infections, ototoxic drugs, and diabetes can be responsible for diminished hearing.

Visual Deficits and Related Nursing Interventions

Cataracts

A cataract is a clouding of the lens or its capsule that causes the lens to lose its transparency. Cataracts are common in the aged, because everyone develops some degree of lens opacity as they age. Researchers at the Johns Hopkins Wilmer Eye Institute have found that exposure to ultraviolet B increases the risk of developing cataracts, and recommend sunglasses to protect the eyes.(Newswatch, 1989) Most aged persons do have some degree of lens opacity with or without the presence of other eye disorders. No discomfort or pain is associated with cataracts. At first, vision is distorted and objects appear blurred. The opacification continues, and eventually lens opacity and vision loss are complete. Glare from sunlight and bright lights is extremely bothersome to the affected person. Nuclear sclerosis develops, causing the lens of the eye to become yellow or yellow-brown; eventually the color of the pupil changes from black to a cloudy white.

Surgery to remove the lens is the only cure for a cataract. Patients with a single cataract may not necessarily undergo surgery if vision in the other eye is good, and these individuals should concentrate on strengthening their existing visual capacity, reducing their limitations, and using the safety measures applicable to any visually impaired person (Fig. 27-3). Sunglasses, sheer curtains over windows, furniture placed away from bright light, and several soft lights instead of a single bright light source minimize annoyance from glare. It is beneficial to place items within the visual field of the unaffected eye, a consideration when preparing a food tray and arranging furniture and frequently used objects. Regular reevaluations of the patient by an ophthalmologist are essential to detect changes or a new problem in the unaffected eye.

Surgery

For most patients, surgery is successful in improving vision. Cataract surgery is an outpatient procedure and the aged withstand it well. Geronto-

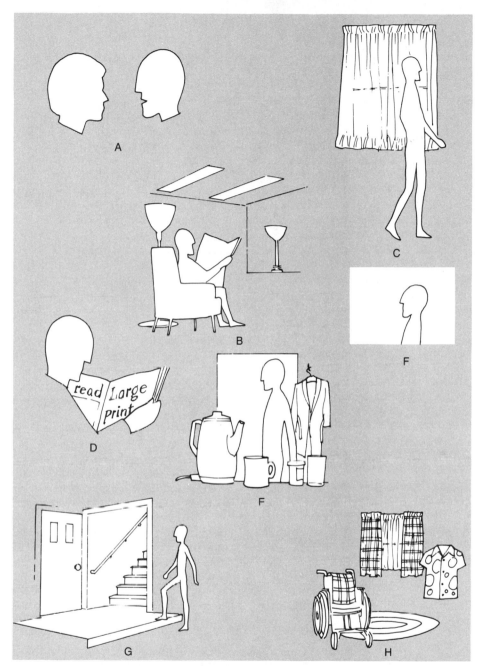

Figure 27-3. Compensating for visual deficits in the aged. (**A**) Face the person when speaking. (**B**) Use several soft indirect lights instead of a single glaring one. (**C**) Avoid glare from windows by using sheer curtains or stained windows. (**D**) Use large-print reading material. (**E**) Have frequently used items within the visual field. (**F**) Avoid the use of low-tone colors and attempt to use bright ones. (**G**) Use contrasting colors on doorways and stairs and for changes in levels. (**H**) Identify personal belongings and differentiate the room and wheelchair with a unique design rather than by letters or numbers.

logical nurses are in a position to reassure older patients and their families that age is no deterrent to cataract surgery. The simple surgical procedure and several weeks of rehabilitation can result in years of improved vision and, consequently, a life of higher quality. Two types of surgical procedures are used for removing the lens. Intracapsular extraction is the surgical procedure of choice for the aged patient with cataracts and consists of removing the lens and the capsule. Extracapsular extraction is a simple surgical procedure in which the lens is removed and the posterior capsule is left in place. A common problem with this type of surgery is that a secondary membrane may form, requiring an additional procedure for discission of the membrane.

The most common method of replacing the surgically removed lens is the insertion of an intraocular lens at the time of cataract surgery. For older patients, this method has been more successful than adjusting to a contact lens or special cataract glasses. The intraocular lens tends to distort vision less than cataract glasses do and does not require the care of a contact lens. Some patients do develop complications with lens implant, such as eye infection, loss of vitreous humor, and slipping of the lens implant.

Glaucoma

Glaucoma ranks after cataracts as a major eye problem in the aged. It tends to have a high incidence between the ages of 40 and 65 years and declines in incidence in old age. Ten percent of all blindness in the United States is a result of glaucoma. Although the exact cause is unknown, glaucoma can be associated with an increased size of the lens, iritis, allergy, endocrine imbalance, emotional instability, and a family history of this disorder. An increase in intraocular pressure occurs rapidly in acute glaucoma and gradually in chronic glaucoma.

Acute Glaucoma

With acute, or closed-angle, glaucoma, the patient experiences severe eye pain, nausea, and vomiting. In addition to the increased tension within the eyeball, edema of the ciliary body and dilation of the pupil occur. Vision becomes blurred, and blindness will result if this problem is not corrected within a day. Diagnosis is confirmed by placing a tonometer on the anesthetized cornea to measure intraocular pressure (Fig. 27-4). The normal pressure is within 20 mmHg. A reading between 20 to 25 mmHg is considered potential glaucoma. Another diagnostic test (*i.e.,* gonioscopy) uses a contact lens and a binocular microscope to allow direct examination of the anterior chamber and differentiate closed-angle from open-angle glaucoma. In the past, if intraocular pressure did not decline within 24 hours, surgical intervention would be necessary. However, medications are now effective in treating the acute attack (*e.g.,* carbonic anhydrase inhibitors, which reduce the formation of aqueous solution; mannitol, urea, or glycerin, which reduce fluid because of their ability to increase osmotic tension in the circulating blood). An iridectomy may be performed after the acute attack to prevent future episodes of acute glaucoma.

Chronic Glaucoma

Chronic, or open-angle, glaucoma is the more common type. It often occurs so gradually that affected individuals are unaware that they have a visual problem. Peripheral vision becomes slowly but increasingly impaired so that people may not realize for a long time why they bump or knock over items at their side. They may need to frequently change eyeglasses. As the impairment progresses, central vision is affected. People may complain of a tired feeling in their eyes, headaches, misty vision, or seeing halos around lights—symptoms that tend to be more pronounced in the morning. The cornea may have a cloudy appearance, and the iris may be fixed and dilated. Although this condition usually involves one eye, both eyes can become affected if treatment is not sought. The same procedures as mentioned with acute glaucoma are used to diagnose this problem. Treatment, aimed toward reducing the intraocular pressure, may consist of a combination of a miotic and a carbonic anhydrous inhibitor or of surgery to establish a channel to filter the aqueous fluid (*e.g.,* iridectomy, iridencleisis, cyclodialysis, corneoscleral trephining).

Care and Prevention

Vision lost due to glaucoma cannot be restored. However, additional damage can be prevented by avoiding any situation or activity that increases intraocular pressure. Physical straining and emo-

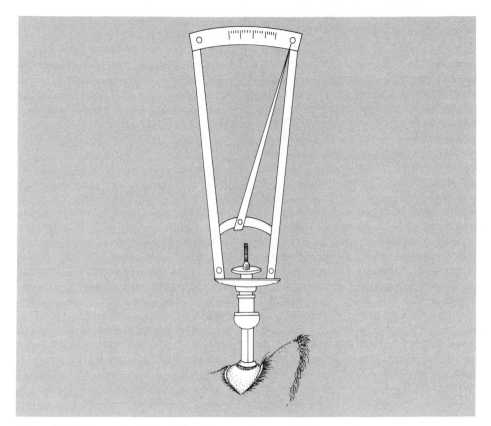

Figure 27-4. *Measuring intraocular pressure by use of a tonometer.*

tional stress should be prevented. Miotics may be instilled into the eye; acetazolamide may be used. Mydriatics, stimulants, and agents that elevate the blood pressure must not be administered. It may benefit patients to carry a card or wear a bracelet indicating their problem to prevent administration of these medications in situations in which they may be unconscious or otherwise unable to communicate. Abuse and overuse of the eyes must also be prevented. Periodic evaluation by an ophthalmologist is an essential part of the continued care of the patient with glaucoma.

Macular Degeneration

Macular degeneration involves damage or breakdown of the macula, which results in a loss of central vision. The most common form is involutional macular degeneration, associated with the aging process, although macular degeneration also can

result from injury, infection, or exudative macular degeneration. Routine ophthalmic examinations can identify macular degeneration, emphasizing the importance of annual eye examinations.

Laser therapy has been used for the treatment of some forms of macular degeneration, but the involutional type does not respond well to this procedure. Magnifying glasses, high-intensity reading lamps, and other aids can prove helpful to patients with this condition.

Detached Retina

The aged may experience detachment of the retina, a forward displacement of the retina from its normal position against the choroid. The symptoms, which can be gradual or sudden, include the perception of spots moving across the eye, blurred vision, flashes of light, and the feeling that a coating is developing over the eye. Blank areas of vision

progress to complete loss of vision. The severity of the symptoms depends on the degree of retinal detachment. Prompt treatment is required to prevent continued damage and eventual blindness. There does not tend to be pain. Initial measures most likely to be prescribed, bed rest and the use of bilateral eye patches, can be frightening to the aged patient who may react with confusion and unusual behavior. The patient should be made to feel as secure as possible; frequent checks and communication, easy access to a call light or other means of assistance, and full, honest explanations will help provide a sense of well-being. After time has been allowed for the maximum amount of "reattachment" of the retina to occur, surgery may be planned.

Several surgical techniques are used in the treatment of detached retina. Electrodiathermy and cryosurgery cause the retina to adhere to its original attachment; scleral buckling and photocoagulation decrease the size of the vitreous space. Eye patches remain on the patient for several days after surgery. Specific routines vary according to the type of surgery performed. The patient needs frequent verbal stimuli to minimize anxiety and enhance psychological comfort. Physical and emotional stress must be avoided. Approximately 2 weeks after surgery, the success of the operation can be evaluated. A minority of patients must undergo a second procedure. It is important for the patient to understand that periodic examination is important, especially because some patients later suffer a detached retina in the other eye.

Corneal Ulcers

Inflammation of the cornea, accompanied by a loss of substance, causes the development of a corneal ulcer. Febrile states, irritation, dietary deficiencies, lowered resistance, and cerebrovascular accident tend to predispose the individual to this problem. Corneal ulcers, which are extremely difficult to treat in the aged, may scar or perforate, leading to destruction of the cornea and blindness. This problem is responsible for 10% of all blindness. The affected eye may appear bloodshot and show increased lacrimation. Pain and photophobia are also present. Nurses should advise clients to seek assistance promptly for any irritation, suspected infection, or other difficulty with the cornea as soon as it is identified. Early care is often effective in preventing the development of a corneal ulcer

and preserving visual capacity. Cycloplegics, sedatives, antibiotics, and heat may be prescribed to treat a corneal ulcer. Sunglasses will ease the discomfort associated with photophobia. It is important that the underlying cause be treated—an infection, abrasion, or presence of a foreign body. Corneal transplants are occasionally done for more advanced corneal ulcers.

Hearing Deficits and Related Nursing Interventions

Most aged have some degree of hearing loss, resulting from a variety of factors other than aging. Exposure to noise such as that of jets, traffic, and guns cause cell injury and loss. The higher incidence of hearing loss in men may be associated with the fact that they are more often employed in occupations that subject them to loud noises (*e.g.,* truck driving, construction, and heavy factory work). Recurrent otitis media and trauma can damage hearing. Certain drugs may be ototoxic, including aspirin, streptomycin, neomycin, and karomycin; the delayed excretion of these drugs in many older persons may promote this effect. Diabetes, tumors of the nasopharynx, other disease processes, and psychogenic factors can also contribute to hearing impairment.

Particular problems affect the ears of the aged person (Fig. 27-5). Vascular problems, viral infections, and, as mentioned, presbycusis are often causes of inner-ear damage. In otosclerosis, an osseous growth causes fixation of the footplate of the stapes in the oval window of the cochlea. This may be a middle ear problem; it is more common among women and can progress to complete deafness. Middle-ear infections are less common in older individuals; they usually accompany more serious disorders such as tumors and diabetes. The external ear can be affected by dermatoses, furunculosis, cerumen impaction, cysts, and neoplasms.

The following diagram briefly outlines the normal transmission of sound through the ear. Interference with the transmission of the physical sound waves causes conduction deafness. Conduction deafness may be due to an easily correctable problem such as infection or cerumen accumulation. Perception deafness is the term used to describe a problem with the nerve endings registering the electrical signals. Degeneration of the

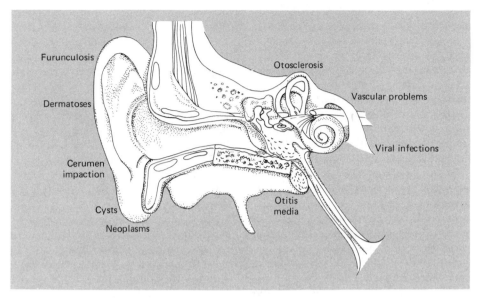

Figure 27-5. *Problems affecting the ears of aged people.*

auditory nerve with age may be a factor in this form of deafness. Some aged individuals possess both conduction and perception deafness.

Normal Transmission of Sound

Sound
↓
External Ear
↓
Middle Ear
↓
Inner Ear
(Here, sound waves are converted from physical waves to electrical signals.)
↓
Auditory Nerve
↓
Brain receives
nerve impulse

The first action in caring for someone with a hearing deficit should be to encourage audiometric examination. Hearing impairment should not be assumed to be a normal consequence of aging and ignored. It would be most sad and negligent if the cause of the hearing problem were easily correctable (*e.g.*, removal of cerumen or a cyst) but allowed to limit unnecessarily the life of the affected individual. The aged should be advised not to purchase a hearing aid without a complete audiometric evaluation. Many older persons invest money for a hearing aid from their limited budget just to discover that their particular hearing deficit cannot be improved by this means.

Sometimes the underlying cause of the hearing problem can be corrected. Frequently, however, the aged must learn to live with varying degrees of hearing deficits. Assisting the aged to live with these deficits is a challenge in gerontological care. It is not unusual for the impaired to demonstrate emotional reactions to their hearing deficits. Unable to hear conversation, patients may become suspicious of those around them and accuse people of talking about them. Anger, impatience, and frustration can result from repeatedly unsuccessful attempts to understand conversation. Patients may feel confused or react inappropriately on receiving distorted verbal communications. Being limited in the ability to hear danger and protect themselves, they may feel insecure. Being self-conscious of their limitation, they may avoid social contact to escape embarrassment and frustration.

Social isolation can be a serious threat because people sometimes avoid the aged person with a hearing deficit due to the difficulty in communication. Even telephone contact may be threatened.

Approximately 10% of the aged have difficulty hearing telephone conversations. Physical, emotional, and social health can be seriously affected by this deficit.

Someone nearby should be alerted to the individual's hearing problem so that he or she can be protected in an emergency. In an institutional setting, such patients should be located near the nurse's station. People with hearing loss should be advised to request explanations and instructions in writing so that the full content is received. Those working with the aged can minimize the limitations caused by hearing deficits. When talking with individuals with high-frequency hearing loss, the speaker should talk slowly, distinctly, and in a low-frequency voice. Raising the voice or shouting will only raise the sounds to a higher frequency and compound the deficit. Methods for promoting more accurate and complete communication include talking into the least impaired ear; facing the individual when talking; using visual speech (*e.g.,* sign language, gestures, and facial expressions); allowing the person to lip-read; and using flash cards, word lists, and similar aids and devices.

Hearing Aids

The otologist can determine if a hearing aid would be valuable for the given individual and recommend the particular aid best suited to the patient's needs. The nurse is in a key position to educate the aged individual on the importance of consult-ing an otologist before purchasing a hearing aid (Fig. 27-6). Patients must understand that, even with a hearing aid, their problems will not be solved. Hearing will not return to normal although it will improve; speech may sound distorted through the aid because when speech is amplified, so are all environmental noises, which can be most uncomfortable and disturbing to the individual. Sounds may be particularly annoying in areas where reverberation can easily occur (*e.g.,* a church or large hall). Some persons never make the adjustment to a hearing aid and choose not to wear the appliance rather than to tolerate these disturbances and distortions.

To facilitate adjustment to a hearing aid, an initial period should be provided for experimentation with the controls. This will help the wearer find the most beneficial setting. It may be useful for the person to wear the hearing aid for short periods at first, increasing the length of time as adjustment is made. To reduce disturbances, the individual may find it useful to sit in the front rows of churches and meeting halls, where there is less reverberation. Lowering the amplification in a noisy environment—such as a train station, airplane terminal, or stadium—may also reduce annoyance and discomfort.

Like any fine instrument, the hearing aid must be well cared for. The ear mold can be separated from the receiver for daily washing with soap and water. The cannula should be checked for patency because cerumen can accumulate in it and inter-

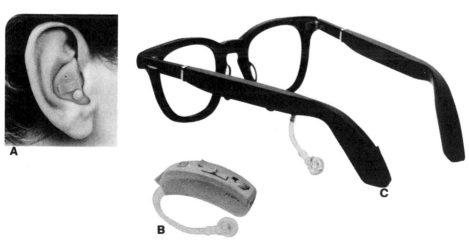

Figure 27-6. *Types of hearing aids.* (**A**) *In-the-ear model.* (**B**) *Behind-the-ear model.* (**C**) *Eyeglass model. (Courtesy of Zenetron, manufacturer of Zenith Hearing Aids.)*

fere with the function of the hearing aid. A pipe cleaner will effectively remove any particles from the cannula. The batteries should be periodically checked; new batteries should be installed before the old ones are expected to wear out. The wearer may find it useful to carry extra batteries in a pocketbook or pocket. Prompt repair is advisable when damaged cords or faulty functioning are detected.

Prevention

Gerontological nurses have a responsibility to help aging persons protect and preserve their hearing. Some hearing deficits in old age can be avoided by good care of the ears throughout life. Such care should include the following.

Prompt and complete treatment of ear infections should be obtained.

Trauma to the ear (*e.g.*, from a severe blow or a foreign object in the ear) should be prevented.

Cerumen or particles should be removed by irrigating the external auditory canal rather than by using cotton-tipped applicators, hairpins, and similar devices. A forceful stream of solution during this procedure can cause perforation of the eardrum.

People should be protected from exposure to loud noises such as those associated with factory and construction work, vehicles, loud music, and explosions. Earplugs or other sound-reducing devices should be used when exposure is unavoidable.

Regular audiometric examinations should be scheduled.

Local chapters of hearing and speech associations and organizations serving the deaf can provide assistance and educational materials to those affected by and interested in hearing problems.

Other Sensory Deficits and Related Nursing Interventions

Sight and hearing are not the only senses affected by the aging process; other sensations are also reduced with age. The number of functioning taste buds may be significantly decreased, especially those responsible for sweet and salty flavors. Pain and pressure are not as easily sensed by the aged. Age-related effects on tactile sensation may also be noted by the difficulty some aged persons have in

discriminating between temperatures. Some loss of olfactory function may be noted.

To compensate for the multiple sensory deficits the aged may experience, special attention must be paid to stimulation of all the senses during part of daily living activities. The diet can be planned to include a variety of flavors and colors. Perfumes, fresh flowers, and scented candles, safely used, can provide interesting fragrances. In an institutional setting, having a pot brewing fresh coffee in the patients' area can provide a pleasant and familiar aroma during the early morning hours; likewise, a table-top oven can allow for cookie baking and other cooking activities in the patients' area, providing a variety of stimuli. Different textures can be used in upholstery and clothing fabrics. Clocks that chime, music boxes, and wind chimes can vary environmental sounds. The design of facilities for the aged should take into consideration the use of different shapes and colors. Intellectual stimulation—through conversation, music, and books, for instance—is also vital.

Touch is not only a means of sensory stimulation but also an expression of warmth and caring. Too frequently, the nurse may inadvertently only touch the patient during specified procedures. It is easy for patients to begin to feel that others perceive them only in terms of tasks rather than as a total human beings. How often are patients referred to as "a complete bath," "a Foley irrigation,"

Sample Care Plan Goals for the Patient With a Sensory Deficit

To develop an effective mechanism for communication

To obtain ophthalmologic or audiometric evaluation or both

To learn special practices to protect self from hazards

To verbalize understanding of deficit and related care

To adapt to the use of a hearing aid, eyeglasses, assistive device

To verbalize a positive self-concept

To be free from injury

To engage in regular satisfying activity

To perform activities of daily living independently and safely

To be free from pain

Resources to Assist Patients With Sensory Deficits

Alexander Graham Bell Association for the Deaf
3417 Volta Pl., N.W.
Washington, DC 20007
(202)337-5220

American Council of the Blind
1211 Connecticut Ave., N.W.
Suite 506
Washington, DC 20036
(202)833-1251

American Humane Association Hearing Dog
  Program
1500 W. Tufts Ave.
Englewood, CO 80110
(303)762-0342

Blinded Veterans Association
1735 DeSales St., N.W.
Washington, DC 20036
(202)347-4010

Design Center for the Deaf
Dept. of Environmental Design
Rochester Institute of Technology
Rochester, NY 14623
(716)464-1653

Guide Dogs for the Blind
P.O. Box 1200
San Rafael, CA 94902
(415)479-4000

Guiding Eyes for the Blind
250 E. Hartsdale Ave.
Hartsdale, NY 10530
(914)723-2223

Helen Keller National Center
111 Middle Neck Rd.
Sand Point, NY 11050
(516)944-8900

Independent Living Aids
11 Commercial St.
Plainview, NY 11803
(516)681-8288

Leader Dogs for the Blind
1039 S. Rochester Rd.
Rochester, MN 48063
(313)651-9011

National Association for the Deaf
814 Thayer Ave.
Silver Spring, MD 20910
(301)587-1788

National Association for Hearing and Speech
  Action
10801 Rockville Pike
Rockville, MD 20852
(301)897-8682

National Association for the Visually Handicapped
305 E. 24th St.
New York, NY 10010
(212)899-3141

National Braille Association
654A Goodwin Ave.
Midland Park, NJ 07432
(201)447-1484

National Center for Law and the Deaf
7th St. and Florida Ave., N.E.
Washington, DC 20002
(202)651-5454

National Eye Institute
Building 31, Rm. 6A-32
Bethesda, MD 20205
(301)496-5248

National Federation of the Blind
National Center for the Blind
1800 Johnson St.
Baltimore, MD 21230
(410)659-9314

National Information Center on Deafness
Gallaudet College
T-6, 800 Florida Ave., N.E.
Washington, DC 20002
(202)651-5109

National Library Service for the Blind
  and Physically Handicapped
Library of Congress
1291 Taylor St., N.W.
Washington, DC 20542
(202)287-5100

Recorded Periodicals
919 Walnut St.
Philadelphia, PA 19107
(215)627-0600

Recordings for the Blind
215 W. 58th St.
New York, NY 10022
(212)751-0860

The Seeing Eye
Morristown, NJ 07960
(201)539-4425

Self-Help for Hard of Hearing People
P.O. Box 34889
Washington, DC 20034

---

or "a feed?" How often are these labels nonverbally communicated when the nurse's only encounters with the patient are for the sake of these activities? To hold a hand, rub a cheek, and pat a shoulder, basic as they may seem, can convey a message to patients that they are still perceived as human beings. Acceptance of the patient's efforts to touch is also important. The universal language of touch can often communicate a friendship, warmth, and caring that overcomes the most severe sensory deficit. Numerous resources that can assist patients with sensory deficits are presented in the Resource List.

Reference

Newswatch: Keep your hat on! Geriatr Nurs 1989; 10(4):176.

Recommended Readings

Burrage RL, Dixon L, Sehy YA. Physical assessment: an overview with sections on the skin, eye, ear, nose and neck. In: Chenitz WC, Stone JT, Salisbury SA, eds. Clinical gerontological nursing. Philadelphia: WB Saunders, 1991:37.

Gulya AJ. Ear disorders. In: Abrams WB, Berkow R, eds. The Merck manual of geriatrics. Rahway, NJ: Merck Sharp & Dohme Research Laboratories, 1990:1083.

Kane RL, Ouslander JG, Abrass IB. Essentials of clinical geriatrics. 2nd ed. New York: McGraw-Hill, 1989:301.

Kupfer C. Ophthalmologic disorders. In: Abrams WB, Berkow R, eds. The Merck manual of geriatrics. Rahway, NJ: Merck Sharp & Dohme Research Laboratories, 1990:1055.

Shields JA. Malignant tumors of the eye in geriatric patients. Geriatrics 1991;46(9):28.

28

Hematological Problems

Hematological problems are common in the elderly; conditions such as lymphosarcoma, chronic lymphocytic leukemia, reticulum cell sarcoma, macroglobulinemia, and multiple myeloma are of high incidence. Anemia occurs with such frequency among older adults that it is often mistakenly considered a normal consequence of growing old. Hematological diseases are significant because they reduce the elderly's capacities to manage stress and protect themselves from serious risks.

Aging and the Hematological System

A variety of factors are believed to be associated with the development of hematological problems in old age. The thymus and lymph nodes atrophy. Cutaneous hyperreactivity is impaired. Less immunoglobulin is produced in response to stress. More lymphocytes are in the bone marrow, and the circulating red-cell mass is reduced. Display 28-1 summarizes the changes to the hematological system that occur with age.

Assessment

General Observations

On first inspection of the patient, hematological problems may be apparent through signs such as pallor, dry skin with poor turgor, atrophy of the tongue, easily breakable fingernails, and thin, brittle hair.

Interview

A history of symptoms should be explored, with special attention to fatigue; edema; weight loss; irritability; confusion; depression; bleeding; enlarged nodes; anorexia; nausea; vomiting; bone pain; and tenderness or pain over the liver, spleen, or lymph nodes.

Physical Examination

The skin should be inspected for pallor, petechiae, and ecchymoses. The oral cavity and conjunctiva often will show pallor when it is less evident on the skin surface. The tongue should be examined for changes that are associated with certain anemias (e.g., smooth, red tongue with vitamin B_{12} deficiency; atrophy of tongue with pernicious anemia). Examination of the lymph nodes can reveal enlarged nodes in the presence of Hodgkin disease.

Evaluation of the blood sample is essential in detecting hematological disorders. Some of the normal laboratory values for the older adult are presented in Display 28-2.

Review of Selected Disorders and Related Nursing Interventions

Anemia

Anemia refers to a decrease in the number of red blood cells and in hemoglobin level. Although anemia is a common problem in the older population,

DISPLAY 28-1   Age-Related Changes of the Hematological System

Decline in amount of marrow space occupied by hematopoietic tissue

Impaired incorporation of iron into red blood cells due to ineffective erythropoiesis

Slight decrease in hemoglobin and hematocrit (although remain within normal range)

DISPLAY 28-2   Normal Blood Values for the Older Adult

Hematocrit: men, 38%–54%
women, 35%–47%
Hemoglobin: men, 14–18 g/dl
women, 12–16 g/dl
Sedimentation rate: men, < 20 mm/hr
women, < 30 mm/hr
Red blood cells: men, 4,600,000–6,200,000/mm³
women, 4,200,000–
5,400,000/mm³
White blood cells (WBC): 5,000–10,000/mm³
Neutrophils: 50%–70% of total WBC count
Eosinophils: 1%–4% of total WBC count
Basophils: 0%–1% of total WBC count
Lymphocytes: 20%–40% of total WBC count
Monocytes: 0%–6% of total WBC count
Platelets: 200,000–350,000/mm³
Total bilirubin: 0.1–1.2 mg/dl
Calcium: 9–11 mg/dl; 4.5–5.5 mEq/L
Bicarbonate: 24–32 mEq/L
Chloride: 350–390 mg/dl; 95–105 mEq/L
Total cholesterol: 150–250 mg/dl
Creatinine: 0.6–1.2 mg/dl
Fibrinogen: 150–300 mg/dl
Glucose: 70–120 mg/dl
Protein-bound iodine: 4–8 μg/dl
Iron: 65–170 μg/dl
Lead: < 40 μg/dl
Lipids (total): 400–1000 mg/dl
PCO₂: 35–45 mmHg
PO₂: 95–100 mmHg
pH: 7.35–7.45
Phosphatase: acid, 0.5–3.5 units; alkaline, 2–4.5 units
Potassium: 18–22 mg/dl; 3.5–5.5 mEq/L
Protein, total: 6–8 g/dl
Protein, albumin: 3.2–4.5 g/dl
Protein, globulin: 2.3–3.5 g/dl
Sodium: 310–340 mg/dl; 135–145 mEq/L
Urea nitrogen: 10–18 mg/dl
Uric acid: men, 2.1–7.8 mg/dl
women, 2–6.4 mg/dl

it is not a normal condition. In addition to the fatigue and pallor that usually accompany this problem, the aged may demonstrate a greater susceptibility to infection, confusion, angina attacks, and episodes of congestive heart failure. Certain problems can contribute to the development of the various types of anemia in the elderly, including the following:

- poor diet
- rheumatoid arthritis
- uremia
- chronic hepatitis
- cirrhosis
- prostatic hypertrophy
- diabetes
- cancer, especially of the hematopoietic organs and digestive tract
- peptic ulcers
- chronic bronchitis
- tuberculosis
- urinary tract infections and other chronic or subacute infections.

Therefore, in addition to treatment, a thorough evaluation of the patient is needed to detect any underlying disease causing the anemia.

Iron-Deficiency Anemia

Iron-deficiency anemia is the most common form of anemia in all age groups. In addition to poor dietary intake of iron, the aged can develop this anemia as a result of hemorrhoidal bleeding, peptic ulcers, or impaired absorption of iron. The clinical manifestations of this impaired tissue nutrition are dry, inelastic skin; headache; dizziness; fatigue; thin, brittle hair; atrophy of the tongue; and thin, brittle, and easily breakable fingernails. Blood tests confirm the diagnosis of iron-deficiency anemia, and a misdiagnosis can result if problems that reduce iron-binding capacity and serum iron are also present, such as rheumatoid arthritis and chronic infection. Hemoglobin and hematocrit values are low, although red blood cells can be normal in size and color until the condition is advanced. Serum iron decreases and total iron-binding

capacity is elevated. Because anemia in the presence of an adequate iron intake can indicate poor absorption, bleeding, or other problems, a complete review of the older person's diet is essential. Therapeutic measures, similar to those used with younger patients, include correcting any underlying cause, maintaining good nutrition, and using iron preparations. The patient should be instructed to administer the iron after meals and preferably not with dairy products.

It is important for the nurse to assist in the prevention of iron-deficiency anemia through the encouragement of a well-balanced diet and a good nutritional status. Helping the older patient obtain food stamps, introducing the patient to lunch programs, encouraging the correction of dental problems, teaching about diet, and providing guidance in the purchase of the best quality foods within limited budgets can be beneficial. The nurse can also discuss with the physician the value of iron supplements as a prophylactic measure.

Pernicious Anemia

Pernicious anemia is found mostly in elderly patients and is usually accompanied by a reduced platelet and white blood cell count. A vitamin B_{12} deficiency is the cause of pernicious anemia, which is frequently associated with cancer of the stomach. Individuals on a vegetarian diet are at high risk of developing this problem.(Sherman, 1991) Accompanying the usual symptoms of anemia are premature graying or whitening of the hair, atrophy of the tongue with flattening of the papillae, and leg edema. Gastrointestinal changes contributing to this disease may cause anorexia, weight loss, diarrhea, constipation, and other related symptoms. The central nervous system may also be involved, depending on the extent of the problem. The treatment plan is the same at all ages. Monthly vitamin B_{12} injections will be required for the remainder of the patient's life. Because gastric cancer is of greater incidence in patients with pernicious anemia, close follow-up and periodic stool examination are essential.

Folic Acid Deficiency

Folic acid deficiency is one of the major causes of nutritional anemia. Persons with limited fruit and vegetable intake are more likely to develop this form of anemia. Although folic acid deficiency is most commonly found in alcoholics, many aged persons risk developing this problem because a limited budget prevents them from including fruits and vegetables in their diet. Treatment consists of folic acid therapy, which, fortunately, can be replaced by good nutrition once the serum folic acid level has returned to normal.

Hodgkin Disease and Multiple Myeloma

Hodgkin disease and multiple myeloma in the aged are associated with anemia, leukopenia, or thrombocytopenia. Because symptomatology, diagnostic measures, and therapy for Hodgkin disease are similar to those described for other age groups, the reader is advised to explore medical–surgical nursing literature for a complete review of this disease, which runs a more rapid and aggressive clinical course in the elderly.

Multiple myeloma, more frequently diagnosed in middle-aged persons, has a decreasing incidence with age. Pathological fractures are a particular risk in aged people with multiple myeloma. Not only are these problems disabling in themselves, but they can pose serious threats to the aged as a result of emboli, pneumonia, and complications resulting from immobility. Confusion, behavioral changes, and coma are threats resulting from hypercalcemia associated with this disease. Many supportive measures to control pain and close observation for signs of complications are required of the nurse.

Leukemias

Leukemias have a higher incidence in aged people, in whom they have an insidious onset, manifest nonspecific symptoms that interfere with early diagnosis, are difficult to manage, and have a complicated course. A review of leukemias, readily available in medical–surgical literature, will not be presented here. However, some factors are unique to the aged. Acute leukemia runs an aggressive course in the aged, is difficult to manage, and has a poor prognosis. Chronic lymphocytic leukemia, which is the most common leukemia in the aged, progresses slowly. With chronic myeloid leukemia, the associated spleen and liver enlargement may not develop in the aged.

Although aged patients with leukemia require the same general care as younger patients, the gerontological nurse must be especially alert for

Table 28-1 Nursing Diagnoses Related to Hematological Problems

NURSING DIAGNOSIS	CAUSE OR CONTRIBUTING FACTOR
Activity intolerance	Anemia (altered O_2 transport), fatigue, pain
Altered bowel elimination: constipation	Low food intake due to anorexia or fatigue, pain, medications (iron, analgesics)
Altered bowel elimination: diarrhea	Pernicious anemia
Pain	Cancer, symptoms of anemia
High risk for infection	Altered leukocytes, anemia
High risk for injury	Fatigue, vertigo, confusion
Altered nutrition: less than body requirements	Anorexia, sore tongue, pain, weakness, medications
Self-care deficit	Pain, fatigue, vertigo
Sensory–perceptual alterations	Anemia, pain
Sexual dysfunction	Fatigue
Impaired skin integrity	Dry, inelastic skin
Altered thought processes	Anemia, cancer, pain

complications. The elderly are already at higher risk of infection than the young, and a disease such as leukemia compounds that risk. Infections must be prevented and promptly treated if they occur. Because the aged do not manage the stress of hemorrhage well, this complication should be prevented; if it occurs, it should be readily detected and promptly treated. Radiation therapy and chemotherapy may cause nausea, vomiting, stomatitis, anorexia, and other problems that threaten the nutritional status of the patient. Careful attention to the prevention of mouth trauma, avoidance of extremes in the temperature and seasoning of food, and the encouragement of a good diet are beneficial. The patient's psychological state may be affected by changes in body image caused by chemotherapy, radiation, or surgery. Maintaining the best possible appearance (e.g., through wigs and attractive clothing) and allowing patients to vent their reactions openly and discuss their disease may help them cope with these difficult adjustments.

Nursing diagnoses and care plan goals associated with hematological problems are presented in Table 28-1 and the Sample Care Plan, respectively.

Sample Care Plan Goals for the Patient With a Hematological Problem

To verbalize understanding of disorder and its management

To ingest a diet that contains prescribed amounts of nutrients

To improve dietary intake of vitamins and minerals

To identify foods rich in vitamins and iron

To be free from infection

To be free from pain

To prevent complications associated with hematological disorder

To regain sufficient energy to independently engage in activities of daily living

To restore normal cognitive function

Reference

Sherman D. Treating anemia in the elderly. Contemporary Long-Term Care 1991;14(4):56,58,87.

Recommended Readings

Freedman ML, Weintraub NT: Anemias. In: Abrams WB, Berkow R, eds. The Merck manual of geriatrics. Rahway, NJ: Merck Sharp & Dohme Research Laboratories, 1990:644.

Freedman ML, Weintraub NT. Malignancies and myelo-proliferative diseases. In: Abrams WB, Berkow R. The Merck manual of geriatrics. Rahway, NJ: Merck Sharp & Dohme Research Laboratories, 1990:655.

Freedman ML, Weintraub NT. Normal aging and patterns of hematologic disease. In: Abrams WB, Berkow R, eds.

The Merck manual of geriatrics. Rahway, NJ: Merck Sharp & Dohme Research Laboratories, 1990:643.

Kane RL, Ouslander JG, Abrass IB. Essentials of clinical geriatrics. 2nd ed. New York: McGraw-Hill, 1989:281.

29

Dermatological Problems

Perhaps the most obvious effects of growing old are the changes that involve the integumentary system. Lines and wrinkles, thicker nails, and graying hair are constant reminders of the aging process. The status of the integument is largely influenced by past health practices; in turn, it will influence the degree of risk to current health because of the problems resulting from an unhealthy integumentary system.

Aging and the Integumentary System

The rate of change to the integument depends on genetic, nutritional, emotional, biochemical, and environmental factors. Drying of the skin occurs until the sixth decade of life, at which time the moisture of the skin stabilizes somewhat. The skin becomes thinner and atrophies, providing less protection to underlying blood vessels. A loss of subcutaneous fat and elasticity, in addition to increased dryness, contributes to a wrinkling of the skin; more profound aging of the skin is noted in skin surfaces frequently exposed to ultraviolet light, a condition known as solar elastosis. In light-skinned persons, the skin may appear gray or pale yellow. Skin pigmentation (*i.e.*, lentigo senilis—commonly called liver spots or age spots) occurs on the dorsal portion of the hands and other exposed areas. Skin circulation is decreased, as evidenced by the ease of skin breakdown and prolonged bruises. There is an increased incidence of

benign skin tags and lesions, as well as a higher rate of malignant ones.

The scalp, axillary, and pubic hair thins. Men may experience significant loss of scalp hair and less facial hair; women may notice the appearance of thick facial hair above their lips and on their chins. Decreased pigmentation causes the hair to lose its color. The nails become thicker and may display longitudinal lines. Display 29-1 summarizes the age-related changes to the integumentary system.

Assessment
General Observations

One of the positive features of assessing the integumentary system is that its status is evident to the naked eye. A quick observation can assist in evaluating skin color, moisture, and cleanliness; the presence of lesions; hair condition and grooming; and the condition of the nails. Signs such as pallor or flushing can provide clues to health problems.

Interview

The patient should be asked about itching, burning sensations on the skin surface, hair loss, increased fragility of nails, and other symptoms associated with integumentary system problems. This opportunity also can be used to review bathing and shampooing practices.

Reduction in skin turgor
Flattening of the dermal–epidermal junction
Reduced thickness and vascularity of dermis
Degeneration of elastin fibers
Clustering of melanocytes, causing skin pigmentation
Thinning and graying of hair on scalp, pubic, and axilla areas
Thickening of hair in nose and ears
Slower growth of fingernails, more brittle nails
Reduction in number of sweat glands

Physical Examination

The entire skin surface should be examined from head to toes, including behind the ears, within skin folds, under the breasts, and between the toes. Bathing and massages are good opportunities to inspect the skin. Lesions should be described as specifically as possible in regard to their color (e.g., purple, black, hypopigmented), configuration (e.g., linear, separate, confluent, annular), size (e.g., measurement of depth and diameter), drainage, and type. Terms used to describe types of lesions include the following.

Macule   a small nonpalpable spot or discoloration

Papule   a discoloration <1/2 cm in diameter with palpable elevation

Plaque   a group of papules

Nodule   a lesion ½ to 1 cm in diameter with palpable elevation; the skin may or may not be discolored

Tumor   a lesion >1 cm with palpable elevation; the skin may or may not be discolored

Wheal   a red or white palpable elevation that may occur in variable sizes

Vesicle   a lesion <1/2 cm in diameter that contains fluid and has a palpable elevation

Bulla   a lesion >1/2 cm in diameter that contains fluid and has a palpable elevation

Pustule   a lesion containing purulent fluid; of variable size and palpable elevation

Fissure   a groove in the skin

Ulcer   an open depression in the skin that may occur in variable sizes.

Skin turgor can be tested by gently pinching various areas of the skin. Skin turgor tends to be poor in most older adults; however, the areas over the sternum and forehead do experience less of an age-related reduction in turgor and are good areas for turgor assessment.

By using the back of the hands and touching various areas, the nurse can obtain a gross assessment of skin temperature. Coldness or temperature inequalities between the extremities should be noted.

Review of Selected Disorders

Senile Pruritus

The most common dermatological problem among the elderly is pruritus. Although atrophic changes alone may be responsible for this problem, senile pruritus can be precipitated by any circumstance that dries the person's skin, such as excessive bathing and dry heat. Diabetes, arteriosclerosis, uremia, liver disease, cancer, pernicious anemia, and certain psychiatric problems also can contribute to pruritus. If not corrected, the itching may cause traumatizing scratching, leading to breakage and infection of the skin. Prompt recognition of this problem and implementation of corrective measures are, therefore, essential. If possible, the underlying cause should be corrected. Bath oils, moisturizing lotions, and massage are beneficial in treating and preventing pruritus. Vitamin supplements and a high-quality, vitamin-rich diet may be recommended. Antihistamines and topical steroids may be prescribed for relief.

Senile Keratoses

Senile keratoses, also referred to as actinic or solar keratoses, are small, light-colored lesions, usually gray or brown, on exposed areas of the skin. Keratin may be accumulated in these lesions, causing the formation of a cutaneous horn with a slightly reddened and swollen base. Freezing agents and acids can be used to destroy the keratotic lesions, but electrodesiccation or surgical excision ensures a more thorough removal. Close nursing observation for changes in keratotic lesions is vital because they are precancerous.

Seborrheic Keratoses

It is not uncommon for aged persons to have several dark, wartlike projections on various parts of their bodies. These lesions, called seborrheic kera-

toses, may be as small as a pinhead or as large as a quarter. They tend to increase in size and number with age. In the sebaceous areas of the trunk, face, and neck and in persons with oily skin, these lesions appear dark and oily; in less sebaceous areas, they are dry in appearance and of a light color. Normally, seborrheic keratoses will not have swelling or redness around their base. Sometimes abrasive activity with a gauze pad containing oil will remove small seborrheic keratoses. Larger, raised lesions can be removed by freezing agents or by a curettage and cauterization procedure. Although these lesions are benign, medical evaluation is important to differentiate them from precancerous lesions. In addition, the cosmetic benefit of removal should not be overlooked for the older patient.

Stasis Dermatitis

Poor venous return can cause edema of the lower extremities, which leads to poor tissue nutrition. As the poorly nourished legs accumulate debris, inadequately carried away with the venous return, the legs gain a pigmented, cracked, and exudative appearance. Subsequent scratching, irritation, or other trauma can then easily result in the formation of a leg ulcer. Stasis ulcers need special attention to facilitate healing. Infection must be controlled, and necrotic tissue removed, before healing will take place. Good nutrition is an important component of the therapy, and a diet high in vitamins and protein is recommended. Once healing has occurred, concern should be given to avoiding situations that promote stasis dermatitis. The patient may need instruction regarding a diet for weight reduction or the planning of high-quality meals. Venous return can be enhanced by elevating the legs several times a day and by preventing interferences to circulation such as standing for long periods, sitting with legs crossed, and wearing garters. Some patients may require ligation and stripping of the veins to prevent further episodes of stasis dermatitis.

Pressure Ulcers

Tissue anoxia and ischemia resulting from pressure can cause the necrosis, sloughing, and ulceration of tissue. This is commonly known as a pressure ulcer, or decubiti. Any part of the body can develop a pressure ulcer, but the most common

sites are the sacrum, greater trochanter, and ischial tuberosities. The aged are high-risk candidates for the following reasons:

> Their skin is more fragile and is damaged more easily.
> They often are in a poor nutritional state.
> They have reduced sensation of pressure and pain.
> They are more frequently affected by immobile and edematous conditions, which contribute to skin breakdown.

Prevention

In addition to developing more easily in older persons, pressure ulcers require a longer period to heal than in younger people. Therefore, the most important nursing measure is to prevent their formation, and to do this, it is essential to prevent unrelieved pressure. Encouraging activity or turning the patient who cannot move independently at least every 2 hours is necessary. Shearing forces that cause two layers of tissue to move across each other should be prevented by not elevating the head of the bed more than 30°, not allowing patients to slide in bed, and lifting instead of pulling patients when moving them. Pillows, flotation pads, alternating-pressure mattresses, and water beds can be used to disperse pressure from bony prominences. It must be emphasized that these devices do not eliminate the need for frequent position changes. While sitting in a chair, patients should be urged to move and assisted with shifting their weight at certain intervals. Lamb's wool and heel protectors are useful in preventing irritation to bony prominences. Sheets should be kept wrinkle free, and the bed should be checked frequently for foreign objects, such as syringes and utensils, which the patient may be lying on unknowingly.

A high-protein, vitamin-rich diet to maintain and improve tissue health is essential in avoiding pressure ulcer formation. Good skin care is another essential ingredient in prevention. Skin should be kept clean and dry, and blotting the patient dry will avoid irritation from rubbing the skin with a towel. Bath oils and lotions, used prophylactically, will help keep the skin soft and intact. Massage of bony prominences and range-of-motion exercises promote circulation and assist in keeping the tissues well nourished. The incontinent patient should be thoroughly cleansed with soap and water and dried after each episode to avoid skin breakdown from irritating excreta.

Treatment

Preventing pressure ulcers from developing is the best treatment for this problem. Once evidence of an ulcer is noted, aggressive intervention is required to avoid the multiple risks associated with this impairment of skin integrity (Display 29-2). It is useful to determine the stage of the pressure ulcer because various treatments are effective for different stages. The various stages of pressure ulcers may be recognized and relieved by the following signs and measures:

Hyperemia. Redness of the skin appears quickly and can disappear quickly if pressure is removed. There is no break in the skin and the underlying tissues remain soft. Relieving the pressure by the use of a square of adhesive foam is useful; it is advisable to protect the skin with a product such as Duoderm (Squibb) or Tegasorb (3M) before applying the adhesive.

Ischemia. Redness of the skin develops from as much as 6 hours of unrelieved pressure and is often accompanied by edema and indura-

---

DISPLAY 29-2 Techniques Used to Treat Pressure Ulcers

Chemical Debriding. Elase (a fibrinolytic enzyme) or Santyl (a collagenase) can be applied to a cleansed wound and dressed with a dry bandage or gauze. Specific instructions and frequency vary according to the agent. These agents facilitate the removal of necrotic tissue, allowing granulation and epithelization of tissue to occur.

Gelfoam With Flotation Therapy. The compressed or powder form of Gelfoam is implanted in the tissue of a clean wound to promote the growth of new cells. The dressing is left undisturbed for 3 to 7 days; tissue granulation is better when the dressing is allowed to remain in place longer. A nonpurulent discharge may occur, but it is no cause for alarm. Flotation pads are used to displace weight.

Insulin. After cleansing and irrigation of the wound, 10 units of U-40 regular insulin are dropped on the wound. The ulcer is then exposed to air to dry, with no dressing applied. This procedure is performed twice daily.

Karaya. After cleansing the wound with pHisoHex and irrigating with a hydrogen peroxide solution, the edges of the wound are massaged. A Karaya ring is then fitted around the wound and Karaya powder is sprinkled directly into the wound. Reston is sometimes used to relieve pressure on the wound. A piece of plastic wrap is attached to the Reston to cover the wound while allowing view of it. This window is changed and additional powder is applied every 8 hours.

Maalox or Sugar. After cleansing and irrigating the wound, Maalox or sugar is applied to promote granulation. Irrigation and reapplication of the substance is repeated every 8 hours.

Oxygen. After debridement of ulcers, the ulcer is irrigated and exposed to high concentrations of oxygen, either through the direct application of a face mask or in a hyperbaric chamber. This promotes oxygen diffusion to areas of poor circulation.

Surgical Debriding. Necrotic tissue can be removed surgically to promote faster debridement and new tissue growth.

Ultrasound. High-intensity and high-frequency sound waves are directed at the sore to break down cellular obstructions and promote circulation.

Wet-to-Dry Dressings. Following cleansing of the ulcer, gauze dressing soaked in normal saline or other prescribed solutions is placed on the wound for 6 to 8 hours (or as specified) and allowed to dry. Some debridment occurs as the dry dressing is removed.

General Measures. Techniques to treat pressure ulcers include the following general procedures: (1) frequent turning to prevent reduced circulation from blocked capillaries, (2) the use of flotation pads, alternating pressure mattresses, water beds, and heel protectors to displace body weight, (3) the use of sheepskin to prevent irritation to the skin and to promote evaporation of skin moisture, (4) using a turn sheet to allow greater weight distribution when lifting or turning the patient and to prevent friction to the skin during these activities, and (5) providing a high-protein, high-vitamin diet to promote a positive nitrogen balance and tissue growth.

tion. It can take several days for this area to return to its normal color, during which the epidermis may blister. Doughnut-shaped adhesive padding is applied to this ulcer, but the skin should be protected with Vigilon, which contains water and is soothing to the area. If the skin surface is broken, it should be cleansed daily with normal saline or the product suggested by your agency.

Necrosis. Unremitting pressure extending over 6 hours can cause ulceration with a necrotic base. This type of sore requires a transparent dressing that protects from bacteria but is permeable to oxygen and water vapor. An adhesive foam doughnut should be placed around the dressing to relieve pressure. Thorough irrigation is essential during dressing changes. Sometimes, topical antibiotics are used. It may take weeks to months for full healing to occur.

Ulceration. If pressure is not relieved, necrosis will extend through the fascia and potentially to the bone. Eschar, a thick, coagulated crust, is frequently present, and bone destruction and infection may occur. Unless eschar is removed, the underlying tissue will continue to break down, so debridement is essential.

A recommended system for describing the stages of ulcers, and one that is used in the Minimum Data Set tool for assessing nursing home residents, is described in Display 29-3.

General Nursing Interventions Related to Dermatological Problems

Facilitating Good Skin Status

Some general measures are used to prevent and manage dermatological problems in the elderly. It is important to avoid drying agents, rough clothing, highly starched linens, and other items irritating to the skin. Good skin nutrition and hydration can be promoted by activity, bath oils, lotions, and massages. Although skin cleanliness is important, excessive bathing may be hazardous to the skin; daily partial sponge baths and complete baths every third or fourth day are sufficient for the average aged person. Early attention to and treatment of pruritus and skin lesions are advisable for preventing irritation, infection, and other problems.

DISPLAY 29-3   *Stages of Pressure Ulcers*

Stage 1

A persistent area of skin redness (without a break in the skin) that does not disappear when pressure is relieved.

Stage 2

A partial thickness loss of skin layers that presents clinically as an abrasion, blister, or shallow crater.

Stage 3

A full thickness of skin is lost, exposing the subcutaneous tissues—presents as a deep crater with or without undermining adjacent tissue.

Stage 4

A full thickness of skin and subcutaneous tissue is lost, exposing muscle, or bone, or both.

Care Planning

Actual or potential problems can be revealed during the assessment of the integumentary system. Assessment data should be reviewed for those problems that fall within the realm of nursing to diagnose and manage, and related nursing diagnoses developed accordingly. Table 29-1 lists some of the major nursing diagnoses that can be related to dermatological problems.

The development of realistic goals guides care and provides a yardstick by which the patient's progress can be measured. Although the goals developed for individual patients will be specific to their unique needs, some possible goals in the care of dermatological problems for older patients are listed in the Sample Care Plan. Patients and their significant others should be active participants in the development of goals and establishment of priorities. See Chapter 18 for more information on planning and providing care.

Promoting Normalcy

Psychological support can be especially important to the patient with a dermatological problem. Unlike respiratory, cardiac, and other disorders, der-

Table 29-1 *Nursing Diagnoses Related to Dermatological Problems*

NURSING DIAGNOSIS	CAUSE OR CONTRIBUTING FACTOR
Anxiety	Altered body appearance
Pain	Pruritus, infection, ulcer
Fluid volume deficit	Excessive wound drainage
High risk for infection	Ulcer, fragile skin
High risk for injury	More fragile skin
Disturbance in self-concept	Age-related changes to skin, hair, and nails; pain
Sexual dysfunction	Altered self-concept due to age-related changes, more fragile vaginal epithelium
Impaired skin integrity	Fragile skin, immobility
Impaired social interactions	Altered self-concept due to age-related changes to integument
Altered tissue perfusion	Pressure sites, ulcers

matological problems are often visibly unpleasant to the patient and others. Visitors and staff may unnecessarily avoid touching and being with the patient in reaction to their skin problems. The nurse can reassure visitors regarding the safety of contact with the patient and provide instruction for any special precautions that must be followed. The most important fact to emphasize is that the patient is still normal, with normal needs and feelings, and will appreciate normal interactions and contact.

Encouraging a Positive Image

All persons should be encouraged to look their best and make the most of their appearance. However, efforts to avoid the normal outcomes of the aging process are for the most part fruitless and frustrating. Money that could be applied to more basic needs is sometimes invested in attempts to defy reality. The nurse should emphasize to persons young and old that no cream, lotion, or miracle drug will remove wrinkles and lines or return youthful skin. While clarifying misconceptions regarding rejuvenating products, the nurse can encourage the use of cosmetics for the purpose of protecting the skin and maintaining an attractive appearance; many benefits may be derived from this practice. Perhaps, as society achieves a greater acceptance and understanding of the aging process, the use of cosmetics will be replaced by an appreciation of the natural beauty of age.

Sample Care Plan Goals for the Patient With a Dermatological Problem

To be free from itching and pain associated with dermatological conditions
To be free from infection
To demonstrate appropriate techniques to prevent spread of infection
To maintain good skin integrity
To be free from pressure ulcers
To have improvement in pressure ulcer from stage to stage
To demonstrate good skin care measures
To verbalize and demonstrate a positive self-concept and body image

---

Recommended Readings

Bergstrom N, Braden BJ, Laguzza A, Holman V. The Braden scale for predicting pressure sore risk. Nurs Res 1987;36:205.

Bolin AK, Kligman AM. Aging and the skin. New York: Raven, 1988.

Braden BJ, Bryant R. Innovations to prevent and treat pressure ulcers. Geriatr Nurs 1990;11(4):182.

Brozena SJ, Waterman G, Fenske NA. Malignant melanoma: management guidelines. Geriatrics 1990;45(6):55.

Duncan C, Fenske NA. Cutaneous signs of internal disease in the elderly. Geriatrics 1990;45(8):24.

Frantz RA, Kinney CK. Variables associated with skin dryness in the elderly. Nurs Res 1986;35:98.

Munro BH, Brown L, Heitman B. Pressure ulcers: one bed or another? Geriatr Nurs 1989;10(4):190.

Pajk M. Pressure sores. In: Abrams WB, Berkow R, eds. The Merck manual of geriatrics. Rahway, NJ: Merck Sharp & Dohme Research Laboratories, 1990:140.

Proper SA, Rose PT. Non-melanomatous skin cancer in the elderly: diagnosis and management. Geriatrics 1990; 45(7):57.

Shenefelt PD, Fenske NA: Aging and the skin: recognizing and managing common disorders. Geriatrics 1990;45 (10):57.

30

Cancer

Cancer, a serious problem at any age, is the second leading cause of death among the older population. The incidence of cancer increases with age until the ninth decade, when a tendency for fewer new cases in proportion to that age group is noted. The primary sites of cancer in later life are the lungs, breasts, prostate, and colorectal areas (Table 30-1). Although the prevalence of most carcinomas is higher among the aged, some forms, such as cervical cancers and sarcomas, are diagnosed less frequently in older persons. Cancer tends to progress more slowly and run a less aggressive course in the aged.

Risks and Detection

The exact etiology of cancer is presently unknown, but several factors have been associated with it. Chronic irritation, from pipe smoking for instance, has been known to promote lesions that can become cancerous. Radiation can alter cellular activity and cause abnormal cell growth. Certain agents, such as air pollutants and some food additives, are carcinogenic. The familial tendency toward certain forms of cancer and the frequent detection of abnormal chromosomal composition of cancer cells raise questions as to the relationship of genes to cancer. Relationships between the incidence of certain forms of cancer and the dietary practices of certain countries can be noted. A viral cause for cancer has been postulated. Although none of these factors is known to be a definite cause of cancer, gerontological nurses can recognize them as predisposing factors in preventive health practices. The nurse should advocate the following practices:

Do not smoke.

Limit alcohol intake.

Follow a well-balanced diet, avoiding extremes in food temperature and seasoning.

Consult a dentist for treatment of poorly fitting dentures or jagged-edged teeth.

Use protection against excessive exposure to sun.

Avoid prolonged exposure to coal dust, asbestos, and other carcinogenic substances.

Be alert to signs and symptoms that might indicate cancer: a sore that does not heal, unexplained weight loss, a painless mass, increasing digestive problems, blood from any body orifice, or a change in bowel habits.

Regularly self-examine breasts or testicles.

Receive a complete physical examination, including a rectal and gynecological examination, regularly.

Early detection of cancer improves the potential for a good prognosis. Approximately one-half of the sites that cancer invades can be directly examined (*e.g.*, the breast, oral cavity, rectum, and skin, for instance) thereby increasing the opportunity for abnormalities to be discovered during a routine physical examination. Unfortunately, people do not

Table 30-1 *Most Common Causes of Cancer Death in Later Life (per 100,000 Population)*

	55–64 Years		65–74 Years		75–84 Years		85 + Years	
	MEN	*WOMEN*	*MEN*	*WOMEN*	*MEN*	*WOMEN*	*MEN*	*WOMEN*
Type of Cancer								
Respiratory	229.2	94.4	423.2	152.0	567.9	146.3	472.9	113.0
Digestive organs	126.6	72.7	268.6	162.5	465.3	303.1	665.0	482.1
Breast	0.5	80.9	1.0	109.9	1.8	136.2	3.1	180.0
Genital organs	25.2	42.4	112.5	71.9	324.4	91.0	637.5	108.4
Lymphatic and hematopoietic tissue	23.9	16.5	55.4	38.3	93.9	67.2	110.8	77.1
Urinary organs	21.8	9.2	49.7	19.0	105.8	39.1	174.8	62.0
Lip, oral cavity, pharynx	15.5	5.6	22.2	8.6	26.4	10.4	37.0	17.2
Leukemia	14.1	9.0	34.0	18.3	71.6	37.6	109.3	61.3

From US Department of Commerce. Statistical abstract of the US. 110th ed. Washington, DC: Bureau of the Census, 1990.

always seek regular checkups, waiting instead until they feel ill. By the time the disease has progressed to the extent that it causes symptoms, valuable treatment time may be lost and the chances of a good prognosis are reduced. Symptoms produced by cancer in a particular site may be confused with other problems; for example, constipation associated with cancer of the colon may mistakenly be attributed to poor peristalsis in the aged. If baseline information has been obtained through the nursing assessment, it can provide comparative data for the nurse to use when changes indicating cancer are suspected. Because the general principles of diagnosis and management are similar for old and young, the nurse should consult medical–surgical texts for more information regarding facts about cancer.

Cancer in Later Life
Lung Cancer

The incidence of lung cancer is increasing among women, particularly smokers, and carcinoma of the lung is the most common fatal malignancy of older men. Symptoms of this problem include dyspnea, fever, weakness, wheezing, cyanosis, and hemoptysis. Because the symptoms of lung cancer can be easily confused with other respiratory dis-

eases, diagnosis can be delayed. Without early detection and treatment, metastasis throughout the entire body can occur. Chest x-ray usually will detect the tumor before any symptoms occur. Persons who are high risk (e.g., smokers and those who have been chronically exposed to asbestos, chromium, uranium, nickel, and other carcinogenic pollutants) should be advised to obtain an annual chest x-ray.

Cancer of the Female Reproductive System

Breast cancer steadily rises in incidence with age (see Table 30-1). The seriousness of this problem warrants that all women understand and practice self-examination of the breasts; review of the patient's knowledge about this procedure is an essential part of the assessment of every woman. If the patient is unfamiliar with the technique for self-examination of the breasts, she should receive instruction and become familiar with the normal contour of her breasts (Fig. 30-1). It can be easier for the patient to remember to perform breast examination if she links the date to a specific day of the month, such as the day her pension check arrives. It must be reinforced that a woman is likely to detect a change in her breasts more quickly than the physician. If the patient is not capable of inde-

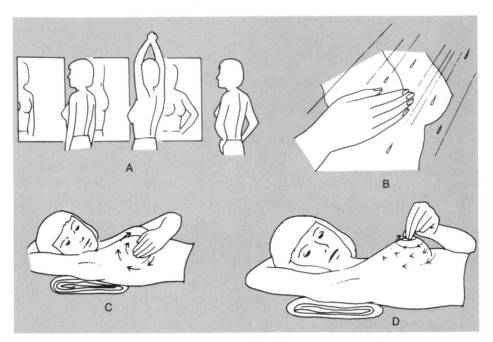

Figure 30-1. *Self-examination of the breasts. (**A**) With the arms straight at the sides, arms over the head, and hands on the hips while flexing the chest muscles, inspect the breasts before a mirror to detect swelling, changes in contour, dimpling, nipple change, or any other differences. (**B**) While in a tub or shower, run the hand over the breast with the fingers flat to detect thickening or lumps. (**C**) Inspect the breasts while lying down, with a folded towel under the shoulder of the side being examined and the arm of that side behind the head. (**D**) With the fingers flat, examine the outer portion of each breast, progressing in a circular motion around the circumference of the breast. Move the fingers 1 inch toward the center and repeat until the entire breast is examined. Then gently squeeze nipple to detect any discharge. (Additional information is available from the American Cancer Society.)*

pendently examining her breasts, arrangements should be made for monthly examination by a caregiver. Any lump, dimpling of the skin, or discharge from the nipples is cause for medical evaluation. Annual mammograms should be done on the older woman; unfortunately, older women are less likely to receive mammograms than younger women (Table 30-2). Gerontological nurses should be advocates for annual mammograms for older women and educate lay and professional persons on the importance of this procedure for this high-risk group.

Although cervical cancer does not occur as frequently among older women as younger women, elderly women should receive regular Pap smears and thorough gynecological examinations. The nurse may need to clarify potential misconcep-

tions (e.g., gynecological exams not being necessary after menopause) to ensure that these women obtain regular examinations.

Cancer of the Male Genitourinary System

Cancer of the prostate gland is a common problem of older men and is the second most common cause of cancer death in men older than 75 years of age. Most patients with this problem are asymptomatic or experience symptoms similar to benign prostatic hypertrophy; therefore, regular examination of the prostate gland is essential for early detection. Digital rectal examination will reveal a firm nodule or induration of the gland in the presence of cancer. A small percentage of benign hypertrophies develop into malignancies; the nurse should

Table 30-2 *Percentage of Women Who Have Had a Mammogram, Breast Physical Exam, or Who Perform Breast Self-Examination*

| AGE (y) | MAMMOGRAM | | BREAST PHYSICAL EXAM | | BREAST SELF-EXAM | |
	Ever	Past year	Ever	Past year	At least once per month	Less than once per month
40–54	42.2	16.8	86.7	39.0	47.3	20.0
55–64	41.1	16.9	83.1	31.9	49.8	18.6
65–74	35.2	12.9	76.8	30.7	46.1	17.2
75+	24.8	8.0	68.2	21.8	34.2	13.1

From US National Center for Health Statistics. Vital and health statistics. Series 10. No. 172. Data for 1987.

emphasize the importance of periodic reevaluation of benign prostatic hypertrophy. Cancer at this site is known to metastasize to the pelvis, vertebrae, and brain.

Hematuria can be an indication of cancer within the genitourinary tract and should receive prompt evaluation. Older men tend to have a higher incidence of bladder cancer than younger men. Cancer within this system can metastasize to the lungs, liver, lymph nodes, and other organs if not discovered and treated.

Colorectal Cancer

Most persons who develop colorectal cancer are aged; the incidence begins to rise in the fourth decade of life and doubles every 5 years thereafter. Colorectal cancer is more common in higher socioeconomic classes and in persons who consume a diet low in fiber and high in refined sugars. Because colon cancer in its early stage is asymptomatic, routine screening measures (*e.g.*, fecal occult blood testing) are beneficial.

Other Gastrointestinal Cancers

The oral cavity is frequently the location of cancerous growths. A squamous cell form of cancer may develop on the lip, primarily involving the lower lip. Exposure to sun and irritation from a pipe, teeth, or dentures are among the contributing factors. Cancer of the lip can metastasize to the cervical lymph nodes. Vitamin-B deficiencies, syphilis, excessive smoking, and pressure from jagged-edged teeth or dentures can promote cancer of the mouth. Cancer of the tongue can metastasize to local lymph nodes, although it does not usually me-

tastasize to other body organs, and the tonsils can develop cancer that affects the surrounding lymph nodes. Because bleeding is a symptom that may indicate cancer in this site, and because this symptom can initially be misjudged as hemoptysis, the nurse should carefully examine the mouth and throat when bleeding occurs to more accurately differentiate the cause of the problem. Cancer of the tonsils may be secondary to breast cancer.

Cancer of the pharynx requires keen observation and assessment for early detection. Associated symptoms are soreness of and bleeding from the throat and a slight deafness. Cancer of the pharynx may be a result of metastasis from cancer of the esophagus, heart, bronchi, or palate.

Gastric cancer increases in incidence with age and is more common in blacks and those in lower socioeconomic groups. Early symptoms can mimic indigestion or peptic ulcer, which can result in delayed diagnosis. As it progresses, the pain increases and is accompanied by anorexia, weight loss, hematemesis, and dysphagia. Surgery is the treatment of choice.

Cancer of the pancreas is the second most common gastrointestinal malignancy and is more prevalent among men. Cigarette smoking, diabetes, and a diet high in animal fat, coffee, and nitrosamines are among the risk factors associated with this disease. Pancreatic cancer is a difficult problem to diagnose and treat in the aged. Symptoms can include anorexia, weakness, weight loss, dyspepsia, epigastric pain radiating to the back, diarrhea, constipation, obstructive jaundice, and depression and other emotional changes. Sometimes venous thrombosis occurs; it is believed to be caused by an elevation in serum trypsin. Because these symptoms can be confused with those of pancre-

atitis and peptic ulcer, diagnosis is often delayed. Unfortunately, surgery and chemotherapy do not offer much success in treatment of pancreatic cancer at this time.

Cancer of the gallbladder is difficult to diagnose and treat. Most persons having this problem are aged. Unlike pancreatic cancer, it tends to have a higher incidence among women. Symptoms of gallbladder cancer include anorexia, weakness, nausea, vomiting, weight loss, pain in the right upper quadrant, jaundice, and constipation. The nature of these symptoms makes early detection difficult. Metastasis to the common duct, peritoneum, lungs, and ovaries can occur, and the prognosis for the patient with gallbladder cancer is poor.

Most malignant neoplasms of the liver result from metastasis from other sites. Symptoms include right upper quadrant or epigastric pain, weight loss, and altered mental status. Other symptoms can be related to metastasis. Treatment is usually unsuccessful and the prognosis is poor.

Leukemia and Lymphoma

The aged have a high incidence of leukemia, lymphosarcoma, and myeloma. Radiation and high-level benzene exposure are believed to be associated with acute leukemia. Often, acute leukemia appears similar to an infectious process (e.g., high fever, acute onset); weakness, delirium, and pallor occur also. Acute leukemia runs an aggressive course in the aged, although chemotherapy is often successful in producing remissions.

Chronic lymphocytic leukemia or myeloma, on the other hand, is not an aggressive disease in the aged. A minority of patients with chronic lymphocytic leukemia are asymptomatic, whereas many experience fatigue and activity intolerance as primary signs. Enlarged lymph nodes and splenomegaly may be present. Prognosis is based on the stage of the disease when it is diagnosed. Multiple myeloma increases in incidence with age and is more common in black individuals. Bone pain is a common symptom, particularly in the lower back or ribs; spontaneous pathologic fracture may occur. Anemia occurs in most patients and can lead to other symptoms, such as fatigue, dyspnea, and palpitations. Hypercalcemia is common and can cause a variety of neurological symptoms. The disease tends to progress slowly and the survival rate with treatment is good, except in poor-risk elderly.

Hodgkin disease peaks between 15 and 35 years of age and again between 50 and 80 years of age. Enlarged lymph nodes in the neck are a common sign, although any nodes can be affected. Survival is good with early treatment; older patients in advanced stages of the disease do not tolerate high radiation and chemotherapy doses and tend to have a poor prognosis.

Other Cancers

Hoarseness may be an early symptom of cancer of the larynx and should be evaluated. Fortunately, metastasis is rare. Cancer of the thyroid gland is rare among the aged. Skin cancer can develop from excessive exposure to the sun or chronic irritation. Sores that do not heal, new lesions, or changes in the appearance of moles in the aged should arouse suspicion. Depending on location and size, a good prognosis can result from the use of excision, radiation, and electrodesiccation and curettage.

Nursing Interventions

As mentioned earlier, treatment of cancer in the aged will be basically similar to treatment methods selected for younger adults, striving toward cure with minimal limitation. Surgery may prove beneficial, but the elderly have a higher surgical risk than do the young. The benefits of chemotherapy must be weighed against the side-effects it may cause in the aged. A therapeutic ratio is usually sought whereby the optimum effect is achieved with the least toxicity. Individualized decisions for cancer management are based on the general health status of the person, the form of cancer, the expected outcome, and the preference of the patient. At no time should treatment be discouraged or withheld based on age alone.

The nurse is a key figure in cancer management. It may be the nurse who first detects a symptom of cancer and who can facilitate a prompt diagnosis. The nurse can offer support and explanations during the diagnostic process. Once a positive diagnosis is made, the nurse can help the patient work through the denial, anger, depression, and other reactions frequently associated with a new diagnosis of cancer. While providing hope, the nurse can also guide the patient toward a realistic understanding of the outcomes of the disease (Table 30-3). If disability and death are to be ex-

Table 30-3 *Nursing Diagnoses Related to Cancer*

NURSING DIAGNOSIS	CAUSE OR CONTRIBUTING FACTOR
Activity intolerance	Depression, bedrest, fatigue, chemotherapy, radiation, pain
Anxiety	Terminal illness, treatments, hospitalization, uncertain future
Altered bowel elimination: constipation	Analgesics, immobility, pain
Altered bowel elimination: diarrhea	Gastrointestinal cancer, surgical intervention of bowel, antibiotics, chemotherapy
Pain	Diagnostic procedures, treatments, organ invasion by tumor
Impaired verbal communication	Tumor of head, neck, spinal cord areas; drugs; surgery
Ineffective individual coping	Loss of body part or function, disfigurement, side-effects of therapies, separation from support system, terminal nature of illness
Ineffective family coping	Terminal illness of patient; changes in roles, responsibilities, caregiving demands
Diversional activity deficit	Hospitalization, depression, change in functional ability
Altered family processes	Changes in roles, responsibilities, grieving, impending death
Fear	Loss of body part or function, pain, treatments, impending death
Fluid volume deficit	Anorexia, fatigue, depression, pain, high-solute tube feeding
Fluid volume excess	Renal failure, liver disease, pleural effusion, inadequate lymphatic drainage
Grieving	Loss of body part or function, terminal illness, pain
Altered health maintenance	Dependency, disability, pain, lack of knowledge
Impaired home maintenance management	Disability, pain, fatigue
High risk for infection	Altered immune system, invasive procedures, chemotherapy, radiation, IV therapy, immobility, malnutrition, drugs
High risk for injury	Altered cerebral function, pain, weakness, drugs
Knowledge deficit	Diagnostic tests, treatments, characteristics of disease
Impaired physical mobility	Pain, weakness, missing limb
Noncompliance	Lack of knowledge, denial
Altered nutrition: less than body requirements	Anorexia, pain, fatigue, nausea, vomiting, effects of therapy
Altered oral mucous membrane	Oral cancer, radiation, malnutrition, chemotherapy
Powerlessness	Dependency, disability, lack of knowledge, hospitalization
Altered respiratory function	Invasion by cancer, pain, fatigue, immobility
Disturbance in self-concept	Loss of body part or function, pain, dependency, terminal nature of illness
Sensory–perceptual alterations	Invasion of sensory organs by cancer, drugs, pain, immobility, radiation, isolation

(Continued)

Table 30-3 Nursing Diagnoses Related to Cancer (Continued)

NURSING DIAGNOSIS	CAUSE OR CONTRIBUTING FACTOR
Sexual dysfunction	Cancer of genitalia or breast, pain, fatigue, depression, anxiety, hospitalization
Impaired skin integrity	Emaciation, radiation, edema, immobility, sedation
Sleep pattern disturbance	Pain, anxiety, depression, drugs
Impaired social interactions	Loss of body part or function, terminal illness, depression
Social isolation	Disfigurement, hospitalization, fear or coping inability of others
Spiritual distress	Terminal illness, hospital barriers to practicing rituals
Altered thought processes	Depression, anxiety, fear, isolation
Altered tissue perfusion	Invasion of organ by cancer, edema, immobility, drugs, invasive lines, malnutrition
Altered pattern of urinary elimination	Malignancy of urinary tract or genitalia, chemotherapy, sedation, toileting deficit

pected, the patient and family may need strong nursing support as they learn to accept and plan for these consequences. On the other hand, patients with a good prognosis should be encouraged not to self-impose limitations or become emotional cripples as a result of having had a diagnosis of cancer. Within a realistic framework, all patients with cancer should be inspired to maintain a normal life-style and maximize their existing capacities.

When the terminal stage of cancer is reached, additional nursing intervention may be required to compensate for the patient's increasing limitations. The relief of pain is a priority for terminally ill patients. Concern as to the reality of the pain or the risk of narcotic addiction should not prevent the administration of analgesics. A low dosage should be administered initially, with periodic reevaluations as to the need for dosage change. To reduce stress and preserve the energy of the terminally ill patient, analgesics should be given to prevent pain, not just to correct it once it has already occurred. The nurse should observe the nature of the pain as the disease progresses; as death approaches, less pain may be sensed, and consequently fewer analgesics are required to provide relief. Small, frequent feedings of foods enjoyed by the patient may compensate for poor appetite and promote a bet-

ter food intake. Vitamin and protein supplements may be beneficial. An ample fluid intake should be maintained.

The skin should be kept clean, dry, and unbroken. Because of the general debilitated state of the patient, skin breakdown may be a greater risk than normal. Frequent skin care can provide cleanliness, comfort, and prevention of breakdown. Comfort is important, both physically and psychologically. Certain forms of cancer produce an unpleasant odor, and the nurse should be sure the patient is kept as attractive as possible, especially in light of any disfigurement, weight loss, jaundice, or other changes that may be occurring. Positioning should provide optimum comfort. Environmental considerations such as adequate ventilation, soft lights, and a clean area mean a great deal to the bedridden patient and the family. Opportunities for conversations should be provided. The terminally ill patient and the family may need to discuss their relationships, feelings, and the impending death. Involvement of the clergy may provide them with valuable support. The skills of the nurse may determine if the patient's death will be an unnecessarily traumatic experience or one of beauty and dignity. Some of the resources to assist patients who have cancer are presented in the Resources List.

Resources for Patients With Cancer

The following organizations provide information, educational materials, and support groups for patients with cancer; local chapters are available:

American Cancer Society
777 Third Avenue
New York, NY 10017
(212)371-2900

Leukemia Society of America
800 Second Avenue
New York, NY 10017
(212)575-8484

Make Today Count
P.O. Box 303
Burlington, IA 52601
(319)753-6251

National Cancer Institute
Office of Cancer Communications
Building 31, Room 10A18
Bethesda, MD 20205
(800)492-6600

National Hospice Organization
301 Tower
Suite 506
301 Maple Avenue
Vienna, VA 22181
(804)243-5900

Recommended Readings

Brozena SJ, Waterman G, Fenske NA. Malignant melanoma: management guidelines. Geriatrics 1990;45(6):55.

Gross JS. Current management modalities for prostate cancer. Geriatrics 1990;45(4):60.

Proper SA, Rose PT. Non-melanomatous skin cancer in the elderly: diagnosis and management. Geriatrics 1990; 45(7):57.

Zensk TV, Coe RM, eds. Cancer and aging. New York: Springer-Verlag, 1989.

31

Emergencies

This chapter will review selected emergencies that may be confronted in gerontological nursing care. The format is intended to provide easy information retrieval if this section needs to be consulted during actual emergencies.

Emergencies in elderly persons are particularly problematic due to the following factors:

They occur more frequently because of the age-related changes that lower resistance and make the body more susceptible to injury and illness.

They often present an atypical picture that complicates diagnosis.

They can be more difficult to treat or stabilize because of the elderly's altered response to treatment.

They carry a greater risk of causing serious complications and death.

By recognizing emergency situations and intervening promptly, nurses can spare considerable discomfort and disability to older patients and, in many situations, save their lives.

Regardless of the type of emergency, the following basic principles should guide nursing actions:

Maintain life functions.

Prevent and treat shock.

Control bleeding.

Prevent complications.

Keep the patient physically and psychologically comfortable.

Observe and record signs, treatments, responses.

Assess for causative factors.

Whenever there is question as to whether or not a true emergency exists, nurses should err on the side of safety. It is far better to obtain an x-ray or electrocardiogram (ECG) that results in a negative finding than to believe it would be an unnecessary bother or expense and have the patient suffer from a delayed diagnosis.

Review of Selected Emergencies

Acute Abdomen

Clinical manifestations: pain, although it may not be severe; abdominal tenderness and rigidity; possible reduction in bowel sounds.

Goal: determine underlying cause.

Review onset, characteristics, pattern of pain, and precipitating or related factors.

Palpate abdomen for muscular rigidity and tenderness.

Auscultate bowel sounds.

Take vital signs. Obtain ECG and urine and blood samples.

Goal: prevent complications.

Observe for signs of shock (*e.g.,* decreased blood pressure; rapid pulse; pallor; cold, moist skin; altered mental status; decreased urine output). Obtain treatment promptly.

Move patient with caution until cause is determined.

Goal: control pain.

Support treatment of underlying problem.

Administer analgesics as prescribed.

Note: an acute abdomen can be caused by appendicitis, liver distention from congestive heart failure, myocardial infarction, ruptured aortic aneurysm, dissecting abdominal aorta, and other disorders. Because of the atypical pattern of pain in the elderly, the severity of pain presented may not be a reliable indicator as to the severity of the problem. It is not uncommon for pain to be referred to another site.

Acute Confusion or Delirium

Clinical manifestations: rapid decline in cognitive function, disturbed intellectual function, disorientation to time and place, diminished attention span, poorer memory, labile mood, meaningless chatter, poor judgment, altered level of consciousness, restlessness, insomnia, personality changes, suspiciousness.

Goal: identify and correct causative factor.

Assess for changes in physical health, stresses, life-style changes, medications taken, dietary intake, other problems.

Obtain blood samples for evaluation.

Monitor vital signs, intake and output, and behaviors.

Support treatment plan, for example, electrolyte replacement, medication change, and fever control.

Goal: protect from injury and complications.

Supervise activities closely.

Remove hazardous substances, medications, and machinery from patient's immediate environment.

Ensure adequate nutritional intake, toileting, and hygiene.

Goal: reduce confusion.

Limit number of staff who provide care. Offer consistency of approach.

Maintain stable, calm environment. Avoid bright lights, excessive noise, and extreme room temperatures.

Offer orienting statements, such as "Mr. Jones, you are in the hospital. It is Tuesday evening. Your wife is at your side."

Clarify misconceptions.

Note: a thorough evaluation is crucial when confusion exists. This problem can result from a wide range of disturbances such as hypoglycemia, hypercalcemia, malnutrition, infection, trauma, and drug reactions.

Aspiration

Clinical manifestations: choking, coughing, respiratory distress, cyanosis.

Goal: restore patency of airway.

Suction. Remove obvious obstructions from oral cavity.

Perform the Heimlich maneuver. Stand behind patient, reach hands around to middle of patient's abdomen below sternum, lock hands, and quickly pull them inward and upward.

Goal: prevent respiratory infection.

Obtain x-ray of lungs.

Administer antibiotics as ordered.

Observe for signs of infection or distress.

Corneal Abrasion

Clinical manifestations: eye pain, increased lacrimation, photophobia, bloodshot eye.

Goal: prevent corneal ulcer.

Promptly remove foreign object from eye.

Prevent patient from rubbing eye.

Goal: provide comfort.

Eliminate bright lights and recommend use of sunglasses to relieve photophobia.

Apply warm compresses.

Dehydration

Clinical manifestations: concentrated urine, decreased or excessive urine output, weight loss, output exceeds intake, increased pulse rate, increased temperature, decreased skin turgor, dry-coated tongue, dry skin and mucous membrane, weakness, lethargy, confusion, nausea, anorexia; thirst may or may not be present.

Goal: restore lost fluids.

Obtain blood sample for analysis of electrolytes.

Force fluids unless contraindicated. Administer intravenous solutions as ordered.

Monitor and record intake and output, weight, and vital signs.

Goal: minimize or eliminate causative factors.

Assess for possible causes (*e.g.,* insufficient intake, fever, vomiting, diarrhea, wound drainage).

Correct underlying cause.

Monitor and encourage good fluid intake.

Note: the reduction in intracellular fluid that occurs with age contributes to less total body fluids; thus, any fluid loss is more significant in older adults. Unless there is a medical need for restriction, fluid intake should range between 2000 ml and 3000 ml daily. Special factors that can lead to dehydration should be assessed in older patients, such as diminished thirst sensations, disabilities that restrict independent fluid intake, altered mental status, and desires to minimize frequency and nocturia.

Detached Retina

Clinical manifestations: complaints of seeing particles or flashes of light in visual field, blurred vision, areas of blank vision progressing to blindness.

Goal: support treatment plan in correcting detachment.

Obtain prompt treatment.

Keep patient in bed. Physician may order bandaging of eyes and restricting position.

Prepare patient for surgery, if ordered.

Goal: reduce patient's anxiety.

Comfort patient. Antianxiety drugs may be ordered.

Explain procedures and activities.

Keep patient oriented.

Provide diversional activities (*e.g.,* music or talking books).

Offer realistic hope. Most patients successfully recover.

Note: prompt identification and treatment of this problem are crucial. Untreated detachments can progress to blindness.

Diarrhea

Clinical manifestations: loose liquid stool, increased frequency of bowel movements, abdominal cramps or pain, signs of potassium depletion (*e.g.,* muscle weakness; confusion; shallow, irregular respirations; arrhythmias).

Goal: determine and treat underlying cause.

Assess for all possible causes (*e.g.,* fecal impaction, laxative abuse, intestinal infection, food poisoning, medications such as colchicine, food allergies, cancer, stress, tube feeding).

Support treatment plan.

Monitor intake and output, weight, and vital signs.

Goal: prevent and promptly identify complications.

Protect skin from breakdown.

Prevent falls during patient's weakened state.

Offer fluids. Observe for dehydration.

Observe for signs of potassium depletion. Have serum electrolytes reviewed.

Note: the reduced fluid reserves and increased sensitivity to stress make the elderly more vulnerable to the serious effects of diarrhea. This problem needs to be corrected promptly.

Fainting

Clinical manifestations: weakness, muscle flaccidity, loss of consciousness.

Goal: ensure that no injury has occurred.

Examine patient for possible fractures, cuts, bruises. Manage accordingly (*e.g.,* immobilize limb, control bleeding).

Goal: determine causative factor.

Obtain blood sample and ECG.

Take vital signs. Observe level of consciousness.

Review events preceding fainting episode (*e.g.,* emotional upset, position change, chest pain, headache).

Goal: support treatment plan to correct cause.

Follow prescribed plan (*e.g.,* treat anemia, manage cardiovascular disease, control diabetes).

Note: fainting episodes are sometimes referred to as "drop attacks" by older persons. With these attacks, the person's legs suddenly experience muscle flaccidity for several minutes to several hours. Consciousness is not lost during these attacks, and their cause is not fully understood.

Falls

Clinical manifestations: patient found on floor or reports falling.

Goal: evaluate and treat injury sustained from fall.

Do not move patient until status is evaluated.

Obtain x-ray if fracture is suspected.

Control bleeding.

Relieve patient's anxiety.

Assess vital signs, mental status, and functional capacity. Note signs and symptoms (*e.g.*, incontinence, tremors, weakness).

Review events preceding fall (*e.g.*, position change, medication administration, pain, dizziness).

Observe and monitor patient's status for the next 24 hours.

Goal: prevent future falls.

Assess and correct factors contributing to falls (*e.g.*, gait disturbances, poor vision, confusion, improper use of assistive device, medications, environmental hazards).

Teach patient how to fall safely (*e.g.*, protect head and face, do not move until checked).

Teach patient how to reduce risk of falls.

Wear safe shoes; avoid long robes.

Sit on edge of bed for a few minutes before rising.

Use rails, particularly in tubs and stairways.

Walk only in well-lighted areas.

Eliminate clutter and loose rugs from environment.

Note: an older person who falls once is at greater risk of falling again; thus, active prevention is necessary. Falls are the second leading cause of accidental death; the morbidity and mortality associated with falls increase with age.

Food Poisoning

Clinical manifestations: nausea, vomiting, abdominal pain, diarrhea, temperature elevation.

Goal: identify and treat causative agent.

Culture feces, urine, and blood. If possible, save sample of vomitus for analysis.

Ask about onset of symptoms in relation to food and fluid intake. Review 24-hour intake.

Review symptoms. Neurological symptoms occur with botulism; diarrhea usually does not. Fever usually accompanies salmonella and fish poisoning.

Goal: Support treatment plan.

Assist with prescribed treatment; for example, induce vomiting, prevent and treat respiratory failure.

Goal: maintain and restore fluid and electrolyte balance.

Review blood chemistry for abnormalities.

Replace lost fluids and electrolytes as ordered. Severe vomiting can cause alkalosis; severe diarrhea can cause acidosis.

Monitor intake and output, weight, and vital signs.

Note: reinforce good food handling techniques to prevent food poisoning; for example, do not ingest raw eggs or use eggs that are cracked, cook meats thoroughly, handle food with clean hands and utensils, protect foods from insects and rodents, and refrigerate foods that require refrigeration.

Frostbite

Clinical manifestations: depends on degree of frostbite.

First degree: edema, hyperemia, skin peeling, mild cyanosis.

Second degree: redness, swelling, vesicles, skin sloughing (*i.e.*, eschars).

Third degree: edema, vesicles, shriveling toes, hard, dry eschars.

Fourth degree: gangrene of affected area.

Goal: increase warmth and circulation to affected extremity.

Remove constricting or cold clothing.

Soak affected extremity in 105°F (41°C) water for several minutes or as ordered.

Allow extremity to be exposed to room temperature air after soaking.

Goal: control pain.

Administer analgesics as prescribed.

Comfort patient.

Goal: prevent further tissue damage.

Elevate and do not use affected part.

Administer antibiotics prophylactically, as ordered.

Inspect affected parts for damage.

Note: poor peripheral circulation and altered pain sensations, which could delay sensation of frostbite, contribute to the high risk of this problem in older individuals.

Heatstroke

Clinical manifestations: increased temperature, possibly to 103°F (39°C) to 106°F (41°C); rapid, weak, and irregular pulse; weakness; headaches; hot, dry skin; muscle cramps; no sweating; loss of consciousness.

Goal: reduce body temperature.

Remove patient's clothing. Move patient to a cool area.

Sponge with room temperature or cool water, as prescribed. Hypothermia blanket may be used.

Administer antipyretics.

Goal: promote circulation.

Massage extremities and back.

Change positions frequently.

Goal: prevent and treat complications.

Administer oxygen if patient is cyanotic.

Monitor intake and output—acute tubular necrosis can occur.

Start IV—usually hypotonic multiple electrolyte solution.

Observe for signs of shock.

Hemorrhage

Clinical manifestations: increased pulse; decreased blood pressure; rapid, deep respirations; pallor; reduced temperature; confusion; apprehension.

Goal: restore and maintain blood supply.

Apply pressure bandage over bleeding site, but do not obstruct circulation; elevate affected part.

Obtain blood sample for typing and cross-matching.

Assist with administration of plasma expanders or whole blood.

Monitor vital signs.

Goal: comfort patient.

Reassure patient.

Administer sedative, analgesic as ordered.

Note: the reduction in functional reserve causes hemorrhage to have a more profound effect on the older patient. Hypovolemia is not well tolerated and can rapidly progress to shock and death.

Myocardial Infarction

Clinical manifestations: acute confusion, dyspnea, reduced blood pressure, pale skin, weakness; chest pain may or may not be present.

Goal: aid in prompt diagnosis.

Identify signs early. Signs may be missed or attributed to other problems.

Even with the slightest suspicion that a myocardial infarction exists, proceed with a diagnostic evaluation.

Obtain an ECG and blood specimen—sedimentation rate will be elevated.

Monitor vital signs.

Goal: reduce cardiovascular stress.

Support prescribed treatment. Administer antiarrhythmics.

Provide oxygen. Monitor blood gases. Observe for signs of carbon dioxide retention.

Support limbs.

Control stress.

Relieve pain and anxiety.

Goal: prevent and promptly identify complications.

Perform range-of-motion exercises. Ensure frequent change of position.

Monitor intake and output. Anuria can develop; straining due to constipation can produce strain on heart.

Evaluate response to medications. Note adverse reactions, for example, bleeding, bradycardia, hypokalemia.

Observe for signs of congestive heart failure (*e.g.,* dyspnea, cough, rhonchi, rales).

Observe for signs of shock (*e.g.,* drop in blood pressure, increased pulse, cool moist skin, decreased urine output, restlessness).

Seizure

Clinical manifestations: involuntary muscle contractions.

Goal: protect from injury.

Maintain patent airway.

Protect head.

Loosen constrictive clothing.

Goal: determine causative factor.

Record length, progression of symptoms, other characteristics of the seizure.

Ask about events preceding seizure (*e.g.,* aura).

Assess symptoms following seizure (*e.g.,* aphasia, confusion, weakness of limbs, incontinence, deep sleep).

Review medications being taken and vital signs.

Goal: support treatment plan.

Address underlying cause (*e.g.,* treat infection, change medication, control epilepsy).

Note: seizures can be a lifelong problem for the elderly or a new problem in old age. Sometimes, seizures are an initial sign of stroke or cardia infarction.

Suicide Attempt

Clinical manifestations: depend on method used (*e.g.,* hemorrhage, poisoning, starvation, overdose).

Goal: sustain life.

Maintain patent airway.

Observe for and treat shock.

Support treatment of injury (*e.g.,* gastric lavage, control of bleeding).

Monitor vital signs and general status.

Goal: prevent future suicide attempts.

Refer for psychiatric treatment as soon as physical condition stabilizes.

Support psychiatric treatment plan.

Note: twenty-five percent of all suicides occur in persons over 65 years of age. The highest rate is among white men 75 years of age and older. Depressed individuals and those in early stages of dementia who are aware of their deficits are at high risk. Inquiries into suicidal thought should be included during every assessment, and threats and attempts should be taken seriously.

- Diverticulitis
- Fecal impaction
- Gallbladder attack
- Heart block
- Hyperglycemia
- Hypertension
- Hypoglycemia
- Hypothermia
- Incontinence
- Ischemic foot lesions
- Malnutrition
- Paroxysmal atrial tachycardia
- Peptic ulcer
- Pneumonia
- Premature contractions
- Pulmonary emboli
- Pyelonephritis
- Rheumatic fever
- Transient ischemic attacks
- Tuberculosis
- Urinary tract infections
- Venous thromboembolism
- Ventricular tachycardia

Other Problems

Other problems that can present as emergency situations or require prompt action are discussed elsewhere in this book. Some of these problems are listed below. The reader should consult the index for easy retrieval.

- Abdominal angina
- Acute bacterial endocarditis
- Acute coronary insufficiency
- Acute glaucoma
- Aneurysm
- Angina
- Appendicitis
- Arrhythmias
- Arterial embolism
- Asthma
- Atrial fibrillation
- Bacterial endocarditis
- Carbon dioxide retention
- Cerebrovascular accident
- Cheyne-Stokes respirations
- Congestive heart failure
- Corneal ulcers
- Depression
- Digitalis toxicity

Recommended Readings

Arie T. Acute confusion. In: Abrams WB, Berkow R, eds. The Merck manual of geriatrics. Rahway, NJ: Merck Sharp & Dohme Research Laboratories, 1990:84.

Besdone RW. Hyperthermia and accidental hypothermia. In: Abrams WB, Berkow R, eds. The Merck manual of geriatrics. Rahway, NJ: Merck Sharp & Dohme Research Laboratories, 1990:35.

Demarest GB, Osler TM, Clevenger FW. Injuries in the elderly: evaluation and initial response. Geriatrics 1990; 45(8):36.

Gerhart TN. Fractures. In: Abrams WB, Berkow R, eds. The Merck manual of geriatrics. Rahway, NJ: Merck Sharp & Dohme Research Laboratories, 1990:69.

Kay AD, Tideiksaar R. Falls and gait disorders. In: Abrams WB, Berkow R, eds. The Merck manual of geriatrics. Rahway, NJ: Merck Sharp & Dohme Research Laboratories, 1990:52.

Lipsitz LA. Sycope. In: Abrams WB, Berkow R, eds. The Merck manual of geriatrics. Rahway, NJ: Merck Sharp & Dohme Research Laboratories, 1990:45.

Pathy MSJ, Finucani P, eds. Geriatric medicine: problems and practice. New York: Springer-Verlag, 1989.

Ross KL. Meningitis as it presents in the elderly: diagnosis and care. Geriatrics 1990;45(8):63.

32

Surgical Care

The improvement of surgical procedures and the increased numbers of persons living to old age account for the fact that nurses now are confronted with many more aged surgical patients. People are no longer denied the benefit of surgery based on their age alone. Surgical intervention has provided many of our aged people not only with more years to their lives, but also with more functional years. Successful surgical management of an older person's health problems depends on the nurse's understanding of the age-related factors that alter normal surgical procedures.

In general, the aged have a smaller margin of physiological reserve and are less able to compensate for and adapt to physiological changes. Infection, hemorrhage, anemia, blood pressure changes, and fluid and electrolyte imbalances are more problematic in the elderly. Unfortunately, inelasticity of blood vessels; malnourishment; increased susceptibility to infection; and reduced cardiac, respiratory, and renal reserves cause complications to occur more frequently in the elderly, especially during emergency or complicated surgical procedures. By strengthening their capacities preoperatively, maintaining these capacities postoperatively, and being alert to early signs of complications, the nurse can help reduce the risk of surgical problems (Table 32-1).

Preoperative Procedures

The gerontological nurse must be sensitive to the fears that many older patients have concerning surgery. Throughout their lifetimes, the aged may

have witnessed severe disability or death in older persons having surgery, and they may be concerned about similar outcomes from their operation. Reassurance should emphasize the increased success of surgical procedures through the following advances:

- better diagnostic tools facilitating earlier diagnosis and treatment
- improved therapeutic measures, including surgical techniques and antibiotics
- increased knowledge concerning the unique characteristics of the aged.

In addition to reassurance, patients and their families should be taught what to expect before, during, and after the operative procedure, including the following information:

- preoperative preparation—scrubs, medications, nothing to eat by mouth (NPO)
- types of reactions expected to anesthesia
- length of the surgery and a brief description
- routine recovery room procedures
- expected pain and its management
- turning, coughing, and deep-breathing exercises
- rationale for and frequency of dressing changes, suctioning, oxygen, catheters, and other anticipated procedures.

Explanations given by the nurse should be communicated to others responsible for care through documentation in the patient's record. Concerns, questions, and fears should be identified by the

Table 32-1 Nursing Diagnoses Related to Surgical Intervention

NURSING DIAGNOSIS	CAUSES OR CONTRIBUTING FACTORS
Activity intolerance	Altered oxygen transport, pain
Anxiety	Fear of death or disability, pain, lack of knowledge
Altered bowel elimination: constipation	Anesthesia, immobility, actual or perceived pain, analgesics
Altered cardiac output: decreased	Shock, fluid and electrolyte imbalances, sepsis, anesthesia
Pain	Diagnostic tests, positioning, tissue trauma, immobility
Impaired verbal communication	Decreased cerebral flood flow, endotracheal intubation, pain, anesthesia, central nervous system depressants
Fear	Concern about loss of body function or part, death, outcome of surgery
Fluid volume deficit	Shock, infection, excessive wound drainage, NPO status, electrolyte imbalance, blood loss
Fluid volume excess	Excessive IV infusion, venous pooling/stasis
High risk for infection	IV therapy, intubation, break in aseptic technique, catheterization
High risk for injury	Altered cerebral function, pain
Knowledge deficit	Of surgical procedure, expected outcome, risks, postoperative care
Impaired physical mobility	Pain, weakness, altered cognition, restrictions
Altered nutrition: less than body requirements	Anorexia, nausea, vomiting, pain, inability to feed self
Altered oral mucous membrane	Trauma from endotracheal tube, NPO status, mouth breathing, inadequate oral hygiene
Powerlessness	Inability to help self, lack of knowledge
Altered respiratory function	Anesthesia, narcotics, immobility, pain, secretions
Self-care deficit	Immobility, weakness, restrictions from IV apparatus
Disturbance in self-concept	Change in body function or part, pain, dependency
Impaired of skin integrity	Immobility, pressure from operating table, edema, dehydration
Sleep pattern disturbance	Immobility, anxiety, pain, new environment, drugs
Altered patterns of urinary elimination	Anesthesia, drugs, confusion, dehydration, indwelling catheter

nurse during assessment and preoperative preparation, and the physician should be made aware of these findings.

The nurse should review with the physician the medications the patient is receiving to determine those that must be continued throughout the hospitalization. Medications that the patient usually takes may need to be administered despite NPO restrictions. Sudden interruption of steroid therapy, for instance, can cause cardiovascular collapse, which must be prevented. The nurse may learn that the patient has been taking antihypertensive, tranquilizing, or other medications before hospitalization. Occasionally, patients forget or are reluctant to tell the physician about these drugs. Because cardiac and pulmonary functions can be altered by certain drugs, it is important to make sure this information is communicated to the physician.

Nurses should ensure that basic preoperative screening has been completed, including the following:

- analysis of blood samples: creatinine clearance, glucose, electrolytes, complete blood counts, total plasma proteins, arterial blood gases, cardiac enzymes, lymphocyte count, serum albumin, hemoglobin, hematocrit, total iron-binding capacity, transferrin
- chest x-ray
- electrocardiogram
- pulmonary function testing—for obese individuals and those with a history of smoking or pulmonary disease
- nutritional assessment: height, weight, mid-arm circumference, triceps skin-fold, diet history
- mental status.

Because of the direct nature of the care they give, nurses may be the only ones to recognize certain problems. They may discover loose teeth, which can become dislodged and aspirated during the surgical procedure, causing unnecessary complications. This problem should be brought to the physician's attention to ensure preoperative dental correction. Another precaution during preparation for surgery is to pad the bony prominences of aged patients to protect them from lying on a hard operating room table and subsequently acquiring decubiti.

Infection control must be at the forefront of the nurse's mind during the entire hospitalization and begins early during the preoperative preparation. Promoting a good nutritional state and correcting existing infections are important preoperative considerations. To further reduce the risk of infection, three preoperative bathings, in the morning and at bedtime on the day before surgery and on the morning of surgery, using an antiseptic is recommended, as is performing preoperative shaving as close to the time of surgery as possible. Although it is the physician's legal responsibility, nurses can ensure that informed consent has been obtained preoperatively.

Operative and Postoperative Procedures

Because anesthesia produces depression of the already compromised functions of the cardiovascular and respiratory systems of the aged patient, it must be carefully selected. Close monitoring by the anesthesiologist during the surgery can detect and prevent difficulties in the patient's vital functions. Prolonged surgery for the aged patient is discouraged. Rough, frequent handling of the tissue during surgery usually is avoided because this stimulates reflex activity, increasing the demand for anesthesia. If inhaled agents are used for anesthesia, the nurse should be aware that the patient may remain anesthetized for a longer time due to the slower elimination of these agents; turning and deep breathing will facilitate faster elimination of inhaled agents.

Hypothermia is one of the major complications older adults face intra- and postoperatively. Factors that contribute to this problem include the lower normal body temperatures possessed by many older persons, the cool temperature of operating rooms, and the use of medications that slow metabolism. The cool environment and shivering that may result can increase cardiac output and ventilation and deprive the heart and brain of necessary oxygen; however, shivering occurs less frequently in the elderly. Further, the slowing of metabolism that occurs with hypothermia delays awakening and the return of reflexes. Close monitoring of body temperature is essential.

Frequent, close postoperative observation and monitoring are extremely important. The decreased ability of the aged to manage stress reinforces the need to detect and treat symptoms of shock and hemorrhage promptly. Although not fully conscious after surgery, the aged patient may demonstrate restlessness as the primary symptom of hypoxia. It is important that this restlessness not be mistaken for pain; administration of a narcotic could deplete the body's oxygen supply even more. Prophylactic administration of oxygen may be a beneficial component of the postoperative therapy. Blood loss should be accurately measured and, if excessive, promptly corrected. Frequent checking of urinary output can help reveal the onset of serious complications. Fluid and electrolyte imbalances can be avoided and detected through strict recording of intake and output. Output should include drainage, bleeding, vomitus, and all other sources of fluid loss.

Routine care in the recovery phase of older patients is similar to that for all other adults. Activity is vital postoperatively; the benefits of surgery will be diminished if the patient becomes debilitated from the complications arising from immobility.

(Text continues on page 300)

Table 32-2 Common Complicating Conditions in Elderly Surgical Patients

COMPLICATING CONDITION	MEDICAL–SURGICAL FACTORS	AGING PROCESSES	NURSING INTERVENTIONS
Fluid and electrolyte imbalance	Blood, fluid losses during surgery, cool operating room, fluids evaporate from tissues, surgery and anesthesia stimulate ADH and aldosterone, overhydration with IV infusion	Decreased renal function—nephron loss, GFR, decreased renal blood flow and creatinine clearance; decreased cardiopulmonary function	Careful monitoring of intake and output, assessment of skin turgor—over sternum or forehead, assess for signs of hypervolemia and hypovolemia, determine urinary status, note nonmeasured fluid losses such as diaphoresis, assess for sacral edema, correct imbalances with isotonic IV infusions and electrolytes
Malnutrition	NPO for test preparations, decreased intake postoperatively, psychosocial influences, operative site, stress of surgery increases nutritional needs	Decreased secretion, motility, and absorption; decreased basal metabolic rate; loss of taste buds; loss of appetite; reduced absorption of iron, B_{12}, calcium; sensory losses	Preoperative nutritional assessment, monitor weight, fluid balance, food intake and laboratory values, preoperative nutritional preparation, calorie and protein increases postoperatively, hyperalimentation if indicated, use of nutritional support team, maintain positive nitrogen balance postoperatively; vitamin/mineral supplements
Pneumonia, atelectasis	Heavy smokers with cough, obesity, bronchitis, chronic pulmonary disease, thoracic or upper abdominal surgery, anesthesia and pain medication reduce functional residual capacity, lung expansion and gas exchange	Reduced bronchopulmonary movement, decreased pulmonary function—tidal volume, vital capacity, increased residual volume, loss of protective airway reflexes	*Preoperatively*—cease smoking for 1 week, weight reduction, pulmonary function testing; if bronchitis present, give antibiotics, expectorants and bronchodilators, teach pulmonary maneuvers; cough (tongue extended to loosen secretions), deep breathing, incentive spirometer *Postoperatively*—position change hourly, monitor blood gases, off ventilator as soon as possible, continue pulmonary maneuver; O_2 to ensure adequate oxygenation, early ambulation, chest physiotherapy

(Continued)

Table 32-2 *Common Complicating Conditions in Elderly Surgical Patients (Continued)*

COMPLICATING CONDITION	MEDICAL–SURGICAL FACTORS	AGING PROCESSES	NURSING INTERVENTIONS
Pressure ulcers	Malnutrition; chronic disease (*e.g.*, diabetes, CHF, PVD); length of time on OR table.	Moisture loss, thinning epidermis, capillary loss in dermis, loss of sensory receptors, loss of subcutaneous fat	Frequent turning, correct positioning, pressure relieving devices, avoidance of shearing forces, early movement and ambulation, good skin hygiene, lotions, gentle massage, nutritional supplements, increase fluid intake, high-protein, high-calorie diet
Wound dehiscence, wound evisceration	Malnutrition; large, sudden weight loss	Delayed immune response, delayed wound healing—slowing of inflammatory response, mitosis, cell proliferation, abnormal collagen formation causing poor tensile strength in wound, decreased muscle strength	1—3 weeks preoperative nutritional preparation, hyperalimentation, vitamin supplements, strict aseptic wound care, encourage rest—slow-wave sleep aids wound healing, inspiratory breathing exercises, coughing only if secretions present, prevent/reduce vomiting; discharge teaching, proper wound care and observation for complications, diet instructions
Incidental hypothermia	Cold operating rooms, room temperature infusions, exposure of skin for draping and preparation, exposure of peritoneum/pleura during surgery, peripheral vasodilation	Impaired thermoregulatory mechanisms, decreased cardiopulmonary reserves, impaired ability to increase basal metabolic rate	Temperature monitoring in OR, careful cardiac monitoring, hyperthermia blanket, warm top blankets after incision closure, warm IV fluids, transfer from OR quickly, thermal top blankets in RR, transfer blankets with patient to surgical unit
Joint stiffness, contractures	Presence of degenerative joint disease, osteoporosis, reduced mobility during preoperative preparation, immobility during surgery, pain limiting motion in postoperative period	Decreased muscle strength and wasting, decreased bone mass, ossification of cartilage in joints, flexion of joints, stooped posture, slowed movement, gait changes	Assess prior functioning level, leg exercises preoperatively, early ambulation, proper positioning and movement in bed, active/passive range of motion, encourage active movement by patient

Table 32-2 Common Complicating Conditions in Elderly Surgical Patients (Continued)

COMPLICATING CONDITION	MEDICAL–SURGICAL FACTORS	AGING PROCESSES	NURSING INTERVENTIONS
Acute, confusional states, delirium	Type of anesthesia, penetration of blood–brain barrier by certain drugs, presence of preexisting depression or dementia, environmental factors, number of medications taken, hypoxemia, psychosocial factors	Loss of neurons, brain atrophy, decreased cerebral blood flow and oxygen consumption, decreased renal function, slowed clearance of drugs from system, sensory losses, decreased cardiopulmonary reserves	*Preoperatively*—baseline assessment of mental status and emotional state, psychological support, allow time for questions and verbalization of fears, provide pastoral care if desired, correct electrolyte imbalances, anemia *Postoperatively*—monitor level of consciousness, avoid restraints, provide calm environment, avoid use of indwelling catheters, orient to environment, progressive mobility, small doses of Haldol if organic causes, reassurance from all staff, need special attention if have hearing loss, monitor electrolytes and fluid balance, ensure adequate oxygenation
Cardiac failure	Existing cardiac disease, hypertension, anesthesia effects on blood pressure, stress of surgery increases metabolic needs and increases workload on heart	Decreased cardiac output, altered O_2 transport, fatty accumulations in heart valves, atherosclerosis and arteriosclerosis of vessels, widening pulse pressure	*Preoperatively*—risk assessment, correct, treat existing conditions; low dosage heparinization; improved nutritional status will improve cardiac function. *Postoperatively*—continuous CVP monitoring, assess JVD and breath sounds hourly; continuous ECG monitoring; close observation of vital signs, level of consciousness and urinary output, maintain infusion rates; check intake and output; observe peripheral circulation, color; maintain cardiovascular functions; careful, early mobilization, rest periods

ADH, antidiuretic hormone; CHF, congestive heart failure; CVP, central venous pressure; ECG, electrocardiogram; GFR, glomerular filtration rate; IV, intravenous; JVD, jugular vein distention; NPO, nothing by mouth; OR, operating room; PVD, pulmonary vascular disease; RR, recovery room.
From Palmer MA. Care of the older surgical patient. In: Eliopoulos C, ed. Caring for the elderly in diverse care settings. Philadelphia: JB Lippincott, 1990:358.

Because the aged patient has a greater risk of developing infections, strict attention must be paid to caring for wounds and changing dressings. A good nutritional status is beneficial to tissue healing and should be encouraged. To conserve the patient's energy and provide comfort, relief of pain is essential. Maintaining regular bowel and bladder elimination, keeping joints mobile, and assisting the patient in achieving a comfortable position can aid in pain control. If medications are used for pain relief, attention should be given to the reduced activity that may result and to the prevention of the ill effects of such immobilization. It is vital to observe the patient for respiratory depression if narcotic analgesics are administered.

Aged patients are particularly subject to several postoperative complications. Respiratory complications include atelectasis, pulmonary emboli, and pneumonia. If pneumonia develops in an aged patient, it is more problematic than it would be for a younger adult and requires a longer period for recovery. Cardiovascular complications include embolus, thrombus, myocardial infarction, and arrhythmias. Cerebrovascular accident and coronary occlusion occur, but they are less common than other complications. Reduced activity and lowered resistance can cause pressure ulcers to develop easily. Postoperative older patients, particularly those with hip repair, tend to have a higher incidence of delirium than the general population. Paralytic ileus, accompanied by fever, dehydration, abdominal tenderness, and distention, is an additional postoperative complication that the aged may experience. Other complications are listed in Table 32-2.

It is not unusual for the positioning on the operating room table and the pulling and moving of the unconscious patient to cause soreness of the aged patient's muscles and bones for several days postoperatively. The nurse should be aware that this is a normal consequence of surgery and take steps to provide comfort. The nurse is in a key position to assist the geriatric patient in achieving the maximal benefit from surgery. The most sophisticated surgical procedure in the world performed by the most skillful surgeon is of little value if poor rehabilitative care causes disability or death from avoidable complications. To combine the principles and practices of surgical nursing with the unique characteristic of the aged patient is an immense challenge to the gerontological nurse. To see the increased capacity and more meaningful life many aged persons derive from the benefits of surgery is an immense satisfaction.

Recommended Readings

Adkins RB, Scott HW. Surgical care for the elderly. Baltimore, MD: Williams & Wilkins, 1988.

Pousada L, Leipzig RM. Rapid bedside assessment of postoperative confusion in older patients. Geriatrics 1990; 45(4):59.

Schafer S, Sampsei D. 33-Day laceration stay. Geriatr Nurs 1989;10(3):124.

Tompkins RG, Welch CE. Surgery: preoperative evaluation and intraoperative and postoperative care. In: Abrams WB, Berkow R, eds. The Merck manual of geriatrics. Rahway, NJ: Merck Sharp & Dohme Research Laboratories, 1990:225.

White HE, Thurston NE, Blackmore KA, Green SE, Hannah KJ. Body temperature in elderly surgical patients. Res Nurs Health 1987; 10:317.

33

Mental-Health Problems

Mental health indicates a capacity to cope with and manage life's stresses in an effort to achieve a state of emotional homeostasis. The elderly have an advantage over other age groups in that they probably have had more experience with coping, problem solving, and crisis management by virtue of the years they have lived. Most older persons have few delusions regarding what they are or what they are going to be. They know where they have been, what they have accomplished, and who they really are. Immigrating to a new country, watching loved ones die from epidemics, fighting in world wars, and surviving the Great Depression may be among the numerous stresses that today's elderly have faced and overcome. Such experiences have provided them with unique strength that should not be underestimated. This is not to imply that psychiatric illness is not a problem among the older population. More people than ever are reaching old age; many bring to their later years the mental-health problems they have possessed throughout their lifetimes. The many losses and challenges of old age may exceed the physical, emotional, and social resources of some persons and promote mental illness. By promoting mental health, detecting problems early, and minimizing the impact of existing psychiatric problems, nurses can aid the elderly in achieving optimal satisfaction and function.

Aging and Mental Health

Many myths are in evidence regarding mental health and the elderly. For instance, many people still believe that loss of mental functioning, senility, or mental incompetence are a natural part of old age. Stereotypes about personality in later life propagate through descriptions of the elderly being childlike, rigid, or cantankerous. Frequently, these misconceptions are so widely accepted that when pathological signs are demonstrated by an older person, it is considered normal and no attempt is made to intervene. Nurses can play a significant role in ensuring that the myths and realities of mental health in old age are understood.

Cognitive function in later life is highly individualized based on personal resources, health status, and the unique experiences of the individual's life. Some age-related structural changes in the cerebrum tend to be universal and include the following:

- decrease in brain weight
- reduction in number of functioning neurons
- increase in neuroglia
- increase in amount of senile plaque and neurofibrillary tangles, usually in the seventh decade and beyond
- accumulation of lipofuscin.

The relationship between these structural changes and mental function is unclear and may be nonexistent.

General changes in intellectual ability do not occur with age, although alterations in specific functions (*e.g.,* memory, speed of psychomotor response) may be noted. Verbal comprehension and arithmetic operations remain unchanged. Crystallized intelligence, which enables the use of past learning and experiences for problem-solving, is maintained throughout adulthood. Fluid intelligence, which controls emotions, retention of non-intellectual information, creative capacities, spatial perceptions, and aesthetic appreciation, is believed to decline in later life. Intellectual decline should be viewed as an indication of a physical or mental-health problem.

The ability to learn is not lost with age; however, more factors interfere with the learning process. Differences in the intensity and duration of physiological arousal could make it more difficult to extinguish previous responses and acquire new information. The early phases of the learning process tend to be more problematic for older adults; but, after a longer early phase, the elderly are able to keep equal pace with the young. Older adults demonstrate some difficulty with perceptual motor tasks.

Vigilance performance (*e.g.,* the ability to retain information longer than 45 minutes) declines in later life. Older adults are more easily distracted by irrelevant information and stimuli and less able to perform tasks that are complicated or require simultaneous performance.

With age, there can be a slowing of retrieval of information from long-term memory, particularly if the information is not frequently called on or used. Some age-related forgetfulness can be improved by the use of memory aids (*i.e.,* mnemonic devices).

Drastic changes in personality do not occur with age. Personality, attitude, morale, and self-esteem tend to be stable through the life span; changes in these characteristics can be associated with health problems or reactions to life events (*e.g.,* reduction in income, death of loved one, retirement).

The incidence of mental illness is higher in the old than the young. It is estimated that approximately one-fourth of the elderly in the community and more than one-half of those in nursing homes have symptoms of serious mental-health problems.

DISPLAY 33-1   *Age-Related Changes in Mental Function*

Slower retrieval from long-term memory
Some decline in fluid intelligence
More difficulty extinguishing previous responses to learn new material
Slower early phase of learning
Difficulty with perceptual motor tasks
Decrease in vigilance performance
Increased ease of being distracted by irrelevant information and stimuli
Reduced ability to perform tasks that are complicated or require simultaneous performance

---

Nearly 10% of the older population has a problem with alcoholism, and 25% of all suicides are committed by persons age 65 years and older. Between 4% and 5% of the elderly are victims of Alzheimer disease. Depression increases in prevalence and intensity with age. Multiple losses; altered sensory function; and alterations, discomforts, and demands associated with illnesses that the elderly frequently encounter set the stage for a variety of mental-health problems. Display 33-1 summarizes changes in mental function associated with aging.

Assessment

Every comprehensive assessment includes an evaluation of mental status. Because patients may be anxious, embarrassed, or insulted by having their mental status reviewed, an explanation of the importance of and the reasons for it can prove useful. The evaluation should be approached in a matter-of-fact manner, not in an apologetic or intimidating one, with reassurance that this evaluation is part of every patient's assessment. Making the patient comfortable and establishing rapport before the assessment can reduce some of the barriers to an effective examination.

General Observations

Assessment of mental status actually begins the moment the nurse meets the patient. The initial observation can yield insight into mental health, and as such, attention should be paid to the following indicators:

Grooming and dress: is clothing appropriate for the season, clean and presentable, appropri-

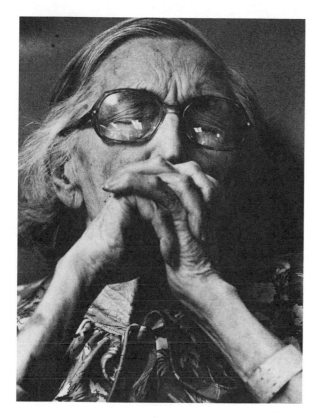

Astute assessment of behavior and cognitive function aids in differentiating symptoms of psychiatric illness from normal reactions to life events. (Photograph by Eric Schenk.)

ately worn? Is the patient clean? Is the hair clean and combed? Are make-up and accessories excessive or bizarre?

Posture: does the patient appear stooped and fearful? Is body alignment normal?

Movement: are tongue rolling, twitching, tremors, or hand wringing present? Are movements hyperactive or hypoactive?

Facial expression: is it masklike or overly dramatic? Are there indications of pain, fear, or anger?

Level of consciousness: does the patient drift into sleep and need to be aroused (*i.e.*, lethargic)? Does the patient offer only incomplete or slow responses and need repeated arousal (*i.e.*, stuporous)? Are painful stimuli the only thing the patient responds to (*i.e.*, semiconscious)? Is there no response, even to painful stimuli (*i.e.*, unconscious)?

While the nurse observes the patient, general conversation can aid in evaluating mental status. The nurse can note the tone of voice, rate of speech, ability to articulate, use of unusual words or combinations of words, and appropriateness of speech. Mood also can be evaluated during this time.

Interview

Through effective questioning, much can be revealed about the patient's mental health. Direct questions can be asked to unveil specific problems, such as the following:

"How do you feel about yourself? Would you say others would say you are a good or bad person?"

"Do you have many friends? How do you get along with people?"

"Do you feel that anyone is trying to harm you? Who? Why?"

"Are you moody? Do you quickly go from laughing to crying or from being happy to sad?"

"Do you have trouble falling asleep or staying asleep? How much sleep do you get? Do you use any drug or alcohol to become sleepy?"

"How is your appetite? How does your appetite

and eating pattern change when you are sad or worried?"

"Do you ever have feelings of being nervous, such as palpitations, hyperventilating, or restlessness?"

"Are there any particular problems in your life or anything you are concerned about now?"

"Do you see or hear things that other people do not? Have you ever heard voices? If so, how do you feel about them?"

"Does life bring you pleasure? Do you look forward to each day?"

"Have you ever thought about suicide? If so, what were those ideas like? How would you do it?"

"Do you feel you are losing any of your mental abilities? If so, describe how."

"Have you ever been hospitalized or had treatment for mental problems? Has any member of your family?"

Listen carefully to the answers and how they are given. It is important to pick up nonverbal clues.

Cognitive Testing

A variety of reliable, validated tools can be used in assessing mental function, such as the Short Portable Mental Status Questionnaire,(Pfeiffer, 1975) the Philadelphia Geriatric Center Mental Status Questionnaire,(Fishback, 1977) Mini-Mental Status,(Folstein et al, 1975) Symptoms Check List 90,(Derogatis et al, 1974) General Health Questionnaire,(Goldberg, 1972) OARS,(Duke University, 1978) and, specifically for depression, the Zung Self-Rating Depression Scale.(Zung, 1965) Most mental status evaluation tools test orientation, memory and retention, the ability to follow commands, judgment, and basic calculation and reasoning. Even without the use of a tool, the nurse can assess basic cognitive function in the following ways.

Orientation: ask the patient his or her name, where he or she is, the date, time, and season.

Memory and retention: at the beginning of the assessment, ask the patient to remember three objects (*e.g.,* watch, telephone, boat). First ask the patient to recall the items immediately after being told; then, after asking several other questions, ask for recall of the three items again; near the end of the assessment, ask what the three items were one last time.

Three-stage command: ask the patient to perform three simple tasks (*e.g.,* "Pick up the pencil, touch it to your head, and hand it to me.")

Judgment: present a situation that requires basic problem solving and reasoning (*e.g.,* "What is meant by the statement 'A bird in the hand is worth two in the bush'?")

Calculation: ask the patient to count backwards from 100 by increments of 5; if this is difficult, ask the patient to count backwards from 20 by increments of 2. Simple arithmetic problems may be asked also, if they are within the realm of the patient's educational experience.

Whenever cognitive function is tested, the unique experiences, educational level, and cultural background of the patient must be considered, as must the role of sensory deficits, health problems, and the stress associated with being examined.

Persons with Alzheimer disease or other cognitive deficits may become overwhelmed by the assessment and react with anger, tears, or withdrawal. This is referred to as a catastrophic reaction. The assessment may need to be discontinued temporarily and the patient reassured and comforted.

Physical Examination

Physical health problems are often at the root of many cognitive disturbances; as such, it is essential that a complete physical examination supplement the mental status evaluation. A complete review of medications being used is crucial. In addition, a variety of laboratory tests may be conducted, including the following:

- complete blood count
- serum electrolytes
- serologic test for syphilis
- blood urea nitrogen
- blood glucose
- bilirubin
- blood vitamin level
- sedimentation rate
- urinalysis.

Depending on the problem suspected, cerebrospinal fluid may be tested, and a variety of diagnostic procedures performed including electroencephalography, computed tomography, magnetic resonance imaging, and position emission tomography scan.

The mental status evaluation often presents only a snapshot of the individual. Cerebral blood flow, body temperature, blood glucose, fluid and electrolyte balance, and the stress to which the patient is subjected can change from one day to the next and cause different levels of mental function to occur. Repeated assessments may be necessary to obtain an accurate evaluation of the patient's mental status.

Review of Selected Disorders

Delirium

A variety of conditions can impair cerebral circulation and cause disturbances in cognitive function (see Potential Causes of Confusion). The onset of symptoms tends to be rapid and can include disturbed intellectual function; disorientation to time and place but usually not of identity; altered attention span; worsened memory; labile mood; meaningless chatter; poor judgment; and altered level of consciousness including hypervigilance, mild drowsiness, semicomatose status). Disturbances in sleep–wake cycles can occur; in fact, restlessness and sleep disturbances may be early clues. The patient may be suspicious, have personality changes, and experience illusions more often than delusions. Physical signs may accompany behavioral changes, such as shortness of breath, fatigue, and slower psychomotor activities.

Nurses can play a significant role in the care of the mental health of the elderly by detecting signs of confusion promptly. A good history and assessment of mental status on initial contact can provide the baseline data to which changes can be compared. Any change in behavior or cognitive pattern warrants an evaluation. Too often, acute confusion is not detected—in fact, nearly 7 in 10 patients who become acutely confused while hospitalized are never recognized by physicians or nurses as having a disturbance.(Foreman, 1990) Acute confusion is reversible, and prompt treatment can prevent permanent damage. Treatment depends on the cause (e.g., stabilizing blood glucose, correcting dehydration, discontinuing a medication). Treating the symptoms rather than the cause or accepting the symptoms as normal and not obtaining treatment can result not only in worsened mental status but also the continuation of a physical condition that could be life-threatening.

During the confusional stage, maintaining stability and minimizing stimulation are primary goals. Consistency in care is important, and the patient benefits from interaction with only a limited number of people. Environmental temperature, noise, and traffic flow should be controlled. Avoid bright lights, but provide ample lighting to enable the patient to adequately visualize the environment. Ensure that the patient does not harm himself or others and that physical care needs are met. Regardless of the level of intellectual function or consciousness, it is important to speak to the patient and offer explanations of activities or procedures being done. Families may need considerable support during this time and realistic explanations to alleviate their anxieties (e.g., "No, he does not have Alzheimer disease. His confusion occurred because the level of glucose, or sugar, in his blood dropped too low. He'll be better as soon as the level is brought back to normal.")

Potential Causes of Confusion

Confusion in the elderly may be caused by the following factors:

- fluid and electrolyte imbalances
- congestive heart failure
- hyperglycemia and hypoglycemia
- hyperthermia and hypothermia
- hypercalcemia and hypocalcemia
- decreased cardiac function
- decreased respiratory function
- decreased renal function
- emotional stress
- malnutrition
- anemias
- infection
- hypotension
- trauma
- medications
- hypoxia
- toxic substances
- azotemia.

Dementia

Senile dementia, arteriosclerotic brain disease, chronic brain disease, and organic brain syndrome are all terms that label the progressive, irreversible decline in cognitive function. It is estimated that 4 million older adults suffer some form of dementia. The symptoms develop gradually. Symptoms have

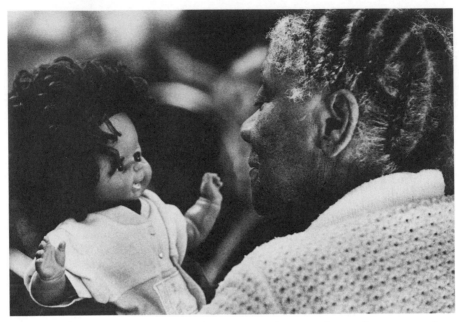

Familiar objects, a stable environment, and consistency of caregivers can reduce some of the behavioral problems associated with dementias. (Photograph by Eric Schenk.)

been grouped according to the stage of dementia, as described below:(Wolanin and Phillips, 1981)

Early
    Declining interest in life
    Has trouble identifying people
    Indifference to courtesies and rituals
    Vague, uncertain, indecisive
    Forgets nouns
Advanced
    Significant decline in memory, recall, retention
    Slow in responding to questions
    Disoriented to time (e.g., confuses day and night)
    Complains of neglect
    Loses important papers, forgets responsibilities and appointments
    Unable to retain simple directions
    Neglects health and hygiene
Later
    Disoriented to place
    Misidentifies people
    Deterioration of motor ability
    Loses sense of time, cannot recall meals
    Major communication problems, incoherent use of nonverbal language

Final or terminal
    Incontinence
    Cannot communicate verbally
    Physical deterioration
    Physiological crisis usually ends life.

Early in the disease, the patient may be aware of changes in intellectual ability and become depressed or anxious or attempt to compensate by writing down information, attempting to structure routines, and simplifying responsibilities. It may take some time for symptoms to be detected, even by those close to the patient.

Dementia may be caused by a variety of pathologies, including the following.

Alzheimer disease. Presenile dementia occurs before 60 years of age; senile dementia of Alzheimer type occurs after 60 years of age. Alzheimer disease causes brain atrophy with widening of sulci, narrow convolutions, lateral ventricular enlargement, reduction in white matter, cortical neuronal loss, senile plaques, and neurofibrillary tangles in the cortex. It is responsible for 50% to 80% of all dementias.

Multi-infarct dementia. This form of dementia results from small cerebral infarctions. Damage to brain tissue can be diffuse or localized, the onset can be rapid or gradual depending on the degree of brain ischemia.

Pick disease. This pathology demonstrates a similar clinical picture to Alzheimer disease, but differs in that its pathological process consists of narrowing of the frontal and temporal lobes, extreme shrinkage of localized cortical areas, and reduction in neurons in the affected areas. Senile plaques, neurofibrillary tangles, and granulovacuolar degeneration, as seen with Alzheimer disease, are unusual with Pick disease.

Creutzfeld–Jacob disease. This dementia has a rapid onset and progression and is characterized by severe neurological impairment that accompanies the dementia. It is believed that this disease can be transmitted through a slow virus; a familial tendency toward the disease is possible. The pathological process displays destruction of neurons in the cerebral cortex, overgrowth of glia, abnormal cellular structure of the cortex, hypertrophy and proliferation of astrocytes, and a spongelike appearance of the cerebral cortex.

Others. Wernicke encephalopathy and Parkinson disease are responsible for a small percentage of dementias. Trauma and toxins are among the other causes of this problem.

The irreversible nature of dementias and their progressive deteriorating course can have devastating effects on affected individuals and their families. A majority of the care needs presented will fall within the scope of nursing practice. One of the foremost considerations is the safety of these patients. Their poor judgment and misperceptions can lead to serious behavioral problems and mishaps. A safe, structured environment is essential. The persons and components of the environment should be consistent. Items to trigger memory are useful to include, such as photographs of the patient or a consistently used symbol (*e.g*, flower, triangle). Noise activity and lighting levels can overstimulate the patient and further decrease function; thus, they need to be controlled. Cleaning solutions, pesticides, medications, and nonedible items that could be ingested accidentally must be stored in locked cabinets. Coverings should be applied to unused sockets, electrical outlets, fans,

motors, and other items into which fingers may be poked. Matches and lighters should not be accessible; if the patient smokes, it must be under close supervision. Windows and doors can be protected with plexiglass, and screens can be placed to avoid falls from windows. Wandering is common among patients with dementia; rather than restrain or restrict them, it is more advantageous to provide a safe area in which they can wander. Protective gates can be installed to prevent patients from wandering away; alarms and bells on doors can signal when they are attempting to exit. With the great risk of patients wandering away and not being able to give their names or residence when found, it is beneficial to have identification bracelets on them at all times.

Various therapies and activities can be offered to the dementia patient, depending on the patient's level of function. Occupational therapy and expressive therapies can benefit those with early dementia. Various degrees of reality orientation ranging from daily groups to reminding the patient who he or she is during every interaction can be used. Even the most regressed patient can maintain contact and derive stimulation through activities such as listening to music and touching various objects. Being touched is also a pleasurable and stimulating experience.

The physical-care needs of patients with dementia are easy to overlook. They may not complain that they are hungry, so no one notices that they have consumed less than one-quarter of the food served; they cannot remember to drink water, so they become dehydrated; they fight their bath so strongly that they are left unbathed, and pressure ulcers on their buttocks go unnoticed; they are not toileted in a timely fashion, fall on their urine puddle, and fracture a hip. These patients need close observation and careful attention to their physical needs. Consideration must be given to the fact that they may be unable to communicate their needs and discomforts; a subtle change in behavior or function, a facial grimace, or repeated touching of a body part may give clues that a problem exists. This reinforces the importance of consistency in caregivers because they will be familiar with a patient's unique behaviors and more quickly recognize a deviation from that individual's norm.

As patients regress, their dignity, personal worth, freedom, and individuality may be jeopardized. Loved ones may view the demented family

member as a stranger living inside the body that once housed the person they knew; staff see another dependent or total-care patient before them with no sense of that person's unique life history. Seen less and less as a normal human being or the same person they have known, the person with dementia may being treated in a dehumanizing manner. Special attention must be paid to maintaining and promoting the following qualities:

Individuality. The personal history and uniqueness of the patient should be learned and added to.

Independence. Even if it takes three times longer to guide patients through dressing than it would take to dress them, they should be afforded every opportunity for self-care.

Freedom. As major freedoms become limited, minor choices and control become especially important. Nurses must be careful that, in the name of efficiency and safety, such severe restrictions to freedom are not imposed that the quality of life becomes minimal.

Dignity. To become angry or laugh at the behaviors of a demented person is no less cruel than reacting in a similar fashion to a stroke victim who falls during ambulation. These patients should be afforded the respect given to any adult, including attractive clothing, good grooming, adult hairstyles, use of their name, privacy, and confidentiality.

Assistance and support to the families of patients are integral parts of nursing persons with dementias. The physical, emotional, and socioeconomic burden of caring for a cognitively impaired relative can be immense. It should not be assumed that family members understand basic care techniques. Basic, specific care techniques need to be reviewed, including lifting, bathing, and controlling inappropriate behaviors. Families should be prepared for the guilt, frustration, anger, depression, and other feelings that normally accompany this responsibility. Helping them plan respite, network with support groups, and obtain counseling may be beneficial. Most states now have chapters of the Alzheimer's Disease and Related Disorders Association.

Depression

Depression is the most frequent problem that psychiatrists treat in the elderly, and it increases in incidence with age. Various estimates have placed the prevalence of depression in the elderly anywhere from 10% to 65%, with the highest prevalence in persons with physical ailments.(Gallagher and Thompson, 1981) The severity of depression is higher in the elderly (Fig. 33-1). Although depressive episodes may have been a lifelong problem for some individuals, it is not uncommon for depression to be a new problem in old age. This is not surprising when one considers the adjustments and losses the elderly face, such as the independence of one's children; the reality of retirement; significant changes or losses of roles; reduced income restricting the pursuit of satisfying leisure activities and limiting the ability to meet basic needs; decreasing efficiency of the body; a changing self-image; the death of family members and friends, reinforcing the reality of one's own shrinking life span; and overt and covert messages from society that one's worth is inversely proportional to one's age. Under these circumstances, it is understandable that many persons become depressed in old age. In addition, drugs can cause or aggravate depression (Display 33-2).

Depression is a complex syndrome and is demonstrated in a variety of ways in older persons. The most common manifestations of this problem are the vegetative symptoms, which include insomnia, fatigue, anorexia, weight loss, constipation, and decreased interest in sex. Depressed persons may express self-depreciation, guilt, apathy, remorse, and feelings of being burdens. They may have problems with their personal relationships and social interactions and lose interest in people. Hygienic practices may be neglected. Physical complaints of headache, indigestion, and other problems may surface. Confusion may be present, caused by malnutrition or other effects of the depression. The symptoms of depression can mimic those of dementia; thus, careful assessment is crucial to avoid misdiagnosis. A decline in intellect and personality are usually indicative of dementia, not depression. Depression can occur in the early stage of dementia as the patient becomes aware of declining intellectual abilities.

The relationship of life events to the depression is essential to explore during the assessment; the approach for the person depressed from the effects of a drug obviously will differ from that for a person who has just become widowed. The underlying problem should be addressed. Although depressions do tend to last longer in the elderly, prompt treatment can hasten recovery. Treatment

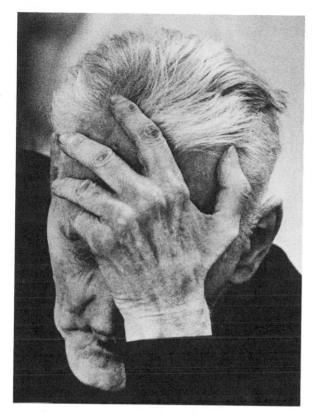

Figure 33-1. *Depression is a complex syndrome that can be exhibited in many ways. (Photograph by Eric Schenk.)*

should not be withheld because it is associated with a serious or terminal illness; alleviating the depression may help the individual cope more effectively and be in a better position to manage other health problems.

Psychotherapy and antidepressants (see Chap. 35) can alleviate many depressions to varying degrees. Electroconvulsive therapy has been shown to be effective in patients who have serious depressions that have been unresponsive to other therapies. In addition to supporting those interventions, nurses need to perform the following functions:

DISPLAY 33-2   Examples of Drugs That Can Cause Depression

Antihypertensives: β blockers, reserpine, methyldopa, spironolactone
Hormones: corticotropin, corticosteroids, estrogens
Sedatives: barbiturates, benzodiazepines
Others: alcohol, cimetidine, L-dopa, rantidine

Help the patient develop a positive self-concept. It must be emphasized that, although the situation may be bad, the person is not. Opportunities for success, regardless of how minor, should be provided, and new goals should be formed.

Encourage the expression of feelings. Anger, guilt, frustration, and other feelings should be vented. Nurses should afford time to listen and guide patients through these feelings. Statements such as "Don't worry, things will get better" or "Don't talk that way; you have a lot to be thankful for" offer little benefit to depressed persons.

Ensure that physical needs are met. Good nutrition, activity, sleep, and regular bowel movements are among the factors that enhance a healthy physical state, which in turn strengthen the patients' capacities to work through depression. Physical-care problems must be aggressively addressed.

Offer hope. While being realistic regarding the individual situation, nurses can, by words

and deeds, convey their belief that the future will have meaning and that the patient's life is of value.

Suicide

Suicide is a real and serious risk among depressed persons. The suicide rate increases with age and is highest among older white men. Twenty-three percent of all suicides are elderly individuals. All suicide threats from the elderly should be taken seriously. In addition to recognizing obvious suicide attempts, nurses must learn to recognize those that are more subtle but equally destructive. Medication misuse, either in the form of overdosages or omission of dosages, may be a suicidal gesture. Self-starvation is another sign and can occur even in an institutional setting if staff members are not attentive to monitoring intake and nutritional status. Engaging in activities that oppose a therapeutic need or threaten a medical problem (*e.g.,* ignoring dietary restrictions or refusing a particular therapy) may indicate a desire to die. Walking through a dangerous area, driving while intoxicated, and subjecting oneself to other risks can be signals of suicidal desires. Suicidal risk can further be assessed by asking the patient about recent losses, life-style changes, new or worsening health problems, new symptoms of depression, changes in or a limited support system, and a family history of suicide.

The suicidal elderly need close observation, careful protection, and prompt therapy. Treatment of the underlying depression should be supported. The environment should be made safe by removing items that could be potentially used for self-harm. Nurses need to convey a willingness to listen to and discuss thoughts and feelings about suicide. Being able to reach out for help by expressing their suicidal thoughts to nursing staff may prevent patients from taking actions to end their lives.

Anxiety

Adjustments to physical, emotional, and socioeconomic limitations in old age, and the new problems that frequently are encountered due to aging, add to the variety of causes for anxiety. Anxiety reactions, not uncommon in older persons, can be manifested in various ways, including somatic complaints, rigidity in thinking and behavior, in-somnia, fatigue, hostility, restlessness, chain smoking, pacing, fantasizing, confusion, and increased dependency. An increase in blood pressure, pulse, respirations, psychomotor activity, and frequency of voiding may occur. Appetite may increase or decrease. Anxious individuals often handle their clothing, jewelry, or utensils excessively and become intensively involved with a minor task (*e.g.,* folding a piece of linen), and have difficulty concentrating on the activity at hand.

Treatment of anxiety depends on its cause. Nurses should probe into the patient's history for recent changes or new stresses (*e.g.,* rent increase, increased neighborhood crime, divorce of child). The consumption of caffeine, alcohol, nicotine, and over-the-counter drugs should be reviewed for possible causes. Interventions specific to the underlying cause should be planned. In addition to drugs, interventions such as biofeedback, guided imagery, and relaxation therapy can prove helpful. Anxious persons need their lives to be simplified and stable, with few unpredictable occurrences. Environmental stimuli must be controlled. Basic interventions that could prove beneficial include the following:

Allow adequate time for conversations, procedures, and other activities.

Prepare the individual for all anticipated activities.

Provide thorough, honest, and basic explanations.

Control the number and variety of persons with whom the patient must interact.

Adhere to routines.

Keep and use familiar objects.

Prevent overstimulation of the senses by reducing noise, using soft lights, and maintaining a stable room temperature.

Paranoia

Paranoid states frequently occur in older persons, which is not surprising considering the following:

Sensory losses, so common in later life, easily cause the environment to be misperceived.

Illness, disability, living alone, and a limited budget promote insecurity.

Ageism within society sends a message of the undesirability of the old.

Older people are frequent victims of crime and unscrupulous practices.

The elderly's mistrust of the world can be viewed as a sensible and normal reaction when these realities are reviewed.

The initial consideration in working with paranoid older individuals is to explore mechanisms that could reduce insecurity and misperception. Corrective lenses, hearing aids, supplemental income, new housing, and a stable environment are potential interventions. Psychotherapy and medications (see Chap. 35) can be used when improvement is not achieved through other interventions. Nurses should ensure that these patients do not become withdrawn from the rest of the world because of self-imposed isolation. Not to be overlooked is the impact of the paranoid state on general health and well-being. Nutritional status can be threatened if the patient refuses to eat because she believes her food is poisoned; sleep deprivation can result if there is suspicion that a stranger is in the house; and health problems may not be diagnosed if the person believes the doctor is an enemy. Honest, basic explanations and approaches to dealing with paranoid misperceptions are beneficial; at no time should delusions be supported.

Hypochondriasis

Hypochondriasis may be a problem of older individuals. Although it commonly is associated with depression, for some elderly it may be an attention-getting mechanism. Often, health professionals reinforce this behavior by reacting to physical complaints promptly but not reinforcing periods of good function and health. Staff members may not respond to a request to sit down and talk with a patient, but they give undivided attention when that same person expresses physical discomfort. Some older people find hypochondriasis an effective means of controlling a spouse or children. Older people may use it as a means of socialization; if they do not have travels, professions, or interests they can share with others, they can count on their peers having similar ailments, which can serve as the common ground for conversation.

Regardless of how unfounded they seem, complaints need to be evaluated for their validity before assuming that they are part of hypochondriasis. Even the complaints of a known hypochondriac deserve evaluation, particularly if a new set of complaints emerges. It is beneficial to help these people find alternatives to their obsession with their bodily functions. Spending time in non–illness-related conversation can demonstrate that one can receive attention without resorting to physical complaints. Family members need to understand the dynamics of this problem so that they can reinforce positive behaviors and not be manipulated. Telling these patients that nothing is wrong is of little help; the underlying reason for this reaction must be addressed.

General Nursing Interventions Related to Mental-Health Problems

Promoting Mental Health

Mental health in old age implies a satisfaction and interest in life. This can be displayed in a variety of ways, ranging from quiet reflection to zealous activity. The quiet individual who stays at home does not necessarily have less mental capacity or mental health than the person who is actively involved in every senior citizen program. There is no single presentation for mental health; attempts to assess an older individual's mental status based on any given stereotype are to be avoided.

Good mental-health practices throughout an individual's lifetime promote good mental health in later life. To preserve mental health, people need to maintain the activities and interests that they find satisfying. They need opportunities to prove their value as a member of society and to have their self-worth reinforced. Security through the provision of adequate income, safe housing, the means to meet basic human needs, and support and assistance through stressful situations will promote mental health. A basic ingredient in the preservation and promotion of mental health that cannot be overstated is the importance of optimum physical health.

Nurses must recognize that there are times in everyone's life when disturbances occur and alter the capacity to manage stress. The same principles guiding the care of physical-health problems can be applied to the care of persons with mental-health problems. The following actions can be used in care.

Strengthen the individual's capacity to manage the problem.

Eliminate or minimize the limitations imposed by the problem.

Act for or do for the individual only when absolutely necessary.

Table 33-1 *Checklist for Documenting Drugs and Behavior*

DATE	A.M. 12	1	2	3	4	5	6	7	8	9	10	11	P.M. 12	1	2	3	4	5	6	7	8	9	10	11
Medications:																								
Disoriented regarding: Self																								
Others																								
Place																								
Day																								
Time																								
Forgetful of: Today's events																								
Past events																								
Inappropriate: Speech																								
Behavior																								
Hallucinations																								
Wandering																								
ADL deficits: Feeding																								
Bathing																								
Dressing																								
Toileting																								
Mobility																								
Incontinence, urinary																								
Pulse																								
Blood pressure																								

Table 33-1 Checklist for Documenting Drugs and Behavior (Continued)

DATE	A.M. 12	1	2	3	4	5	6	7	8	9	10	11	P.M. 12	1	2	3	4	5	6	7	8	9	10	11
Bowel movement																								
Sleeping/napping																								

Other symptoms:

FOOD INTAKE:	100%	75%	50%	25%	0%	COMMENTS
Breakfast						
Lunch						
Dinner						
Snacks						

Use back to describe specific problems/changes

Efforts that strengthen the patient's capacity to manage an emotional problem include improvement of physical health, good nutrition, increasing knowledge base, meaningful activity, income supplements, and socialization. Efforts to eliminate or minimize limitations include providing consistency in care, not fostering hallucinations, reality orientation, correction of physical problems, and modifying the environment to compensate for deficits. Efforts to act for or do for include selecting an adequate diet, bathing, managing finances, and directing activities for the patient.

Mental-health problems must be seen in the perspective of the patient's total world. The elderly confront many problems that challenge their emotional homeostasis, such as the following.

Illness: acceptance, management, pain, altered function or body image.
Death: friends, family, significant support person.
Retirement: loss of status, role, income, sense of purpose.
Increased vulnerability: crime, illness, disability, abuse.
Social isolation: lack of transportation, funds, health, friends.
Sensory deficits: decrease in or loss of function of hearing, vision, taste, smell and touch.

Greater awareness of own mortality: increased number of deaths of peers.
Increased risk of institutionalization, dependency: loss of self-care capabilities to varying degrees.

With these factors in mind, some of the symptoms displayed may be revealed to be normal reactions to the circumstances at hand. Before labeling the patient with a psychiatric diagnosis, there should be an attempt to explore the relationship of such factors to the patient's behavior and to address the cause of the problem rather than its effects alone.

Monitoring Medications

Medications used to treat psychiatric disorders can bring significant improvement to patients, but they also can have profound adverse effects in older adults. Some of the adverse effects of these medications can lead to anorexia, constipation, falls, incontinence, anemia, lethargy, sleep disturbances, and confusion. See Chapter 35 for information about specific drug groups. The lowest possible dosage should be used, and any reactions should be observed closely. It may be useful to initiate a checklist for problem identification, as shown in Table 33-1, to track the impact of medi-

Table 33-2 *Understanding and Managing Common Behavioral Problems*

BEHAVIOR	POSSIBLE CAUSES	NURSING ACTIONS
Physically abusive (*e.g.*, hitting, kicking, biting others)	Dementia Paranoia Misinterpretation of actions of others Anger Feeling powerless Anxiety Fatigue	Avoid putting resident in situations that promote abusive behavior Recognize warning signs (*e.g.*, cursing, pacing) Get help to protect self and others Speak to resident in calm, quiet manner Move resident to area away from other residents
Verbally abusive (*e.g.*, insulting, accusing, threatening)	Dementia Feeling powerless Anger	Avoid arguing, reasoning, reacting to comments Distract with activities Reinforce positive behaviors Allow maximum decision-making and participation
Resisting care	Dementia Misinterpretation of actions, objects, environment Depression	Prepare for activities Break activities into single, simple steps Use alternatives if possible (*e.g.*, sponge bath instead of tub bath) Monitor hygiene, nutritional status, intake and output, elimination
Undressing	Dementia Soiled clothing Irritation from clothing Feeling too warm	Ensure clothing is clean, dry; replace as necessary Examine clothing for irritation, poor fit Inspect skin for irritation Redress Use clothing that is difficult to undo Comment on appearance when resident remains dressed
Repetitive actions	Dementia Agitation Anxiety Boredom	Ignore Distract with other activities Replace with a more acceptable repetitive activity (*e.g.*, folding laundry, stacking papers)
Wandering	Dementia Boredom Restlessness Anxiety	Schedule times for supervised ambulation Provide activities Safeguard environment (*e.g.*, alarm doors, install door locks that require punching in code to open, ensure window screens cannot be removed) Ensure resident is wearing some form of identification Familiarize resident with environment; orient
Night wandering and restlessness	Dementia Excess daytime sleeping Misinterpretation of environment Sundowner syndrome Medications (*e.g.*, sedatives, hypnotics, diuretics, laxatives)	Provide daytime activities Provide late day exercise Toilet before bedtime Keep night light on in bedroom and bathroom Reassure and orient when resident awakens Provide safe environment

Table 33-2 *Understanding and Managing Common Behavioral Problems (Continued)*

BEHAVIOR	POSSIBLE CAUSES	NURSING ACTIONS
Inappropriate sexual behavior	Dementia, leading to poor judgment, loss of inhibition Misinterpetation of actions and messages from others	Relocate resident to private area Distract with other activities Set limits and remind of acceptable behaviors Review medications for those that can cause reduced inhibitions (*e.g.,* antianxiety agents) or that increase libido (*e.g.,* L-dopa) Provide acceptable means of touch, human contact
Suspiciousness	Paranoid state Dementia Suspicious personality Medications (*e.g.,* anticholinergics, L-dopa, tolbutamide)	Assess cause Don't react to behavior; depersonalize Protect from harm Provide explanations; prepare for activities, changes Afford maximum decision-making Do not try to explain to resident that suspicions are unfounded or wrong; this will not be helpful

From Eliopoulos C. Common behavioral problems. Long-Term Care Educator 1991;2(5):5.

cations on behavior and function. Of course, drugs complement and do not substitute for other forms of treatment.

Promoting a Positive Self-Concept

The importance of promoting a positive self-concept in all older adults cannot be overemphasized. All people need to feel that their lives have had meaning and that there is hope. A sense of meaninglessness and hopelessness threaten mental health and minimize the pleasures that the last segment of life can bring. Nurses should take a sincere interest in the lives and accomplishments of their elderly patients. It must be remembered that the disabled or frail person who now presents to the nurse may once have demonstrated the courage to venture from a native country to America, risked his life to save fellow soldiers in a war, scrubbed floors at night to support a family during the Great Depression, or developed a successful business from scratch. Struggles and accomplishments exist in every life and can be recognized to aid in promoting self-esteem. Activities such as life-review discussions, taping oral histories, and compiling a scrapbook of life events not only help older adults feel a sense of worth about the lives they have lived but also provide a sense of history and legacy for younger generations. In addition to the past, the present and future should hold meaning for the elderly, and this can be promoted by helping patients participate in relevant activities, engage in meaningful social interactions, have opportunities to do for others, exercise the maximal amount of control possible over their lives, maintain religious and cultural practices, and be respected as individuals.

Managing Behavioral Problems

Behavioral problems are actions that are annoying, disruptive, harmful, or generally deviate from the norm, and that tend to be recurrent in nature, such as physical or verbal abuse, resistance to care,

repetitive actions, wandering, restlessness, suspiciousness, and inappropriate sexual behavior and undressing. These problems can occur in persons with altered cognitive status who are incapable of thinking rationally and making good judgments. Any type of illness that lowers the patient's ability to cope with changes and stress can contribute to these problems. Medications, environmental factors, a loss of independence, and insufficient activity can cause problematic behaviors, also.

Assessment of the cause of the behavior is the first step in assisting the patient who displays behavioral problems. Factors associated with the behavior should be closely observed and documented and include the following information: (Eliopoulos, 1991)

- time of onset
- where it occurred
- environmental conditions
- persons present
- activities that preceded
- pattern of behavior
- signs and symptoms present
- outcome
- measures that helped or worsened behaviors.

The underlying cause of the problem should be corrected or changed whenever possible. Likewise, factors that precipitate the behavioral problem should be avoided (e.g., if it is identified that the patient becomes agitated when seated in a busy hallway, it can be beneficial to avoid seating the patient in this area). Staff or caregivers should learn to identify signs and symptoms that precipitate the behavior and intervene in a timely manner. Environmental considerations that can decrease behavioral problems include maintaining a room temperature between 70°F (21°C) and 75°F (24°C), avoiding wall coverings and linens that have busy patterns, limiting traffic flow, controlling noise, preventing dramatic transitions from daylight to nighttime darkness (Display 33-3), and installing safety devices for monitoring, such as alarms on doors and video cameras. A review of some of the major behaviors, their causes, and related nursing interventions are presented in Table 33-2.

Care Planning

Actual or potential problems can be revealed during the mental status assessment. Assessment data should be reviewed for those problems that fall

---

DISPLAY 33-3   *Sundowner Syndrome*

Nursing home and hospital staff may witness agitation, disorientation, wandering, and a general worsening of behavior in some patients "after the sun goes down." This condition, called sundowner syndrome or nocturnal confusion, occurs most frequently in persons with impaired cognitive function. Although research in this area has been limited, factors that have been associated with sundowner syndrome include delirium, short period of time in institution, recent relocation within an institution, change in circadian rhythms (persons experiencing sundowner syndrome had higher oral temperatures and lower blood pressures in the afternoon), dehydration, sensory overload or deprivation, use of restraints, and conditions that interrupt sleep (e.g., sleep apnea).* Nursing staff can find the following measures beneficial in preventing and managing sundowner syndrome:

Turn on lights before dark and keep some form of lighting in room; use night lights.
Frequently check on and orient patient; use touch.
Provide afternoon activity without overexerting the patient.
Place familiar objects and personal possessions within the patient's view.
Ensure adequate fluid intake; offer fluids in the evening.
Provide toileting assistance during evening and night as needed.

---

*Evans, L. The sundown syndrome: a nursing management problem. In: Chenitz WC, Stone JT, Salisbury SA, eds. Clinical gerontological nursing: a guide to advanced practice. Philadelphia: WB Saunders, 1991:345.

From Eliopoulos C. Common behavioral problems. Long-Term Care Educator 1991;2(5):10.

---

within the realm of nursing to diagnose and manage, and related nursing diagnoses developed accordingly. Table 33-3 lists some of the major nursing diagnoses that can be related to mental-health problems.

The development of realistic goals guides care and provides a yardstick by which the patient's progress can be measured. Although the goals developed for individual patients will be specific to their unique needs, some possible goals in the care of patients with mental-health problems are listed

Table 33-3 *Nursing Diagnoses Related to Mental-Health Problems*

NURSING DIAGNOSIS	CAUSES OR CONTRIBUTING FACTORS
Activity intolerance	Depression, lack of motivation, sensory overload, fatigue, medications
Anxiety	Threat to self-concept, losses
Altered bowel elimination: constipation	Psychomotor slowing, medications, inactivity, lack of recognition of need to defecate
Altered bowel elimination: diarrhea	Anxiety, medications, stress
Pain	Hyperactivity, sensory overload, suicidal attempt
Impaired verbal communication	Impaired cerebral function, anxiety, suspiciousness
Ineffective individual coping	Stress, altered body function, low self-esteem, dependency, sensory overload, loss of significant other
Ineffective family coping	Patient dependency; history of poor family relationships
Diversional activity deficit	Physical, mental, or social limitations
Fear	New or misperceived environment, losses
Grieving	Loss of body part, function, role, significant other
Altered health maintenance	Cognitive impairment, lack of motivation, misperceptions
Impaired home maintenance management	Cognitive impairment, misperceptions, lack of motivation
High risk for infection	Medications, inactivity, inability to protect self
High risk for injury	Cognitive impairment, fatigue, medications, suicidal attempt
Impaired physical mobility	Medications, fatigue
Noncompliance	Cognitive impairment, lack of motivation or capacity, suicidal attempt
Altered nutrition: less than body requirements	Depression, anxiety, stress, paranoia, cognitive impairment, suicidal attempt
Altered nutrition: more than body requirements	Depression, anxiety, cognitive impairment, inactivity
Powerlessness	Paranoia, depression, disability, stress
Self-care deficit	Cognitive impairment, lack of motivation, knowledge, skill
Disturbance in self-concept	Altered body image or function, losses, ageism
Sensory–perceptual alterations	Cognitive impairment, medications, paranoia, sensory deficits, isolation, stress
Sexual dysfunction	Depression, anxiety, paranoia, guilt, stress, altered self-concept, medications
Impaired skin integrity	Cognitive impairment (inability to protect self), malnutrition
Sleep pattern disturbance	Anxiety, paranoia, depression, confusion, medications
Impaired social interactions	Altered body part or function, cognitive impairment, anxiety, depression, misperceptions, paranoia, hypochondriasis
Social isolation	Anxiety, depression, paranoia, cognitive impairment
Altered thought processes	Cognitive impairment, fear, depression, anxiety, stress, isolation
Altered patterns of urinary elimination	Cognitive impairment, anxiety, depression, medications
High risk for violence	Cognitive impairment, paranoia, stress, misperceptions, fear, suicidal attempt

Sample Care Plan Goals for the Patient With a Mental Health Problem

To engage in activities of daily living with highest possible level of independence

To regain normal cognitive function

To be free from signs of mental illness

To be free from injury

To maintain weight at desired level

To be free from signs of malnutrition and fluid and electrolyte imbalance

To be free from elimination-related problems

To communicate effectively

To be able to make needs known

To perceive environment accurately

To be oriented to person, place, and time

To have a reduction in the number of incidents of _____ (behavioral problem)

To verbalize an interest in life and a positive self-concept

To learn effective means to manage stress

To learn effective means to cope with grief

To increase social activities to specific times per week

To be free from adverse effects of medications used to treat mental illness

Resources to Assist Patients With Mental Health Problems

Alcoholics Anonymous
P.O. Box 459
Grand Central Station
New York, NY 10017
(212)686-1100
(Local chapters are available)

Alzheimer's Disease and Related Disorders Association, Inc.
919 N. Michigan Ave.
Suite 1000
Chicago, IL 60611
(800)272-3900
(Local chapters are available)

Mental Health Association
1800 North Kent St.
Arlington, VA 22209
(703)528-6405

Respite Programs for Caregivers of Alzheimer's Disease Patients (Hotline)
(800)648-COPE

in the Sample Care Plan. Patients and their significant others should be active participants in the development of goals and establishment of priorities. See Chapter 18 for more information on planning and providing care. Resources that can assist patients and their caregivers are presented in the Resources List.

References

Derogatis RS, Lipma K, Rickels EH, Uhlenhuth EH, Covi L. The Hopkins symptom checklist: a measure of primary symptom dimensions. Pharmacopsychiatry 1974; 7:79.

Duke University Center for the Study of Aging. Multidimensional functional assessment: the OARS methodology. Durham, NC: Duke University, 1978.

Eliopoulos C. Common behavioral problems. Long-Term Care Educator 1991; 2(5):4.

Fishback DB. Mental status questionnaire for organic brain syndrome, with a new visual counting test. Am Geriatr Soc 1977; 25:167.

Folstein MF, Folstein S, McHugh PR. Mini-mental state: a practical method for grading the cognitive state of patients for the clinician. J Psychiatry Res 1975; 12:189.

Foreman MD. Complexities of acute confusion. Geriatr Nurs 1990; 11(3):136.

Gallagher D, Thompson LW. Depression in the elderly: a behavioral treatment manual. Los Angeles: University of Southern California, 1981:2.

Goldberg D. The detection of psychiatric illness by questionnaire. London: Oxford University, 1972.

Pfeiffer E. A short portable mental status questionnaire for the assessment of organic brain deficit in elderly patients. J Am Geriatr Soc 1975; 23(10):433.

Wolanin MO, Phillips LRF. Confusion: prevention and care. St Louis: CV Mosby, 1981.

Zung WWK. A self-rating depression scale. Arch Gen Psychiatr 1965; 12:63.

Recommended Readings

Abraham AL, Neundorfer MM. Alzheimer's: a decade of progress, a future of nursing challenges. Geriatr Nurs 1990; 11(3):116.

Blixen CE. Aging and mental health care, J Gerontol Nurs 1988; 14(11):11.

Brock CD, Simpson WM: Dementia, depression or grief? The differential diagnosis. Geriatrics 1990; 45(10):37.

Buckwalter KC. How to unmask depression. Geriatr Nurs 1990; 11(4):179.

Burckhardt CS. The effect of therapy on the mental health of the elderly. Res Nurs Health 1987; 10:277.

Duffy LM, Hepburn K, Christensen R, Brugge-Wiger P. A research agenda in care for patients with Alzheimer's disease. Image: Journal of Nursing Scholarship 1989; 21:254.

Ebersole P. Caring for the psychogeriatric client. New York: Springer-Verlag, 1989.

Foreman MD. Complexities of acute confusion. Geriatr Nurs 1990; 11(3):136.

Foreman MD. Reliability and validity of mental status questionnaires in elderly hospitalized patients. Nurs Res 1987; 36:216.

Foreman MD. Confusion in the hospitalized elderly: incidence, onset and associated factors. Res Nurs Health 1989; 12:21.

Gomez G, Gomez EA. Dementia or delirium? Geriatr Nurs 1989; 10(3):141.

Harvis K, Rabins P. Dementia: helping family caregivers cope. J Psychosocial Nurs 1989; 27:7.

Hoch CC, Reynolds CF, Houck PR. Sleep patterns in Alzheimer, depressed, and healthy elderly. West J Nurs Res 1988; 10:239.

Hogstel MO, ed. Geropsychiatric nursing. St. Louis: CV Mosby, 1990.

Johnson FL, Foxall MJ, Kelleher E, Kentopp E, Mannlein EA, Cook E. Comparison of mental health and life satisfaction in five elderly ethnic groups. West J Nurs Res 1988; 10:613.

Mace NL. Dementia care: patient, family and community. Baltimore: Johns Hopkins University, 1989.

Norberg A, Athlin E. Eating problems in severely demented patients: issues and ethical dilemmas. Nurs Clin North Am 1989; 24:781.

Raskin AJ. Replication of factors of psychopathology of hospitalized depressives. J Nerv Ment Dis 1960; 148:87.

Reed PG. Mental health of older adults. West J Nurs Res 1989; 11:143.

Teng EL, Chui HC. The modified mini-mental state (3MS) examination. J Clin Psychiatry 1987; 48(8):314.

34

Rehabilitative Aspects of Care

Throughout this book, the high prevalence of chronic illness and disability among the elderly has been discussed. Many older persons must learn to live with limited mobility, pain, impaired communication, and multiple risks to their safety and well-being. As growing numbers of people achieve old age and survive once-fatal conditions with residual disabilities, the prevalence of disabled elderly also will grow. Increasingly, the emphasis on saving lives will be replaced by an emphasis on preserving the quality of the lives that have been saved. The advantages of modern technology in diagnosing and treating disease and improving life expectancy may be minimized if older adults must live with disabilities that result in discomfort, dependency, and distress.

Confronting Disability

An accident or stroke may have brought sudden disability to a previously independent, functional adult; or perhaps a chronic condition has progressively worsened and its disabling impact is more acutely realized. Whatever the circumstances, few of us are prepared to deal with disability. It is difficult to accept in ourselves or our loved ones. Relationships, roles, and responsibilities are disrupted; disfigurement and dysfunction alter body image and self-concept. Losses and limitations cause a new vulnerability to emerge and make death seem more real and close. Concern occurs over potential physical and emotional pain, and frustration in wanting to eliminate the cause of the problem and

knowing we cannot. Disability can be an extremely difficult and devastating mountain to climb.

The severity of the disability is usually less important to rehabilitation efforts than the attitude and coping capacity of the disabled patients and their families. Nurses may have witnessed situations in which someone with a mild cardiac problem confines himself to his home, becomes preoccupied with his illness, and demands to be waited on, yet a hemiplegic returns to independent living in his modified apartment, finds a job, and cultivates new friends and interests. Previous attitudes, personality, and life-style have a strong influence on reactions to disability. A person who has always felt that life has dealt him a bad hand could view a disability as the last straw and give up all hope. On the other hand, an optimistic person who has approached problems as new challenges to overcome may be determined not to allow a disability to control his life. Individuals who relish independence and never let illness slow their life-styles will respond to disability differently than those who use real or exaggerated ills for other gains. The family's response to the disabled person also will influence that person's reactions. Families that reinforce sick role behaviors and insist on doing everything for the disabled person can cripple him physically and psychologically, whereas families that promote self-care and treat the disabled person as a responsible family member can help him to feel like a normal, useful human being.

Many losses may accompany disability, such as the loss of function, role, income, status, independence, or, perhaps, a body part. Disabled persons

mourn these losses, often demonstrating the same reactions experienced during the stages of dying. They may deny their disabilities by making unrealistic plans and not complying with their care plans. They may have angry outbursts and become impatient with those who are trying to help them. They may shop for medical advice that will offer them a more optimistic outlook or invest their hopes in any faith healer they can find. On one day they may optimistically state that their disability has given them a new perspective on life, whereas the very next day they tearfully question what they have to live for. These reactions can fluctuate; it is the rare individual who accepts a disability without some periods of regret or resentment.

Rehabilitative Nursing

Most of the disabilities possessed by older adults cannot be eliminated or, in many cases, significantly improved. Damaged lungs, amputations, diseased heart muscle, partial blindness, presbycusis, and deformed joints may accompany patients for the remainder of their lives. Often these chronic disabilities receive the least intervention; reimbursement and aggressive attention are given to restore the function of someone who has suffered a stroke or fracture, but those with no rehabilitation potential often are overlooked in their need to maintain function and prevent further decline through rehabilitation efforts.

Rehabilitation must be defined broadly in geriatric care. It may be considered as those efforts that help individuals gain ways to improve their functional capacity so that they can better cope, be maximally independent, have a sense of well-being, and enjoy a satisfying life. The principles guiding gerontological nursing care are of particular significance in rehabilitation and include the following actions:

Increase self-care capacity.
Eliminate or minimize self-care limitations.
Act for or do for when the person is unable to do for self.

Efforts to increase self-care capacity could include building the patient's arm muscles to enable better transfer to and propelling of a wheelchair or teaching the patient how to inject insulin with the use of only one hand. Relieving pain and having a ramp installed for easier wheelchair mobility are efforts that minimize or eliminate limitations. Ob-

taining a new prescription from the pharmacy and performing range-of-motion exercises demonstrate ways in which nurses act or do for the patient. Whenever nurses do or act for patients, they need to question what could be done to enable patients to perform this act independently. Patients will always be dependent on others for some activities, but for others actions patients can assume responsibility with sufficient education, time allocation, encouragement, and assistive devices. The following information should be remembered in rehabilitative nursing:

Know the unique capacities and limitations of the individual. Assess the patient's self-care capacity, mental status, level of motivation, and family support.
Emphasize function rather than dysfunction.
Provide time and flexibility. At times, institutional routines (e.g., having all baths completed by 9 A.M., collecting all food trays 45 minutes after delivery) cause caregivers to do tasks for patients so that they may be completed efficiently. Staff needs for efficiency and orderliness should never supersede the patient's need for independence.
Recognize and praise accomplishments. Seemingly minor acts, such as combing hair or wheeling themselves to the hallway, can be the result of tremendous effort and determination on the part of disabled persons.
Do not equate physical disability with mental disability. Treat the disabled as mature, intelligent adults.
Prevent complications. Recognize potential risks (e.g., skin breakdown, social isolation, or depression) and actively prevent them.
Demonstrate hope, optimism, and a sense of humor. It is difficult for disabled persons to feel positive about rehabilitation if their caregivers appear discouraged or defeated.
Keep in mind that rehabilitation is a highly individualized process, requiring a multidisciplinary team effort for optimal results.

Assessing Functional Capacities

A determination of individual levels of independence in meeting the activities of daily living (ADL) and instrumental activities of daily living (IADL) is essential to understanding the rehabilitation needs of the patient. An assessment of ADLs explores the

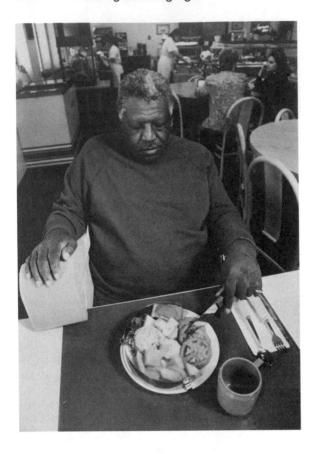

Assistive devices can facilitate independence and maintain dignity in persons with disabilities. (From Birchenall, JM. Care of the older adult. 3rd ed. Philadelphia: JB Lippincott, 1993.)

skills possessed by the patient in meeting basic requirements such as eating, hygiene, dressing, toileting, and moving. IADL assessment examines those skills beyond the basics that enable the individual to function independently in the community, such as the ability to prepare meals, shop, use a telephone, safely use medications, clean, travel in the community, and manage finances. Persons can be totally independent, partially independent, or dependent in their ability to perform these activities (Table 34-1). Tools such as the Katz Index of Independence in Activities of Daily Living can serve as guidelines for assessing ADL.

When a deficit in ADL capacity exists, its specific cause must be identified so that appropriate interventions can be planned. For example, a person who is partially dependent in bathing because he needs to have a basin of water brought to him will have different nursing requirements than one who forgets what he is doing as he bathes and needs to be reminded of the next action to take.

Proper Positioning

Correct body alignment facilitates optimal respiration, circulation, and comfort and prevents complications such as contractures and pressure ulcers. When patients are unable to position their bodies independently, nurses must be attentive to keeping their bodies properly aligned. Figure 34-1 demonstrates proper alignment in various positions.

Range-of-Motion Exercises

Exercise is an essential component of the health maintenance and promotion plan of every adult and is particularly significant for the elderly. The benefits of exercise are many, including the promotion of joint motion and muscle strength, stimulation of circulation, maintenance of functional capacity, and prevention of contractures and other complications. Exercises can be done in the following degrees:

Table 34-1 *Assessing Capacity to Perform Activities of Daily Living*

TOTAL INDEPENDENCE	PARTIAL INDEPENDENCE	DEPENDENCE
Eating		
Uses all utensils	Needs tray set up	Needs to be fed
Cuts meats	Cannot cut foods or butter bread	
Butters bread	Needs encouragement, reminders to eat	
Drinks from cup or glass		
Hygiene		
Transfers in or out of tub or shower	Reaches some body parts to cleanse	Needs complete bathing assistance
Reaches and bathes all body parts	Unable to brush teeth, dentures	
Brushes teeth or dentures	Unable to turn faucets or flush toilet	
Brushes or combs hair	Needs assistance transferring in or out of tub or shower	
Cleanses self after toileting	Needs assistance to comb or brush hair	
Turns faucets, flushes toilet	Must have basin brought	
	Needs reminders, encouragement to bathe	
Dressing		
Selects appropriate garments	Needs assistance with some garments, zippers, buttons, snaps	Needs to be fully dressed
Puts on all clothing	Unable to select appropriate garments	
Slips on shoes, socks, stockings	Needs encouragement, reminders to dress	
Ties shoelaces		
Able to manage zippers, buttons, snaps		
Continence		
Continent of bladder and bowels	Incontinent less than once daily	Total incontinent
Toileting		
Uses bedpan or toilet without assistance	Needs to be taken to toilet or have bedpan brought or taken	Needs assistance getting on or off bedpan or commode
Able to reach or transfer to and from bedpan or toilet	Needs encouragement or reminders to toilet	Unable to use bedpan or commode
Manages ostomy or catheter independently	Needs assistance with ostomy or catheter care	Unable to perform ostomy or catheter care
Mobility		
Ambulates with no assistance	Ambulates with assistance	Bedbound
Turns corners	Climbs stairs with assistance	Needs to be pushed in wheelchair
Climbs stairs	Transfers with assistance	Unable to transfer
Sits or lifts from chair and bed	Propels wheelchair but needs to be assisted in and out	Unable to climb stairs
Uses wheelchair, cane, walker with no assistance	Wanders in limited area	Wanders away if not supervised

Active: independently by patients.
Active assistive: with assistance to the patient.
Passive: with no active involvement of the patient.

During the assessment, all joints should be put through a full range of motion to determine the degree of movement possible actively, with active assistance, and passively. The most significant concern is the degree to which range of motion is sufficient to participate in the activities of daily living.

Patients should be encouraged to put all joints through a full range of motion at least once daily.

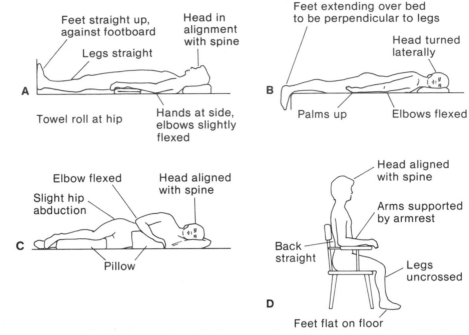

Figure 34-1. (**A**) *Supine position.* (**B**) *Prone position.* (**C**) *Lateral position.* (**D**) *Chair position.*

When nurses need to assist patients with these exercises, the following points must be remembered:

Offer support below and above the joint being exercised.

Move the joint slowly and smoothly, exercising it at least three times.

Do not force the joint past the point of resistance or pain.

Record joint mobility.

Some of the terms used in describing joint motion are listed below.

Flexion   bending
Extension   straightening
Hyperextension   extending beyond normal range
Abduction   moving away from body
Adduction   moving toward body
Pronation   rotating down, toward back of body
Supination   rotating up, toward front of body
Internal rotation   turning limb inward, toward center
External rotation   turning limb outward, from center

Inversion   turning joint inward
Eversion   turning joint outward
Circumduction   moving in a circular manner

Figure 34-2 demonstrates basic range-of-motion exercises that should be incorporated into the older adult's daily activities. Table 34-2 offers a tool that can be used to document the patient's range of motion.

Use of Mobility Aids

Wheelchairs, canes, and walkers can make the difference between older persons living a full life or being confined to their immediate environments. Mobility aids can enable patients to independently fulfill their universal needs and enhance functional capacity. If misused, however, these aids can present significant safety risks; thus, nurses must ensure that these pieces of equipment are used properly.

The first principle in using mobility aids is to only use them if necessary. Using a wheelchair

(Text Continues on page 328)

SHOULDER

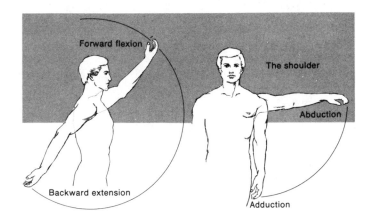

ELBOW

FOREARM

WRIST

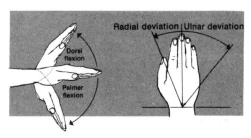

Figure 34-2. *Range-of-motion exercises.*

(continued)

HIP

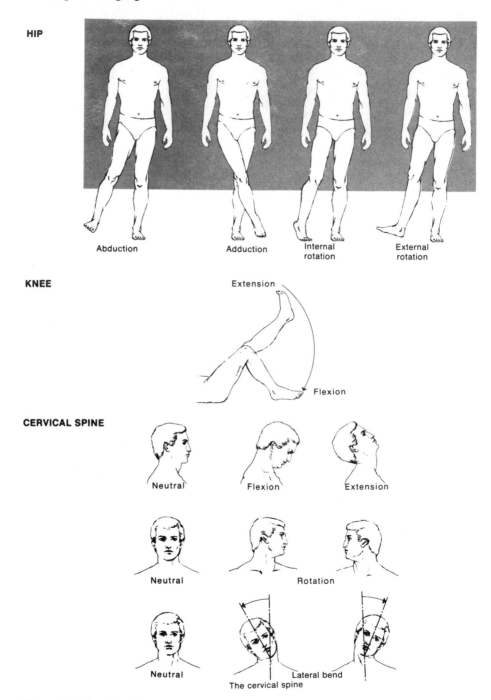

Abduction   Adduction   Internal rotation   External rotation

KNEE

Extension

Flexion

CERVICAL SPINE

Neutral   Flexion   Extension

Neutral   Rotation

Neutral   Lateral bend

The cervical spine

Figure 34-2. (continued)

THUMB

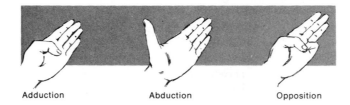

Adduction   Abduction   Opposition

FINGERS

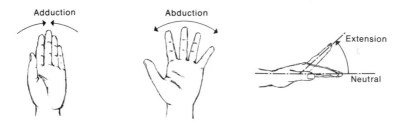

Adduction   Abduction   Extension / Neutral

ANKLE   **FOOT**

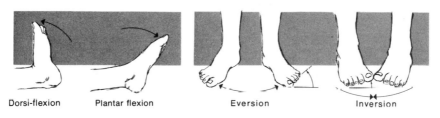

Dorsi-flexion   Plantar flexion   Eversion   Inversion

TOES

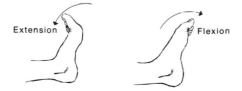

Extension   Flexion   Adduction   Abduction

Figure 34-2. (continued)

Table 34-2 *Tool for Assessing Range of Motion*

JOINT	NORMAL RANGE	PATIENT'S RANGE
Shoulder	Flexion 160° Extension 50°	
Elbow	Flexion 160° Extension from 160° to 0°	
Wrist	Flexion 90° Extension 70° Abduction 55° Adduction 20°	
Hip	Flexion (bent knee) 120° Flexion (straight knee) 90° Abduction 45° Adduction 45°	
Knee	Flexion 120°	
Neck	Extension 55° Flexion 45° Lateral bending 40° Rotation 70°	
Ankle	Dorsiflexion 20° Plantar flexion 45° Inversion 30° Eversion 20°	
Great Toe	Distal phalange: Flexion 50° Proximal phalange: Flexion 35° Extension 80°	
Finger	Proximal phalange: Flexion 90° Extension 30° Middle phalange: Flexion 120° Distal phalange: Flexion 80°	
Thumb	Proximal phalange: Flexion 70° Distal phalange: Flexion 90°	

© From Eliopoulos C. Range of motion exercises. Long-Term Care Educator 1991;2(9):3.

because it is quicker or easier can result in unnecessary dependency and decline of functional capacity. The true need for the aid must be evaluated. If a mobility aid is deemed necessary, it must be individually selected according to the following criteria:

> Canes are used to provide a wider base of support and should not be used for weight bearing.

> Walkers offer a broader base of support than canes and can be used for weight bearing.

> Wheelchairs provide mobility for persons unable to ambulate due to various disabilities such as paralysis or severe cardiac disease.

These aids are individually fitted based on the patient's size, need, and capacities. Patients should be fully instructed in their proper use. Physical therapists are excellent resources for sizing and in-

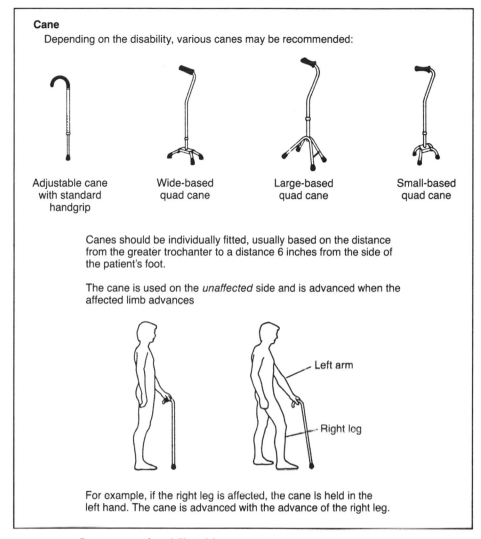

Cane

Depending on the disability, various canes may be recommended:

Adjustable cane with standard handgrip | Wide-based quad cane | Large-based quad cane | Small-based quad cane

Canes should be individually fitted, usually based on the distance from the greater trochanter to a distance 6 inches from the side of the patient's foot.

The cane is used on the *unaffected* side and is advanced when the affected limb advances

Left arm

Right leg

For example, if the right leg is affected, the cane is held in the left hand. The cane is advanced with the advance of the right leg.

Figure 34-3. *Proper use of mobility aids.*

(continued)

structing patients for cane, walker, or wheelchair use. Figure 34-3 shows some of the considerations involved in using these aids.

Bowel and Bladder Training

Incontinence can have a profound impact on the elderly's general health and well-being. Skin breakdown can result from the moisture and irritation to which the skin is subjected. Urine or feces on the floor can cause falls. Soiled, odorous clothing can lead to embarrassment and social isolation.

Infections, fractures, depression, altered self-concept, anorexia, and other problems can stem from poor bladder and bowel control.

The physical and mental capacity of the patient to achieve continence must be evaluated before a training program is begun. Some patients may not have the functional capacity to control their elimination despite good intentions; to initiate a training program with them would be unrealistic and frustrating. If the patient has the capacity to be continent, training should begin as early as possible (Displays 34-1 and 34-2). Consistency is a cru-

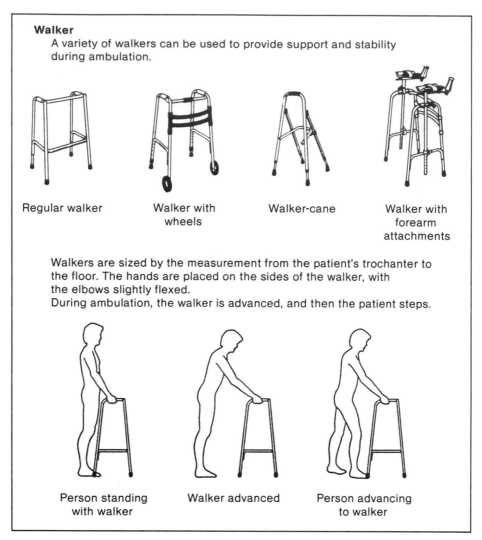

Walker

A variety of walkers can be used to provide support and stability during ambulation.

Regular walker   Walker with wheels   Walker-cane   Walker with forearm attachments

Walkers are sized by the measurement from the patient's trochanter to the floor. The hands are placed on the sides of the walker, with the elbows slightly flexed.
During ambulation, the walker is advanced, and then the patient steps.

Person standing with walker   Walker advanced   Person advancing to walker

Figure 34-3. (continued)

cial factor in training programs; the gains of the day shift in keeping the patient continent are lost if the evening and night shifts do not toilet the patient at the appropriate intervals. Success should be recognized and praised; patients should not be chastised for accidents, but the reasons for the incontinent episodes should be discussed with them. Encouraging patients to wear street clothes promotes a positive self-image and normality and often discourages regression. Results should be documented and regularly reviewed to determine the effectiveness of the plan.

Maintaining and Promoting Mental Function

The function of muscles and joints is only one aspect of rehabilitation. Equally important are efforts to restore, promote, or maintain mental function. In institutional settings where the main contact patients have with staff revolves around illness-related issues, or in their own homes where they may be socially isolated, healthy mental stimulation may be sorely lacking. Like any other function, mental function can deteriorate if not exercised;

Appropriate use of the walker for transfer activities is

When lowering to seat:
back walker to seat

When lifting from seat:
push on arms of seat
to a standing position;
walker should not be used
to pull to a standing position.

Hand should be
on chair arm as
person is lifting

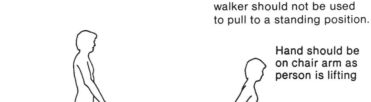

Chair

Walker

Wheelchair

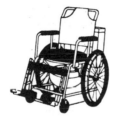

A wheelchair should be individually fitted to the patient. The seat
should be slightly larger than the patient's width to prevent pressure
and friction; the patient's arms should be able to reach the wheels
easily; footrests should be adjusted to support the patient's foot
in a flat position.

Removable or fold-down armrests facilitate transfer.

Wheelchairs should be checked routinely for ease of wheeling, function
of brakes, jagged edges, tears in upholstery, and broken or missing
hardware.

Figure 34-3. (continued)

thus, all rehabilitative efforts include the promotion of mental activity.

Mental stimulation is a highly individualized process, based on the unique intellectual and educational level of the patient. Some people enjoy reading the classics; others are barely interested in reading the local newspaper. Some people thrive on large social events, whereas others could spend days alone solving a crossword puzzle. Some people want to make things happen; others derive pleasure from watching them happen. This diversity, present in all age groups, reinforces the need to gear mental activities to the unique capacities and interests of the individual.

Patients can partake of a wide range of intellectual, recreational, and social activities. Some activi-

DISPLAY 34-1   Care Plan for Altered Urinary Elimination Pattern: Incontinence

Overview

Urinary incontinence is a condition in which urine is lost involuntarily due to factors such as weak supporting pelvic muscles, urinary tract infection, prostatic hypertrophy, tumors of the bladder or pelvic region, bladder neck obstruction, medications (e.g., sedatives, diuretics), cerebral cortex lesions, disturbances along the neural path, altered cognition, and toileting dependency.

Goal

To reestablish control over micturition

Actions

Ensure patient has been thoroughly evaluated to determine that restoration of bladder function is possible.

Record and evaluate the voiding pattern. Usually 2-hour intervals during the day and 4-hour intervals during the night are scheduled to check continence unless the patient's individual pattern indicates a greater frequency of checks.

One-half hour before anticipated voiding time, having the patient drink a glass of water.

Tell the patient to make a conscious efort not to void.

Sit patient on commode at schedule time.

Have patient rock back and forth or prop feet on stool to increase intraabdominal pressure.

Instruct patient to massage over bladder area.

Encourage voiding by running water.

Record results.

Reinforce desired behaviors. Give positive feedback for successes. When incontinent episodes do occur the patient should not be chastised, nor should the incident be ignored; instead, discuss the causes for the incontinence with the patient and establish goals for improvement.

As continence improves, the interval between voiding times can be increased.

It is essential that the schedule be rigidly followed.

DISPLAY 34-2   Care Plan for Altered Bowel Elimination: Incontinence

Overview

Bowel incontinence refers to the inability to voluntarily control the passage of stool. It can result from decreased anal muscle tone, disturbances in the neural innervation of the rectum, loss of cortical control, rectal prolapse, diarrhea, constipation with overflow related to impaction, or altered cognition.

Goal

To control bowel elimination

Actions

Record and evaluate patient's bowel elimination pattern.

Establish consistent time to toilet based on pattern.

Position patient in best physiological position for bowel movement: sitting with normal posture.

Have patient lean forward or prop feet on stool to increase intraabdominal pressure.

Instruct patient to bear down and attempt to defecate.

Record results; ensure that patient does not develop fecal impaction.

If necessary, stimulate anorectal reflex with glycerin suppository 30 to 45 minutes before scheduled bowel movement.

Supplement toilet activities with exercise and good fluid and roughage intake.

ties have specific therapeutic aims, one of which is reminiscence. Butler and Lewis have described reminiscence, or the life review, as a means of validating existence, resolving past conflicts, and finding meaning in remaining life.(Butler and Lewis, 1982) Nurses can guide patients in reminiscing through individual or group miens. Often, patients can supply meaningful themes for reminiscence. For example, the patient may comment, "Kids today have it a lot easier than I did when I was young," which could lead the nurse to explore the patient's youth and feelings associated with that

period of his life. Knowing something of the patient's personal history can aid nurses in finding relevant topics for reminiscence, such as the patient's immigration to America, development of a business, or efforts to assist the country during wartime. As the patient discusses the topic, questions can be asked and comments made to encourage greater exploration, for instance, "Really? Tell me more." "What was that like?" "How did that make you feel?" "That must have been very difficult for you." If the patient begins to ramble aimlessly, he can be redirected to the topic by comments such as, "Yes, you've mentioned that before . . . I can tell it was important to you. Now tell me what happened after that." Themes can be selected for group reminiscing, including playing old records and asking participants what their lives were like when those records were popular, showing old photographs and asking participants what memories arise, and asking them to describe the important pieces of history they have witnessed. Perhaps the most important skill for nurses to use in reminiscing activities is listening.

Patients with moderate to severe memory loss, confusion, or disorientation demand therapeutic efforts to keep them mentally integrated with the world around them. For these patients, reality orientation is an effective tool. Reality orientation frequently is assumed to be special group sessions that review day, date, weather, next meal, and next holiday. Actually, reality orientation encompasses much more; it is a total approach to keeping the patient oriented. Every nurse–patient contact can enhance orientation. For example, when passing medications, the nurse can state, "Hello Mr. Richards, I'm Nurse Jones with your medicine. How are you on this sunny Tuesday? It's very warm for March 10th, isn't it?" This simple exchange adds no more time to the act of administering the medications but provides helpful orientation. Misinformation and misperceptions of the patient should be clarified simply, for instance: "No, your son will not be visiting today. He comes on Sunday and today is Wednesday." Chastising or becoming frustrated with the patient for not remembering serves no therapeutic value. Clocks, calendars, holiday theme decorations, and reality boards enhance, but do not substitute for, staff interactions. Consistency is crucial to promoting orientation; it makes little sense for the day shift to reinforce to a patient

that he is in a nursing home while the evening shift agrees with the patient's claim that he is on his grandfather's farm.

Resources

Every community has its unique resources for persons with rehabilitative needs, which can provide education, support, and various forms of assistance to the disabled and their caregivers. Social workers, physical therapists, occupational therapists, speech and hearing therapists, and rehabilitation and vocational counselors are among the professionals who can offer guidance in locating appropriate resources. Local libraries, health departments, and information and referral services for the elderly can provide valuable assistance also. Some national organizations that can be contacted are listed below.

Alcoholism

Alcoholics Anonymous
P.O. Box 459
Grand Central Station
New York, NY 10017
(212)686-1100

National Clearinghouse for Alcohol Information
P.O. Box 2345
Rockville, MD 20852
(301)468-2600

Alzheimer's Disease

Alzheimer's Disease and Related Disorders
   Association, Inc.
919 N. Michigan Ave.
Chicago, IL 60601
(312)272-3900

Amputations

Accent on Living Publications
P.O. Box 700
Bloomington, IL 61701
(309)378-2961

National Amputation Foundation
12-45 150th St.
Whitestone, NY 11357
(212)767-0596

Arthritis

Arthritis Foundation
3400 Peachtree St.
Suite 1101
Atlanta, GA 30326
(404)266-0795

Arthritis Information Clearinghouse
P.O. Box 34427
Bethesda, MD 20034
(301)881-9411

Asthma

Asthma and Allergy Foundation of America
19 W. 44th St.
New York, NY 10036

Cancer

American Cancer Society
777 Third Ave.
New York, NY 10017
(212)371-2900

Make Today Count
P.O. Box 303
Burlington, IA 52601
(319)753-6521

National Cancer Institute
Office of Cancer Communications
Bldg. 31, Rm. 10A18
Bethesda, MD 20205
(800)492-6600

Diabetes

American Diabetes Association
2 Park Ave.
New York, NY 10016
(212)683-7444

Diabetes Education Center
4959 Excelsior Blvd.
Minneapolis, MN 55416
(612)927-3393

Head Injuries

National Head Injury Foundation
280 Singletary Lane
Framingham, MA 01701
(617)879-7433

Hearing Impairments

American Humane Association
Hearing Dog Program
1500 W. Tufts Ave.
Englewood, CO 80110
(303)762-0342

Design Center for the Deaf
Dept. of Environmental Design
Rochester Institute of Technology
Rochester, NY 14623
(716)464-1653

National Institute of Neurological and
Communicative Disorders
Bethesda, MD 20014
(202)496-4000

National Association for the Deaf
814 Thayer Ave.
Silver Spring, MD 20910
(301)587-1788

Organization for Use of the Telephone
P.O. Box 175
Owings Mills, MD 21117
(301)655-1827

Self-Help for Hard of Hearing People
P.O. Box 34889
Washington, DC 20034

Heart Disease, Stroke

American Heart Association
7320 Greenville Ave.
Dallas, TX 75231
(214)750-5551

International Association of Pacemaker Patients
P.O. Box 54305
Atlanta, GA 30308
(800)241-6993

The Mended Hearts
7320 Greenville Ave.
Dallas, TX 55231
(214)750-5442

Lung Disease

American Lung Association
1740 Broadway
New York, NY 10019
(212)245-8000

Emphysema Anonymous
P.O. Box 66
Fort Myers, FL 33902
(813)334-4226

Mental Illness

Alzheimer's Disease and Related Disorders
  Association, Inc.
919 N. Michigan Ave.
Suite 1000
Chicago, IL 60601
(800)272-3900

Mental Health Association
1800 N. Kent St.
Arlington, VA 22209
(703)528-6405

Neurological Diseases

American Parkinson's Disease Association
116 John St.
New York, NY 10038
(212)732-9550

Epilepsy Concern
1282 Wynnewood Dr.
West Palm Beach, FL 33409
(305)967-7616

Epilepsy Foundation of America
4351 Garden City Dr.
Landover, MD 20785
(301)459-3700

Myasthenia Gravis Foundation
15 E. 26th St.
New York, NY 10010
(212)889-8157

National Huntington's Disease Association
128A E. 74th St.
New York, NY 10021
(212)744-0302

National Multiple Sclerosis Society
205 E. 42nd St.
New York, NY 10017
(212)986-3240

National Parkinson Foundation
1501 NW 9th Ave.
Miami, FL 33136
(305)547-6666

Ostomies

United Ostomy Association
2001 W. Beverly Blvd.
Los Angeles, CA 90057
(213)413-5510

Spinal Cord Disorders

National Spinal Cord Injury Foundation
369 Elliot St.
Newton Upper Falls, MA 02164
(617)964-0521

Paralyzed Veterans of America
4350 East-West Hwy.
Suite 900
Washington, DC 20014
(301)652-2135

Visual Impairments

American Foundation for the Blind
15 W. 16th St.
New York, NY 10011
(212)620-2000

Blinded Veterans Association
1735 DeSales St., N.W.
Washington, DC 20036
(202)347-0410

Guide Dogs for the Blind
P.O. Box 1200
San Rafael, CA 94902
(415)479-4000

Guiding Eyes for the Blind
250 E. Hartsdale Ave.
Hartsdale, NY 10530
(914)723-2223

Helen Keller National Center
111 Middle Neck Rd.
Sand Point, NY 11050
(516)944-8900

Leader Dogs for the Blind
1039 S. Rochester Rd.
Rochester, MN 48063
(313)651-9011

National Association for the Visually
  Handicapped
305 E. 24th St.
New York, NY 10010
(212)899-3141

National Braille Association
654A Goodwin Ave.
Midland Park, NJ 07432
(201)447-1484

National Eye Institute
Bldg. 31, Rm. 6A-32
Bethesda, MD 20205
(301)496-5248

National Federation of the Blind
National Center for the Blind
1800 Johnson St.
Baltimore, MD 21230
(301)659-9314

National Library Service for the Blind and
Physically Handicapped
Library of Congress
1291 Taylor St., N.W.
Washington, DC 20542
(202)287-5100

National Public Radio Service for Print
Handicapped
2025 M St., N.W.
Washington, DC 20036
(202)822-2000

Recordings for the Blind
215 E. 58th St.
New York, NY 10022
(212)751-0860

General

Accent on Living
P.O. Box 726
Bloomington, IL 61701

Disabled American Veterans
P.O. Box 14301
Cincinnati, OH 45214
(606)441-7300

General Services Administration
18th and F Sts., N.W.
Washington, DC 20405
(202)655-4000

National Rehabilitation Information Center
Catholic University of America
4407 8th St., N.E.
Washington, DC 20017
(202)635-5822

Office for Handicapped Individuals
Room 338D, Hubert H. Humphrey Bldg.
200 Independence Ave., S.W.
Washington, DC 20201
(202)245-1961

Sister Kenny Institute
Abbott-Northwestern Hospital
2727 Chicago Ave.
Minneapolis, MN 55407
(612)874-4175

Reference

Butler RN, Lewis MI. Aging and mental health. St Louis: CV Mosby, 1982:58.

Recommended Readings

DiDomenico RL, Ziegler WZ. Practical rehabilitative techniques for geriatric aides. Rockville, MD: Aspen, 1989.

Hartigan JD, Connolly TJ: Is "wheelchair wrist drop" a new syndrome to watch for? Geriatrics 1990;45(6):63.

Heexhen SJ. Getting a handle on patient mobility. Geriatr Nurs 1989;10(3):146.

Lee MHM, Itoh M. General concepts of geriatric rehabilitation. In: Abrams WB, Berkow R, eds. The Merck manual of geriatrics. Rahway, NJ: Merck Sharp & Dohme Research Laboratories. 1990:249.

Mumma C, ed. Rehabilitation nursing: concepts and practice. 2nd ed. Evanston, IL: Rehabilitation Nursing Foundation, 1987.

Phipps MA, Kelly-Hayes M.: Rehabilitation of older adults. In: Murrow E, ed. Perspectives on gerontological nursing. Newbury Park, CA: SAGE, 1991:357.

35

Geriatric Pharmacology

The many health problems of the elderly cause this group to use a large number and variety of medications. Although they account for only 12% of the total population, the elderly consume nearly one-third of all prescription drugs and spend over $3 billion per year on medications. The average community-based older adult has 11 prescriptions filled yearly; an average of eight drugs are prescribed for each nursing home resident (Fig. 35-1). At least 90% of all elderly use at least one drug daily, with the more typical situation involving the use of several drugs daily. The most commonly used drugs by the older population include the following:

- cardiovascular agents
- antihypertensives
- analgesics
- antiarthritic agents
- sedatives
- tranquilizers
- laxatives
- antacids.

The drugs on this list can cause adverse effects (*e.g.*, confusion, dizziness, falls, fluid and electrolyte imbalances) that threaten the elderly's quality of life. Further, when taken together, some of these drugs can interact and cause serious adverse effects (Table 35-1).

In addition to the types and large numbers of drugs used by the older population, age-related differences in pharmacokinetics and pharmaco-

dynamics heighten the risks associated with drug therapy in this age group. Pharmacokinetics refer to the absorption, distribution, metabolism, and excretion of drugs; pharmacodynamics refers to the biological and therapeutic effects of drugs at the site of action or on the target organ. Drugs behave differently in older adults and require careful dosage adjustment and monitoring. To minimize the risks associated with drug therapy and ensure that medications do not create more problems than they solve, close supervision and adherence to sound principles of safe drug use are essential in gerontological nursing.

Pharmacokinetics

Absorption

Generally, older people have fewer problems in the area of drug absorption than with distribution, metabolism, and excretion of drugs. A variety of factors can alter the absorption of drugs, such as the following:

Age-related changes: decreased intracellular fluid, increased gastric pH, decreased gastric blood flow and motility, reduced cardiac output and circulation, and slower metabolism can slow drug absorption.

Route of administration: drugs given intramuscularly, subcutaneously, orally, or rectally are not absorbed as efficiently as drugs that are

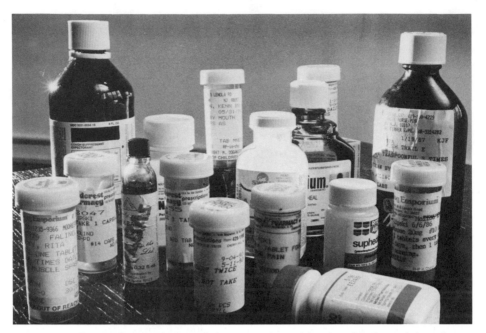

Figure 35-1. *The high prevalence of drugs consumed by the elderly and the complexity of drug dynamics in old age require gerontological nurses to regularly evaluate the continued need, appropriateness of dosage, and intended and adverse effects of every drug given to older individuals. (Photograph by Eric Schenk.)*

inhaled, applied topically, or instilled intravenously.

Concentration and solubility of drug: drugs that are highly soluble (*e.g.,* aqueous solutions) and in higher concentrations are absorbed with greater speed than less soluble and concentrated drugs.

Diseases and symptoms: conditions such as diabetes mellitus and hypokalemia can increase the absorption of drugs, whereas pain and mucosal edema will slow absorption.

Although nurses cannot change many of the underlying factors responsible for altered drug absorption, they can use measures to maximize the absorption of drugs. Exercise will stimulate circulation and should be encouraged. Massage and heat likewise will increase blood flow at the absorption site. Prevention of fluid volume deficit, hypothermia, and hypotension is beneficial in facilitating absorption. Preparations that neutralize gastric secretions should be avoided if a low gastric *p*H is required for drug absorption. Drug–drug

and drug–food interactions should be monitored (Table 35-2). Consideration should be given to using the most effective administration route for the drug.

Distribution

Although it is difficult to predict with certainty how drug distribution will differ among older adults, it is known that changes in circulation, membrane permeability, body temperature, and tissue structure can modify this process. For example, adipose tissue increases compared to lean body mass in the elderly, and occurs to a greater extent in women; drugs stored in adipose tissue (*i.e.,* lipid-soluble drugs) will have increased tissue concentrations, decreased plasma concentrations, and a longer duration in the body. Decreased cardiac output can raise the plasma levels of drugs while reducing their deposition in reservoirs; this is particularly apparent with water-soluble drugs. Reduced serum albumin levels can be problematic if several protein-bound drugs are consumed and

Table 35-1 Interactions Among Popular Drug Groups

	ANTACIDS	ANTIANXIETY	ANTICOAGULANTS	ANTIDIABETICS	ANTIDEPRESSANTS	ANTI-HYPERTENSIVES	ANTI-INFLAMMATORY	ANTIPSYCHOTICS	DIGITALIS PREPARATIONS	LAXATIVES	SALICYLATES	SEDATIVES	THIAZIDE DIURETICS	TRICYCLIC ANTIDEPRESSANTS
Antacids			↓			↓		↓						
Antianxiety			↑			↑								
Anticoagulants (oral)				↑										
Antidiabetics														
Antidepressants		↑	↑			↓						↑		
Antihypertensives				↑								↑	↑	
Anti-inflammatory			↑	↑										
Antipsychotic												↑		
Digitalis preparations														
Laxatives									↓					
Salicylates														
Sedatives			↑											
Thiazide diuretics				↓	↑						↓			
Tricyclic antidepressants		↑	↑			↓						↑		

Arrows indicate the effect of drugs listed in the left-hand column on those listed across the top.
Adapted from Eliopoulos C. Safe drug use in the elderly. In: Eliopoulos C, ed. Caring for the elderly in diverse care settings. Philadelphia: JB Lippincott, 1990: 90.

compete for the same protein molecules; the unbound drug concentrations will rise and the effectiveness of the drugs will be threatened. Highly protein-bound drugs include acetazolamide, amitriptyline, cefazolin, chlordiazepoxide, chlorpromazine, cloxacillin, digitoxin, furosemide, hydralazine, nortriptyline, phenylbutazone, phenytoin, propranolol, rifampin, salicylates, spironolactone, sulfisoxazole, and warfarin. When monitoring the blood levels of medications, it also is important to evaluate the serum albumin level; for instance, raising the dosage of phenytoin because the blood level is low can lead to toxicity if the serum albumin also is low.

Conditions such as dehydration and hypoalbuminemia decrease drug distribution and result in higher drug levels in the plasma. When these conditions exist, lower dosage levels may be necessary.

Table 35-2 *Examples of Food and Drug Interactions*

DRUG	POTENTIAL INTERACTIONS
Acetaminophen	Accumulation to toxic level if more than 500 mg vitamin C supplements are ingested daily
Allopurinol	Impairs iron absorption leading to iron deficiency anemia Combined with alcohol or simple carbohydrates can increase blood uric acid level
Aluminum antacids	Depletes phosphate and calcium Decreases absorption of vitamins A, C, and D, and magnesium, thiamine, folacin, and iron
Antihistamines	Ingestion of large amounts of alkaline foods (*e.g.,* milk, cream, almonds, alcohol) can prolong action
Aspirin	Can cause iron deficiency anemia as a result of gastrointestinal bleeding Causes vitamin C deficiency (12 + aspirin tablets daily) Causes thiamine deficiency
Calcium carbonate antacids	Cause deficiencies of phosphate, folacin, iron, thiamine
Calcium supplements	Combined with large doses of vitamin D can cause hypercalcemia Absorption decreased by foods rich in oxalate (*e.g.,* spinach, rhubarb, celery, peanuts), phytic acid (*e.g.,* oatmeal and other grain cereals), phosphorous (chocolate, dried beans, dried fruit, peanut butter)
Chlorpromazine HCl	Large amounts of alkaline foods can delay excretion Can increase blood cholesterol
Cimetidine	Reduces iron absorption
Clonidine HCl	Effectiveness reduced by tyramine-rich foods (*e.g.,* chicken and beef livers, bananas, sour cream, meat tenderizers, salami, yeast, chocolate) Can cause sodium and fluid retention
Colchicine	Effectiveness decreased by caffeine Some herbal teas contain phenylbutazone, which can increase blood uric acid and decrease effectiveness of antigout drugs
Dicumarol	Effectiveness reduced by foods rich in vitamin K (*e.g.,* cabbage, broccoli, asparagus, spinach, turnip greens)
Digitalis	Can cause deficiencies of thiamine, magnesium, and zinc Calcium supplements increase risk of toxicity
Estrogen	Hastens breakdown of vitamin C
Ferrous supplements	Absorption decreased by antacids, increased by vitamin C
Furosemide	Increases excretion of calcium, magnesium, potassium, and zinc
Hydralazine	Can cause vitamin B_6 deficiency
Levodopa	Effectiveness reduced by high-protein diet Can cause deficiencies of potassium, folacin, and vitamins B_6 and B_{12}
Magnesium antacids	Can deplete phosphate and calcium
Magnesium-based laxatives	30 ml contains nearly four times the average daily intake of magnesium; toxicity can result
Mineral oil	Decreases absorption of vitamins A, D, and K
Phenobarbital	Increases breakdown of vitamins D and K Impairs absorption of vitamins B_6 and B_{12} and folic acid

Table 35-2 *Examples of Food and Drug Interactions (Continued)*

DRUG	POTENTIAL INTERACTIONS
Phenylbutazone	Inhibits absorption of iodine
Phenytoin	Increases breakdown of vitamins D and K Reduces absorption of folacin
Potassium supplements	Absorption decreased by dairy products Impairs absorption of vitamin B_{12}
Probenecid	Effectiveness decreased by coffee, tea, or cola
Spironolactone	Increases excretion of calcium Decreases excretion of potassium leading to potassium toxicity
Theophylline	Effectiveness reduced by high-carbohydrate diet
Thiazides	Increases excretion of calcium, potassium, magnesium, zinc Can decrease blood glucose level
Thioridazine	Excretion delayed by high-alkaline diet
Warfarin	Effectiveness reduced by large amounts of vitamin K in diet

From Eliopoulos C. Safe drug use in the elderly. In: Eliopoulos C, ed. Caring for the elderly in diverse care settings. Philadelphia: JB Lippincott, 1990: 94.

Metabolism, Detoxification, and Excretion

The renal system is primarily responsible for the body's excretory functions, and among its activities is the excretion of drugs. Drugs follow a path through the kidneys similar to that of most constituents of urine. After systemic circulation, the drug filters through the walls of glomerular capillaries into the Bowman capsule. The drug continues down the tubule, where substances beneficial to the body will be reabsorbed into the bloodstream through proximal convoluted tubules and where waste substances excreted through the urine will flow into the pelvis of the kidney. Capillaries surrounding the tubules reabsorb the filtered blood and join to form the renal vein. It is estimated that almost 10 times more blood circulates through the kidneys than through similarly sized body organs to promote this filtration process.

The reduced efficiency of body organs with advanced age affects the kidneys as well, complicating drug excretion in the elderly. Nephron units are decreased in number, and as much as 64% of the nephrons can be nonfunctional in older individuals. The glomerular filtration rate is reduced by 46% between 20 and 90 years of age, along with a reduction in tubular reabsorption. Decreasing cardiac function contributes to the almost 50% reduction in blood flow to the kidneys. The implications of reduced kidney efficiency are important. Drugs are not as quickly filtered from the bloodstream and are present in the body longer. The biological half-life, or the time necessary for one-half of the drug to be excreted, can increase as much as 40%. These factors lead to a risk of adverse drug reactions.

The liver also has many important functions that influence drug detoxification and excretion. Carbohydrate metabolism in the liver converts glucose into glycogen and releases it into the bloodstream when needed. Protein metabolism in the parenchymal cells of the liver is responsible for the loss of the amine groups from amino acids, which aid in the formation of new plasma proteins, such as prothrombin and fibrinogen, as well as in the conversion of some poisonous nitrogenous by-products into nontoxic substances such as vitamin B_{12}. Also important is the liver's formation of bile, which serves to break down fats through enzymatic action and to remove substances such as bilirubin from the blood. Although no significant

effects have been reported, the liver's decrease in size and function with age could interfere with the formation of certain necessary body substances such as prothrombin; albumin; and vitamins A, D, and B$_{12}$.

Certain enzymes may not be secreted, which interferes with the metabolism of drugs that require enzymatic activity. Most importantly, the detoxification and conjugation of drugs may be significantly reduced, so that the drug stays in the bloodstream longer. Some evidence indicates larger drug concentrations at administration sites in older persons.

Conditions such as dehydration, hyperthermia, immobility, and liver disease can decrease the metabolism of drugs. As a consequence, drugs can accumulate to toxic levels and cause serious adverse reactions. Careful monitoring is essential. Along this line, the extended biological half-life of many of the drugs consumed by the elderly warrants close evaluation of drug clearance. Estimated creatinine clearance must be calculated based on the age, weight, and serum creatinine level of the individual because serum creatinine levels alone may not reflect a reduced creatinine clearance level.

Pharmacodynamics

Information on pharmacodynamics in the older population is limited and will grow as increased research is done in this area. At this point, some of the differences in older adults' response to drugs include the increased myocardial sensitivity to anesthesias and increased central nervous system receptor sensitivity to narcotics, alcohol, and bromides.

Adverse Reactions

The risk of adverse reactions to drugs is high in the elderly. The following are some general factors to remember in regard to adverse reactions:

   The signs and symptoms of an adverse reaction to a given drug may differ in older persons.

   A prolonged time may be required for an adverse reaction to become apparent in older adults.

   An adverse reaction to a drug may be demonstrated even after the drug has been discontinued.

   Adverse reactions to a drug that has been used over a long period without problems can develop suddenly.

Varying degrees of mental dysfunction often are early symptoms of adverse reactions to commonly prescribed medications for the elderly such as codeine, digitalis, methyldopa, phenobarbital, L-dopa, valium, and various diuretics. Any medication that can promote hypoglycemia, acidosis, fluid and electrolyte imbalances, temperature elevations, increased intracranial pressure, and reduced cerebral circulation also can produce mental disturbances. Even the most subtle changes in mental status could be linked to a medication and should be reviewed with the physician. The elderly easily may become victims of drug-induced mental illness. Unfortunately, mental and behavioral dysfunction in the elderly is sometimes treated symptomatically (*i.e.*, with medications but without full exploration of the etiology). This will not correct a drug-related problem, and it can predispose the individual to additional complications from the new drug.

Promoting Safe Drug Use

The scope of drug use and significant adverse reactions that can result necessitate that gerontological nurses ensure drugs are used selectively and cautiously. Nurses should review all prescription and nonprescription medications used by patients and ask themselves the following questions:

   Why is the drug ordered? Consider whether the drug is really needed. Perhaps warm milk and a back rub could eliminate the need for the sedative; maybe the patient had a bowel movement this morning and now does not need the laxative. Perhaps the medication is prescribed because it has been prescribed for years and no one has thought to have it discontinued.

   Is the smallest possible dose ordered? The elderly usually require lower dosages of most medications because of the delayed time for excretion of the substance. Larger dosages increase the risk of adverse reactions.

   Is the patient allergic to the drug? Sometimes the physician may overlook a known allergy, or perhaps the patient neglected to share an allergy problem with the physician. The

nurse may be aware of a patient's sensitivities to certain drugs. Consideration must also be given to new signs that could indicate a reaction to a drug that has been used for a long period without trouble.

Can this drug interact with other drugs that are being used? It is useful to review resource material to identify potential interactions—they are too numerous for anyone to commit to memory!

Are there any special instructions that accompany the administration of the drug? Some drugs should be given on empty stomachs, others with meals. Some times of the day may be better for drugs to be given than others.

Is the drug prescribed for the most effective route of administration? A person who cannot swallow a large tablet may do better with a liquid form. Suppositories that are expelled due to ineffective melting or oral drugs that are lost due to vomiting obviously will not have the therapeutic effect of the drug given in a different manner.

Nurses must go through a mental checklist of these questions when administering medications and teach elderly who are responsible for their own medication administration, as well as their caregivers, to do the same.

The most common way to administer drugs is orally. Oral medications in the form of tablets, capsules, liquids, powders, elixirs, spirits, emulsions, mixtures, and magmas are used either for their direct action on the mucous membrane of the digestive tract (*e.g.*, antacids) or for their systemic effects (*e.g.*, antibiotics and tranquilizers). Although administration is simple, certain problems can interfere with the process. Dry mucous membranes of the oral cavity, common in older individuals, can prevent capsules and tablets from being swallowed. If they are then expelled from the mouth, there is no therapeutic value; if they dissolve in the mouth, they can irritate the mucous membrane. Proper oral hygiene, ample fluids for assistance with swallowing and mobility, proper positioning, and an examination of the oral cavity after administration will ensure the patient receives the full benefit of the medicine during its travel through the gastrointestinal system. Some elderly may not even be aware that a tablet is stuck to the roof of their dentures or under their tongue.

Because enteric-coated and sustained-release tablets should not be crushed, the nurse should consult with the physician for an alternate form of the drug if a tablet is too large to be swallowed. As a rule, capsules are not to be broken open and mixed. Medications are put into capsule form so that unpleasant tastes will be masked or the coating will dissolve when it comes into contact with specific gastrointestinal secretions. Breaking the capsule defies the purposes of using it; perhaps another form of the drug should be prescribed if the patient has a swallowing problem. Some vitamin, mineral, and electrolyte preparations are bitter, and even more so for older persons, whose taste buds for sweetness are lost long before those for sourness and bitterness. Combining the medication with foods and drinks such as applesauce and juices can make them more palatable and prevent gastric irritation, although there may be a problem if the full amount of food is not ingested. Individuals should be informed that the food or drink they are ingesting contains a medication. Oral hygiene after the administration of oral drugs will prevent an unpleasant aftertaste.

Drugs prescribed in suppository form for local or systemic action are inserted into various body cavities and act by melting from body heat or dissolving in body fluids. Because circulation to the lower bowel and vagina is decreased and the body temperature is lower in many older individuals, a prolonged period may be required for the suppository to melt. If no alternative route can be used and the suppository form must be given, a special effort must be made to ensure that the suppository is not expelled.

Intramuscular and subcutaneous administration of drugs is necessary when immediate results are sought or when other routes are not able to be used, either because of the nature of the drug or the status of the individual. The upper, outer quadrant of the buttocks is the best site for intramuscular injections. Frequently, the older person will bleed or ooze after the injection because of decreased tissue elasticity; a small pressure bandage may be helpful. Alternating the injection site will help to reduce discomfort. Medication should not be injected into an immobile limb because the inactivity of the limb will reduce the rate of absorption. A person receiving frequent injections should be checked for signs of infection at the injection site; reduced subcutaneous sensation in older per-

sons or absence of sensation, as that experienced with a stroke, may prevent the person from being aware of a complication at the injection site.

Occasionally, intravenous administration of drugs is essential. In addition to observing the effects of the medication, the nurse needs to be alert to the amount of fluid in which the drugs is administered. Declining cardiac and renal function make the elderly more susceptible not only to dehydration but also to overhydration. Signs of circulatory overload must be closely monitored, including elevated blood pressure, increased respirations, coughing, shortness of breath, and symptoms associated with pulmonary edema. Intake and output balance, body weight, and specific gravity are useful to monitor. Of course, patients should be observed for complications associated with intravenous therapy in any age group, for example, infiltration, air embolism, thrombophlebitis, and pyrogenic reactions. Decreased sensation may mask any of these potential complications, emphasizing the necessity for close nursing observation.

Because so many elderly are responsible for self-medication, nurses should promote self-care capacity in this area. A detailed description—verbal and written—should be given to the elderly and their caregivers, outlining the drug's name, dosage schedule, route of administration, action, special precautions, incompatible foods or drugs, and adverse reactions. A color-coded dosage schedule can be developed to assist persons who have visual deficits or who are illiterate. Medication labels with large print and caps that can be easily removed by weak or arthritic hands should be provided. During every patient–nurse visit, the patient's medication schedule should be reviewed and new symptoms explored. A variety of potential medication errors can be prevented or corrected by close monitoring. Some of the classic self-medication errors include incorrect dosage, noncompliance arising from misunderstanding, discontinuation or unnecessary continuation of drugs without medical advice, and using medications prescribed for previous illnesses.

Review of Selected Drugs

Some of the major drug groups used by older adults are reviewed in the remainder of this chapter. This review is not intended to be all-inclusive, but rather to be used as a highlight of some of the main concerns associated with selected drugs. Nurses are advised to obtain more complete information from pharmacology literature and pharmacologists.

——————— Analgesics ———————

Examples

Narcotics
  Alphaprodine
  Codeine
  Hydromorphone (Dilaudid)
  Meperidine (Demerol)
  Morphine
  Oxycodone (in Percodan and Tylox)
Non-narcotic
  Acetaminophen (Datril, Panadol, Tylenol)
  Salicylates (Aspirin)

Overview

The elderly are affected by many health problems that cause pain and discomfort to be common complaints. Nurses must not assume that because pain is a frequent occurrence that it is normal or should be taken lightly. Pain indicates that something is wrong; rather then merely treat the symptom of pain, it is more beneficial to identify the cause so that it can be eliminated or improved. For example, a low environmental temperature, awkward position, infection, constipation, or a fracture can each cause pain; more will be accomplished by providing warmth, repositioning, attacking the infection, facilitating bowel elimination, or aligning the bone than would be if the only intervention were to administer an analgesic. By asking about precipitating factors, intensity, duration, frequency, and what relieves the pain, the source of the problem may be identified. When pain is present, non-medication relief measures including massages, warm soaks, relaxation exercises, touch therapy, and position changes should be attempted first before analgesic administration. Administering a medication may be faster and easier, but it carries greater risks for older persons.

Aspirin remains one of the major drugs consumed by the elderly and is popular because of its relatively low cost and effectiveness as an analgesic, antipyretic, and anti-inflammatory agent. When used for arthritic conditions, aspirin re-

duces pain and swelling, which promotes joint mobility. Of the various side-effects of this drug, gastrointestinal bleeding is one of the most serious. Iron-deficiency anemia in older adults should suggest an assessment of aspirin consumption to explore the existence of gastrointestinal hemorrhage. Using buffered or enteric-coated aspirin preparations and avoiding aspirin ingestion on an empty stomach are helpful measures in preventing gastrointestinal irritation and bleeding. Because older people are likely to prescribe and take aspirin on their own, they should be taught to avoid excessive dosages. This can happen subtly as the 2 aspirin tablets taken every 4 hours gradually get increased to 3 tablets every 4 hours and then 3 tablets every 2 to 3 hours. It can be easily missed during assessment if the nurse asks "Are you still taking your aspirin?" instead of exploring the issue through asking "Tell me how many aspirins you take at what times." Because a tolerance for aspirin can develop, the continued effectiveness of the drug must be evaluated, and the patient must be advised not to increase the dosage without consulting the physician.

Occasionally, disturbances of the central nervous system develop when persons with decreased renal function use salicylates. Because renal function may be reduced in some older persons, the patient should be observed for symptoms of central nervous system problems, including changes in mental status (most commonly confusion), dizziness, tinnitus, and deafness. Acetaminophen, a nonsalicylate antipyretic and analgesic with a low incidence of adverse reactions, may be used instead to bring relief.

Codeine is sometimes prescribed as a mild analgesic. Two effects of this drug are significant for the elderly. First, codeine therapy may result in drowsiness, predisposing the elderly to accidents. Elderly people should be cautioned about this effect and advised against driving, climbing a ladder, or engaging in any other activity that could pose a risk. Second, constipation sometimes results from codeine use. Because of reduced peristalsis and an often limited intake of bulk foods, constipation is already a common problem for the elderly; thus, the probability of constipation while on codeine therapy is high. The ingestion of fruit juices and bulk foods should be encouraged as a preventive measure, and bowel habits should be noted to detect constipation early.

Narcotic analgesics are prescribed for the relief of severe pain of short duration, such as that which may accompany postoperative periods, a myocardial infarction, or the terminal phase of an illness. Narcotics must be used with extreme caution in older adults. Morphine sulfate, an opium derivative used for the relief of severe pain, produces euphoria, mild disorientation, reduced peristalsis, slower respirations, increased sphincter muscle tone, and a slightly reduced heartbeat while increasing the force of the beat, in addition to its analgesic effect. Dulled sensations and depressed respirations compound the problems that elderly persons with these functions already possess. It is believed that a lower dosage of morphine should be prescribed for the elderly to compensate for their more severe reaction to the drug's depressant effects; the recommendation is that persons in their 60s receive one-half the usual adult dosage and that morphine use be avoided, if possible, in persons 70 years of age and older.

Meperidine is a narcotic analgesic for mild to severe pain and has actions similar to morphine but without the severe side-effects associated with morphine. Unlike morphine, meperidine does not produce deep sedation or respiratory depression, although these effects will be seen if the drug is administered with other central nervous system depressants. In the elderly especially, meperidine is known to cause hypotension, dizziness, nausea, and impaired mental and physical functioning.

Interactions

Aspirin can increase the effects of oral anticoagulants, oral antidiabetics, cortisonelike drugs, penicillins, and phenytoin.

Aspirin can decrease the effects of probenecid, spironolactone, and sulfinpyrazone.

Aspirin's effects can be increased by large doses of vitamin C and decreased by antacids, phenobarbital, propranolol, and reserpine.

Acetaminophen's effects can be decreased by phenobarbital.

Narcotic analgesics can increase the effects of antidepressants, sedatives, tranquilizers, and other analgesics.

The effects of narcotics can be increased by antidepressants and phenothiazines. Nitrates can increase the action of meperidine.

Meperidine can decrease the effects of eye drops used for the treatment of glaucoma.

Nursing Guidelines

If nonmedicinal means of pain relief are not effective and pharmacological intervention is required, begin with the weakest type and dose of analgesic and gradually increase if necessary.

Use narcotics discriminately in older persons. The administration of non-narcotic analgesics with the narcotic can decrease the amount of narcotic that is needed, thereby minimizing side-effects. Some of the side-effects to observe for include weakness, dizziness, fainting, confusion, decreased respirations, nausea, and vomiting.

Administer analgesics regularly to maintain a constant blood level.

Observe for signs of infection other than fever when the patient is taking aspirin or acetaminophen. The antipyretic effect of these drugs can mask fevers associated with infection.

Because bleeding and a slower clotting time can result from long-term aspirin use, observe for anemia, altered hemoglobin and prothrombin time, and other signs of bleeding.

Note signs of salicylate toxicity (e.g., dizziness, vomiting, tinnitus, hearing loss, sweating, fever, confusion, burning in mouth and throat, convulsions, and coma). The risk of aspirin toxicity is greater when the drug is taken with furosemide and para-aminosalicylic acid.

Aspirin can alter glycosuria readings; thus, urine testing may be unreliable for persons on long-term use.

Hypoglycemic reactions can be promoted when diabetic individuals combine aspirin with sulfonylureas.

———————— Antacids ————————

Examples

Aluminum carbonate gel (Basaljel)
Aluminum hydroxide gel (Amphojel)
Aluminum hydroxide and magnesium hydroxide (Maalox)
Aluminum hydroxide, magnesium hydroxide and simethicone (Di-Gel, Gelusil, Mylanta)
Aluminum phosphate gel (Phosphajel)
Calcium carbonate (Alka-2, Tums, Chooz)

Dihydroxyaluminum sodium carbonate (Rolaids)
Magaldrate (Riopan)
Magnesium hydroxide (Milk of Magnesia)
Sodium bicarbonate (Soda Mint, baking soda)
Sodium bicarbonate acetaminophen, citric acid (Bromo-Seltzer)

Overview

Decreased gastric acid secretion and increased intolerance to fatty and fried foods make indigestion a common problem in old age. It is important, however, that nurses assess the reason for antacid use. What patients believe to be indigestion actually could be gastric cancer or ulcer; also, cardiac disorders can present with atypical symptomatology that resembles indigestion. Chronic antacid use could warrant the need for a diagnostic evaluation.

The easy availability and widespread use of antacids can cause some individuals to minimize the seriousness of these drugs. Antacids are drugs and they do interact with other medications. For example, aluminum hydroxide and sodium bicarbonate can decrease the absorption of tetracycline, sodium bicarbonate can increase the serum level of aspirin, and excess use of calcium-based antacids can increase the heart to the effects of digoxin and lead to digitalis toxicity.

Antacids can cause fluid and electrolyte imbalances, for instance, by promoting diarrhea (e.g., magnesium hydroxide combinations), hypernatremia (e.g., sodium bicarbonate), hypercalcemia (e.g., calcium carbonate), and metabolic acidosis (e.g., sodium bicarbonate). Prolonged use of calcium-based antacids can lead to renal problems. The serious outcomes of excess or prolonged use emphasize the importance of only using antacids for occasional relief.

Interactions

Aluminum hydroxide can increase the effects of meperidine and pseudoephedrine.

Magnesium hydroxide can increase the effects of dicumarol.

· Most antacids can decrease the effects of barbiturates, chlorpromazine, digoxin, iron preparations, isoniazid, nitrofurantoin, oral antico-

agulants, para-aminosalicylic acid, penicillins, phenytoin, phenylbutazone, salicylates, sulfonamides, tetracycline, and vitamins A and C.

Nursing Guidelines

Routinely ask patients about antacid use while collecting their medication history. Some patients do not consider antacids serious medications and may omit contributing information about their use.

Chronic use of antacids may be related to symptoms of a problem other than indigestion, such as gastric cancer, ulcer, or cardiac disease. Refer the patient for diagnostic evaluation as needed.

Avoid administering other medications within 2 hours of administration of an antacid, unless otherwise ordered, to prevent other drugs from having reduced absorption.

Monitor bowel elimination. Constipation can result from the use of aluminum hydroxide and calcium antacids; diarrhea can occur when magnesium hydroxide combinations are used.

Advise patients who are on sodium-restricted diets to avoid using sodium bicarbonate as an antacid.

Avoid combining the administration of calcium carbonate antacids with milk or vitamin-D–rich foods; this can cause hypercalcemia and gastric hypersecretion (i.e., acid rebound). Likewise, milk–alkali syndrome, demonstrated by nausea, vomiting, headache, delirium, can occur when calcium carbonate or sodium bicarbonate is administered with milk or foods rich in vitamin D.

————— Antianxiety Drugs —————

Examples

Benzodiazepines
  Chlordiazepoxide (Librium)
  Clorazepate dipotassium (Tranxene)
  Diazepam (Valium)
  Halazepam (Paxipam)
  Lorazepam (Ativan)
  Oxazepam (Serax)
  Prazepam (Centrax)

Barbiturates
  Amobarbital (Amytal)
  Mephobarbital (Mebaral)
  Phenobarbital

Overview

Financial concerns, deaths, crime, illness, and many of the other problems commonly faced by older adults give legitimate cause for anxiety. Financial aid, counseling, self-care instruction, and other interventions can yield better long-term effects in treating situational anxiety than a medication will alone, and the use of these measures may also prevent additional problems arising from drug therapy complications. When tranquilizers are required to control anxiety associated with neurosis or mild depression, they should be coupled with other therapeutic approaches. The longer biological half-life of these drugs necessitates that lower than normal adult doses be used to avoid accumulation and toxicity. Older adults are more prone to the side-effects of tranquilizers such as drowsiness, dizziness, confusion, slurred speech, constipation, unsteadiness, dry mouth, gastrointestinal upset, double vision, photosensitivity, impaired bladder control, and decreased resistance to infection. Antianxiety drugs are contraindicated in persons who have acute alcohol intoxication; myasthenia gravis; blood dyscrasias; acute narrow-angle glaucoma; and severe pulmonary, hepatic, or renal disease. Because tranquilizers can cause physical and psychological dependency, they should not be discontinued abruptly.

Interactions

Antianxiety drugs can increase the effects of anticonvulsants, antihypertensives, oral anticoagulants, and other central nervous system depressants.

The effects of antianxiety drugs can be increased by tricyclic antidepressants.

Nursing Guidelines

Ensure that nonpharmacological means of treating the anxiety have been attempted. Even if these measures once proved ineffective, the patient may be in a better position to benefit from treat-

ments after drug therapy is initiated, and they should be tried again.

Advise patients to change positions slowly and to avoid operating a car or machinery that requires mental alertness and fast reactions.

Incorporate foods in the diet to prevent constipation. Monitor bowel elimination to detect this potential side-effect early.

Note nutritional status, including periodic weight measurements, to ensure that food intake is not jeopardized by lethargy or gastrointestinal upset.

Consult with the physician to have the dose decreased or discontinued if incontinence develops.

Observe for fever, sore throat, cellulitis, or other signs of infection and arrange prompt treatment.

Store drug in tightly closed container, away from light.

Be aware that several days of administration may be necessary before clinical effects are seen and that effects will continue several days after the drug is discontinued.

Be alert for drug interactions.

Anti-infectives

Examples

Aminoglycosides (Garamycin, Kantrex)
Antituberculars (INH, Rifampin)
Cephalosporins
Penicillins
Sulfonamides
Tetracyclines

Overview

The treatment of infections in the elderly is more difficult and complicated and carries more risks than with younger adults. It takes more time for the elderly to respond to antibiotic therapy. Adverse reactions occur more frequently, and allergic reactions can develop even if the patient has taken the drug before without a problem. It is important that the nurse be familiar with the unique profile of each antibiotic and special factors associated with their use:

Oral ampicillin remains stable in the presence of gastric acid. The frequent use of antacids can change the acidity of gastric contents and reduce the drug's potency.

Gentamicin has a high potential for toxicity in the elderly and should be used with extreme caution, particularly in persons with impaired renal function.

The risk of ototoxicity from gentamicin therapy is compounded when potent diuretics are also being used because they contribute to ototoxicity as well.

Plasma prothrombin activity can be depressed during tetracycline therapy, necessitating an adjustment if anticoagulants are also being used.

Antituberculars carry a high risk for hepatotoxicity in older adults.

Hypokalemia may develop during carbenicillin therapy because of the drug's high sodium content.

Doxycycline will alter the results of Clinitest.

Kanamycin carries a high risk of nephrotoxicity and ototoxicity.

Nitrofurantoin therapy may cause the urine to become brown, which is of no significance, and create false glycosurias.

Sulfisoxazole can cause crystals to form in the urine unless it is taken with ample fluids; the urine may also become brown, which is not significant. Vitamin C deficiencies can occur during sulfisoxazole therapy but should not be treated until after therapy is discontinued because vitamin C can contribute to crystal formation in the urine.

Ampicillin, carbenicillin, erythromycin, and tetracycline should not be taken with meals.

Interactions

Penicillins are protein-bound drugs. When taken with other highly protein-bound drugs, the effects of penicillin can be reduced, and penicillin can, in turn, reduce the effects of other protein bound drugs.

The effects of ampicillin and carbenicillin can be decreased by antacids, chloramphenicol, erythromycin, and tetracycline.

The effects of doxycycline can be decreased by aluminum-, calcium-, or magnesium-based laxa-

tives; antacids; iron preparations; phenobarbital; and alcohol.

The effects of sulfisoxazole can be increased by aspirin, oxyphenbutazone, probenecid, sulfinpyrazone, and trimethoprim and decreased by paraldehyde and para-aminosalicylic acid. It can increase the effects of alcohol, oral anticoagulants, oral antidiabetic agents, methotrexate, and phenytoin.

Probenecid delays the excretion of most antibiotics, thereby increasing their effects.

Nursing Guidelines

Ensure that cultures are obtained before initiating therapy. Different antibiotics are effective for different infections.

Administer antibiotics regularly to maintain a constant blood level. Emphasize to patients that they should not skip doses. A medication chart or calendar may be used to assist older persons in remembering to administer their drugs, or whether they have already administered them.

Observe for signs of superinfections, which may develop from long-term antibiotic therapy.

Note any indication of adverse reactions. The reduced efficiency of kidneys in old age makes it easier for toxic doses to accumulate.

Anticoagulants

Examples

Coumarins (Dicumarol, Phenprocoumon, Warfarin)
Heparin

Overview

Anticoagulants are used with caution in the elderly because of the higher risk of bleeding in this age group. There is a greater possibility of producing a lowered prothrombin time in atherosclerotic individuals, many of whom are in the geriatric population. Absorption of these drugs can be slow and erratic in older persons. Some physicians discourage anticoagulant therapy in persons older than 70 years of age; others believe cautious use of these agents can be of great benefit to the elderly.

Heparin is usually prescribed for rapid anticoagulation, followed by coumarin for prolonged results. Heparin does not dissolve existing clots but inhibits the formation of clots by preventing the conversion of fibrinogen to fibrin. The same general principles applied to heparin therapy in the general population are also relevant to the elderly. Heparin is known to block the eosinophilic response to adrenocorticotropic hormone and insulin. Osteoporosis and spontaneous fractures are known to occur in persons who have used heparin for a long time. Older women need particularly close observation while on heparin therapy because they tend to be at greater risk of bleeding.

Warfarin also may be prescribed for anticoagulant therapy. It inhibits fibrin clotting but has no effect on established thrombus nor does it reverse tissue damage. It is highly protein-bound and difficult to prescribe in an accurate dose in the elderly. Receptor sensitivity is increased. Caution is necessary when this drug is administered in the presence of infectious disease, trauma, hypertension, and moderate to severe hepatic or renal insufficiency.

Interactions

Anticoagulants can increase the effects of phenytoin and hypoglycemic agents.

Anticoagulants can decrease the effects of cholestyramine.

The effects of anticoagulants can be increased by alcohol, amiodarone, broad-spectrum antibiotics, chloral hydrate, chlorpromazine, cimetidine clofibrate, colchicine, ethacrynic acid, mineral oil, phenylbutazone, phenytoin, probenecid, reserpine, salicylates, steroids, thyroxine, tolbutamide, and tricyclic antidepressants.

The effects of anticoagulants can be decreased by antacids, barbiturates, carbamazepine, chlorpromazine, cholestyramine, rifampin, and vitamins C and K.

Heparin's effects can be partially counteracted by digitalis, antihistamines, nicotine, and tetracyclines.

Nursing Guidelines

Administer the anticoagulant at the same time each day to maintain a constant blood level of

the drug. This should be reinforced in patients who are self-administering anticoagulants.

Ensure that older adults have appropriate dosage adjustments (*e.g.,* warfarin is usually started at one-half the normal adult dose in older persons).

Monitor prothrombin time carefully.

Promote a stable nutritional intake of vitamin K of about 300 μg/day. A deficiency of this vitamin increases the risk of bleeding, whereas large amounts can lower prothrombin time.

Keep vitamin K (*i.e.,* menadiol sodium diphosphate or phytonadione) readily available as an antidote whenever caring for patients on anticoagulant therapy.

Ensure that the patient receives nutritional instruction about foods that can interfere with the effectiveness of anticoagulants (*e.g.,* turnip greens, broccoli, cabbage, spinach, and liver).

Avoid aspirin use if possible; acetylsalicylic acid can interfere with platelet aggregation and cause bleeding. Three grams or more of salicylates are sufficient to result in hemorrhage, and this level could be reached by older persons taking aspirin for arthritic pain. Alternative analgesics should be explored.

Observe and instruct patients to observe closely for any indication of bleeding or hemorrhage, including headaches, dizziness, bleeding gums, bleeding wounds, hemoptysis, vomiting coffee-ground–like material, bloody or tarry stools, fatigue, fever, and chills.

Note fever. Higher doses of an anticoagulant may be required when the patient is febrile.

———— Anticonvulsants ————

Examples

Barbiturates (Amobarbital, phenobarbital, primidone)
Benzodiazepines (Clonazepam, Diazepam)
Hydantoins (Phenytoin, Mephenytoin)
Oxazolidinediones (Paramethadione, Trimethadione)
Succinimides (Methsuximide, Phensuximide)

Overview

Seizures in the elderly can result from a history of epilepsy, injury, hypoglycemia, infection, electro-lyte imbalance, or a drug reaction. Anticonvulsants are used, singularly or in combination, to sustain a blood level that will control seizures with the fewest adverse reactions. Older people have a higher risk of toxicity from these drugs, necessitating that they be used cautiously. Phenobarbital is not as popular in treating the elderly as it is with younger adults because it can cause emotional disturbance, delirium, disorientation, ataxia, and coma. Mysoline, of lesser toxicity, is the drug of choice for long-term anticonvulsant therapy in older adults. Dilantin is widely used to treat seizure disorders; a common side-effect of this drug is gingival hyperplasia, which can be minimized and controlled by regular, thorough oral hygiene. Other drugs, such as sulthiame and carbamazepine, may be used also.

Most oral anticonvulsants cause some degree of gastric irritation. Administering these drugs with food or immediately after a meal may reduce this problem. Alcohol also should be avoided during anticonvulsant therapy.

Interactions

Anticonvulsants can increase the effects of analgesics, antihistamines, propranolol, sedatives, and tranquilizers.

Anticonvulsants can decrease the effects of cortisone.

The effects of anticonvulsants can be increased by isoniazid.

Coumarin anticoagulants will decrease the effects of phenobarbital and increase the effects of mephenytoin and phenytoin.

Anticonvulsants and digitalis preparations taken concurrently significantly increase the risk of toxicity from both drugs.

Nursing Guidelines

Observe for side-effects, including the following:
Change in bowel habits (*e.g.,* diarrhea from phenobarbital, constipation from phenytoin)
Abnormal bruising, pallor, weakness, bleeding gums, jaundice, dark urine, and other signs of blood disorders
Muscle and joint pain, leg cramps
Nausea, vomiting, anorexia
Ataxia, dizziness, syncope

Blurred vision, diplopia

Decreased body temperature

Confusion, agitation, slurred speech, hallucinations

Arrhythmia

Hypotension

Sleep disturbances

Tinnitus

Urinary retention, glycosuria.

These signs should be reviewed with the physician to determine the need for a dosage reduction.

Promote exercise and activity to compensate for the depressed psychomotor activity caused by the anticonvulsant.

Ensure that periodic evaluations of the blood level of the drug are performed.

Antidepressants

Examples

Lithium carbonate

Lithium (Eskalith, Lithonate)

Monoamine oxidase inhibitors

Isocarboxazid (Marplan)

Phenelzine sulfate (Nardil)

Tranylcypromine (Parnate)

Tricyclic compounds

Amitriptyline HCl (Elavil, Amitril)

Amoxapine (Ascendin)

Desipramine HCl (Norpramin, Pertofrane)

Doxepin HCl (Adapin, Sinequan)

Fluoxetine (Prozac)

Imipramine pamoate (Trofanil-PM)

Maprotiline (Ludiomil)

Nortriptyline HCl (Aventyl)

Overview

The incidence of depression increases with age, making it the major mental-health problem treated in the elderly; therefore, antidepressants are widely used in geriatric practice. Tricyclic antidepressants are the drugs most preferred because they are safer than other antidepressants and have a good benefit-to-risk ratio. It is not uncommon for some sedation to occur during the first few days after therapy is initiated; it can take approximately 1 month before therapeutic effects are noted and mood is elevated. Antidepressants tend to be more effective in newly depressed rather than chronically depressed persons.

Interactions

Antidepressants can increase the effects of anticoagulants, atropinelike drugs, antihistamines, sedatives, tranquilizers, narcotics, and levodopa.

Antidepressants can decrease the effects of clonidine, phenytoin, and various antihypertensives.

The effects of antidepressants can be increased by alcohol and thiazide diuretics.

Nursing Guidelines

Evaluate possible causes of depression. Persons who have experienced retirement or death of a loved one should not be placed on antidepressants when other interventions may prove beneficial (e.g., widows' coping group, counseling, involvement in a local senior organization).

Use other therapies in addition to antidepressants; this will be particularly useful during the early stage of therapy before the drug's effects are present.

Ensure that the plasma level of the drug is monitored. Dosage adjustment may be required.

Observe for side-effects, including the following:

Dry mouth

Diaphoresis

Urinary retention

Indigestion

Constipation

Hypotension

Blurred vision

Drowsiness

Increased appetite, weight gain

Blurred vision, photosensitivity

Fluctuating blood glucose levels.

Administer the drug at bedtime, if possible, so that most of the uncomfortable side-effects can occur while the patient is sleeping.

Identify and monitor high-risk patients carefully, including persons with cardiac arrhythmias, glaucoma, and prostatic hypertrophy.

Be alert to anticholinergic symptoms (Display 35-1) when antidepressants are used. Amitriptyline, amoxapine, doxepin, imipramine, maprotiline and nortriptyline carry a moderate to strong risk for this side-effect.

DISPLAY 35-1 *Anticholinergic Symptoms*

Dry mouth
Constipation
Urinary retention
Blurred vision
Insomnia
Restlessness
Fever
Confusion
Disorientation
Short-term memory loss
Hallucinations
Agitation
Picking behaviors

——————— Antidiabetic Drugs ———————

Examples

Sulfonylureas
    Acetohexamide (Dimelor, Dymelor)
    Chlorpropamide (Chloronase, Diabinese)
    Tolazamide (Tolinase)
    Tolbutamide (Orinase, Tolbutone)
Second-generation sulfonylureas
    Glipizide (Glucotrol)
    Glyburide (DiaBeta)
Biguanides
    Metformin (Diabexyl)
Insulins
    Insulin globin zinc (PZI)
    Insulin injection (Crystalline zinc, Regular)
    Insulin isophane (Humulin-N, NPH)
    Insulin protamine zinc (Intermediate)
    Insulin zinc (Lente)
    Insulin zinc, extended (Ultralente)
    Insulin zinc, prompt (Semilente)

Overview

Perhaps more so than any other drug group, antidiabetic drugs require careful dosage adjustment based on the individual's weight, diet, and activity level. Oral antidiabetic agents are used when some endogenous insulin production still exists; tolbutamide is the drug of choice in these circumstances. Chlorpropamide has seven times the half-life of tolbutamide and is much more hazardous to the elderly. When insulin is necessary, small dosages are begun and then gradually increased until an effective level without adverse effects is obtained.

Hypoglycemia is a more probable and serious problem to older diabetic patients than ketosis. The classic signs of hypoglycemia are frequently absent in the elderly, and confusion and slurred speech may give the first clues.

Interactions

The effects of antidiabetic drugs can be increased by alcohol, oral anticoagulants, isoniazid, phenylbutazone, sulfinpyrazone, and large doses of salicylates.

The effects of antidiabetic drugs can be decreased by chlorpromazine, cortisonelike drugs, furosemide, phenytoin, thiazide diuretics, and thyroid preparations.

Nursing Guidelines

Teach diabetic persons and their caregivers about the proper use and storage of medications and recognition of hypoglycemia and hyperglycemia.

Ensure that diabetic persons wear an identifying device to alert others of their condition in the event they are found confused or unconscious.

Review the need for dosage adjustments of antidiabetic drugs when patients can have nothing by mouth or are altering their diet or activity pattern.

Examine injection sites regularly. Local redness, swelling, pain, and nodule development at the injection site can indicate insulin allergy. A sunken area at an injection site can be caused by atrophy and hypertrophy, a harmless although unattractive condition known as insulin lipodystrophy.

Chapter 23 provides more information on the management of diabetes in older adults.

——————— Antihypertensives ———————

Examples

α-Adrenergic blocking agents
    Phentolamine (Regitine)
    Prazosin (Hypovase, Minipress)
Antiadrenergic/adrenergic neuron-blocking agents

Guanethidine (Ismelin, Visutensil)
Reserpine (Eskaserp, Hydropres, Serpasil)
β-Adrenergic blocking agents
Metopropol (Betaloc, Lopressor)
Nadolol (Corgard, Corzide)
Propranolol (Inderal, Panadol)
Calcium channel blockers
Diltiazem (Cardizem)
Isradipine (DynaCirc)
Nicardipine (Cardene)
Nifedipine (Procardia, Adalat)
Central-acting α-adrenergic agonists
Clonidine (Catapres, Dixarit)
Methyldopa (Aldomet, Dopamet, Presinol)
Vasodilators
Diazoxide (Hyperstat, Proglycem)
Hydralazine (Apresoline, Lopress, Nor-press)

Overview

Good circulation becomes more difficult to achieve in later life because of reduced elasticity of peripheral vessels and the accumulation of deposits in the lumen of vessels. To compensate for increased peripheral resistance, systolic blood pressure may rise. Likewise, the diastolic blood pressure may rise in response to an age-related reduction in cardiac output. Higher blood pressures may be needed to meet the circulatory demands of older adults; lowering the blood pressure to normal levels for a younger adult population could prove harmful to the elderly. A careful evaluation is crucial before the diagnosis of hypertension is made, and then the benefits *versus* the risks of antihypertensive therapy must be considered. Because of the potential risks associated with antihypertensive drug therapy, other treatment measures should be tried first, such as dietary restriction of sodium, weight reduction, exercise, and relaxation techniques.

Thiazide diuretics frequently are the first pharmacological means of managing hypertension in the elderly (see Diuretics), and sometimes they are used effectively in combination with other medications. Reserpine is one such drug, which can be used with a diuretic or alone in the management of mild hypertension. In addition to lowering blood pressure, reserpine carries a high risk of causing serious depression in the elderly; nurses must be alert to the most subtle indications of this problem, closely noting any withdrawal, agitation,

lack of interest in activities or self-care, or new questions or conversations about death. It is not uncommon for this depression to continue for weeks after reserpine is discontinued. Obviously, reserpine is not recommended in persons with a history of depression. Other side-effects include confusion, nightmares, orthostatic hypotension, gastrointestinal bleeding, increased appetite, weight gain, decreased libido, and impotence.

Methyldopa may be prescribed for sustained moderate to severe hypertension. Hematocrit and hemoglobin levels should be evaluated frequently when this drug is used; hemolytic anemia may develop. The breakdown of methyldopa or its metabolites may cause urine to darken when exposed to air; it is helpful to prepare patients and their caregivers to expect this harmless condition. Close observation of individuals with angina pectoris is required because methyldopa can aggravate this problem. The elderly tend to experience a high incidence of hepatitis from methyldopa therapy. Reversible liver damage, depression, changes in cognition, edema, weight gain, and orthostatic hypotension are other potential side-effects from this drug. Tolerance to methyldopa can develop when it is used for several months, emphasizing the need to continually evaluate the effectiveness of the drug.

Propranolol and nadolol, β-adrenergic blocking agents, tend to produce fewer side-effects than other antihypertensives and are often prescribed for older adults with hypertension. Therapeutic effects of these drugs are usually noted within 1 week after therapy is initiated. They do not cause the postural hypotension and drowsiness that other antihypertensives do, although in some persons they can cause insomnia, nightmares, nausea, vomiting, diarrhea, fatigue, hallucinations, dizziness, and psychotic behaviors. Often, the extremities of persons taking these antihypertensive drugs will feel unusually cold as a result of reflex vasoconstriction caused by the drugs. Special care is required when using these drugs in diabetic patients because they are known to mask signs of hypoglycemia and increase sensitivity to tolbutamide. In patients with angina, the sudden discontinuation of these drugs can precipitate attacks, possibly leading to myocardial infarctions. These drugs can worsen congestive heart failure and bradycardia and may be contraindicated or used with extreme

caution in persons having those conditions. Absorption is increased when these drugs are administered on a full stomach; to maintain an even absorption rate, all doses should be taken in the same manner (*i.e.*, all with or all without meals but not inconsistently).

The long-acting forms of calcium channel blockers are becoming increasingly popular in the treatment of elderly hypertensive patients. Because they are vasodilators with a mild diuretic effect, they are beneficial for patients who have hypertension as a result of increased peripheral resistance, and, due to their peripheral and coronary vasodilating effects, are particularly beneficial for hypertensive individuals who also have angina, supraventricular tachycardia, claudication, or Raynaud disease. Calcium channel blockers are relatively safe, with the most common adverse effects being headaches, tachycardia, palpitations, flushing, ankle edema, and constipation. One of the main problems associated with this group of antihypertensive agents is the high cost, which can be several hundreds of dollars more than other agents.

Interactions

Antihypertensive drugs can increase the effects of barbiturates, insulin, oral antidiabetics, sedatives, and thiazide diuretics.

The effects of antihypertensives can be decreased by amphetamines, antihistamines, and tricyclic antidepressants.

The effects of propranolol can be increased by phenytoin, and propranolol can decrease the effects of antihistamines and anti-inflammatory drugs.

The use of β-blockers and verapamil can slow the heart rate.

Verapamil can increase the blood digoxin level.

Nifedipine can have increased effects from cimetidine.

Nursing Guidelines

Evaluate blood pressure carefully. Obtain readings with the patient in lying, sitting, and standing positions.

Advise patients to change positions slowly to avoid falls from the orthostatic hypotension that these drugs may cause.

Observe patients' reactions to therapy. Be aware of symptoms and level of function at various blood pressure levels.

Ensure that blood studies are done periodically to detect the potential reduction in white blood cells and platelets, which can occur during therapy.

Monitor mental status.

Prepare patients and caregivers for possible side-effects.

Reinforce the need to adhere to the antihypertensive therapy plan, even when symptoms are not present.

———— Anti-inflammatory Drugs ————

Examples

Antigout
   Allopurinol (Lopurin, Zyloprim)
   Colchicine (Colsalide)
   Probenecid (Benemid, Probalan)
   Sulfinpyrazone (Anturane)
Indole acetic acid derivatives
   Sulindac (Clinoril)
   Tolmetin (Tolectin)
Prednisone (Cortan, Deltasone)
Propionic acid derivatives
   Fenoprofen (Fenopron, Nalfon)
   Ibuprofen (Advil, Motrin, Nuprin)
Pyrazolones
   Oxyphenbutazone (Oxalid, oxybutazone, tandearil)
   Phenylbutazone (Azolid, Butazolidin, Phenbutazone)
Remittive agents
   Gold sodium thiomalate
   Penicillamine (Cuprimine, Depen Titratabs)
Salicylates
   Aspirin (Anacin, A.S.A., Bayer, Ecotrin, Zorprin)

Overview

Among the musculoskeletal problems in the elderly for which anti-inflammatory drugs are used, arthritic conditions are the most common. The salicylates (see Analgesics) are the most popularly chosen anti-inflammatory drugs. A growing number of other drugs that produce fewer gastrointes-

tinal side-effects are being used in the treatment of arthritis and other joint inflammations (e.g., fenoprofen, tolmetin). Fenoprofen is a phenylpropionic acid derivative that requires several weeks of therapy for effects to be noted. Drowsiness, dizziness, tinnitus, and blurred vision are potential side-effects, as is impaired coagulation due to fenoprofen's inhibitory effect on platelet aggregation. Tolmetin is an indomethacin derivative that has effects after the first week of therapy. Side-effects from this drug include hyperthermia, prolonged bleeding time, dizziness, visual disturbances, sodium retention, and reversible renal failure.

Gold salts are prescribed for the treatment of rheumatoid arthritis when salicylate therapy is not effective. These injections can take months for therapeutic effects to be noted. Often, patients receiving gold salts will complain of a metallic taste, which could indicate the side-effect of stomatitis. This drug also can cause thrombocytopenia, aplastic anemia, agranulocytosis, bradycardia, nephritis, hepatitis, corneal ulcers, and anaphylactic shock; close observation and regular evaluation of urine and blood samples are necessary. Dimercaprol is used to treat acute toxicity from gold salts and should be available when these injections are administered. Gold-salt therapy is contraindicated in persons with uncontrolled diabetes, serious hypertension, systemic lupus erythematosus, heart failure, and renal or liver disease.

In the treatment of gout, colchicine proves effective. It must be used cautiously in persons with cardiac, liver, renal, or gastrointestinal disease, and all persons taking colchicine should have regular complete blood counts. The elderly can experience an acute overdosage indicated by nausea, vomiting, diarrhea, anorexia, muscle weakness, peripheral neuritis, confusion, and convulsions.

Oxyphenbutazone and phenylbutazone are extremely potent drugs that are effective within days after therapy is started. They carry a high risk of adverse reactions, and persons taking these drugs must be monitored closely. Some of the problems associated with these drugs include sodium and fluid retention, confusion, hypertension, visual disturbances, hearing impairment, hepatitis, renal failure, respiratory alkalosis, metabolic acidosis, hemolytic anemia, bone marrow depression, and leukopenia. These drugs are contraindicated in persons with blood disorders; temporal arteritis; dementia; gastrointestinal ulcers; glaucoma; and

cardiac, renal, thyroid, or hepatic disease and those on anticoagulant therapy. Long-term therapy is discouraged.

For severe problems or when other drugs have proven ineffective, steroids may be prescribed. Steroids produce serious side-effects and must be used with caution in older adults. Dosage should be low and the drug should be discontinued as soon as possible. Steroids have profound metabolic effects; they modify the body's immune response. Resistance to infection may occur, and symptoms of infection may be masked. Sodium and fluid retention is common. Demineralization of the bones may result from steroid therapy, predisposing the older person to pathologic fractures. Patients with ocular herpes simplex who receive prednisone may experience corneal perforation; prolonged use of steroids can cause glaucoma, with possible damage to the optic nerve, and posterior subcapsular cataracts.

Interactions

Anti-inflammatory drugs can increase the effects of oral anticoagulants, insulin, oral antidiabetics, penicillins, and sulfa drugs.

Oxyphenbutazone can decrease the effects of antihistamines, barbiturates, and digitoxin.

Prednisone can increase the effects of sedatives and decrease the effects of coumarin anticoagulants, pilocarpine, insulin, and oral antidiabetic drugs. Aspirin and indomethacin can increase the effects of prednisone; some antihistamines, chloral hydrate, phenylbutazone, phenytoin, and propranolol can decrease the drug's effects.

Nursing Guidelines

These drugs have a narrowed therapeutic window and toxic levels accumulate much easier and at lower doses in older adults. Observe for side-effects closely and note gastrointestinal symptoms, hearing acuity, and indications of central nervous system disturbances.

Ensure that blood evaluations are performed regularly.

Administer oral anti-inflammatory agents with meals or a glass of milk—unless specifically contraindicated—to reduce gastrointestinal irritation.

———— Antipsychotics ————

Examples

Butyrophenones
  Haloperidol (Haldol)
Phenothiazines
  Acetophenazine (Tindal)
  Chlorpromazine (Thorazine)
  Fluphenazine (Prolixin)
  Loxapine (Loxitane)
  Mesoridazine (Serentil)
  Molindone (Moban)
  Perphenazine (Trilafon)
  Thioridazine (Mellaril)
  Thiothixene (Navane)
  Trifluoperazine (Stelazine)

Overview

Antipsychotics, or major tranquilizers, are widely used in the older population in the treatment of chronic schizophrenia, psychotic paranoid states, agitation, and manic–depressive disorders. The effectiveness of antipsychotics in controlling symptoms has proved useful in improving the quality of life and function of many individuals; however, their profound adverse effects necessitates careful prescription and close monitoring.

A thorough physical and mental health evaluation should be performed before using antipsychotics to derive an accurate understanding of the patient's problem. When possible, other interventions should be attempted prior to the use of antipsychotics, and certainly adjunct therapies should be considered during their use. Antipsychotics are to be used for the treatment of psychotic disorders and not as a means to manage problem behaviors (*i.e.*, chemically restrain patients). Symptoms of psychoses can develop in nonpsychotic patients who are given these drugs.

The elderly are more sensitive to the anticholinergic effects of antipsychotic medications (see Display 35-1); chlorpromazine and thioridazine are particularly problematic in this regard. The risk of injury is high in the elderly who use antipsychotic drugs because of the hypotensive and sedative effects that commonly occur.

Interactions

The effects of antipsychotics can be reduced by anticholinergics and antacids.

DISPLAY 35-2   Extrapyramidal Symptoms

Tardive dyskinesia

Thrusting movements of tongue
Lip smacking, puckering, or chewing movements
Abnormal limb movements

Parkinsonism

Tremors
Postural unsteadiness
Rigidity of muscles in limbs, neck, trunk
Pill-rolling motion with fingers
Shuffling gait

Akinesia

Decrease in spontaneous movements

Dystonia

Holding neck or trunk in rigid, unnatural position

Antipsychotics can increase the effects of sedatives and decrease the effects of levodopa.

Nursing Guidelines

Antipsychotic medications have a longer biological half-life in the elderly; therefore, the smallest possible dosage should be prescribed and gradually increased if necessary. The longer half-life increases the risk of adverse reactions.

A high therapeutic index can cause these drugs to have unpredictable and varying effects among patients. Close monitoring is necessary. During therapy, it can be beneficial to maintain a flow sheet on which behaviors and side-effects can be documented. The response to therapy should be monitored; if one drug is ineffective, another antipsychotic may prove more useful. Night administration is advised so that the sedative and other effects of these drugs can occur as patients sleep.

Nurses should be aware of the anticholinergic and extrapyramidal symptoms associated with these drugs and promptly report these symptoms to the physician (see Display 35-1; Display 35-2 and Table 35-3).

During the initial weeks of therapy, antipsychotics

Table 35-3 Commonly Prescribed Psychotropics and Related Side-Effects

GENERIC NAME	BRAND NAME	SEDATION	HYPOTENSION	ANTICHO-LINERGIC SYMPTOMS	EXTRAPYRA-MIDAL SYMPTOMS
Acetophenazine	Tindal	Mild	Mild	Moderate	Mild
Chlorpromazine	Thorazine	Marked	Marked	Marked	Mild
Fluphenazine	Prolixin	Mild	Mild	Mild	Marked
Haloperidol	Haldol	Minimal	Minimal	Mild	Marked
Loxapine	Loxitane	Mild	Mild	Moderate	Moderate
Mesoridazine	Serentil	Marked	Moderate	Mild	Minimal
Molindone	Moban	Mild	Mild	Moderate	Moderate
Perphenazine	Trilafon	Mild	Mild	Moderate	Moderate
Thioridizine	Mellaril	Marked	Marked	Marked	Mild
Thiothixene	Navane	Mild	Mild	Mild	Marked
Trifluoperazine	Stelazine	Mild	Mild	Mild	Marked

From Eliopoulos C. Resident assessment handbook. Glen Arm, MD: Health Education Network, 1991: 77.

can cause severe sedation and orthostatic hypotension that increase patients' risk of falls. Close supervision and protection from falls are important nursing measures.

Constipation can be a side-effect that can lead to serious complications, such as bowel obstruction. Patients' bowel elimination should be monitored, and fiber should be included in the diet.

Urinary retention and hesitancy can occur in older men with prostatic hypertrophy when they use antipsychotics. Patients should be instructed to monitor urinary symptoms and promptly report problems.

Drug holidays from antipsychotics are recommended.

Gradual weaning rather than abrupt withdrawal from antipsychotics is recommended.

Digitalis Preparations

Examples

Digitoxin (Cardigin, Crystodigin, Purodigin)
Digoxin (Lanoxin, Natigoxine, Winoxin)

Overview

Digitalis preparations are used in the treatment of congestive heart failure, atrial flutter and fibrillation, supraventricular tachycardia, and extrasystoles to increase the force of myocardial contraction through direct action on the heart muscle. The resulting improvement in circulation helps to reduce edema as well. These drugs are absorbed from the intestinal tract within 2 hours after administration, reaching their peak in 1 to 12 hours. The most popularly used drug in this group is digoxin. The biological half-life of digoxin is normally 34 hours but may extend to 45 hours in the elderly; therefore, the elderly require a lower dose of the drug and have a greater risk of adverse reactions. Toxicity to digitalis preparations is a serious threat, requiring prompt recognition and correction. Signs of toxicity are shown in Display 35-3.

DISPLAY 35-3   Indications of Digitalis Toxicity

Anorexia, nausea, vomiting, abdominal pain, diarrhea (most common symptoms)

Delirium, memory loss, personality changes, agitation, hallucinations

Impaired color vision, blurred vision, scotomas, seeing green or yellow halos around lights

Headache

Restlessness, insomnia, nightmares

Dizziness

Aphasia, ataxia, seizures

Muscle weakness and pain

Bradycardia, extrasystoles, cardiac arrhythmias

High serum drug levels: >2 ng/ml digoxin, > 30 ng/ml digitoxin (although toxicity can occur in presence of normal serum levels)

Hypokalemia will make patients more susceptible to toxicity. Digitalis is less effective in persons who have anemia, rheumatic carditis, subacute bacterial endocarditis, and hypocalcemia and those on antibiotic therapy.

Interactions

The effects of digitalis preparations can be increased by guanethidine, phenytoin, propranolol, and quinidine.

The effects of digitalis preparations can be decreased by antacids, cholestyramine, colestysol, kaolin-pectin, laxatives, neomycin, phenobarbital, phenylbutazone, and rifampin.

The risk of toxicity is increased when digitalis preparations are taken with cortisone, diuretics, parenteral calcium, reserpine, and thyroid preparations.

Nursing Guidelines

Check apical–radial pulse for rate, rhythm, and regularity before administering digitalis preparations.

Instruct patients and caregivers in taking pulse and in identifying adverse reactions and interactions.

Encourage a good intake of potassium-rich food. Ensure that serum potassium is evaluated regularly and that hypokalemia is corrected early.

Ensure that a baseline electrocardiogram, pulse, blood pressure, serum creatinine, electrolytes, and blood urea nitrogen are obtained and evaluated regularly.

Obtain prompt medical attention for indications of toxicity. The drug should be discontinued until an evaluation is done.

Instruct patients and caregivers that various forms of digitalis are not interchangeable.

Store the drug in a tightly closed container, away from light.

Diuretics

Examples

Benzothiadiazines or thiazides
  Bendroflumethiazide (Aprinox, Centyl, Naturetin)
  Chlorothiazide (Diupres, Diuril, SK-Chlorothiazide)
  Chlorthalidone (Hygroton, Igroton, Uridon)
  Hydrochlorothiazide (Esidrix, Hydrodiuril, Unipres)
  Quiethazone (Aquamox, Hydromox)
Loop
  Ethacrynic acid (Edecrin, Hydromedin, Taladren)
  Furosemide (Lasix, Neo-Renal, Uritol)
Potassium-sparing
  Amiloride (Midamor, Maduretic)
  Spironolactone (Aldactone)
  Triamterene (Dyrenium, Dytac)
Quinazolines
  Metolazone (Diulo, Zaroxolyn)

Overview

Diuretics are used in the treatment of a variety of cardiovascular disorders such as hypertension and congestive heart failure. They act to reduce body fluid in the following ways:

Thiazide diuretics inhibit sodium reabsorption in the cortical diluting site of the ascending loop of Henle and increase the excretion of chloride and potassium.

Loop diuretics inhibit reabsorption of sodium and chloride at the proximal portion of the ascending loop of Henle.

Spironolactone, known as a potassium-sparing diuretic, antagonizes aldosterone in the distal tubule, which causes water and sodium, but not potassium, to be excreted.

Under normal circumstances, older adults are at greater risk of developing fluid and electrolyte imbalances; diuretic therapy increases this risk considerably. Special attention must be paid to recognizing signs of imbalances early and correcting the problem promptly. Signs to recognize include dryness of the oral cavity, confusion, thirst, weakness, lethargy, drowsiness, restlessness, muscle cramps, muscular fatigue, hypotension, oliguria, nausea, vomiting, slow pulse rate, and gastrointestinal disturbances. Hypokalemia can sensitize the heart to the toxic effects of digitalis; thus, potassium depletion can be a serious problem when both digitalis and diuretics are being used. Thiazide diuretics may increase blood glucose levels, which may alter insulin requirements for diabetic persons on diuretics. Latent diabetes mellitus sometimes is manifested during thiazide therapy. Loop diuretics can cause transient ototoxicity; vertigo

and tinnitus associated with this adverse reaction can be masked by antihistamines and phenothiazines. Other side-effects associated with diuretics include headache, orthostatic hypotension, diarrhea, photosensitivity, aplastic anemia, agranulocytosis, leukopenia, thrombocytopenia, and tinnitus.

Interactions

Diuretics can increase the effects of antihypertensives.

Diuretics can decrease the effects of allopurinol, digitalis preparations, oral anticoagulants, oral antidiabetics, insulin, and probenecid.

The effects of diuretics can be increased by analgesics and barbiturates.

The effects of diuretics can be decreased by cholestyramine and large quantities of aspirin. Administer these drugs at least 1 hour before a diuretic.

Nursing Guidelines

Plan administration times in accordance with the individual's schedule (e.g., do not administer the diuretic one-half hour before the person is to leave for a long bus trip). Morning administration is usually preferable.

Monitor intake and output, and ensure that adequate fluids are ingested. Fluid intake should not be restricted during diuretic therapy.

Observe for side-effects.

Ensure that serum electrolytes, glucose, and blood urea nitrogen are evaluated periodically.

--- Laxatives ---

Examples

Bulk-forming
  Bran
  Methylcellulose (Cologel, Hydrolose)
Lubricants and stool softeners
  Docusate sodium (Colace, Dual Formula Feen-A-Mint)
  Mineral oil (Agoral, Haley-s M-O)
Saline
  Magnesium hydroxide (Milk of Magnesia)
  Magnesium sulfate (Epsom Salt, Mag-S)
Stimulant and irritant
  Bisacodyl (Dulcolax)
  Cascara sagrada (Amlax, Biolax)

Castor oil (Alphamul, Ricifruit)
  Glycerin (Agoral, Glyrol)
Miscellaneous
  Senna (Senokot)

Overview

A reduction in peristalsis, activity, and bulk and fluids in the diet are among the causes of constipation in the elderly. In addition, many elderly believe that a daily bowel movement is essential; as such, it is easy to understand why laxatives are so widely used, and abused, in the older population. Measures to promote elimination without the use of laxatives should be implemented before resorting to the use of medications. When laxatives are necessary, they should be selectively chosen and used. Various types of laxatives can be used, and include the following:

Bulk formers (e.g., methylcellulose) absorb fluid in intestines and create extra bulk, which distends intestines and increases peristalsis. These compounds should not be used when there is any indication of intestinal obstruction. They usually take effect in 12 to 24 hours. Bulk formers should be mixed with large amounts of water.

Stool softeners (e.g., docusate sodium) collect fluid in the stool, which makes the mass softer and easier to move. These products do not affect peristalsis. They take effect in 24 to 48 hours.

Hyperosmolars (e.g., glycerin) pull fluid into the colon, causing bowel distention, which increases peristalsis. They take effect in 1 to 3 hours. They are contraindicated with fecal impaction.

Stimulants (e.g., cascara sagrada) irritate the smooth muscle of the intestines and pull fluid into colon, which causes peristalsis. They take effect in 6 to 10 hours. Stimulants can cause intestinal cramps and excessive fluid evacuation.

Lubricants (e.g., mineral oil) coat fecal material, which facilitates its passage. They take effect in 6 to 8 hours. These compounds are not recommended for use by the elderly.

Interactions

Laxatives can reduce the effectiveness of oral medications by increasing the speed of their passage through the gastrointestinal system.

Chronic use of mineral oil can decrease the effectiveness of fat-soluble vitamins (vitamins A, D, K, E) and substances.

Nursing Guidelines

Prevent development of constipation.

Validate complaints of constipation.

Promote bowel elimination with nonlaxative means first.

Select the laxative best suited to the reason for the constipation and monitor its effectiveness.

Educate the elderly and their caregivers in the realities of constipation and preventive measures. Emphasize that a laxative is a drug and that its use should be weighed, as one would weigh the use of any drug.

Nitrates

Examples

Amyl nitrate

Nitroglycerin (Angised, Cardabid, Nitro-Bid, Nitro-Dur, Nitrobon, Nitrodisc, Nitrol, Nitrospan, Nitrostat, Susadrin, Transderm-Nitro, Tridil)

Overview

Nitroglycerin and the long-acting organic nitrates are prescribed for acute angina pectoris episodes in persons with coronary insufficiency, coronary heart disease, coronary occlusion, and subacute myocardial infarction. These drugs relax vascular smooth muscle, causing vasodilation, which decreases venous return and cardiac output. Antianginals come in a variety of forms, and patients should be thoroughly instructed in the correct administration and precautions associated with each type.

Interactions

Nitrates can increase the effects of atropinelike drugs and tricyclic antidepressants.

Nitrates can decrease the effects of cholinelike drugs (*e.g.*, neostigmine [Prostigmin]).

The hypotensive effects of nitrates can be increased by alcohol and propranolol.

Nursing Guidelines

Know and teach patients the proper use of the nitrate prescribed.

Amyl nitrate comes in vapor form and is rapid act-ing, with effects noted in less than 1 minute. This drug comes in ampule form, which is crushed in a gauze pad or cloth and inhaled. It is not unusual for weakness and dizziness to occur after inhalation, so the individual should be sitting during administration to prevent a fall. The effects last approximately 8 minutes. The ampule is flammable, so it should not be used near fire or cigarettes.

Sublingual nitroglycerin has a rapid effect that lasts 20 minutes or less. It is important that the older person understand that the tablet be placed under the tongue and not swallowed. Because the drier mucous membrane of the oral cavity of older adults can interfere with absorption, the elderly should be advised to take a few seconds to accumulate saliva. Normally, there will be a burning sensation from the tablet; the lack of this sensation can indicate that the drug has lost its potency. If no improvement is noted within several minutes, the dosage can be repeated in 5 to 15 minutes; if three doses do not bring relief, medical attention is warranted. Nitroglycerin should be used only when necessary because tolerance to the drug can develop. The tablets should be stored in a closed dark container, away from heat, and not used if over 6 months old because potency is reduced over time.

It is wise to instruct the patient to use a nitroglycerin tablet to prevent attacks by taking the drug several minutes before engaging in an activity known to precipitate an attack.

Timed-release nitroglycerin capsules should be administered at least 1 hour before or 2 hours after meals, but not with them. The effects of the capsules usually last 8 to 12 hours.

Nitroglycerin ointment is absorbed through the skin and takes effect within 30 minutes. It continues to be absorbed for approximately 4 hours; the patch should not be disturbed during that time. Absorption will be best if the ointment is applied to a hairless area of the body. After the patch is removed, all residual ointment should be thoroughly removed. Sites of application should be rotated.

Nitroglycerin patches are popular because they can be applied once daily. The practice had been to apply and leave in place for 24 hours. New research has shown, however, that the patches work best when worn for 12 to 14 hours

during the day and removed at bedtime. By removing the patch the patient can avoid developing a tolerance.(Newswatch, 1990)

Advise patients to sit or lie down for a short period following the administration of a nitrate to avoid falls caused by the dizziness, orthostatic hypotension, flushing, and cranial throbbing that often occur.

Because a tolerance to these drugs can develop, regular assessment of the ongoing effectiveness of antianginals is important. This also supports the need to use nitroglycerin only when absolutely necessary.

Nitrates can cause an increase in intraocular pressure, a serious concern with individuals who have glaucoma. If this condition exists, discuss the implications with the physician and monitor the patient closely.

Observe for signs of adverse reactions, such as irregular and rapid pulse, hypotension, decreased respirations, blurred vision, muscular weakness, and mental confusion.

——————— Sedatives, Hypnotics ———————

Examples

Chloral hydrate (Chloralex, Somnos)
Ethchlorvynol (Placidyl, Serensil)
Flurazepam (Dalmane, Novoflupam)

Overview

Hypnotics and sedatives often are prescribed for older persons for the treatment of insomnia, nocturnal restlessness, anxiety, acute confusional states, and related disorders. The dose prescribed will determine if the same drug will serve as a hypnotic or sedative. Unlike sedatives, hypnotics do not suppress mental activity, limit attention span, or diminish the ability to concentrate. Because a tolerance to sedatives can develop after several weeks of use, continued evaluation of their effectiveness is necessary. It is not unusual for restlessness, insomnia, and nightmares to occur after sedatives are discontinued. Many of these drugs produce hypotension, drowsiness, and impaired coordination, which can lead to injury.

Chloral hydrate and ethchlorvynol are among the more popular sedatives used in the elderly. They tend to produce less toxic and residual effects, to not modify REM sleep, and to be excreted more rapidly than other sedatives. Tolerance to and dependence on these drugs can develop with long-term use.

Barbiturates are not recommended for use with older persons due to the elderly's increased sensitivity to these drugs. Barbiturates are stored in adipose tissue, and the increased proportion of adipose tissue in the older adult's body can cause these drugs to accumulate and reach toxic levels. Because they are detoxified in the liver, they should be used cautiously if there is known impairment of liver function. Their depressant action warrants caution in use with persons with respiratory difficulties. Activities may need to be adjusted to compensate for the lower basal metabolic rate, blood pressure, and mental activity, that are typically experienced. Barbiturates reduce peristalsis; therefore, special attention must be directed to preventing constipation. The serious consequences of barbiturate use warrant that they be used discriminately.

Interactions

Hypnotics and sedatives can increase the effects of oral anticoagulants, antihistamines, and analgesics.

Hypnotics and sedatives can decrease the effects of cortisone and cortisonelike drugs.

The effects of hypnotics and sedatives can be increased by alcohol, antihistamines, and phenothiazines.

Nursing Guidelines

Investigate sleep problems thoroughly. Correcting a cold, warm, or uncomfortable position or noise problem may be all that is needed to promote sleep. Ask specifically about sleep pattern: some people who claim to have insomnia because they awaken at 4 A.M. each day may not have a sleep problem when it is considered that they sleep for 4 hours on the sofa before retiring to their bed at 11 P.M.

Use alternatives to drugs to promote relaxation and sleep, such as warm milk, back rubs, and music.

Encourage daytime activity to promote rest and sleep.

Observe daytime function. Note if the person is drowsy, mentally dull, or poorly coordinated.

Evaluate the quality and quantity of sleep. There is no reason to continue administering a sedative if the person is awake and active all night.

Reference

Newswatch. Don't wear your patch all day (and night). Geriatr Nurs 1990:11(6);112.

Recommended Readings

Farrell TA. Minimizing the systemic effects of glaucoma medications. Geriatrics 1991;46(5):61.

Ferrell BR, Ferrell BA. Easing the pain. Geriatr Nurs 1990;11(4):175.

Fong LN. Balancing anticoagulant therapy. Geriatr Nurs 1991;12(1):15.

Jeste DV, Krull AJ, Kilbourn K. Tardive dyskinesia: managing a common neuroleptic side effect. Geriatrics 1990;45(12):49.

Lipton HL, Lee PL. Drugs and the elderly: clinical, social and policy perspectives. Stanford, CA: Stanford University, 1988.

Lowenthal DT. Clinical pharmacology. In: Abrams WB, Berkow R, eds. The Merck manual of geriatrics. Rahway, NJ: Merck Sharp & Dohme Research Laboratories, 1990:181.

Maletta G, Mattox K, Dysken M. Guidelines for prescribing psychoactive drugs in the elderly, parts 1 and 2. Geriatrics 1991;46(9):40.

Miller C. When medication harms as well as helps. Geriatr Nurs 1990;11(6):301.

Todd B. Diuretics' dangers. Geriatr Nurs 1989; 10(4):212.

unit IV

Gerontological Care Issues

36

Coping With Chronic Illness

Illness is never an easy situation to accept. Even a common cold disrupts our lives and makes us uncomfortable, irritable, and unmotivated to work and play. When sick, our basic activities of daily living can become a chore, our appearance may be the least of our worries; and our lives may revolve around the medications, treatments, and doctor's visits that will make us feel better. Fortunately, for most people illness is an unusual and temporary event; we recover and return to life as usual. But some illnesses will accompany people for the remainder of their lives—the chronic diseases. Potentially every aspect of one's existence can be affected by chronic illness. The success to which a chronic disease is managed can make the difference between a satisfying life-style in which control of the illness is but one routine component and a life controlled by the demands of the illness.

Chronic Illness and the Elderly

Medical technology has helped more people survive illnesses that once would have killed them; greater numbers of people are reaching old age, when the incidence of chronic disease is higher. Thus, it should be no surprise that more than 80% of the elderly possess at least one chronic disease. In Chapter 1, Table 1-12 lists the rates of chronic illness for various age groups and shows the profound increase in the rate of most chronic illnesses with age. From that list, the major chronic problems for the elderly can be derived

(Table 36-1). Based on those rates, the following can be determined:

> Nearly one-half of the elderly suffer from arthritis.
> More than one-third of the elderly have hypertension.
> Nearly one-third of the elderly have a hearing impairment.
> More than one-fourth of the elderly have a heart condition.
> More than one of every eight elderly people has a visual impairment.
> Nearly another one in eight elderly people has a deformity or orthopedic impairment.
> Almost 10% of the elderly have diabetes.
> Hemorrhoids and varicose veins affect approximately 1 in 12 elderly people.

These are profound numbers, particularly considering the impact of these diseases on the individual elderly person who is affected. When some of the potential nursing diagnoses that can be associated with these major chronic conditions are considered (Table 36-2), the disruption to physical, emotional, and social well-being can be realized fully.

Chronic-Care Goals

Most health professionals were educated in the acute-care model, in which care activities focus on diagnosis, treatment, and cure of illness. Nursing

(Text continues on page 368)

Table 36-1 Major Chronic Problems of the Elderly (per 1000 Population)

PROBLEM	65–74 YEARS OF AGE	75+ YEARS OF AGE
Arthritis	463.6	511.9
Hypertension	392.4	337.0
Hearing impairment	264.7	348.0
Heart condition	284.7	322.2
Cataracts	105.2	252.0
Chronic sinusitis	154.0	131.4
Deformity or orthopedic impairment	154.9	182.0
Hernia (abdominal cavity)	154.9	182.0
Diabetes	98.3	98.2
Visual impairment	56.3	111.2
Varicose veins	82.5	64.8
Hemorrhoids	74.1	73.1

Table 36-2 Potential Nursing Diagnoses Associated With Ten Major Chronic Problems of the Elderly

	ARTHRITIS	HYPERTENSION	HEARING IMPAIRMENT	HEART CONDITION	CATARACTS	CHRONIC SINUSITIS	VISUAL IMPAIRMENT	DEFORMITIES, ORTHOPEDIC IMPAIRMENT	HERNIA	DIABETES	VARICOSE VEINS	HEMORRHOIDS
Activity intolerance	✔	✔		✔	✔			✔	✔	✔	✔	✔
Anxiety	✔	✔	✔	✔	✔	✔	✔	✔	✔	✔	✔	✔
Alterations in bowel elimination: constipation									✔		✔	
Alterations in cardiac output: decreased												
Impaired verbal communication			✔									
Ineffective individual coping	✔	✔	✔	✔	✔	✔	✔	✔	✔	✔	✔	✔
Ineffective family coping	✔	✔	✔	✔		✔	✔	✔		✔	✔	✔
Diversional activity deficit	✔	✔	✔	✔	✔	✔	✔	✔	✔	✔	✔	✔
Alterations in family processes	✔	✔	✔	✔	✔	✔	✔	✔		✔	✔	✔
Fear	✔	✔	✔	✔	✔	✔	✔	✔		✔	✔	✔
Fluid volume deficit								✔				
Fluid volume excess				✔								
Grieving												

Table 36-2 *Potential Nursing Diagnoses Associated With Ten Major Chronic Problems of the Elderly (Continued)*

	ARTHRITIS	HYPERTENSION	HEARING IMPAIRMENT	HEART CONDITION	CATARACTS	CHRONIC SINUSITIS	VISUAL IMPAIRMENT	DEFORMITIES, ORTHOPEDIC IMPAIRMENT	HERNIA	DIABETES	VARICOSE VEINS	HEMORRHOIDS
Alterations in health maintenance	✔	✔	✔	✔	✔	✔	✔	✔		✔	✔	✔
Impaired home maintenance management	✔	✔	✔	✔	✔	✔	✔	✔		✔	✔	✔
High risk for infection				✔		✔			✔	✔	✔	✔
High risk for injury	✔	✔	✔	✔	✔	✔	✔			✔		
Knowledge deficit	✔	✔	✔	✔	✔	✔	✔	✔	✔	✔	✔	✔
Impaired physical mobility	✔	✔		✔	✔			✔	✔	✔	✔	
Noncompliance	✔	✔	✔	✔	✔	✔	✔	✔	✔	✔	✔	✔
Alterations in nutrition: less than body requirements	✔					✔	✔	✔	✔	✔		
Alterations in nutrition: more than body requirements	✔	✔		✔	✔					✔		
Alterations in oral mucous membrane										✔		
Pain	✔	✔		✔		✔	✔	✔	✔		✔	✔
Powerlessness	✔		✔	✔	✔		✔	✔				
Alterations in respiratory function				✔		✔		✔				
Self-care deficit	✔	✔	✔	✔	✔	✔	✔	✔		✔	✔	✔
Disturbance in self-concept	✔	✔	✔	✔	✔	✔	✔	✔		✔	✔	✔
Sensory–perceptual alterations	✔		✔				✔	✔				
Sexual dysfunction	✔	✔		✔				✔		✔		
Impairment of skin integrity				✔				✔		✔	✔	✔
Sleep pattern disturbance	✔	✔		✔		✔		✔	✔	✔	✔	✔
Impaired social interactions	✔	✔	✔	✔	✔	✔	✔	✔		✔		
Social isolation	✔	✔	✔	✔	✔		✔	✔				
Spiritual distress												
Alterations in thought processes		✔	✔	✔			✔			✔		
Alteration in tissue perfusion				✔								
Alteration in patterns of urinary elimination				✔						✔		

Increase self-care capacity
Delay deterioration and decline
Promote highest possible quality of life
Support in dying with comfort and dignity

actions are based on interventions that would cure patients, and success is judged on how quickly and totally patients are able to recover. Chronic illness is an entirely different situation. Patients will not recover from their disease, and care measures will focus on helping patients effectively manage, rather than cure, the illness. Professionals who seek success through the number of patients who recover will be frustrated and disappointed when working with the chronically ill; they must re-orient themselves to a new set of care goals (Display 36-1). The following goals are appropriate to chronic care:

Increase self-care capacity. Chronic illness often places additional demands on people. They may need to eat special diets, modify their activities, administer medications, perform treatments, or learn to use assistive devices or equipment. A variety of measures may be required for these demands to be met, and nurses may need to assist patients in increasing their abilities to engage in these measures. Actions toward achieving this goal include education about the disease and its management, stabilization and improvement of health status, promotion of interest and motivation for self-care, use of assistive devices, and provision of periodic assistance with care.

Delay deterioration and decline. The difference as to whether a diabetic patient lives an active life or becomes a blind amputee is largely determined by the extent to which treatment plans are followed and complications are actively prevented. By their nature, chronic diseases will progressively worsen. A conscious effort must be made to reinforce the importance of care measures and identify problems early. Complications must be prevented because they risk weakening self-care capacity, increasing disability, and hastening decline.

Promote the highest possible quality of life. Sitting in bed attached to an oxygen tank may keep the body functioning but offers little stimulation to the mind and soul. Consideration should be given to helping chronically ill patients participate in activities that bring pleasure and reward. The extent to which recreational, social, spiritual, emotional, sexual, and family needs are met should be assessed, and assistance should be provided to fulfill those needs (e.g., introduction to new hobbies, counseling for alternate positions for intercourse, provision of transportation by specially equipped vehicles, arrangements for home visits by clergy). A positive self-concept needs to be promoted. Health professionals should periodically evaluate the extent to which treatment of the problem promotes or prohibits a satisfying life-style.

Support in dying with comfort and dignity. As health status declines and patients face their final days of life, they will need increasing physical and psychosocial support. Relief of pain, preservation of energy, provision of comfort, and assistance in meeting basic needs become crucial. Nurses also must be sensitive to the importance of listening and talking to dying persons, anticipating their needs, and, most important, instilling a feeling that the nurse can be depended on for support through this period.

The goals of chronic care are such that success must be measured differently. A deterioration of a patient from ambulatory to wheelchair status can be judged a success if, without nursing intervention, that patient may have become bedridden or died. Likewise, a physically and emotionally comfortable death that left positive memories for the patient's survivors can be a significant accomplishment. These determinants of success are different from those of acute care but are no less important.

Assessing Chronic-Care Needs

There will be much diversity in the self-care capacities among chronically ill persons. There also will be variation of self-care capacity within the same chronically ill individual at different times throughout the course of the illness. Keen assessment and reassessment are necessary. The same framework as discussed in Chapters 17 and 18 is used in assessing the care needs of the chronically ill. The capacity of the individual to fulfill each of the universal requirements should be reviewed as well as the capacity to meet the demands imposed by illness (e.g., medication administration, dressings, special exercises). From this, deficits in fulfilling care needs can be determined.

Most chronically ill persons will be managing their illness in a community setting, most likely with family support or involvement; therefore, assessment must consider not only the capacity of the individual to fulfill the care demands but also the capacity of the family unit to fulfill the patient's needs. For instance, a diabetic man may have severe arthritis in his hands and not be able to manipulate a syringe for his insulin injections, but his wife may be able to give him injections; thus, he does not have a deficit in this area. Likewise, an Alzheimer victim may not be able to protect herself from safety hazards, but if she lives with a daughter who supervises her activities, this patient may not have a deficit in her ability to protect herself. Within this framework, the family is the patient, and the capacities and limitations of the total family unit must be evaluated. Remember that family is not limited to relatives but can include a variety of significant others. Nurses cannot assume, however, that the presence of family members guarantees compensation of the patient's care deficits. Sometimes, the caregivers may not have the physical, mental, or emotional abilities to meet the patient's care needs; the patient's caregiver daughter may be a frail older adult herself. Likewise, the family may not want to provide care because of the imposition on their life-style or their feelings toward the patient. These factors must be considered before care is delegated to family members.

Once identified, care needs should be reviewed with the patient and family members. This not only helps to validate data but also promotes an understanding by all parties involved as to what the care needs actually are. Methods of meeting care needs should be identified jointly (e.g., the daughter will assist with bathing, the son will provide transportation to the clinic for monthly visits, the daughter-in-law will call twice daily to remind the patient to take medications). The family should be informed of the services available in their community to supplement their efforts. In fairness to the family, the costs and limitations of community services must be included in this discussion.

Setting goals is important in helping patients and their families understand the realistic direction of care. For instance, a long-term goal of restoring ambulation sets a different tone from a goal of preventing complications as function deteriorates. Acceptance of long-term goals may require acceptance of the realities of the condition, which is not an easy task for patients and their families. It may take time and considerable nursing support for families to come to the understanding that the patient's physical or mental status will decline over time. This is not to suggest that hope should be destroyed, but rather that it be tempered with a realistic sense of what the future may hold. Short-term goals offer a means of evaluating ongoing efforts and serve as benchmarks in care; these goals can be set on a daily, weekly, or monthly basis, depending on the situation.

Written care plans are beneficial to patients and their families. Having the plans in writing avoids discrepancies between what patients thought they were told and what they were really told. It also prevents directions from being forgotten and ensures that anyone who participates in the patient's care will have the same understanding.

Following the Course of Chronic Care

Anyone who has gone on a diet can appreciate the difficulty in sustaining the initial weight-loss behaviors (e.g., diet, exercise) on a long-term basis without regular reinforcement and support. The same is true for the new behaviors associated with managing a chronic illness. Chronically ill persons cannot be given their instructions for care, discharged, and forgotten. They will need periodic contact and reevaluation of their capacity, resources, and motivation to manage their conditions.

A variety of factors can change patients' abilities to manage their illnesses. The status of the illness may change, placing more or different demands on the patient. The status of the patient may change, reducing self-care ability. The status of the care giver may change, limiting the degree to which the patient's deficits can be compensated. All the factors affecting the patient's ongoing care must be evaluated regularly.

The life-style changes, frustrations, and losses commonly experienced by the chronically ill may cause certain reactions to emerge, which could disrupt the flow of care. These reactions are defense mechanisms, used when the situation at hand may be too much for the patient to cope with, and include the following:

Denial   making statements or taking actions that are not consistent with the realities of the illness (e.g., abandoning a special diet, discontinuing medications independently, committing to responsibilities that cannot be fulfilled)

Anger acting hostile to others, having violent outbursts

Depression making statements regarding hopelessness of situation, refusing to engage in self-care activities, withdrawing

Regression becoming increasingly dependent unnecessarily, abandoning self-care behaviors

These and other reactions are indications that the patient's ego strength is threatened and that extra support is needed. Rather than reacting to the patient's reactions, caregivers need to understand their origin and aid the patient in working through them (e.g., by providing an opportunity to vent frustrations and offering respite from the routines of care by doing for the patient until the individual feels psychologically able to resume self-care).

As mentioned earlier, in the home management of a chronic illness, the family is the patient. In evaluating care, the impact on the total family must be considered. The patient with Alzheimer disease may be well-groomed, well-nourished, and free from complications; looking at the patient in isolation, an evaluation could be made that her home care has been successful. However, the patient's status may have been achieved at great cost to the total family, (e.g., her husband may have had to forfeit his job to care for her during the day, her daughter's family life may have been disrupted because she needed to sleep at her parents' home to assist her father in controlling her mother's night wandering, the son's plans to expand his business may have been postponed because he began subsidizing his parents' income). Some sacrifices and compromises are common when family members assume caregiver roles, but serious disruption to their health or their lives should not result. Families may be so embroiled in the situation that they are unable to see the full impact that the caregiving situation is having on their own lives; sometimes, they feel that they must be a "bad" spouse or child to feel that the patient's care is a burden. Nurses can assist by helping family members realistically evaluate their caregiving responsibilities and identify when other caregiving options should be considered. For instance, the family may sense that it is in the patient's best interest to enter a nursing home, but they need the health-care professional to introduce the suggestion and help them through the process of making this difficult decision.

Staff members who provide chronic care in long-term care settings cannot be forgotten, either. Their work is physically and emotionally demanding. Often, particularly if they are direct-care providers, they will be the recipient of patients' displaced feelings. They will develop close relationships with many of these patients as they care for them over an extended time and be affected by patients' declines and deaths. Under the circumstances, it is easy for staff to experience burnout, leading to many ill consequences for themselves. Special efforts to prevent, identify, and manage burnout should be incorporated into the care of staff and could include reducing or rotating work load, providing opportunities for respite from routine work assignments, developing support systems on the job, incorporating mental-health days into the sick leave policy, and conducting stress management programs.

Effective chronic care is not an easy nursing challenge. It requires knowledge and skills related to the management of multiple medical problems, skilled assessment and planning, individualized promotion of self-care capacity, monitoring of family health, and a variety of other demands. The chronically ill person's comfort, independence, and quality of life are largely influenced by the type of services rendered; in chronic care, most of those services will fall within the scope of nursing. Perhaps this type of care, more than any other, provides an opportunity for nursing to demonstrate its facets of independent practice and full leadership potential.

Recommended Readings

Ahroni J. A description of the health needs of elderly home care patients with chronic illness. Home Health Care Services Quarterly 1989;10:77.

Baines EM, Oglesby FM. Conceptualization of chronicity in aging. In: Murrow E, ed. Perspectives on gerontological nursing. Newbury Park, CA: SAGE, 1991:251.

37

Death and Dying

Death is an inevitable, unequivocal, and universal experience, common to all humans. It is difficult for human beings to face—perhaps the most difficult and painful reality of all. Although a certainty, the cessation of life is often dealt with in terms of fury, fear, and flight. Mortals are very reluctant to accept their mortality.

It is difficult for the gerontological nurse to avoid facing the reality of death because more than 80% of all who die are aged. It is not only the final event of death the gerontological nurse must learn to deal with; it is the entire dying process—the complex of experiences that dying individuals, their family, their friends, and all others involved with them must go through. It is far from easy to work with this complicated process, and it requires a fine blend of sensitivity, insight, and knowledge about the complex topic of death (Table 37-1).

What is Death?

The final termination of life, the cessation of all vital functions, the act or fact of dying. These are definitions the dictionary offers concerning death—attempts at succinct explanations of this complex experience. But we human beings are often reluctant to accept such simple descriptions of this in-

escapable thief of life. For example, the world of literature contains many eloquent words on the topic, including the following:

> Now I am about to take my last voyage, a great
>   leap in the dark.
>   THOMAS HOBBES

> Do not go gentle into that good night,
> Old age should burn and rave at close of day;
> Rage, rage against the dying of the light.
>   DYLAN THOMAS

> Down, down, down into the darkness of the grave,
> Gently they go, the beautiful, the tender, the kind;
> Quietly they go, the intelligent, the witty, the
>   brave.
> I know. But I do not approve.
> And I am not resigned.
>   EDNA ST. VINCENT MILLAY

> Death hath this also, that it
> openeth the gate to good fame,
> and extinguisheth envy.
>   FRANCIS BACON

> Each person is born to one
> possession which outvalues
> all the others—his last breath.
>   MARK TWAIN

> The night comes on that knows not morn,
> When I shall cease to be all alone,
> To live forgotten, and love forlorn.
>   ALFRED LORD TENNYSON

> For so the game is ended
> That should not have begun.
>   A. E. HOUSMAN

More information on memorial societies can be obtained by contacting the Continental Association of Funeral and Memorial Societies, 59 East Van Buren Street, Chicago, IL 60605.

Table 37-1 *Nursing Diagnoses Related to Death and Dying*

NURSING DIAGNOSIS	CAUSE OR CONTRIBUTING FACTOR
Activity intolerance	Depression, fatigue, pain, treatments, immobility
Anxiety	Separation from loved ones, loss of body function or part, realization of impending death, concern about treatment prior to and at death
Altered bowel elimination: constipation	Narcotics, immobility, diet, stress
Altered bowel elimination: diarrhea	Stress, antibiotics, tube feedings, cancer, fecal impaction
Altered cardiac output: decreased	Congestive heart failure, cardiogenic shock, anemia, fluid and electrolyte imbalances, drugs, stress
Pain	Cancer, diagnostic tests, poor positioning, overactivity
Impaired verbal communication	Pain, drugs, fatigue
Ineffective individual coping	Changes in body integrity, separation from loved ones, ineffective family coping, helplessness, powerlessness
Ineffective family coping	Impending death of loved one, lack of knowledge or support
Diversional activity deficit	Hospitalization, treatment demands, depression
Altered family processes	Loss of family member, changes in roles, care costs
Fear	Treatments, pain, death
Fluid volume deficit	Shock, fever, infection, anorexia, inability to drink independently, depression
Grieving	Loss of body function or part, pain, separation from family
High risk for infection	Cancer, renal failure, treatments, immobility, lowered resistance, drugs (*e.g.,* antibiotics, steroids), malnutrition
High risk for injury	Altered ability to protect self, pain, drugs, fatigue
Knowledge deficit	Diagnostic tests, treatments, drugs, pain management
Impaired physical mobility	Weakness, pain, bedrest
Noncompliance	Denial, lack of knowledge, impaired functional capacity
Altered nutrition: less than body requirements	Anorexia, depression, pain, treatments, nausea, vomiting
Altered oral mucous membrane	Cancer, infection, drugs, malnutrition, dehydration, mouth breathing, poor hygiene
Powerlessness	Dependency, disability, institutional constraints, inability to reverse condition
Altered respiratory function	Thick secretions, pain, anxiety, drugs, immobility, decreased lung elasticity and activity, mouth breathing
Self-care deficit	Pain, weakness, disability
Disturbance in self-concept	Loss of body function or part, institutionalization, pain
Sensory–perceptual alterations	Metabolic alterations, pain, immobility, isolation, drugs
Sexual dysfunction	Separation from partner, pain, fatigue, depression, drugs, treatments, hospitalization
Impaired skin integrity	Immobility, infections, edema, dehydration, emaciation
Sleep pattern disturbance	Immobility, pain, anxiety, depression, drugs, new environment

Table 37-1 Nursing Diagnoses Related to Death and Dying (Continued)

NURSING DIAGNOSIS	CAUSE OR CONTRIBUTING FACTOR
Impaired social interactions	Loss of body function or part, depression, anxiety
Social isolation	Hospitalization, disability, deformity, discomfort of others
Spiritual distress	Loss of body function or part, barriers imposed by treatments or hospitalization, feelings toward dying process
Altered thought processes	Depression, anxiety, fear, isolation

For as we well wot, that
a young man may dye
soon: so be we very sure
that an olde man cannot
live long.
    SIR THOMAS MORE

Thou shalt come to thy grave
in a full age, like as a shock
of corn cometh in his season.
    JOB 5 :26

The silence of that dreamless sleep
I now envy too much to weep.
    LORD BYRON

Death is fortunate for the
child, bitter to the youth,
too late to the old.
    PUBLILIUS SYRUS

Death is the mother of beauty.
    WALLACE STEVENS

Throughout Shakespeare's voluminous works there is a recurrent mention of death:

. . . death—
The undiscover'd country, from whose bourne
No traveller returns.
    HAMLET

The stroke of death is as a lover's pinch,
Which hurts, and is desir'd.
    ANTONY AND CLEOPATRA

A man can die but once:
We owe God a death.
    HENRY IV

Dramatic or amusing, the descriptions of death offered in popular literature have done little to enhance our knowledge of its true meaning. Current scientific literature does not provide much more in the way of specific definitions of death. The United Nations Vital Statistics definition says that death is the permanent disappearance of every vital sign. However, terms such as brain death, death of brain cells determined by a flat electroencephalogram (EEG); somatic death, determined by the absence of cardiac and pulmonary functions; and molecular death, determined by the cessation of cellular function confuse the issue. The controversy lies in deciding at which level of death a person is considered dead. There are situations in which an individual with a flat EEG still has cardiac and respiratory functions; could this individual be said to be dead? There are also situations in which individuals with flat EEGs and no cardiopulmonary functions still have living cells that permit their organs to be transplanted; are individuals really dead if they possess living cells? The answers to these questions are not easy or simple. Much current thought and investigation are focused on the need for a single criterion in the determination of death.

The Realization of Mortality

At one time, most births and deaths occurred in the home. In extended family living, more older persons were part of the household and could be naturally observed as they grew old and died. Direct contact with births and the dying process was common. Viewed as natural processes, these events were managed by familiar faces in familiar surroundings. Intimate encounters with the beginning and end of life were rich experiences that provided insights and helped foster understanding of these realities. Perhaps the family felt a certain comfort and closeness by being with and doing for the person whose life was about to begin or end. And who

can determine the benefit to the infant or the dying individual of being comforted and cared for by close loved ones? A high mortality rate also made experiences with the dying process more common in the past (Fig. 37-1). Not only were living conditions poor, health-care facilities inadequate, disease control techniques limited, and technologies to fight and control nature's elements unheard of, but there were fewer numbers of hospitals and other institutions in which people could die.

As Figure 37-1 indicates, the mortality rate has decreased over the years. Health and medical care are now more available and accessible, and new medications and therapeutic interventions increase the possibility of surviving an illness. Sophisticated and widespread lifesaving technologies and improved standards of living have also lowered the number of deaths in the population. The declining mortality rate is among several factors that have limited our experience with the dying process. Another factor is that our more mobile nuclear families are frequently composed of young members, with older parents and grandparents living in different households, often in different parts of the country. The funeral of the older family members may be the only part of the dying process shared by other age groups. Aged persons in the family or community will most likely not die in their familiar environment. With a majority of deaths occurring in an institutional setting, and over one-half in a hospital setting, rarely do family and friends remain with the individual or witness the dying process.(Butler, 1975)

The separation of individuals from their loved ones and their familiar surroundings during the dying process seems discomforting, stressful, and unjust. "The final indignity in hospitals is to isolate the old when they are dying."(Butler, 1975) How inhumane to remove dying persons from intimate involvement with their support systems at the time of their greatest need for support. As our direct experiences with dying and death are lessened, death becomes a more impersonal and unusual event. Its reality is difficult to internalize; it is held at arm's distance. Perhaps this explains why many persons have difficulty accepting their own mortality. Avoiding discussions about death and not making a will or other plans related to one's own death are clues to the lack of internalization of one's mortality. Although the topic of death can be confronted on an intellectual level, it is often this internalization of life's finiteness that remains difficult.

To assist the dying and their families effectively, nurses should analyze their own attitudes toward death. Denying their own mortality or feeling angry about it, nurses may tend to avoid dying persons, discourage their efforts to deal realistically with their death, or instill false hopes in them and their families. The difficult process of confronting and realizing one's own mortality need not be viewed as depressing by the nurse; it can provide a fuller appreciation of life and the impetus for making the most of every living day. Nurses who understand their own mortality are more comfortable helping individuals through their dying process. A special book that may be helpful to nurses is *Gramp*, which depicts an aged man's dying experience narratively and photographically.(Jury and Jury, 1976) With honesty and sensitivity, the family supports this dying man in his familiar surroundings as his life declines. The children, grandchildren, and great-grandchildren who share Gramp's dying experience do so with extraordinary warmth, love, and naturalness. One cannot help but marvel at how these individuals learn to accept their own mortality by sharing this process.

Supporting the Dying Individual

For a long time, nurses were more prepared to deal with the care of a dead body than with the dynamics involved with the dying process. Not only was open discussion of an individual's impending death rare, but it was not unusual for the dying person to be moved to a separate and often isolated location during the last few hours of life. If the family was present, they were frequently left alone with the dying person, without benefit of a professional person. Rather than planning for additional staff support for the dying person and the family, nurses were concerned with whether a patient would live until their next shift and require postmortem care. When death did occur, the body was removed from the unit in secrecy so that other patients would not be aware of the event. Nurses were discouraged from showing emotion when a patient died. A detached objectivity was promoted as part of nursing the dying patient.

Nursing has now moved toward a more humanistic approach to caring for the dying patient. Em-

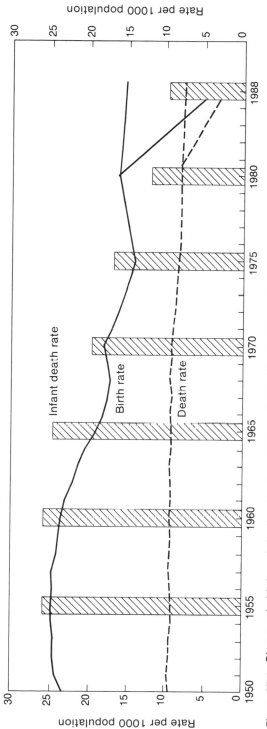

Figure 37-1. Changes in birth and death rates from 1950 to 1985. (Modified from the US Bureau of the Census: Statistical astract of the United States. 1990:57.

DISPLAY 37-1   Hospice

Hospice is a way of caring for the terminally ill and their families. It aids in putting quality and meaning into the remaining period of life.

The first hospice program was St. Christopher's Hospice in London. In 1974, the first hospice in the United States began at Hospice, Inc., in New Haven, Connecticut.

The National Hospice Organization has developed standards for hospice care to guide local hospice programs; however, individuality and autonomy of each program are encouraged.

Hospice care uses interdisciplinary efforts to address physical, emotional, and spiritual needs, including:

- pain relief
- symptom control
- coordinated home care and institutional care
- bereavement follow-up and counseling.

For more information, contact the National Hospice Organization, 1901 North Fort Meyer Drive, Suite 402, Arlington, VA 22209, (703)243-5900.

phasis on meeting the total needs of the patient has stimulated greater concern for the psychosocial care of the dying. There is now recognition that family and significant others play a vital role in the dying process and must be considered by the nurse. Knowledge has increased in the field of thanatology (*i.e.*, the study of death and dying), and more nurses are exposed to this body of knowledge. Hospice care has developed into a specialty (Display 37-1). The nursing profession has come to realize that professionalism does not negate human emotions in the nurse–patient relationship. These factors have contributed to increased nursing involvement with the dying individual. Because the dying process is unique for every human being, individualized nursing intervention is required. Previous experiences with death, religious beliefs, philosophy of life, age, and health status are among the multitude of complex ingredients affecting the dying process. The nurse must carefully assess the particular experiences, attitudes, beliefs, and values that all individuals bring to their dying process. Only through this assessment can the most therapeutic and individualized support be given to the dying person.

Coping Mechanisms and Related Nursing Interventions

Although the dying process varies in each individual, common reactions that have been observed to occur provide a basis for generalizations. Elisabeth Kübler-Ross, after several years of experiences with dying patients, developed a conceptual framework outlining the coping mechanisms of dying in terms of five stages.(Kübler-Ross, 1969) It behooves the nurse to be familiar with these stages and to understand the most therapeutic nursing interventions during each stage. Not all dying persons will progress through these stages in an orderly sequence. Neither will every dying person experience all of these stages. However, an awareness of Kübler-Ross' conceptual framework can assist the nurse in supporting dying individuals as their many complex reactions to death are demonstrated. A brief description of these stages is provided below, along with pertinent nursing considerations.

Denial and Isolation

On becoming aware of their impending death, most individuals initially react by denying the reality of the situation. "It isn't true" and "there must be some mistake" and "they're wrong, not me" are among the comments reflective of this denial. Patients sometimes "shop" for a physician who will suggest a different diagnosis or invest in healers and fads that promise a more favorable outcome. Denial serves several useful purposes for the dying person. It is a shock absorber after learning the difficult and shocking news that one has a terminal condition; it provides an opportunity for people to test the certainty of this information; it allows people time to internalize this information and mobilize their defenses.

Although the need is strongest during the early stages, dying persons may use denial at various times throughout their illness. They may fluctuate between wanting to discuss their impending death and denying its reality. The nurse must be sensitive to the person's need for defenses while also being ready to participate in dialogues on death when the person needs to do so. Contradictions may occur, and although these can be confusing, the nurse should try to accept the dying person's use of defenses rather than focus on the conflicting messages. An individual's life philosophy, unique coping mechanisms, and the knowledge of the condition will determine when denial will be

replaced by less radical defense mechanisms. Perhaps the most important nursing action during this stage is to accept the dying individual's reactions and provide an open door for honest dialogue.

Anger

The stage of denial is gradually replaced, and the "No, not me" reaction is substituted for one of "why me?" The second stage, anger, is often extremely difficult for individuals surrounding the dying person because they are frequently the victims of displaced anger. In this stage, the dying person expresses the feeling that nothing is right. Nurses don't answer the call lights soon enough; the food tastes awful; the doctors don't know what they're doing; and visitors either stay too long or not long enough. Seen through the eyes of the dying person, this anger is understandable. Why wouldn't people resent not having what they want when they want it when they won't be wanting it very much longer? Why wouldn't they be envious of those who will enjoy a future they will never see? Their unfulfilled desires and the unfinished business of their life may cause outrage. Perhaps their complaints and demands are used to remind those around them that they are still living beings.

During this time, the family may feel guilt, embarrassment, grief, and anger as a result of the dying person's anger. They may not understand why their intentions are misunderstood or their actions unappreciated. It is not unusual for them to question whether they are doing things correctly. The nurse can help the family gain insight into the individual's behavior, which will relieve their discomfort and, thereby, create a more beneficial environment for the dying person. If the family can be brought to a realization that the person is reacting to impending death and not to them personally, it may facilitate a supportive relationship and prevent guilt feelings.

The nurse should also guard against responding to the dying person's anger as a personal affront. The best nursing efforts may receive criticism for not being good enough; cheerful overtures may be received with scorn; the call light goes on the minute the nurse leaves the room. It is important that the nurse assess such behavior and understand that it may reflect the anger of the second stage of the dying process. Instead of responding to the anger, the nurse should be accepting, implying to the dying person that it is fine to vent these feelings. Anticipating needs, remembering favorite things, and maintaining a pleasant attitude can counterbalance the anticipated losses that are becoming more apparent to the dying individual. It may be useful for nurses to discuss their feelings about the patient's anger with an objective colleague who can serve as a sounding board and to validate that the nurse–patient relationship continues to be therapeutic.

Bargaining

After recognizing that denial and anger do not change the reality of impending death, dying persons may attempt to negotiate a postponement of the inevitable. They may agree to be a better Christian if God lets them live through one more Christmas; they may promise to help themselves more if the physician initiates aggressive therapy to prolong life; they may promise anything in return for an extension of life. Most bargains are made with God and usually kept a secret. Sometimes such agreements are shared with members of the clergy. The nurse should be aware that dying persons may feel disappointed at not having their bargain honored or guilty over the fact that having gained time, they want an additional extension of life even though they agreed that the request would be their last. It is important that these often covert feelings be explored with the dying person.

Depression

When a patient is hospitalized with increasing frequency and experiences declining functional capacity and a greater prevalence of symptoms, the reality of the dying process is emphasized. The aged patient may already have had many losses and experienced depression. Not only may lifetime savings, pleasurable pastimes, and a normal lifestyle be gone, but bodily functions and even bodily parts may be lost. All this understandably leads to depression. Unlike other forms of depression, however, the depression of the dying person may not benefit from encouragement and reassurances. Urging dying persons to cheer up and look at the sunny side of things implies that they should not contemplate their impending death. It is unrealistic to believe that dying people should not be deeply saddened by the most significant loss of all—their life.

The depression of the dying person is usually a silent one. It is important for the nurse to understand that cheerful words may be far less meaning-

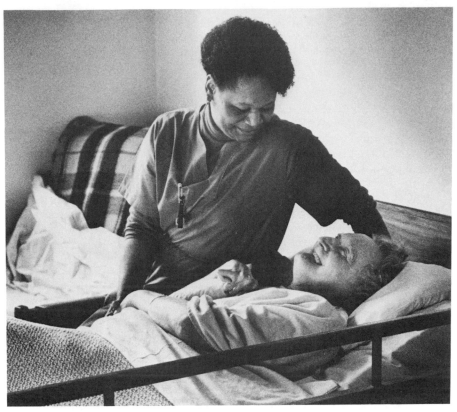

Figure 37-2. *Touching, comforting, and being near the dying individual are significant nursing actions. (Photograph by Eric Schenk.)*

ful to dying individuals than holding their hand or silently sitting with them (Fig. 37-2). Being with the dying person who openly or silently contemplates the future is a significant nursing action during this stage. The nurse may have to help the family understand this depression, explaining that their efforts to cheer the dying person can hinder the patient's emotional preparation rather than enhance it. The family may require reassurance for the helplessness they feel at this time. The nurse may emphasize that this type of depression is necessary for the individual to be able to approach death in a stage of acceptance and peace. An interest in prayer and a desire for visits from clergy are commonly seen during this stage. The nurse should be particularly sensitive to the dying person's religious needs and facilitate the clergy–patient relationship in every way possible.

Acceptance

For many dying persons, a time comes when struggling ends and relief ensues. It is as though a final rest is being taken to gain the strength for a long journey. This acceptance should not be mistaken for a happy state; it implies that the individual has come to terms with death and found a sense of peace. During this stage, patients may benefit more from nonverbal than verbal communication. It is important that their silence and withdrawal not result in isolation from human contact. Touching, comforting, and being near the person are valuable nursing actions. An effort to simplify the environment may be required as the dying person's circle of interests gradually shrinks. It is not unusual for the family to need a great deal of assistance in learning to understand and support their loved one during this stage.

Hope During the Five Stages of Dying

Significantly, hope commonly permeates all stages of the dying process. Hope can be used as a temporary but necessary form of denial, as a rationalization for enduring unpleasant therapies, and as a source of motivation. It may provide a sense of having a special mission to comfort an individual through the last days. A realistic confrontation of impending death does not negate the presence of hope.

Physical Care Needs

Pain

Concern as to the degree of pain that will be experienced and its management may be a considerable source of distress for dying individuals; nurses are in a position to reassure them with realistic information regarding pain. Cancer patients are more likely to experience severe pain than persons dying from other causes, and even among terminally ill cancer patients, only one-half have substantial pain. (Carroll and Lynn, 1990)

Gerontological nurses must be aware that patients will perceive and express pain differently based on their cultural background, medical diagnosis, emotional state, cognitive function, and other factors. Complaints of pain or discomfort, nausea, irritability, restlessness, and anxiety are common indicators of pain; however, the absence of such expressions of pain does not mean pain does not exist. Some patients may not overtly express their pain; in these individuals, signs such as sleep disturbances, reduced activity, diaphoresis, pallor, poor appetite, grimacing, and withdrawal may provide clues to the presence of pain. Confusion can be associated with pain in some circumstances. The presence of pain must be regularly reassessed because it can increase or decrease over time. Patients should be encouraged to report their pain in a timely manner and openly discuss their concerns about pain. It can be useful for patients to rate their pain on a scale of 0 to 10 (0 = no pain, 10 = most severe pain); nursing staff can record patients' self-appraisal of pain along with other factors on a flow sheet, such as that shown in Figure 37-3, to aid in pain assessment.

For the dying patient, the goal of pain management is to prevent pain from occurring rather than treating it once it does occur. Pain prevention not only helps patients avoid discomfort but ultimately reduces the amount of analgesics used by patients. After the pattern of pain has been assessed, a schedule for administration of analgesics can be

Time	Patient's self-assessment (0=no pain, 10=severe pain)	Type of pain (dull, sharp, throbbing)	Precipitating factors	Relief interventions type/effectiveness	Comments

Figure 37-3. An example of a pain record.

developed. The type of analgesic used will depend on the intensity of the pain, ranging from aspirin or acetaminophen for mild pain, to codeine or oxycodone for moderate pain, to morphine or hydromorphone for severe pain. Brompton's cocktail—a combination of morphine or methadone, ethyl alcohol, cocaine, and hydrochloride syrup—may be used for pain control in some patients. Meperidine and pentazocine are contraindicated for pain control in the elderly because of their high incidence of adverse effects, particularly psychosis, at relatively low dosages. Nurses should note and patients should be instructed to report indications of ineffectiveness of analgesic or their schedule of administration, overdosage, and adverse reactions.

Alternatives to medications should be included in the pain control program of dying patients. Such measures could include guided imagery, hypnosis, relaxation exercises, massage, acupressure, acupuncture, and the application of heat or cold.

Respiratory Distress

Respiratory distress is a common problem in dying patients. In addition to the physical discomfort resulting from dyspnea, patients can experience tremendous psychological distress associated with the fear, anxiety, and helplessness that results from the thought of suffocating. The causes of respiratory distress can range from pleural effusion to deteriorating blood gas levels. Interventions such as elevating the head of the bed and administering oxygen can prove beneficial. Atropine or furosemide may be administered to reduce bronchial secretions; narcotics may be used for their ability to control respiratory symptoms by blunting the medullary response.

Poor Nutritional Intake

Many dying patients experience anorexia, nausea, and vomiting that can prevent the ingestion of even the most basic nutrients. Additionally, fatigue and weakness can make the act of eating a monumental task. Serving small-portioned meals that have appealing appearances and smells can stimulate the appetite, as can providing foods that are patient's favorites. An alcoholic drink before meals can boost the appetite in some persons. The sense of taste is sometimes improved by administering steroids in low dosages. Nausea and vomiting can be controlled with the use of antiemetics and antihistamines. Also useful are basic nursing measures, such as assisting with oral hygiene, offering a clean and pleasant environment for dining, providing pleasant company during mealtime, and assisting with feeding as necessary.

Constipation

Reduced food and fluid intake, inactivity, and the effects of medications cause constipation to be a problem for most dying patients—a problem that can add to the discomfort these patients already are experiencing. Knowing that the risk for this problem is high, nursing staff should take measures to promote regular bowel elimination in terminally ill patients. Laxatives usually are administered regularly, and bowel elimination patterns should be recorded and assessed. It must be remembered that what may appear to be diarrhea may actually be seepage of liquid wastes around a fecal impaction.

Signs of Imminent Death

When death is near, bodily functions will slow and certain signs and symptoms noted, including the following:

- decline in blood pressure
- rapid, weak pulse
- dyspnea and periods of apnea
- slower or no pupil response to light
- profuse perspiration
- cold extremities
- bladder and bowel incontinence
- pallor and mottling of skin
- loss of hearing, vision.

By identifying that death is approaching, nursing staff can ensure that family are notified and given the opportunity to share the last minutes of the patient's life. If the family is unavailable, a staff member should remain with the patient. Depending on the wishes of the patient and family, clergy may be called to visit the patient at this time. It is important that the patient not be alone during this period; even if it appears that the patient is unresponsive, the patient should be spoken to and touched.

Spiritual Needs

Americans represent a diversity of religious beliefs. Each religion has its own practices related to death, and nursing staff must respect these practices to promote the fulfillment of patients' spiritual needs. Because it is likely that the importance

Table 37-2 Religious Beliefs and Practices Related to Death

RELIGION	BELIEFS AND PRACTICES RELATED TO DEATH
Baptist	Prayer, communion
Buddhist	Last rites by Buddhist priest
Catholic	Prayer, last rites by priest
Church of Christ	Visit from Christian Science reader
Episcopal	Prayer, communion, confession, last rites
Friends (Quakers)	Individual communicates with God directly, no belief in afterlife
Greek Orthodox	Prayer, communion, last rites by priest
Hindu	Visit by priest to perform ritual of tying thread around neck or wrist, water put in mouth, family cleanses body after death, cremation accepted
Judaism	After death, body washed by religious person, no belief in afterlife
Lutheran	Prayer, last rites
Mormon	Baptism and preaching to deceased
Muslim	Confession, family prepares body after death, deceased must face Mecca
Pentecostal	Prayer, communion
Presbyterian	Prayer, last rites
Russian Orthodox	Prayer, communion, last rites by priest
Scientologist	Confession, visit with pastoral counselor
Seventh-Day Adventist	Baptism, communion
Unitarian	Prayer, cremation accepted

of religion in patients' lives as they are dying will be a reflection of the role of religion throughout their lives, assessment should explore not only their religious affiliation, but also, their individual religious practices.

Table 37-2 lists some basic differences among religions in beliefs and practices related to death. Nursing staff must be sensitive to differences and ensure that they do not inadvertently disrespect the religious beliefs of patients and their families. Clergy and congregation members of the religious group to which the patient belongs should be invited to be actively involved with the patient and family, according to their wishes.

Supporting Family and Friends

Thomas Mann's comment that "a man's dying is more the survivors' affair than his own" is a reminder that the family and friends of the dying person should be considered in the nursing care of that person. They too may have needs requiring therapeutic intervention during the dying process of their loved one. Offering the appropriate support throughout this process may prevent unnecessary stress and provide immense comfort to those involved with the dying person. Just as dying persons experience different reactions as they cope with the reality of their impending death, so may the family and friends pass through the stages of denial, anger bargaining, and depression before they are ready to accept the fact that a special person in their lives is going to die. The reactions described below may be demonstrated by family and friends.

Denial and Isolation   This stage may involve discouraging patients from talking or thinking about death; visiting patients less frequently; stating that patients will be better as soon as they return home, start eating, have their intravenous tube removed, and so forth; and shopping for a doctor or hospital to find a special cure for the terminal illness.

Anger　Reactions may include criticizing staff for the care they are giving; reproaching a family member for not paying attention to the patient's problem earlier; and questioning why someone who has led such a good life should have this happen.

Bargaining　People may tell the staff that if they could take patients home they know they could improve their condition. Through prayers or open expression they may agree to take better care of the patient if given another chance. They may consent to take some particular action (*e.g.*, go to church regularly, volunteer for good causes, give up drinking) if only the patient could live to a particular time.

Depression　Family and friends may become more dependent on the staff. They may begin crying and limiting contact with the patient.

Acceptance　In this stage, people may react by wanting to spend a great deal of time with the dying person; telling the staff of the good experiences they have had with the patient and how they are going to miss the person. They may request the staff to do special things for the patient (*e.g.*, arrange for favorite foods, eliminate certain procedures, provide additional comfort measures). They may frequently remind the staff to be sure to contact them "when the time comes." They may begin making specific arrangements for their own lives without the patient (*e.g.*, change of housing, plans for property, strengthen other relationships for support).

Obviously, the type of nursing support will vary depending on the stage a family member or friend is assessed to be in. Although the nursing actions described for the dying individual during each stage may be applicable for family and friends, the stages experienced by those involved with the dying person may not coincide with the patient's own timetable for these stages. For instance, patients may already have worked through the different stages, come to accept the reality of death, and be ready to openly discuss the impact of their death and make plans for their survivors. However, family members and friends may be at different stages and not be able to deal with the patient's acceptance. The nurse must be aware of these discrepancies in states and provide individualized therapeutic interventions. While providing appropriate support to family and friends as they pass through the stages, the nurse can offer opportunities for dying people to discuss their death openly with a receptive party.

Helping the Family After a Death

When patients die, the nurse should be available to provide any needed support to the family. Some people wish to have several minutes in private with deceased patients to view and touch them. Others want the nurse to accompany them as they visit the deceased. Still others may not want to enter the room at all. The personal desires of the family and friends must be respected; nurses should be careful not to make value judgments of the family's reaction based on their own attitudes and beliefs. It is beneficial to encourage the family and friends to express their grief openly. Crying and shouting may help people cope with and work through their feelings about the death more than suppressing their feelings to achieve a calm composure. Unfortunately, public figures have often been presented as reacting in a composed and stoical manner to a death, thus providing poor role models.

Funeral and burial arrangements may require guidance by a professional. The survivors of the deceased may be experiencing grief, guilt, or other reactions that place them in a vulnerable position. At this time they are especially susceptible to sales pitches equating their love for the deceased to the cost of the funeral. Funerals may be arranged costing thousands of dollars more than survivors can actually afford, either depleting any existing savings or leaving a debt that will take years to repay. The family may need to have the extravagant plans presented by a funeral director counterbalanced by realistic questions concerning the financial impact of such a funeral. Someone must take the role of reminding the family that life does go on and that their future welfare must be considered. Whether it be the nurse, a member of the clergy, or a neighbor, it is valuable to identify some person who can be an advocate for the family at this difficult time and prevent them from being taken advantage of. Rather than waiting for a death to occur before thinking through reasonable funeral plans, people should be encouraged to learn about the funeral industry and plan in advance for funeral arrangements. In addition to books on the topic, a number of memorial societies can assist individuals in their planning.

In addition to assisting the family through the funeral, someone should be available to check on family members several weeks after the death. After the excitement of the funeral has diminished and fewer visitors are calling to pay their respects, the full impact of the death may first be realized. Gorer has described the three stages of mourning as a period of shock during the first few days following the death, a period of intense grief lasting 6 to 8 weeks, and a period of reawakening of interest in life.(Gorer, 1965) As can be noted, intense grief occurs during that letdown period when fewer resources may be available to provide support. Several studies have revealed higher mortality rates in widowers, especially during the first year following the death. Because there are potential threats to the mourning individual's well-being, planned interventions may prove valuable. The gerontological nurse can arrange for a visiting nurse, a church member, a social worker, or someone else to contact the family members several weeks following the death to make sure they are not experiencing any crisis. Widow-to-widow and similar groups can support individuals through their grieving process. It may also be beneficial to provide the phone number of a person whom the family can contact if assistance is required.

Edwin Schneidman, who has done considerable "postventive" work with survivors, offers the following concise guidance in working with the family and friends of the deceased:(Schneidman, 1976)

Total care of a dying person needs to include contact and rapport with the survivors-to-be.

In working with survivor–victims of dire deaths, it is best to begin as soon as possible after the tragedy, within the first 72 hours if possible.

Remarkably little resistance is met from survivor–victims; most are willing to talk to a professional person, especially one who has no ax to grind and no pitch to make.

The role of negative emotions toward the deceased—irritation, anger, envy, guilt—needs to be explored, but not at the beginning.

The professional plays the important role of reality tester—not so much the echo of conscience as the quiet voice of reason.

Medical evaluation of the survivors is crucial. One should be alert for possible decline in physical health and in overall mental well-being.

Supporting the Nurse

The staff members working with the dying individual have their own set of feelings regarding this significant experience. It may be extremely difficult for nurses not only to accept a particular patient's death but also to come to terms with the whole issue of death. As was discussed earlier in this chapter, some nurses share the difficulty that many persons have in realizing their own mortality. Nurses' experiences with death may be limited, as may their exposure to the subject through formal education. In a health profession in which the emphasis is primarily on "curing," death may be viewed as a dissatisfying failure. Nurses may feel powerless as they realize that their best efforts can do little to overcome the reality of impending death.

It is not unusual for a nurse who is involved with a dying patient to also experience the stages of the dying process described by Elisabeth Kübler-Ross. Nurses are commonly observed to avoid contact with dying patients, tell a patient to "cheer up" and not think about death, continue to practice "heroic" measures although a patient is nearing death, and grieve at the death of a patient. Nurses may be limited in their ability to support patients and their families if they are at a different stage from them. For example, the nurse may be unable to accept that the patient is dying; avoidance of the topic and unrealistic plans for the patient's future reflect this denial. The patient, however, may be at the point of accepting the reality of the dying process and may want to discuss personal feelings. Recognizing that the nurse is still denying, the patient may avoid an open discussion of death and be deprived of an important therapeutic activity.

The nurse working with a dying patient requires a great deal of support. Colleagues should help nurses explore their own reactions to dying patients and recognize when those reactions interfere with a therapeutic nurse–patient relationship. The attitude of colleagues and the climate of the environment should be such that nurses can retreat from a situation that is not therapeutic either for them or the patient. To encourage the nurse to cry or show emotions in other forms may be extremely beneficial. The use of thanatologists, hospice staff, and other resource people may also be valuable in providing support to nurses as they assist an individual through the dying process.

References

Butler RN. Why survive? Being old in America. New York: Harper & Row, 1975.

Carroll BJ, Lynn J. Care of the dying patient. In: Abrams WB, Berkow R, eds. The Merck manual of geriatrics. Rahway, NJ: Merck Sharpe & Dohme Research Laboratories, 1990:289.

Gorer G. Death, grief and mourning. New York: Doubleday, 1965.

Jury M, Jury D. Gramp. New York: Grossman, 1976.

Kübler-Ross E. On death and dying. New York: Macmillan, 1969.

Shneidman ES. Postvention and the survivor-victim. In: Schneidman ES, ed. Death: current perspectives. New York: Aronson Jason, 1976.

Recommended Readings

Benoliel JQ. Multiple meanings of death for older adults. In: Murrow E, ed. Perspectives on gerontological nursing. Newbury Park, CA: SAGE Publications, 1991:141.

Gass KA. The health of conjugally bereaved older widows: the role of appraisal, coping and resources. Res Nurs Health 1987;10:39.

Gass KA, Chang AS. Appraisals of bereavement, coping, resources, and psychosocial health dysfunction in widows and widowers. Nurs Res 1989;38:31.

Herth K. Relationship of hope, coping styles, concurrent losses, and setting to grief resolution in the elderly widow(er). Res Nurs Health 1990;13:109.

Rhymes JA. Clinical management of the terminally ill. Geriatrics 1991;46(2):57.

38

Legal Aspects of Nursing Care

Nurses in every specialty must be cognizant of the legal aspects of their practice, and gerontological nurses are no exception. In fact, legal risks may be intensified and legal questions may often arise when working in geriatric-care settings. Frequently, gerontological nurses are in highly independent and responsible positions in which they must make decisions without an abundance of professionals with whom to confer; they often are responsible for supervising nonprofessional staff and ultimately are accountable for the actions of these subordinates. Gerontological nurses are likely to face difficult situations in which their advice or guidance may be requested by patients and families, such as ways to protect the assets of the wife of an Alzheimer victim, how to write a will, what can be done to cease life-sustaining measures, and who can give consent for the patient. The multiple problems faced by older adults, their high prevalence of frailty, and their lack of familiarity with laws and regulations may make them easy victims to unscrupulous practices. Advocacy is an integral part of gerontological nursing; nurses may be particularly concerned about protecting the rights of their elderly patients. To fully protect themselves, the patients, and their employers, nurses must have knowledge of basic laws and ensure that their practice falls within legally sound boundaries.

Laws are generated from several sources (Display 38-1). Because many laws are developed at the state and local levels, variation exists among the states. This necessitates that nurses be familiar with the unique laws within their specific states, particularly those governing professional practice, labor relations, and regulation of health-care agencies.

There are both public and private laws. Public law involves relationships between private parties and the government and includes criminal law and regulation of organizations and individuals engaged in certain practices; the scope of nursing practice and the requirements for being licensed as a home health agency would fall under enforcement of public law. Private law governs relationships between individuals and organizations and involves contracts and torts (*i.e.*, wrongful acts against another party, including assault, battery, false imprisonment, and invasion of privacy). These laws set standards of conduct, which, if violated, can result in liability of the wrongdoer. Some of the general acts that could make nurses liable for violating the law are reviewed in Display 38-2.

Legal Risks

Most nurses do not commit wrongful acts intentionally; however, certain situations can increase the nurse's risk of liability. Such situations could include working without sufficient resources, not checking with agency policy or procedure, bending a rule, giving someone a break, taking shortcuts, or trying to work when physically or emotion-

DISPLAY 38-1   Sources of Laws

Constitutions

State basic rights, grant powers, and place limits on government agencies that guide laws development by those agencies (*e.g.,* the right to the freedom of speech)

Court Decisions

Establish precedents from cases heard in state or federal courts (*e.g.,* the right to discontinue life-support measures)

Statutes

Laws established by local, state, and federal legislation (*e.g.,* nurse practice acts)

Regulations

Laws enacted by state and federal administrative agencies that specifically define the methods to achieve goals and objectives of statutes (*e.g.,* conditions of participation for agencies to receive reimbursement from Medicare or Medicaid)

Attorney General Opinions

Laws derived from the opinions of the chief attorney for the state or federal government (*e.g.,* decisions as to whether or not a case reflects a violation of law prior to filing a lawsuit for that case)

ally stressed. Not only repeated episodes of carelessness but also the chance that is taken just this once can result in serious legal problems. Nurses must assess all the potential legal risks in their practice and make a conscious effort to minimize them. Some of the issues that could present legal risks for nurses are presented below.

Malpractice

It is expected that nurses will provide services to patients in a careful, competent manner according to a standard of care. The standard of care is considered the norm for what a reasonable individual in a similar circumstance would do. When performance deviates from the standard of care, negligence, or malpractice, can be charged. Examples of situations that could lead to malpractice include the following:

Administering the incorrect dosage of a medication to a patient, thereby causing the patient to experience an adverse reaction.

Identifying respiratory distress in a patient, but not informing the physician in a timely manner.

Leaving an irrigating solution at the bedside of a confused patient, who then drinks that solution.

Forgetting to turn an immobile patient during the entire shift, resulting in the patient developing a pressure ulcer.

Having a patient fall from bed because the staff forgot to raise the side rails.

DISPLAY 38-2   Acts That Could Result in Legal Liability for Nurses

Assault

A deliberate threat or attempt to harm another person that the person believes could be carried through (*e.g.,* telling a patient that he will be locked in a room without food for the entire day if he does not stop being disruptive).

Battery

Unconsented touching of another person in a socially impermissible manner or carrying through an assault. Even a touching act done to help a person can be interpreted as battery (*e.g.,* performing a procedure without consent).

Defamation of Character

An oral or written communication to a third party that damages a person's reputation. **Libel** is the written form of defamation; **slander** is the spoken form. With slander, actual damage must be proven, except when:

Accusing someone of a crime
Accusing someone of having a loathsome disease
Making a statement that affects a person's professional or business activity
Calling a woman unchaste.

Defamation does not exist if the statement is true and made in good faith to persons with a legitimate reason to receive the information. Stating on a reference that the employee was fired from your agency for physically abusing patients is not defamation if, in fact, the employee was found guilty of those charges. On the other hand, stating on a reference that the employee was a thief because narcotics were missing every time she was on duty can be considered defamation if the employee was never proven guilty of those charges.

False Imprisonment

Unlawful restraint or detention of a person. Preventing a patient from leaving a facility is an example of false imprisonment, unless it is shown that the patient has a contagious disease or could harm himself or others. Actual physical restraint need not be used for false imprisonment to occur: telling a patient that he will be tied to his bed if he tries to leave can be considered false imprisonment.

Fraud

Willful and intentional misrepresentation that could cause harm or cause a loss to a person or property (*e.g.*, selling a patient a ring with the claim that memory will be improved when it is worn).

Invasion of Privacy

Invading the right of an individual to personal privacy. Can include unwanted publicity, releasing the medical record to unauthorized persons, giving patient information to an improper source,

or having one's private affairs made public. (The only exceptions are reporting communicable diseases, gunshot wounds, and abuse). Allowing a visiting student to look at a patient's pressure ulcers without permission can be an invasion of privacy.

Larceny

Unlawful taking of another person's possession (*e.g.*, assuming that a patient will not be using his personally owned wheelchair anymore and giving it away to another patient without permission).

Negligence

Omission or commission of an act that departs from acceptable and reasonable standards, which can take several forms:

Malfeasance Committing an unlawful or improper act (*e.g.*, a nurse performing a surgical procedure)

Misfeasance Performing an act improperly (*e.g.*, including the patient in a research project without obtaining consent)

Nonfeasance Failure to take proper action (*e.g.*, not notifying the physician of a serious change in the patient's status)

Malpractice Failure to abide by the standards of one's profession (*e.g.*, not checking that a nasogastric tube is in the stomach before administering a tube feeding)

Criminal negligence Disregard to protecting the safety of another person (*e.g.*, allowing a confused patient, known to have a history of starting fires, to have matches in an unsupervised situation)

The fact that a negligent act occurred, in itself, does not warrant that damages be recovered; instead, it must be demonstrated that the following conditions were present:

Duty: a relationship between the nurse and the patient in which the nurse has assumed responsibility for the care of the patient.
Negligence: failure to conform with the standard of care (*i.e.*, malpractice).

Injury: physical or mental harm to the patient, or violation of the patient's rights resulting from the negligent act.

The complexities involved in caring for older adults, the need to delegate responsibilities to others, and the many competing demands on the nurse contribute to the risk of malpractice. As the responsibilities assumed by nurses increase, so will the risk of malpractice. Nurses should be

aware of the risks in their practice and actively prevent malpractice (Display 38-3). Also, it is advisable for nurses to carry their own malpractice insurance and not merely rely on the insurance provided by their employers.

Consent

Patients are entitled to know the full implications of procedures and make an independent decision as to whether or not they choose to have them performed. This may sound simple enough, but it is easy for consent to be overlooked or improperly obtained by health-care providers. For instance, certain procedures may become so routine to staff that they fail to realize patient permission must be granted, or a staff member may obtain a signature from a patient who has a fluctuating level of mental competency and who does not fully understand what is being signed. In the interest of helping patients and delivering care efficiently, or from a lack of knowledge concerning consent, staff members can subject themselves to considerable legal headaches.

Consent must be obtained before performing any medical or surgical procedure; performing procedures without consent can be considered battery. Usually, when they enter a health-care facility patients sign consent forms that authorize the staff to perform certain routine measures (e.g., bathing, examination, care-related treatments, and emergency interventions). These forms, however, do not qualify as carte blanche consent for all procedures. Even blanket consent forms that patients may sign, authorizing staff to do anything required for treatment and care, are not valid safeguards and may not be upheld in a court of law. Consent should be obtained for anything that exceeds basic, routine care measures. Particular procedures for which consent definitely should be sought include any entry into the body, either by incision or through natural body openings; any use of anesthesia, cobalt or radiation therapy, electroshock therapy, or experimental procedures; any type of research participation, invasive or not; and any procedure, diagnostic or treatment, that carries more than a slight risk. Whenever there is any doubt as to whether consent is necessary, it is best to err on the safe side.

Consent must be informed. It is unfair to the patient and legally unsound to obtain the patient's signature for a myelogram without telling the patient what that procedure entails. Ideally, a written consent that describes the procedure, its purpose, alternatives to the procedure, expected consequences, and risks should be signed by the patient, witnessed, and dated. It is best that the person performing the procedure (e.g., the physician or researcher) be the one to explain the procedure and obtain the consent. Nurses or other staff members should not be in the position of obtaining consent for the physician because they may not be able to answer some of the medical questions posed by

the patient. Nurses can play an important role in the consent process by ensuring that it is properly obtained, answering questions, reinforcing information, and making the physician aware of any misunderstanding or change in desire of the patient. Nurses should not influence the patient's decision in any way.

Every conscious and mentally competent adult has the right to refuse consent for a procedure. To protect the agency and staff, it is useful to have the patient sign a release stating that consent is denied and that the patient understands the risks associated with refusing consent. If the patient refuses to sign the release, this should be witnessed, and both the professional seeking consent and the witness should sign a statement that documents the patient's refusal for the medical record.

Competency

Increasingly, particularly in long-term care facilities, nurses are confronting patients who are confused, demented, or otherwise mentally impaired. Persons who are mentally incompetent are not able to give legal consent. Often in these circumstances, staff will turn to the next of kin to obtain consent for procedures; however, the appointment of a guardian to grant consent for the incompetent individual is a responsibility of the court. When the patient's competency is questionable, staff should encourage family members to seek legal guardianship for the patient or request the assistance of the state agency on aging in petitioning the court for appointment of a guardian.

Various forms of guardianship can be granted (Display 38-4), each with its own restrictions. The guardian is monitored by the courts to ensure that he or she is acting in the incompetent individual's best interest; in the case of guardian of property, the guardian must file financial reports with the court.

Guardianship differs from power of attorney in that the latter is a mechanism used by competent individuals to appoint someone to make decisions for them. Usually, a power of attorney becomes invalid if the individual granting it becomes incompetent, except in the case of durable power of attorney. A durable power of attorney allows competent individuals to appoint someone to make decisions on their behalf in the event that they become incompetent; this is a recommended procedure for individuals with dementias and other disorders in

DISPLAY 38-4 Types of Decision-Making Authority That Individuals Can Legally Possess Over Patients

Guardianship

Court appointment of an individual or organization to have the authority to make decisions for an incompetent person. Guardians can be granted decision-making authority for specific types of issues:

Guardian of property (conservatorship): this limited guardianship allows the guardian to take care of financial matters but not make decisions concerning medical treatment.

Guardian of person: decisions pertaining to the consent or refusal for care and treatments can be made by persons granted this type of guardianship.

Plenary guardianship (committeeship): all types of decisions pertaining to person and property can be made by guardians under this form.

Power of Attorney

Legal mechanism by which competent individuals appoint parties to make decisions for them; this can take the form of:

Limited power of attorney: decisions are limited to certain matters (e.g., financial affairs) and power of attorney becomes invalid if the individual becomes incompetent.

Durable power of attorney: provides a mechanism for continuing or initiating power of attorney in the event the individual becomes incompetent.

which competency can be anticipated to decline. To ensure protection of patients' rights, nurses should recommend that patients and their families seek legal counsel for guardianship and power of attorney issues, and when such appointment has been made, clarify the type of decision-making authority that the appointed parties possess.

Staff Supervision

In many settings gerontological nurses are responsible for supervising other staff, many of whom may be nonprofessional. In these situations, nurses are responsible not only for their own ac-

tions but also for the actions of the staff for whom they are responsible. This falls under the doctrine of respondent superior, the old master–servant rule. Nurses should understand that if a patient is injured by one of their subordinates while their employee is working within the scope of the applicable job description, they can be liable. The type of situations that can create risks for nurses include the following:

Permitting unqualified or incompetent persons to deliver care.
Failing to follow-up on delegated tasks.
Assigning tasks to staff members for which they are not qualified or competent.
Allowing staff to work under conditions with known risks (*e.g.*, short staffed, improperly functioning equipment).

These are considerations that nurses need to keep in mind when they accept responsibility for covering the house, or sending an aide into a home to deliver care without knowing the aide's competency, or allowing registry or other employees to work without fully orienting them to agency policies and procedures.

Drugs

Nurses are responsible for the safe administration of prescribed medications. Preparing, compounding, dispensing, and retailing medications fall within the practice of pharmacy, not nursing, and, when performed by nurses, can be interpreted as functioning outside their licensed scope of practice. An act as seemingly benign as going into the agency's pharmacy after hours, pouring some tablets into a container, labeling that container, and taking it to the unit so that the patient can receive a drug that is urgently needed is illegal.

Restraints

The Omnibus Budget Reconciliation Act heightened awareness of the serious impact of restraints by imposing strict standards on their use in long-term care facilities. This increased concern regarding and sensitivity to the use of chemical and physical restraints has had a ripple effect on other practice settings.

Anything that restricts a patient's movement (*e.g.*, protective vests, trays on wheelchairs, safety belts, geriatric chairs) can be considered a re-

straint. Improperly used restraining devices cannot only violate regulations concerning their use, but also result in litigation for false imprisonment and negligence.

Alternatives to restraints should be used whenever possible. Measures that can assist with management of behavioral problems and protection of the patient include alarmed doors, wristband alarms, bed alarm pads, beds and chairs close to the floor level, and increased staff supervision and contact. Specific patient behavior that creates risks to the patient and others should be documented. Assessment of the risk posed by the patient not being restrained and the effectiveness of alternatives should be included.

When restraints are deemed absolutely necessary, a physician's order for the restraints must be obtained, stating the specific conditions for which the restraints are to be used, the type of restraints, and the duration of use. Agency policies should exist for the use of restraints and should be followed strictly. Detailed documentation should include the times for initiation and release of the restraints, their effectiveness, and the patient's response. The patient requires close observation while restrained.

At times, staff may assess that restraint use is required, but the patient or family objects and refuses to have a restraint used. If counseling does not help the patient and family understand the risks involved in not using the restraint, the agency may wish to have the patient and family sign a release of liability statement that states the risks of not using a restraint and the patient's or family's opposition. Although this may not free the nurse or agency from all responsibility, some limited protection may be afforded, and, by signing the release, the patient and family may realize the severity of the situation.

Telephone Orders

In home health and long-term care settings, nurses often do not have the benefit of an on-site physician. Changes in the patient's condition and requests for new or altered treatments may be communicated over the telephone, and in response, physicians may prescribe orders accordingly. Accepting telephone orders predisposes nurses to considerable risks in that the order can be heard or written incorrectly or the physician can deny that the order was given. It may not be realistic or advantageous to patient care to totally eliminate

telephone orders, but nurses should minimize their risks in every way possible by using the following precautions:

Do not involve third parties in the order (*e.g.,* do not have the order communicated by a secretary or other staff member for the nurse or the physician).

Communicate all relevant information to the physician, such as vital signs, general status, and medications administered.

Do not offer diagnostic interpretations or a medical diagnosis of the patient's problem.

Write down the order as it is given and immediately read it back to the physician in its entirety.

Place the order on the physician's order sheet, indicating it was a telephone order, the physician who gave it, time, date, and the nurse's signature.

Obtain the physician's signature within 24 hours.

Tape-recorded telephone orders may be a helpful way for nurses to validate what they have heard, but they may not offer much protection in the event of a lawsuit unless the physician is informed that the conversation is being recorded or unless special equipment with a 15-second tone sound is used.

No-Code Orders

There is a high prevalence of terminally ill patients in the caseloads of many gerontological nurses. It may be understood by all parties involved that these patients are going to die and that resuscitation attempts would be inappropriate; however, unless an order specifically states that the patient should not be resuscitated, failure to attempt to save that person's life could be viewed as negligence. Nurses must ensure that no-code orders are legally sound, remembering the following points:

No-code orders are medical orders and must be written and signed on the physician's order sheet to be valid. DNR (*i.e.,* do not resuscitate) placed on the care plan or a special symbol at the patient's bedside are not legal without the medical order.

Unless it is detrimental to the patient's well-being or the patient is incompetent, consent for the no-code decision should be obtained; if the patient is unable to consent, family consent should be sought.

Every agency should develop a no-code policy to guide staff in these situations; this could be an excellent item for an ethics committee to review.

Death and Dying

A variety of issues surrounding patients' deaths pose legal concern for nurses. Some of these issues arise long before death occurs, when patients choose to execute a living will. Living wills are advance directives that express the desires of competent adults regarding terminal care, life-sustaining measures, and other issues pertaining to their dying and death. States vary in their acceptance of living wills; there may even be variation among agencies as to the conditions under which this document will be entered into the medical record. Nurses can aid by making physicians and other staff aware of the presence of a patient's living will, informing patients of any special measures they must take to have the document be accepted into the medical record, and, unless contraindicated, following the patient's wishes. Readers are advised to check the status of living will legislation in their individual states.

Wills are statements of individuals' desires for the management of their affairs after their death. For wills to be valid, the person making one must be of sound mind, legal age, and not coerced or influenced into making the will. The will should be written—although under certain conditions, some states recognize oral, or nuncupative, wills, signed, dated, and witnessed by persons not named in the will. The required number of witnesses may vary among the states. To avoid problems, such as family accusations that the patient was influenced by the nurse because of his dependency on her, nurses should avoid witnessing a will. Nurses should assist patients in obtaining legal counsel when they wish to execute or change a will. If a patient is dying and wishes to dictate a will to the nurse, the nurse may write it exactly as stated, sign and date it, have the patient sign it if possible, and forward it to the agency's administrative offices for handling. It is useful for gerontological nurses to encourage persons of all ages to develop a will to avoid having the state determine how their property will be distributed in the event of their deaths. Legal aid agencies and local schools of law can be sources of assistance for older adults wishing to write their wills.

The pronouncement of death is another area of concern. Nurses often are placed in the position,

and are capable of, determining when a patient has died and notifying the family and funeral home; the physician may be notified of the death by telephone and sign the death certificate at a later time. This rather common and benign procedure actually is illegal for nurses because the act of pronouncing a patient dead falls within the scope of medical practice, not nursing. Nurses should safeguard their licenses by either holding physicians responsible for the pronouncement of death or lobbying to have the law changed so that nurses are protected in these situations.

Postmortem examinations of deceased persons can be useful in learning more about the cause of death and contributing to medical education. In some circumstances, such as when the cause of death is suspected to be associated with a criminal act, malpractice, or an occupational disease, the death may be considered a medical examiner's case and an autopsy may be mandatory. Unless it is a medical examiner's case, consent for autopsy must be obtained from the next of kin, usually in the order of spouse, children, parents, siblings, grandparents, aunts, uncles, and cousins.

Abuse

Elder abuse can occur in the elderly's homes or in health-care facilities by loved ones, caregivers, or strangers. Particularly in long-term caregiving relationships, in which family members or staff burnout, abuse may be an unfortunate consequence.

Abuse can assume many forms including inflicting pain or injury; stealing; mismanaging funds; misusing medications; causing psychological distress; withholding food or care; or sexually abusing, exploiting, or confining a person. Even threatening to commit any of those acts is considered abuse. All cases of known or suspected abuse should be reported. States vary regarding reporting mechanisms; specific state laws should be consulted.

Other Issues

Other situations can cause nurses to be liable for negligence, including the following:

Failure to take action (e.g., not reporting a change in the patient's condition or not notifying the administration of a physician's incompetent acts)

Contributing to patient injury (e.g., not providing appropriate supervision of confused patients or leaving side rails down)

Failing to report a hazardous situation (e.g., not letting anyone know that the fire alarm system is inoperable or not informing anyone that a physician is performing procedures under the influence of alcohol)

Handling patient's possessions irresponsibly

Failing to follow established policies and procedures.

Legal Safeguards

Good common sense can be the best ally of sound nursing practice. It can never be forgotten that patients, visitors, and employees do not forfeit their legal rights or responsibilities when they are within the health-care environment. Laws and regulations impose additional rights and responsibilities in patient–provider and employee–employer relationships. Nurses should protect themselves in the following ways:

Familiarize yourself with the laws and rules governing your specific care agency, their state's nurse practice act, and labor relations.

Become knowledgeable about your agency's policies and procedures and adhere to them strictly.

Function within the scope of nursing practice.

Ensure for yourself the competency of employees for whom you are responsible.

Check the work of employees under your supervision.

Obtain administrative or legal guidance when in doubt about the legal ramifications of a situation.

Report and document any unusual occurrence.

Refuse to work under circumstances that create a risk to safe patient care.

Carry liability insurance.

Recommended Readings

Adelman RD, Breckman R: Mistreatment. In: Abrams WB, Berkow R, eds. The Merck manual of geriatrics. Rahway, NJ: Merck Sharp & Dohme Research Laboratories, 1990:1135.

Bahr RT. Selected ethical and legal issues in aging. In Murrow E, ed. Perspectives on gerontological nursing. Newbury Park, CA: SAGE, 1991:373.

Bernzweig EP. Nurses' liability for malpractice. 5th ed. St. Louis: CV Mosby, 1990.

Cournoyer CP. The nurse manager and the law. Rockville, MD: Aspen, 1989.

Eliopoulos C. Legal risks in the long-term care facility. Glen Arm, MD: Health Education Network, 1991.

Regan JL. Your legal rights in late life. Glenview, IL: Scott, Foresman, 1989.

Stevenson C, Capezuti E. Guardianship: protection vs. peril. Geriatr Nurs 1991;12(1):10.

Wolf RS, Pellemer KA: Helping elderly victims: the reality of elder abuse. New York: Columbia University Press, 1989.

39

Ethical Considerations

Professional ethics has become a popular phrase in nursing circles. The concept of principles guiding right and wrong conduct is not new to nursing, but changes within the profession and the entire health-care delivery system have heightened the significance of ethics to nursing practice.

Expanded Role of Nurses

Nurses have gone beyond the confines of simply following doctors' orders and providing basic comfort and care. They are now performing sophisticated assessments, diagnosing nursing problems, monitoring and giving complicated treatments, and, particularly in geriatric-care settings, increasingly making independent judgments about patients' status. The wider scope of functions, combined with higher salaries and status, have increased the accountability and responsibility of nurses for the care of patients.

Medical Technology

Artificial organs, wonder drugs, computers, lasers, ultrasound, and other innovations have increased the ability to diagnose and treat problems and to save lives that once would have been given no hope. However, new problems have accompanied these advances, such as determining on whom, when, and how this technology should be used.

New Fiscal Constraints

In the past, the major concern of health-care providers and agencies was to provide quality services to help people maintain and restore health. Now, competing with and sometimes overriding that concern are those of being cost effective, minimizing bad debts, and developing alternate sources of revenue. Patients' needs are weighed against economic survival, resulting in some difficult decisions.

Greater Numbers of Older Adults

The impact of entitlement programs and services to the aged was not felt so severely when only a small portion of the population was old, but with growing numbers of people spending more years in old age and the ratio of dependent individuals to productive workers increasing, society is beginning to feel burdened. Although the elderly's problems and needs are more evident, the ability and responsibility of society to support those needs are in question.

What Are Ethics?

The word ethics originated in ancient Greece, where *ethos* were those beliefs that guided life. Most current definitions of ethics revolve around the concept of accepted standards of conduct and

moral judgment. Basically, ethics aid us in determining right and wrong courses of action. As simple as this sounds, different philosophies disagree as to what constitutes right and wrong.

Utilitarian   This philosophy holds that good acts are those from which the greatest number of people will benefit and gain happiness.

Egoism   At the opposite pole from utilitarianism, egoism proposes that an act is morally acceptable if it is of the greatest benefit to oneself and that there is no reason to perform an act that benefits others unless one will personally benefit.

Relativism   This can be referred to as situational ethics, in that right and wrong are relative to the situation. Within relativism are several subgroups of thinking—some relativists believe that there can be individual variation in what is ethically correct, whereas others feel that the individual's beliefs should conform to the overall beliefs of society for the given time and situation.

Naturalism   There are two schools of thought among naturalists. One holds that something is good if there are positive attitudes or interests in it. The other theorizes that something is good if the ideal, objective person has a positive attitude or interest in it.

To exemplify how these different philosophies would approach an ethical decision, consider the hypothetical situation of four poor old men who share a household. One day, one of these men finds a lottery ticket in the mailbox while checking the household's mail. The ticket holds the winning number for a $1 million prize. Ethically, does he owe his housemates any of the winnings?

A utilitarian would propose that he should split the winnings with his housemates because that would bring good to the greatest number of people.

An egoist would encourage him to keep the winnings because that would do him the most good personally.

A relativist would say that normally he should keep the winnings but, in this situation he would have more money than he will need, so he should share the earnings.

A naturalist would say that he should share the money only if his housemates thought this was the right thing to do.

Consider the different philosophical approaches to the issue of federal subsidies to the elderly.

A utilitarian could say that 12% of the population should not use one-third of the gross national product and that the money instead should be equally allocated on a per capita basis.

An egoist would say that the individual old person should take whatever he feels he needs, regardless of the impact on others.

A relativist would say that the elderly could use that proportion of the budget unless more was needed for dependent children or defense, at which point it would no longer be right to do so.

A naturalist would say that as long as most of society and its leadership felt positive about spending so much of the budget on the elderly, it is right to do so.

Other philosophies exist, but those few that have been briefly described demonstrate the diversity of approaches to ethical thinking and reinforce the fact that deciding right and wrong actions can be a complicated endeavor.

Ethics in Nursing

Professions such as nursing require codes of ethics on which practice can be based and evaluated. A professional code of ethics is accepted by those who practice the profession as the formal guidelines for their actions and should be compatible with individual value systems. The Code for Nurses (Display 39-1) was developed by the American Nurses Association and outlines the broad values of the profession. These are not the only values that direct nursing practice. Federal, state, and local standards, in the form of regulations, guide practice. Standards for specific practitioners and care settings have been developed by various voluntary organizations such as the Joint Commission for the Accreditation of Healthcare Organizations. Individual agencies have philosophies, goals, and objectives that support a specific level of nursing practice. Most importantly, individual nurses possess values that they have developed throughout their lives that will largely influence ethical

DISPLAY 39-1   *Code for Nurses*

1. The nurse provides services with respect for human dignity and the uniqueness of the patient, unrestricted by considerations of social or economic status, personal attributes, or the nature of health problems.
2. The nurse safeguards the patient's right to privacy by judiciously protecting information of a confidential nature.
3. The nurse acts to safeguard the patient and the public when health care and safety are affected by the incompetent, unethical, or illegal practice of any person.
4. The nurse assumes responsibility and accountability for individual nursing judgments and actions.
5. The nurse maintains competence in nursing.
6. The nurse exercises informed judgment and uses individual competence and qualifications as criteria in seeking consultation, accepting responsibilities, and delegating nursing activities to others.
7. The nurse participates in activities that contribute to the ongoing development of the profession's body of knowledge.
8. The nurse participates in the profession's efforts to implement and improve standards of nursing.
9. The nurse participates in the profession's efforts to establish and maintain conditions of employment conducive to high quality nursing care.
10. The nurse participates in the profession's effort to protect the public from misinformation and misrepresentation and to maintain the integrity of nursing.
11. The nurse collaborates with members of the health professions and other citizens in promoting community and national efforts to meet the health needs of the public.

Courtesy of American Nurses Association, Kansas City, MO. Developed and published by the American Nurses Association.

thinking. Ideally, a nurse's individual value system meshes with that the profession, society, and employer; conflict can arise when value systems are incompatible. Several ethical principles are used to guide health care including the following.

Beneficence   to do good for patients
Nonmaleficence   to avoid harm to patients
Justice   to be fair and give patients the service they need
Fidelity   to respect our words and duty to patients
Autonomy   to respect patients' freedoms and rights

Few nurses would argue with the value of these principles, and in fact, practices that reinforce these principles are widely promoted, such as ensuring patients receive the care they need, respecting the rights of patients to consent to or deny consent for treatment, preventing incompetent staff from caring for patients, and following acceptable standards of practice. Actual nursing practice is seldom simple, however, and situations emerge that add new considerations to the application of moral principles to patient care. Ethical dilemmas can emerge when other circumstances interfere with the clear, basic application of ethical principles.

Ethical Dilemmas

Everyday nursing practice carries its share of situations that could produce conflicts between nurses' values and external systems affecting their decisions, and the rights of patients and nurses' responsibilities to those patients. Consider the following examples:

While working in an outreach program to bring services to community-based elderly, you meet Mr. Brooks, a 68-year-old homeless man. Mr. Brooks asks your opinion about respiratory symptoms that he has been experiencing over the past several months. He reports a chronic cough, hemoptysis, and dyspnea. He appears thin and admits to having lost weight. He states he has smoked at least one pack of cigarettes daily over 50 years and has no intention of changing his smoking habit. Although he is not cognitively impaired, he strongly resists efforts to find him housing and arrange for medical evaluation and treatment. You are convinced that without intervention, Mr. Brooks will not survive much longer.

Do you respect Mr. Brooks' right to make his own decisions about his life, even if those decisions

run contrary to what is best for his health and well-being?

You are the new director of nursing for a nursing home and were pleased to get the job because yours has become the sole source of income for your family. Ten cases of diarrhea develop among the residents and you know that the regulations require that you report five cases or more. You bring this to the attention of the medical director and administrator, who direct you not to "cause trouble by putting the health department on their backs." The medical director assures you that the problem is not serious and will pass in a few days. You know you should notify the health department, but you also know that the administrator fired the last nursing director for opposing him on a similar issue.

Do you allow a regulation to be violated or risk losing a job that you may badly need?

Insurance coverage expires tomorrow for 76-year-old Mrs. Brady, and the physician has written an order for her discharge. Because Mrs. Brady continued to be weak and slightly confused, she was not able to be instructed in the safe use of home oxygen and medication administration during her hospitalization. Her 80-year-old husband, who is expected to be her primary caregiver, is weak and in poor health himself. The social worker tells you that arrangements have been made for a nurse to visit the home daily but that the couple does not qualify for 24-hour home-care assistance. You and other nursing staff members firmly believe that Mrs. Brady's health will be in jeopardy if she is discharged tomorrow. The physician tells you that you are probably right, but "the hospital cannot be expected to eat the bills that Medicare does not want to pay."

Do you increase the hospital's financial risks by insisting that nonreimbursed care be provided?

Seventy-nine-year-old Mr. Adams lies in his bed in a fetal position, unresponsive except to deep painful stimuli. He has multiple pressure ulcers, recurrent infections, and must be fed with a nasogastric tube. His wife and children express concern over the quality of his life and state that Mr. Adams would never have wanted to survive in this state. The children privately tell the multidisciplinary team that if their father's care expenses continue, their mother will be destitute, and they beg the staff to remove the tube. The family expresses that they do not have the emotional or financial resources to take the issue to court. The physician is sympathetic, but states he feels compelled to continue the feedings and antibiotics because he does not condone euthanasia; however, privately, the physician tells you that he will close his eyes and keep quiet if you want to pull the tube without anyone knowing.

Do you exceed your authority and discontinue a life-sustaining measure to grant the family's request?

Mrs. Smith is dying of cancer and being cared for at home by her husband. The couple has been married for 63 years and has never been apart during that time. They are highly interdependent and each one's world revolves around the other. During your home nursing visit, the couple openly discusses their plans with you. They tell you that they have agreed that when Mrs. Smith's pain becomes too severe to tolerate, they will both ingest sufficient medication, which they have accumulated, to kill themselves, and die peacefully in each other's arms.

Do you ignore your responsibility to report suicidal intent to respect a couple's wish to end their lives together?

As part of a research project, a new drug is being used to improve the function of Alzheimer victims. Half the patients are receiving the test drug and half a placebo. The group receiving the drug is noted to have significant improvements. You discuss your observations with the research team and suggest that all the patients in the study receive the test drug. The team objects, stating that this would interfere with the study and contaminate the findings.

Do you prevent a group of patients from deriving the benefits of the test drug or respect research protocols that could have wider implications?

You are asked to orient a new staff nurse. Within her first week of employment, you detect that she is inept at administering medications, vio-

lates aseptic technique, and handles patients roughly. She refuses to change or accept constructive criticism. You recommend to the director of nursing that this nurse be dismissed during probation. You are told that the agency has been criticized for discriminatory hiring practices and because this new nurse is a member of a minority group, she will help to dissolve that criticism; thus, she has to be kept.

Do you accept an incompetent nurse to spare your employer labor-relations problems?

You are working with a senior citizen group that is trying to obtain more funding from the state government for long-term care. To provide this funding, some prenatal and well-baby health-care services will have to be discontinued. Government officials argue that a majority of the state's health-care budget is currently spent on long-term care and that the elderly receive a disproportionate amount of services as compared to other age groups. The seniors state that "after paying taxes all their lives, they deserve not to be impoverished by nursing home care and that other groups will just have to make do."

Do you advocate for these older adults, even if it is at the expense of other age groups?

You observe another nurse stealing a hospice patient's narcotic and report it to your supervisor. You are told that this nurse has been suspected of this before and that an undercover agent will be placed on the unit as an orderly to investigate and build a case against the nurse. You suggest that the patient and family be informed but are told to tell no one, as this would jeopardize the investigation.

Do you respect the patient's right to be informed of a situation potentially threatening his care, even if it means that insufficient evidence will be gathered to prove the nurse committed an illegal act?

A new reimbursement system has given a strong financial incentive to nursing homes to admit very ill patients with highly technical needs. You observe that nursing homes without adequate skill or resources are admitting patients to take advantage of this extra revenue and that patient care is suffering as a result. You contact one of the health policy makers who drafted this new reimbursement plan and share your concerns about increased patient morbidity and mortality. He responds, "So what if they die sooner . . . doesn't that end up saving the system money?"

Do you work within a system that knowingly reimburses in a manner that could threaten patients' well-being?

These are typical of the decisions facing nurses every day and for which there are no easy answers. It is easy to say that nurses should always follow the regulations, adhere to principles, and do what is best for the patient. But can nurses be expected to follow these guidelines 100% of the time, even if it means they may lose the income on which their families depend, violate the rights of individuals to decide their own destinies, cause problems for co-workers or their employers, or be labeled as a troublemaker? Is it all right to knowingly violate a regulation or law if no real harm will result? Do nurses need to limit how much of an advocacy role they can assume? Should nurses base their decisions on what is right for themselves, their patients, or their employers? To whom are nurses really most responsible and accountable?

Making Ethical Decisions

Although guidelines exist, no solid answers can solve all of the ethical dilemmas that nurses will face. Nurses should, however, minimize their struggles in making ethical decisions by following measures such as those listed below:

> *Know thyself.* One's personal value system should be reviewed. The influences of religion, cultural beliefs, and personal experiences should be explored to understand one's unique comfort zone with specific ethical issues.
> *Read.* Review the medical literature for discussions and case experiences of other nurses to gain a wider perspective into the types of ethical problems confronted within nursing and strategies for managing them. Literature outside the field of nursing can help to add new facets to one's thinking.
> *Discuss.* In formal education programs or informal coffee breaks, talk about issues with other health-team members. Members of the clergy,

attorneys, ethicists, and others can provide interesting perspectives.

Form an ethics committee. Bringing together various members of the health team, clergy, attorneys, and lay persons to study ethical problems within the specific care setting, clarify legal and regulatory boundaries, develop policies, discuss ethical problems that surface, and investigate charges of ethical misconduct can be an asset to any agency.

Share. When faced with an uneasy ethical decision, consult others and seek guidance and support.

Evaluate decisions. Even the worst decision holds some lessons.

Gerontological nursing holds its share of ethical questions: Should resources be spent for a heart transplant for an octogenarian? . . . Should an affluent child rather than public funds pay for a parent's care? . . . How much sacrifice must a family endure to care for a relative at home? . . . How much compromise in care can nurses accept to keep an agency's budget healthy? The questions will become more numerous and more complicated. Nurses must be active participants in the process of developing ethically sound policies and practices affecting the care of the elderly. The choice between being a leader or an ostrich in this arena can significantly determine the future status of gerontological nursing practice.

Recommended Readings

Bahr RT. Selected ethical and legal issues in aging. In: Murrow E, ed. Perspectives on gerontological nursing. Newbury Park, CA: SAGE, 1991:373.

Bandman EL, Bandman B. Nursing ethics through the lifespan. 2nd ed. Norwalk, CT: Appleton & Lange, 1990.

Calfee BE. Are you restraining your patient's right? Nursing 1988;88(5):148.

Callahan D. Setting limits: medical goals in an aging society. New York: Simon & Schuster, 1987.

Callahan D. What kind of life: the limits of medical progress. New York: Simon & Schuster, 1990.

Henderson ML, McConnell ES. Ethical considerations. In: Matteson MA, McConnell ES, eds. Gerontological nursing. Philadelphia: WB Saunders, 1988.

Kane RA, Caplan AL, eds. Everyday ethics: resolving dilemmas in the nursing home. New York: Springer-Verlag, 1990.

McConnell LT, Lynn J, Moreno JD: Ethical issues. In: Abrams WB, Berkow R, eds. The Merck manual of geriatrics. Rahway, NJ: Merck Sharp & Dohme Research Laboratories, 1990:1155.

Norberg A, Athlin E. Eating problems in severely demented patients: issues and ethical dilemmas. Nurs Clin North Am 1989;24:781.

Shelley SI, Zahorchak RM, Gambrill CDS: Aggressiveness of nursing care for older patients and those with do-not-resuscitate orders. Nurs Res 1987;36:157.

Waymack MH, Taler GA.: Medical ethics and the elderly: a case book. Chicago: Pluribus, 1988.

40

Matching Services to Needs

The needs of the aging population are diverse and multitudinous, and the needs of any one aged individual are dynamic—these needs fluctuate at different periods of time as the individual's capacities and life demands change. A wide range of services is essential to meet the complex and changing needs of the elderly. The continuum of care for the aged takes several factors into consideration.

Physical, emotional, and social factors. Services must be available to meet the unique physical, emotional, and social needs of this group. These services should be planned to deal with whatever problems the aged are most likely to develop and implemented in a manner relevant to the unique characteristics of the aged. For instance, a local health department interested in meeting the unique needs of the aged would add screening programs for hearing, vision, hypertension, and cancer to their existing services. Likewise, a social service agency may decide that a widow's group and retirement counseling services are more relevant for the aged than marriage counseling services.

Individual differences. Flexibility is necessary to provide physical, emotional, and social care services according to the individual's needs at a given time, recognizing that priorities are not fixed. An aged individual may be attending a clinic for hypertension control. During a clinic visit, the individual may express concern regarding a recent increase in rent. Unless assistance is obtained to provide additional income or lower-cost housing, the potential effects of this social problem—such as stress and dietary sacrifices—may have deleterious effects on the individual's hypertension problem. Ignoring this individual's need for particular social services can minimize the effectiveness of the health services provided.

Flexibility. An opportunity must exist for the aged individual to move along the continuum of care, depending on his capacities and limitations at different times. Perhaps an elderly woman lives with her children and attends a senior citizen recreational program during the day. If this woman fractures her hip, she may move along the continuum to hospitalization for acute care and then to nursing-home care for convalescence. As her condition improves and she becomes more independent, she may then move along the continuum to home care and then possibly to a geriatric day-care program.

Matching needs to services. Individualization must be practiced to match the unique needs of the individual with specific services. Just as it is inappropriate to assume that at the age of 65 years all people need nursing home placement, it is equally inappropriate to assume that all aged persons would benefit from counseling, sheltered housing, home-delivered meals, a geriatric day care program, or any other service. Aged individ-

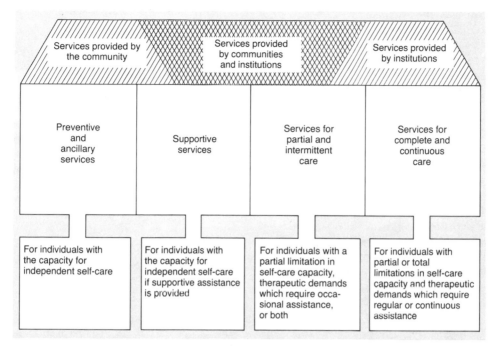

Figure 40-1. Continuum of care services for the aged.

uals' unique capacities and limitations, and most importantly their preferences, are assessed to identify the most appropriate services for them.

The continuum of care provides for community care services, institutional care services, or a combination of both. Figure 40-1 depicts this continuum. The nurse working with the aged must have an understanding of the various forms of care available for this age group to plan effectively. Although services may vary from one area to another, some general forms of geriatric-care delivery can be briefly described.

Preventive and Ancillary Services

The services in this category provide assistance to individuals with independent self-care capacity in an effort to maintain their capacity and prevent physical, emotional, and social problems from developing. The services described below are planned to meet the unique interests and concerns of the aged and may be free or of nominal cost.

Banking Services

By completing a direct-deposit form at their bank, the elderly can have the Social Security Administration mail Social Security and Supplemental Security Income checks directly to the bank. This service saves the aged from having to travel to the bank and serves as a protection from theft. Many banks offer free checking accounts and other special services to senior citizens. Reverse annuity mortgages can be arranged through banking institutions to allow older adults to use the equity in their homes to remain in the community. It is advisable for older persons to explore the details of such services with their individual banks.

Burial Services

Various agencies provide financial assistance for burial and funeral expenses. For instance, wartime veterans are eligible for some assistance from the Veterans Administration (VA), and the Social Security Administration will provide some payment for

burial expenses to those who have been insured by that program; local offices of these administrations should be contacted for information. Social service agencies and religious organizations often provide services for persons with insufficient funds to pay for burial expenses.

Consumer Services

The elderly are frequent victims of unscrupulous people who profit by making convincing, but invalid, promises. It is important that they investigate cure-alls, retirement villages, and get-rich-quick schemes before investing their funds. Local offices of the Better Business Bureau can provide useful information to prevent fraud and deception and offer counseling if these problems do occur. Consumer counseling groups also provide a variety of services to older persons, ranging from money management to assistance in filing suit for fraud.

Counseling Services

Financial problems, the need to find new housing, strained family relationships, death, adjusting to a chronic illness, and retirement are among the situations that may necessitate professional counseling. Local departments of social services, religious organizations, and private therapists are among the resources that may offer assistance.

Educational Services

Some public schools offer literacy, high school equivalency, vocational, and personal interest courses for older adults. Many colleges have free tuition for the elderly. Individual schools should be contacted for more details.

Employment Services

State employment services and the Over-60 Employment Counseling Service conduct programs that provide employment counseling and job placement. Various states also have foster grandparent programs, older businessmen associations, and senior aide projects. Local offices on aging can direct older persons to employment programs and opportunities in their vicinity.

Financial Aid Services

The Social Security Administration may be able to assist the aged in obtaining retirement income, disability benefits, supplemental security income, and Medicare or other health insurances. The district office of the Social Security Administration can provide direct assistance and information. The VA can provide financial aid to aged veterans and their families; the aged should be directed to the local VA office. Various communities offer discounts to senior citizens at department stores, pharmacies, theaters, concerts, and restaurants and for bus and taxicab services. Lists of such discounts may be obtained from local offices on aging.

Food, Health, Housing, and Transportation Services

Departments of social services can supply information and applications for food stamps to help the elderly purchase an adequate diet within the constraints of their budget. These departments may also provide shopping services and nutrition classes. Many senior citizen clubs and religious organizations offer a lunch program that combines socialization with a nutritious meal. The local office on aging or health department may be able to direct persons to the sites of such programs.

The aged should be encouraged to engage in preventive health practices for the purposes of preventing illness and detecting health problems at an early stage. Health services for the aged are provided by health departments, hospital clinics, and private practitioners. In addition to health services, these providers may assist the elderly in obtaining transportation and financial assistance for their health care. Aged persons should inquire about such services at their nearest health-care office.

Local departments of social services and departments of housing and community development can assist aged persons in locating adequate housing at an affordable cost. These agencies also may be able to direct the aged homeowner to resources to assist in home repairs and provide information regarding property tax discounts. A variety of life-care communities, villages, mobile-home parks, and apartment complexes, specifically designed for older persons, are available throughout the country. Some of these housing complexes include special security patrols, trans-

portation services, health programs, recreational activities, and architectural aids (*e.g.*, low cabinets, grab bars in bathrooms, tinted windows, slopes instead of curbs or stairs, and a call bell for emergencies). There may be one initial purchase price or a monthly fee. The aged person exploring retirement housing should be advised that sound facts are more important to decision-making than exciting promises. Visits to the housing complex and a full investigation of benefits and costs prior to a contractual commitment are essential.

Information and Referral Services

Local offices on aging, commissions on retirement education, libraries, and health departments usually provide assistance to the aged in learning about available services. Older persons should be encouraged to use these resources for any questions and problems and for any form of help needed. The Silver Pages telephone directory for older adults also is a useful resource.

Legal and Tax Services

Local legal aid bureaus and lawyer referral services of the Bar Association may help older persons obtain competent legal assistance at a nominal cost. The Internal Revenue Bureau can help older persons prepare federal tax returns and the state comptroller's office can assist with state tax returns; local offices should be called for additional information. Various colleges and law schools should be investigated for free legal and tax services that they may offer for senior citizens.

Recreational Services

Bureaus of recreation, religious organizations, and other groups may sponsor clubs and activities expressly for senior citizens. Local commissions or offices on aging may be able to provide information related to the availability of such programs, their activities, meeting dates, and persons to contact for more details. Local chapters of the American Association of Retired Persons (AARP) can provide valuable information on services that keep older persons active and independent—ranging from creative leisure endeavors at home to discount travel opportunities. Information on leisure pur-

suits is just one of the many services provided by the AARP.

The Young Men's (or Women's) Christian Association offers recreational activities for persons of all ages; the aged should explore the opportunities available at their nearest association. Art museums, libraries, theaters, concert halls, restaurants, and travel agencies should be explored for special programs offered to senior citizens.

Services by Mail

Persons who are homebound or geographically isolated from services may find it useful to obtain services by mail. Shopping by mail services have a long tradition and may reduce the inconveniences and risks associated with traveling to a shopping district, maneuvering in stores, handling large sums of money in public, and carrying packages. The postage and handling charge for this service may be no greater than the transportation costs, not to mention the energy costs, expended for direct shopping. Many libraries have a service by which books can be borrowed by mail; the aged should be encouraged to inquire about such services at their local branch. The United States Postal Service provides a service at a nominal fee by which stamps can be ordered by mail. Order blanks for stamps by mail can be obtained by contacting the local postal station.

Transportation Services

Older persons are often given discounts for bus, taxicab, subway, and train services; individual agencies should be contacted for more information. Commissions or offices on aging, health departments, departments of social services, and local chapters of the American Red Cross may be able to direct persons to services accommodating wheelchairs and other special needs. Various health and medical facilities provide transportation for persons using their services; individual facilities should be explored for specific details.

Volunteer Services

The wealth of knowledge and experiences possessed by older persons makes them especially good at volunteer work. Not only do older volun-

teers provide valuable services to other persons, but they may achieve a sense of self-worth from their contributions to society. Communities offer numerous opportunities for senior volunteers in hospitals, nursing homes, organizations, schools, and other sites. The aged should be encouraged to inquire about volunteer opportunities at the agency in which they are interested in serving. Frequently, agencies without a formal volunteer program are able to use a volunteer's services if contacted. National programs also provide meaningful volunteer services in which older persons can participate. The American National Red Cross, Service Corps of Retired Executives, and Retired Senior Volunteer Program are a few such programs. Local offices of these programs should be consulted for details.

Supportive Services

The services in this category offer assistance to individuals who are capable of self-care if aided but who are at risk of physical, emotional, and social problems without some planned intervention.

Chore Services

Departments of social services, health departments, private homemaker agencies, and religious organizations have services for older persons, which help them remain in their homes and maintain independence. These services include light housekeeping, minor repairs, errands, and shopping. Local agencies should be contacted for specific information.

Day-Care Programs

Geriatric day-care programs provide services to persons with moderate physical or mental handicaps who live alone or with families in the community. Individuals attend the program for a portion of their day and enjoy a safe, pleasant, therapeutic environment under the supervision of qualified personnel. The programs attempt to maximize the existing self-care capacity of aged individuals while preventing further limitations. Although the primary focus is social, there usually is some health component to these programs. Rest periods and meals accompany the planned thera-

peutic activities. Older persons attending day-care programs are provided with transportation to the site, and usually the buses are equipped with lifts and adjusted for wheelchairs.

In addition to helping the aged person avoid further limitations and institutionalization, day-care programs are extremely beneficial to the families of the individual. Families interested in caring for their aged relative may be able to continue their routine life-style (e.g., maintaining a job), knowing that the older person is safe and cared for. They may also be comforted knowing that they and the aged person have some respite from each other. Because day-care programs vary in their schedule, activities, costs, and sponsoring agency, individual programs should be contacted for specific information. Health departments, departments of social services, and commissions or offices on aging may be able to provide lists of geriatric day-care programs.

Foster Care and Group-Home Services

Adult foster care and group-home programs offer services to individuals who are capable of self-care but who require supervision to protect them from harm. Older persons placed in these homes may need someone to direct their self-care activities (e.g., remind them to bathe and dress and encourage and provide good nutrition); they may also need someone to oversee their judgments (e.g., financial management). Foster care and group living serve as short- or long-term alternatives to institutionalization for older persons unable to manage independently in the community. The local department of social services can supply details about these programs.

Home-Delivered Meal Services

Persons unable to shop and prepare meals independently may benefit from having meals delivered to their homes. Such a service not only facilitates good nutrition but also provides an opportunity for a social contact. Meals-on-Wheels is the most popularly known program for home delivery of meals although various community groups provide a similar service. If a local Meals-on-Wheels is not available, departments of social

services, health departments, and commissions or offices on aging should be consulted for alternative programs.

Home Monitoring

Some hospitals, nursing homes, and commercial services provide home monitoring systems whereby by the older adult can wear a small remote alarm that can be pressed if the person falls or experiences another type of need for help. The alarm triggers a central monitoring station to call predesignated contact persons or the police to assist the individual. This type of service can be located by calling the local agency on aging or looking in the telephone directory under listings such as Medical Alarms.

Sheltered Housing

Sheltered housing, frequently in the structure of an apartment complex, supplements independent living with special services that maximize an individual's capacity for self-care. The housing complex is adjusted to meet the needs of older or handicapped persons (e.g., wide doors, low cabinets, grab bars in bathroom, and a call-for-help light). A guard, hostess, or resident screens and greets visitors in the lobby. Residents are encouraged to develop mutual support systems; one example is a system by which residents check on each other every morning to ensure that no one needs help. Tenant councils may determine policies for the facility. Some facilities have a health professional on call or on duty during certain hours; social programs and communal meals may also be available. The local office of the Department of Housing and Urban Development may be able to direct interested persons to such facilities.

Telephone Reassurance Programs

Aged persons who are homebound, handicapped, or lonely may benefit from a telephone reassurance program. Those who participate in the program receive a daily telephone call—usually at a mutually agreed on time—to provide them with a social contact and ensure that they are safe and well. Local chapters of the American Red Cross and other health or social service agencies should be consulted for the telephone reassurance programs they may conduct.

Services for Partial and Intermittent Care

The services in this category provide assistance to individuals with a partial limitation in self-care capacity and a therapeutic demand for which occasional assistance is required. Either due to the degree of the self-care limitation or the complexity of the therapeutic action required, the individual would be at risk of institutionalization if some assistance were not provided at periodic intervals. Such services can be for day treatment or home care.

Day treatment offers social and health programs, with a primary focus on the latter. Assistance is provided with self-care activities (e.g., bathing and feeding) and therapeutic needs (e.g., medication administration, dressing change, and vital signs monitoring). Physicians, nurses, occupational therapists, and physical therapists are among the care providers affiliated with programs for day treatment. Like geriatric day-care programs, geriatric day hospitals usually provide transportation services for the participants. Day hospitals can be used as alternatives to hospitalization and nursing homes. In addition, earlier discharge from an institution may be facilitated if an individual has an opportunity for continued therapeutic supervision in this type of program. These programs are sponsored by hospitals, nursing homes, or other agencies. The local commission or office on aging can guide persons to programs of day treatment in their community.

Home care is for persons who are confined to their homes but in need of therapeutic assistance. The programs vary, and services can include bedside nursing, home health aides, physical therapy, health education, family counseling, and medical services. Visiting nurse associations have a long reputation of providing care in the home and are able to assist many aged persons to remain in their homes rather than enter an institution. Offices or commissions on aging, health departments, and social work agencies may be able to answer inquiries about other available programs for home care.

Hospice

Hospices actually can be listed under partial- and intermittent-care services or complete- and continuous-care services because the nature of the pa-

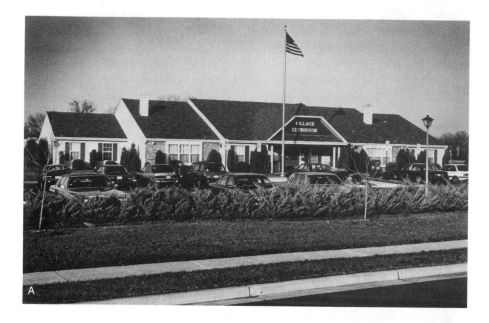

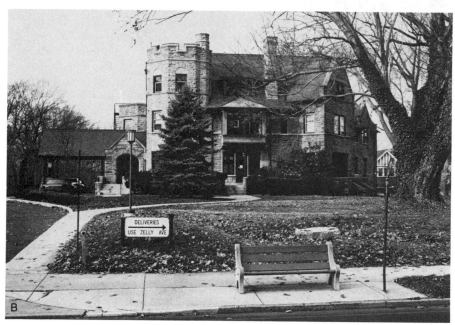

Figure 40-2. (**A**) *Retirement and life-care communities can provide an independent lifestyle for the aged person with the benefits of supervision and security.* (**B**) *Housing options for older adults come in a variety of styles and settings. (Photographs by Eric Schenk.)*

tient's needs will determine the level at which this service will be provided. Rather than a site of care, hospice is a philosophy of caring for dying individuals. Hospice provides support and palliative care to patients and their families. Typically, an interdisciplinary team assists patients and families in meeting physical, emotional, social, and spiritual needs. The focus is on the quality of remaining life rather than life extension. Survivor support also is an important component of hospice care. Although hospice programs can exist within institutional settings, most hospice care is provided in the home. Health care and social service agencies can be consulted for information on hospice programs in a specific community.

Services for Complete and Continuous Care

The services in this category provide regular or continuous assistance to individuals with some limitation in self-care capacity whose therapeutic needs require 24-hour supervision by a health professional. These services provide hospital care or long-term institutional care.

Hospital care for older persons may be required when diagnostic procedures and therapeutic ac-

tions indicate a need for specialized technologies or frequent monitoring. Increasingly, hospitals are establishing special services for older adults, such as geriatric assessment centers, hot lines, and long-term care units. Local medical societies and state hospital associations can answer inquiries about specific hospitals.

Long-term institutional care varies from one region to another and differs in the quality and quantity of medical, nursing, and other services provided (Fig. 40-2). State health departments may be able to answer inquiries about specific long-term care facilities. Hospitals for chronic diseases and rehabilitation, nursing homes, hospices, and facilities for extended and intermediate care provide long-term institutional care. Although this form of care for the aged with health problems is not the only kind available, it is appropriate and beneficial for some aged persons. The unique needs of the aged individual must be matched with the particular services offered by a long-term care facility. Older persons and their families should be actively involved with the selection of the facility. It is important to examine the costs, services, and quality of the institution before admission. Guidelines for choosing a nursing home are presented in Display 40-1.

DISPLAY 40-1   *Factors to Consider in Selecting a Nursing Home*

Cost

- per diem rate
- type of health care insurance accepted
- out-of-pocket costs necessary to supplement health care insurance
- services covered and excluded in daily rate
- charge for services not covered in daily rate
- policy regarding care of resident if or when reimbursement limits are reached

Philosophy of Care

- custodial versus restorative/rehabilitative
- promotion of independence and individuality
- encouragement of residents and families to be active participants in care

Administration

- organizational structure
- ownership
- accessibility and availability of administrator, director of nursing, medical director, department heads
- existence of regularly scheduled meetings between administration and residents and families

Special Services

- availability of podiatry, speech therapy, occupational therapy, physical therapy, transportation, beauty/barber shop
- cost for special services
- conditions and arrangements for transfer to hospital

Continued on next page

Staff

- amount of caregivers available on typical shift
- ratio of RNs, LPNs, nursing assistants
- number of supervisory staff on duty on typical shift
- frequency and type of in-service education offered to staff
- appearance, image portrayed by staff
- quality of staff–resident interactions
- courtesy, helpfulness of staff

Residents

- cleanliness, grooming, general appearance
- type of clothing worn (pajamas, streetclothes, clean, wrinkled)
- activity level
- ease of interaction with staff and other residents

Physical Facility

- cleanliness, attractiveness, fresh-smelling
- ease of use for disabled and frail
- lighting
- noise control
- safe areas for walking
- general fire and safety precautions
- proximity of bathrooms, dining rooms, activity rooms, nursing stations, and exits to residents' rooms
- visibility of residents to staff

Meals

- meal schedule
- type of food served
- attractiveness, temperature of food served
- availability of staff to assist residents at mealtime
- location where residents dine (*e.g.*, bedroom, communal dining hall)
- availability of dietitian or nutritionist for consultation
- range of special diets
- ability to have meal substitutions

Activities

- posted activity schedule
- range and frequency of activities
- ability of families and visitors to participate in activities with residents
- existence of resident council
- mechanisms for residents to have input into planning and evaluation of activities
- opportunity of residents to engage in activities off facility grounds

Care

- basic daily care provided
- frequency of contact with licensed staff
- management of special problems: incontinence, confusion, wandering, immobility
- efforts to increase mobility and function
- dignity, privacy, individuality afforded residents
- frequency at which complications develop (*e.g.*, pressure ulcers, dehydration)
- management of unusual incidents, emergencies
- evaluations by regulatory agencies

Family Involvement

- preadmission preparation offered to families
- orientation and ongoing support to families
- frequency of family conferences
- mechanisms for communicating with families, involving families in care
- visitation policies

Spiritual Needs

- religious affiliation of facility, if any
- availability of chapel, synagogue, meditation room
- visitations from clergy
- measures to assist residents in meeting spiritual needs

Recommended Readings

Eliopoulos C, ed. Caring for the elderly in diverse care settings. Philadelphia: JB Lippincott, 1990.

Eliopoulos C. Caring for the nursing home patient: clinical and managerial challenges for nurses. Rockville, MD: Aspen, 1989.

Hing E. Use of nursing homes by the elderly: preliminary data from the 1985 National Nursing Home Survey. In: Advance data from vital and health statistics. no. 135. DHHS pub. no. 87-1250. Hyattsville, MD: Public Health Service, 1987.

Kane RA, Kane RL. Long-term care: principles, programs and policies. New York: Springer-Verlag, 1987.

Matteson MA, McConnell ES, Calhoon M, Henderson ML, Lekan-Rutledge D. Context of services: network of care. In: Matteson MA, McConnell ES, eds. Gerontological nursing: concepts and practice, Philadelphia: WB Saunders, 1988:652.

Naylor MD. Comprehensive discharge planning for hospitalized elderly: a pilot study. Nurs Res 1990;39:156.

O'Brien CL. Adult day care: a practical guide. Monterey, CA: Wadsworth Health Sciences, 1982.

Resnick BM. Care for life. Geriatr Nurs 1989; 10(3):130.

41

Gerontological Nursing in Diverse Care Settings

The facts are all around us. The media reports the spiraling costs of Medicare and Social Security. Our banks advertise reverse annuity mortgage programs aimed toward helping persons age in their own homes. We drive by the construction of a new retirement community. A major corporation initiates a benefit of parent-care leave. A circular arrives from the local hospital announcing new services for senior citizens. Our church sponsors a caregiver support group.

Even if we weren't nurses, we couldn't help but notice that older adults are having a great impact on all segments of society. As nurses, we are increasingly aware that the elderly are major users of virtually all health-care services. Consider the following facts:

Growing numbers of Americans are interested in wellness programs that help them stay youthful, active, and healthy for a longer period of time.

More than one-third of all surgical patients are over 65 years of age.

The prevalence of mental-health problems increases with age.

Chronic diseases occur at a rate four times greater in old age than at other ages.

Approximately 40% of all elderly will spend some time in a nursing home during their lives.

Most beds in acute medical hospitals are filled by elderly patients.

Older adults are the most significant users of home health services.

Regardless if they work in nursing homes, mental-health clinics, health maintenance organizations (HMOs), recovery rooms, medical–surgical hospital units, hospice programs, rehabilitation centers, or private practice, nurses are likely to be involved in gerontological nursing.

The diversity of the aging population creates the need for a wide range of nursing services. The functions of the gerontological nurse are varied and multifaceted and address the following goals (Display 41-1):

Educate persons of all ages in practices that promote a positive aging process.

Assess and provide interventions for nursing diagnoses.

Identify and reduce risks.

Promote self-care capacity and independence.

Collaborate with other providers in the delivery of services.

Maintain health of the aging family.

Protect the rights of older adults.

Advocate for the use of ethics and standards in the care of older adults.

Help the elderly live their final days in peace, comfort, and dignity.

Guide persons of all ages toward a healthy aging process

Eliminate ageism

Respect the rights of older adults and ensure others do the same

Oversee and promote the quality of service delivery

Notice and reduce risks to health and well-being

Teach and support caregivers

Open channels for facing developmental tasks

Listen and support

Offer optimism and hope

Generate, support, implement, and participate in research

Implement restorative and rehabilitative measures

Coordinate services

Assess, plan, implement, and evaluate care in an individualized manner

Link services with needs

Nurture future gerontological nurses for advancement of the specialty

Understand the unique assets of each older individual

Recognize and encourage the appropriate management of ethical concerns

Support and comfort through the dying process

Educate to promote self-care and independence

As the presence of older adults in diverse health-care settings continues to increase, there will be a crucial need in those settings for nurses with gerontological nursing expertise. These nurses must understand normal aging, unique presentations and management of geriatric health problems, pharmacodynamics and pharmacokinetics in later life, psychological challenges, socioeconomic issues, family dynamics, unique risks to health and well-being, and available resources. By possessing gerontological nursing knowledge and skills, nurses can promote efficient, effective, and appropriate health-care services to older adults in a variety of settings (Fig. 41-1).

Although the review is hardly all-inclusive, the following pages will describe some of the roles and responsibilities of gerontological nurses in major-care settings.

Long-Term Care Facilities

The nursing-home setting, which had been regarded as a low-status area for nursing practice, is emerging as a complex, dynamic care site. Because earlier hospital discharges shift extremely sick individuals from the acute to long-term care setting and changing reimbursement patterns require that residents be in need of more than custodial care, long-term care facilities now possess a population with greater needs. Consumers, armed with media portrayals of a small minority of facilities with scandalous nursing home conditions, are more informed of the standards of good nursing-home care and have higher expectations of providers in this setting. Further, the Omnibus Budget Reconciliation Act of 1987 (OBRA), also known as the nursing home reform law, has put new demands on facilities for competent resident assessment, care planning, quality assurance, and protection of resident rights. The increased demands and complexities of long-term care facilities necessitate that highly competent nurses be employed in this setting.

Most care in the nursing home setting is delivered by unlicensed nursing personnel. This imposes greater demands on licensed staff; not only must nurses oversee the status of residents, but they also must monitor the competency and performance of the unlicensed caregivers. Staff education, role modeling, good supervision, performance evaluation, and correction of performance problems become responsibilities of most long-term care nurses that are superimposed on their major clinical or administrative duties.

Nurses have increasing opportunities for role variety in the long-term care facility. They can fill administrative and management roles as director of nursing, assistant director of nursing, supervisor, unit nurse coordinator, or charge nurse. They can fill specialized roles, such as staff development coordinator, quality assurance coordinator, infec-

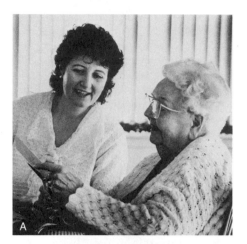
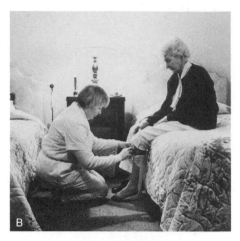
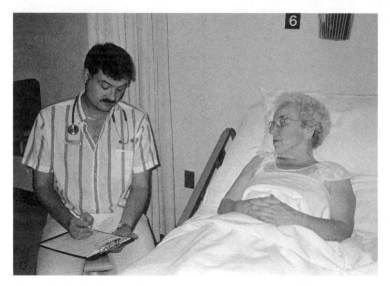

Figure 41-1. (**A**) *In adult day-care centers, gerontological nurses assist older adults in preserving and improving function and provide family caregivers important respite.* (**B**) *Home health services provide the periodic interventions that enable the ill elderly to manage in their homes. (Photographs by Eric Schenk.)* (**C**) *Gerontological nursing assessment skills are applicable in a wide range of clinical settings. (From Farrell J. Nursing care of the older person. Philadelphia: JB Lippincott, 1990:46.)*

tion control coordinator, geropsychiatric nurse specialist, or rehabilitative nurse. Of course, nurses can be direct care providers to residents.

Nurses influence the quality of care provided for long-term care residents in a variety of ways.

Some of their major responsibilities include the following:

Assist residents and their families in the selection and adjustment to the facility.

Assess and develop an individualized care plan based on assessment data.

Monitor residents' health status.

Incorporate rehabilitative and restorative care techniques as possible.

Evaluate the effectiveness and appropriateness of care.

Identify changes in residents' conditions.

Communicate and coordinate care with the interdisciplinary team.

Protect residents' rights.

Promote a high quality of life for residents.

Unlike many other clinical settings, the average long-term care facility does not have physicians and other professionals on-site at all times. Although this places a greater burden on nurses for assessment and management of problems, it does offer the opportunity for nurses to function independently and use a wide range of knowledge and skills. The independence of nursing practice and the ability to develop long-term relationships with residents and their families are among the exciting features of nursing in this setting.

Hospitals

Older adults can be patients on virtually all acute hospital services except pediatrics and obstetrics. Although the diagnostic problem or procedure for which they seek care from the hospital will dictate many of their service needs, the following are some basic measures that should be considered in caring for older patients:

Perform a comprehensive assessment. It is not uncommon for the patient's diagnostic problem to be the primary and sometimes only concern during the hospitalization. However, the patient being treated for a myocardial infarction or hernia also may show depression, caregiver stress, hearing deficit, or other problems that significantly affect health status. By capitalizing on the contact with the patient during a hospitalization and conducting a comprehensive evaluation, nurses can reveal risks and problems that affect health status and may not have been detected before. Broader problems, other than those for which the patient was admitted to the hospital, should be explored.

Recognize differences. Older patients are not the same as younger individuals. Different norms may be used to interpret laboratory tests and clinical findings. The signs and symptoms of disease can appear atypically. More time is needed for care activities. Drug dosages must be adjusted. The priorities of older patients can differ from those of younger patients. Nurses must be able to differentiate normal from pathology in older adults and understand the adjustments that must be made in caring for this population.

Reduce risks. The hospital experience can be traumatic for older patients if special protection is not afforded. The elderly require more time to recover from stress; therefore, procedures and activities must be planned to provide adequate rest. Altered function of major systems and decreased immunity make it easy for infections to develop. Reduced ability of the heart to manage major shifts in fluid load demand close monitoring of intravenous infusion rates. Lower normal body temperature, the lack of shivering, and reduced capacity to adapt to severe changes in environmental temperature require that older patients receive special protection against hypothermia. Differences in pharmacodynamics and pharmacokinetics in the elderly alter their response to medications and heighten the need for close monitoring of drug therapy. The strange environment, sensory deficits, and effects of illness and medications cause falls to occur more easily and make injury prevention a priority. Confusion often emerges as a primary sign of a complication, challenging staff to detect this disorder promptly and identify its cause. Nurses should ensure that measures are taken to reduce patients' risks and recognize complications promptly when they do occur.

Maintain and promote function. Priorities addressing the primary reason for admission usually take the forefront during a patient's hospitalization. For example, the arrhythmia must be corrected, the infection controlled, the fracture realigned. In the midst of diagnostic procedures and treatment activities, consideration of factors that will ensure the patient's optimal function and independence

can be lost. Although management of the acute problem is an urgent goal, the maintenance and promotion of functional abilities are significantly important. An injustice is done to the patient if ambulation is threatened due to imposed immobility during the hospitalization, continence is lost due to the unnecessary insertion of a catheter, or self-care deficits arise due to staff's perception that the patient may not be able to perform activities competently or quickly enough. Functional ability should be assessed, maintained, and, if possible, increased (see Chap. 34).

Prepare for discharge early. Promoting and maintaining function is part of assisting the patient with discharge from the health-care facility. Throughout the hospitalization, the patient should be instructed in the procedures that will need to be performed, the medications that must be administered, and any special measures that should be followed. This information should be reinforced, and opportunities provided for return demonstrations and evaluation of the patient's knowledge. As needed, family members or other caregivers who will assist the patient after discharge should be included in the instruction. Referrals for other service needs (*e.g.*, financial aid, participation in adult day care, housing, home health care) should be generated as early in the hospital stay as possible (see Chap. 40). With the shorter length of hospital stays and brief notice that often accompanies discharge, early preparation is crucial to avoid overloading the older patient with information at the time of discharge from the health-care facility.

Nurses can practice and advance gerontological nursing in the hospital setting through a variety of roles. Increasingly, clinical specialists in gerontological nursing provide consultation, leadership, and selected intervention to hospital staff. Subspecialization of gerontological clinical specialists is emerging through roles such as the geriatric nurse rehabilitation specialist and geropsychiatric nurse specialist. Staff development educators can have an impact on gerontological care by providing educational experiences that enhance knowledge about aging and geriatric care, compiling a library of resources relevant to the care of older patients, and communicating to staff current research and legislative activities pertaining to older adults. Of course, all nurses who have direct contact with older patients can demonstrate gerontological nursing expertise in their specialized approach to the care of the aging and aged.

Home Health

Home health nursing frequently makes the difference between older adults remaining independent in the community or requiring institutional care. Home health nurses serve as care providers, motivators, teachers, counselors, and advocates for older adults; they also function as advisors, respite providers, and tremendous sources of support for family caregivers. Some responsibilities that home health nurses fulfill with older patients include the following:

Increase self-care capacity. By promoting positive health practices, instructing in care techniques, and arranging for the use of adaptive/assistive equipment, nurses can minimize or eliminate patients' self-care deficits.

Perform environmental assessment and modification. Features of the home environment can enhance or prohibit independent living. Home health nurses need to evaluate home safety, state of repair, cleanliness, ease of use, and accessibility of kitchens, bathrooms, telephones, laundry facilities, and frequently used items. Nurses may recommend the need for correction of an electrical problem, educate patients about safe food storage, or advise family members in alternate ways to arrange furniture to accommodate disabilities of patients. Referrals to low-cost home-repair services or better housing may be warranted.

Coordinate with the health team. Home health nurses are a vital link between patients and their professional caregivers. Nurses must be aware of changes in status and the need for revision of the care plan and communicate this information to other disciplines involved in patients' care. In addition, nurses can reinforce and explain the care prescribed by other disciplines to promote patients' compliance.

Monitor family health. Many older patients are assisted in home care by family caregivers. Caregiving can be a challenging, stressful task

for family members and can threaten their physical, emotional, and socioeconomic well-being. Home health nurses must assess the family's caregiving capabilities, guide family members in realistically evaluating their capacities for home care, instruct caregivers in the performance of specific procedures and tasks, inform families of resources that can ease their caregiving burdens, encourage the use of respite services, monitor the ongoing ability of family caregivers to provide necessary care, and identify risks to the health status of patients and family caregivers that arise from the caregiving experience (*e.g.,* elder abuse associated with caregiver burnout, declining health of the caregiver arising from the physical care demands of the patient). Home health nurses are in an ideal position to assess the impact of a patient's health on the total family unit. Often, family caregivers can more easily explore the use of alternative care measures if the recommendation comes from a health-care professional.

Provide a link with community resources. Home health nurses are aware of health and social services that can meet patients' specific needs, and can assist with referral of patients to these resources (see Chap. 40).

Educate about reimbursement benefits. Many health professionals become confused working through the maze of reimbursement policies and procedures, so it is not surprising that many older patients have difficulty understanding insurance coverages. Home health nurses are in an ideal position to educate patients about services that are covered or excluded from insurance policies. Further, nurses can prevent unnecessary expenditures for older patients by reviewing their policies and ensuring that they are not paying for duplicate or unnecessary insurance.

Home health nursing services can be provided for a limited period, until health status and self-care capacity improve, or on a long-term basis. Because alterations in the status of medical problems, response to therapy, and self-care capacity are likely to change in older patients, nurses are challenged with regularly evaluating the appropriateness of home health care and arranging for other services as needed.

Adult Day Care

Although adult day care has existed in various forms for several decades, recent years have seen a dramatic growth in the number of these programs for older adults. Adult day care is a program that helps people with physical or mental impairments remain in the community. The typical program arranges for or provides transportation to the center, offers activities to promote socialization, monitors health problems, supervises or provides medication administration, and assists participants with the use of other resources. Families are afforded respite while participants are in attendance.

As adult day care has shifted from a social to health focus, the need for nursing services in these programs has grown. Day care nurses assess and monitor health status, provide education to participants and their families, locate and refer to services that can further assist participants, support, and counsel. Regular communication between day-care nurses and participants' physicians facilitates compliance with prescribed measures and evaluation of the effectiveness of these measures.

Continued-Care Communities

Retirement and life-care communities are growing throughout the country in response to the increased number of elderly who wish to maintain independent living in a supervised environment and have the financial means to do so. For a fee, residents purchase housing and a variety of other services, which could include meals, health-care services, housekeeping, laundry, recreational activities, transportation, and long-term care. Because each community differs in the resident population and services offered, nurses are developing unique roles in various communities. Some of the services nurses can provide in these settings include the following:

Initially assess for appropriateness of placement and identification of service needs.
Periodically reassess for appropriateness of living arrangements and service needs.
Monitor health problems and self-care ability.
Recognize problems such as isolation, depression, malnutrition, and cognitive alterations.
Provide health-screening programs.
Educate and counsel.

Resources of Interest to Gerontological Nurses in Diverse Settings

GENERAL

American Association of Retired Persons
1909 K St., N.W.
Washington, DC 20049
(202)872-4700

American Geriatrics Society
770 Lexington Ave., Suite 400
New York, NY 10021
(212)308-1414

American Health Care Association
1200 15th St., N.W.
Washington, DC 20005
(202)833-2050

American Nurses Association, Inc.
Council on Gerontological Nursing
2420 Pershing Rd.
Kansas City, MO 64108

American Society on Aging
833 Market St., Suite 512
San Francisco, CA 94103
(415)543-2617

Association for Gerontology in Higher Education
600 Maryland Ave., S.W.
West Wing 204
Washington, DC 20024
(202)484-7505

Design for Aging
American Institute of Architects
1735 New York Ave., N.W.
Washington, DC 20006

Gerontology Society of America
1411 K St., N.W.
Suite 300
Washington, DC 20005
(202)393-1411

National Association for Spanish Speaking Elderly
2025 I St., N.W.
Suite 219
Washington, DC 20006
(202)293-9329

National Caucus of the Black Aged
1424 K St., N.W.
Suite 500
Washington, DC 20005
(202)797-8227

National Council on the Aging, Inc.
600 Maryland Ave., S.W.
West Wing 100
Washington, DC 20024

National Council on Senior Citizens
925 15th St., N.W.
Washington, DC 20005

National Gerontological Nursing Association
11501 Georgia Ave.
Suite 203
Wheaton, MD 20902

National Hospice Organization
301 Maple Ave., West
Suite 506
Vienna, VA 22180
(703)938-4449

National Institute on Aging
9000 Rockville Pike
Bethesda, MD 21205
(301)496-1752

National Institute of Mental Health
Mental Disorders of Aging Research Branch
Room 11C-03
5600 Fishers Lane
Rockville, MD 20857
(301)443-1185

Older Women's League
1325 G St., N.W.
Lower Level B
Washington, DC 20005

Veterans Administration
810 Vermont Ave., N.W.
Washington, DC 20420
(202)233-4000

NURSING HOMES

American Association of Homes for the Aging
1129 20th St., N.W.
Suite 400
Washington, DC 20036
(202)296-5960

American College of Nursing Home
  Administrators
4650 East-West Highway
Washington, DC 20014

American Nurses Association, Inc.
Council on Nursing Home Nurses
2420 Pershing Rd.
Kansas City, MO 64108

National Association of Directors of Nursing
  Administration in Long Term Care
10999 Reed Hartman Hwy.
Suite 234
Cincinnati, OH 45242
(800)222-0539

HOME HEALTH/COMMUNITY HEALTH

American Public Health Association
Section on Gerontological Health
1015 18th St., N.W.
Washington, DC 20036

International Senior Citizens Association, Inc.
11753 Wilshire Blvd.
Los Angeles, CA 90025

National Association of Home Care
205 C St., N.E.
Washington, DC 20002

National Association of Home Health Agencies
426 C St., N.E.
Suite 200
Washington, DC 20002
(202)547-1717

National Association for Senior Living Industries
125 Cathedral St.
Annapolis, MD 21401

National Home Caring Council
235 Park Ave. South
New York, NY 10003

National League of Nursing
Council of Community Health Services
10 Columbus Circle
New York, NY 10019
(212)582-1022

ADULT DAY CARE

National Association of Adult Day Care
180 East 4050 South
Murray, UT 84107
(801)262-9167

National Institute on Adult Day Care
600 Maryland Ave., S.W.
Washington, DC 20024
(202)479-1200

SUPPORT GROUPS
(National headquarters that can direct inquiries to local chapters)

Alcoholics Anonymous World Services
P.O. Box 459
Grand Central Station
New York, NY 10017
(212)686-1100

Alzheimer's Disease and Related Disorders
  Association, Inc.
919 N. Michigan Ave.
Suite 1000
Chicago, IL 60611
(800)272-3900

American Diabetes Association
2 Park Ave.
New York, NY 10016
(212)683-7444

Arthritis Foundation
3400 Peachtree Rd.
Suite 1101
Atlanta, GA 30326
(404)266-0795

Asthma and Allergy Foundation of America
19 W. 44th St.
New York, NY 10036
(212)921-9100

Emphysema Anonymous
P.O. Box 66
Fort Myers, FL 33902
(813)334-4226

Make Today Count (cancer)
P.O. Box 303
Burlington, IA 52601
(319) 753-6521

Mended Hearts (heart surgery)
7320 Greenville Ave.
Dallas, TX 55231
(214)750-5442

National Huntington's Disease Association
128A East 74th St.
New York, NY 10021
(212)744-0302

National Multiple Sclerosis Society
205 E. 42nd St.
New York, NY 10017
(212)986-3240

Continued on next page

Parkinson's Disease Foundation
William Black Medical Research Bldg.
640-650 W. 168th St.
New York, NY 10032
(212)923-4700

Phoenix Society (burn victims)
11 Rust Hill Rd.
Levittown, PA 19056
(215)946-4788

United Ostomy Association
2001 W. Beverly Blvd.
Los Angeles, CA 90057
(213)413-5510

Nurses also serve as advocates for the older residents by ensuring that residents are included in planning and decision-making and that their rights are respected.

Support Groups

Support groups exist to assist patients and their families with a wide range of health problems. Alzheimer disease, widowhood, mastectomy, and ostomy are among the themes of some of these groups in which persons meet to learn from and help each other cope with their shared problem. Nurses function in support groups to provide the following services:

> Identify the need for a support group and stimulate its development.
> Lead or facilitate the leadership of the group.
> Increase the community's awareness of the group and its purpose.
> Provide education, support, and counseling.

By combining group leadership skills with the broad knowledge base they already possess, nurses can serve as important resources in support groups.

Senior Centers

Community senior citizen centers are sites that attract independent elderly people for socialization experiences and, sometimes, congregate meals. These individuals benefit from nursing services that assist them in optimizing their self-care abilities, and nurses meet this demand by providing health screening, education, and monitoring of health problems. Regular consultation and health checks by the nurse can prevent small problems from becoming major ones.

This discussion has barely scratched the surface of various types of gerontological nursing practice. Gerontological nursing is an exciting, challenging specialty that offers nurses a rare opportunity to create and develop innovative roles in a wide range of clinical settings. The Resources List presents numerous groups with information available for the gerontological nurse. Also, with many of the health problems of the elderly falling within the realm of nursing to diagnose and manage, gerontological nursing can provide independence in practice that few other clinical specialties can afford. It is indeed an exciting time to be part of this growing specialty!

Recommended Readings

Brooke V. Nursing home life: your helping hand. Geriatr Nurs 1989;10(3):126.

Burns-Tisdale S, Goff W. The geriatric nurse practitioner in home care: challenges, stressors, and rewards. Nurs Clin North Am 1989; 24:809.

DeWitt SC, Matre M. Nursing careers working with the elderly. West J Nurs Res 1988;10:335.

Eliopoulos C, ed. Caring for the elderly in diverse care settings. Philadelphia: JB Lippincott, 1990.

Eliopoulos C. Caring for the nursing home patient: clinical and managerial challenges for nurses. Rockville, MD: Aspen, 1989.

Fulmer TT, Walker MK. Lessons from the elder boom in ICUs. Geriatr Nurs 1990:11:120.

Mezey MD, Lynaugh JE, Cartier MM, eds. Nursing homes and nursing care: lessons from the teaching nursing home. New York: Springer-Verlag, 1989.

Naylor MD. Comprehensive discharge planning for hospitalized elderly: a pilot study. Nurs Res 1990;39:156.

Oliver DB, Tureman S. The human factor in nursing home care. Binghamton, NY: Haworth, 1988.

Resnick BM. Care for life. Geriatr Nurs 1989;10(3):130.

42

Challenges of the Future

Historically, nursing has always carried a significant responsibility for geriatric care. Long before it was popular or profitable for other disciplines to become involved in this specialty, nursing personnel were the major caregivers to the elderly. However, on close examination, it can be noted that the power and leadership of the nursing profession in the gerontological care arena did not equal the responsibility and workload assumed. Not only did health professionals other than nurses influence the course of this specialty, but persons with no health background whatsoever influenced geriatric services. The tales are many: entrepreneurs who become millionaires by owning substandard nursing homes, bureaucrats who developed policies with no understanding of their clinical impact, and reimbursement programs that favored highly technical acute services over the chronic and rehabilitative ones that were most needed. Rather than aggressively lobbying to effect changes that could have made long-term care settings more attractive to fine nurses, the nursing community harbored sentiments that nurses who were employed in institutional settings were inferior to the rest. Schools of nursing not only omitted gerontological nursing courses in their programs but also did little to bridge the severe gap between the significant educational and research needs of geriatric-care settings and academic resources. One must wonder why gerontological nurses were not entrepreneurial enough to own and control nursing homes and

other service agencies, why they allowed others to mandate practices that diluted quality nursing care, and why they were not assertive enough to demand that their colleagues be constructive problem-solvers rather than critics of the status of geriatric care. Whatever the reasons, one thing is certain: gerontological nursing must never take a back seat to other specialities again.

Since gerontological nurses have begun to advocate advancement of the specialty, tremendous advances have been made. Dynamic professionals are selecting gerontological nursing as a specialty that offers a multitude of opportunities to use a wide range of knowledge and skills and presents many problems that can be independently addressed within the realm of nursing practice. Excellent research for and by nurses is growing to provide a strong scientific foundation for practice. Increasing numbers of nursing schools are adding specialization in gerontological nursing. New opportunities for gerontological nurses to develop practice models are emerging in acute hospitals, health maintenance organizations, life-care communities, adult day care, and other settings. The future of gerontological nursing is challenging and exciting.

Research

The growing complexity of and demand for gerontological nursing services are exciting and challenging, but they are accompanied by the require-

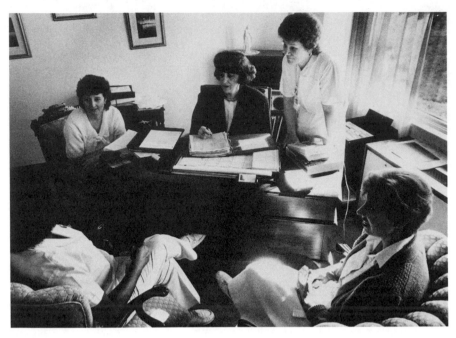

Opportunities for gerontological nurses to develop new practice models are emerging in a variety of settings. (Photograph by Eric Schenk.)

ment for a strong knowledge base on which those services can be built. There is no room for the trial and error that flavored nursing actions in the past: the elderly's delicately balanced health status and lower margin for error, increased consumer expectations, the risk of litigation, and the requisites of being a professional demand scientific foundations for nursing practice. Fine nursing research is being conducted on a variety of issues, and gerontological nurses must encourage and support these efforts through the following actions:

Learn about and communicate with nurse researchers. Local academic institutions, teaching hospitals, and nursing homes may be conducting research that can be relevant to various geriatric settings or in which a service agency can participate. Those researchers can be important resources by meshing their research skills with a service setting to solve clinical problems.

Support research efforts. Support of research comes in many forms. As funding is being sought for research projects, letters of support and testimony can help funding agen-

cies understand the full benefit of the effort. Regular contact with leaders who influence the allocation of funds can provide opportunities to educate those persons on the value of supporting research. No less significant to the support of research efforts is the assurance that protocols be followed. The efforts of researchers can be facilitated or thwarted by colleagues in clinical settings.

Keep abreast of new findings. Gerontological nursing knowledge is continuously expanding, disproving past beliefs and offering insights never before considered. Independent study, formal courses, and continuing education programs are among the mechanisms that nurses can use to keep current. Equally important to acquiring knowledge is implementing it to improve the care of older adults.

Education

Be it the nursing director, a family member who delivers personal care to an elderly relative, a health aide who has more frequent contact with

the patient than the professional nurse, or the physician who only occasionally has an older person in the caseload, caregivers at every level require competency in providing services to the elderly. Gerontological nurses can influence the education of caregivers by doing the following:

Assist nursing schools in identifying relevant issues for inclusion in curricula.

Participate in classroom and field experience of students.

Evaluate educational deficits of personnel and planning education experiences to eliminate deficits.

Promote interdisciplinary team conferences.

Attend and participate in continuing education programs.

Read current nursing literature and share information with colleagues.

Serve as a role model by demonstrating current practices.

With increasing numbers of family members providing more complex care in the home setting than ever before, it is essential that the education of this group not be overlooked. It should not be assumed that because the family has had contact with other providers or has been providing care that they are knowledgeable in correct care techniques. Their knowledge and skills must be evaluated and reinforced periodically.

Developing New Roles

As geriatric subspecialties and settings for care grow, so will the opportunities for nurses to carve new roles for themselves. Nurses can demonstrate creativity and leadership as they break from traditional roles and settings and develop new models of practice, which may include the following:

- geropsychiatric nurse specialist in the nursing home setting
- case manager for community-based chronically ill patients
- preadmission assessor for hospitals
- owner/director of elder women's health-care center, geriatric day-care program, respite agency, caregiver training center
- preretirement counselor/educator for industry
- consultant/educator/case manager for geriatric surgical patients.

This list only begins to describe opportunities awaiting gerontological nurses. It will be important for gerontological nurses to identify nontraditional roles, approach them creatively, test innovative practice models, and share their successes and failures with colleagues to aid them in their development of new roles. Nurses must appreciate that their knowledge of biopsychosocial sciences, clinical competencies, and human-relations skills gives them a strong competitive edge over other disciplines in affecting a wide range of services.

Balancing Priorities

The growing number of older adults in society is placing demands for greater amounts and diversity of services than ever before. At the same time, third-party reimbursers are trying to control the constantly escalating cost of services. Earlier hospital discharges, limited home health visits, more complex nursing-home patients, and greater out-of-pocket payment for services by patients demonstrate some of the effects of changes in reimbursement policy. Some health care professionals suspect that, as a result of these changes, patients are discharged from hospitals prematurely and suffer greater adverse consequences, nursing homes are confronting patients with complex problems for whom they are not adequately prepared or staffed, families are being strained by considerable caregiving burdens, and patients are being deprived of needed but unaffordable services. Such charges are disconcerting and may cause nurses to feel overwhelmed, frustrated, or dissatisfied. Unfortunately, more cost-cutting is likely to occur. Rather than experience burnout or consider a change in occupation, nurses should become involved in cost-containment efforts so that a balance between quality services and budgetary concerns can be achieved. Efforts toward this goal can include the following:

Test creative staffing patterns. Maybe six nurses can be more productive than three nurses and six nonprofessionals. Perhaps some of the high nonproductive time costs associated with nonprofessionals is related to poor hiring and supervision practices; improved management techniques may increase the cost-effectiveness of these workers.

Use lay caregivers. Neighbors assisting each other, a family member rooming-in during hospitalizations, and other methods to increase the resources available for service provision can be explored.

Drop ritual practices. Why must nurses spend time administering medications to patients who have successfully administered them before admission and who will continue to administer them after discharge, or take vital signs every 4 hours on patients who have shown no abnormalities, or bathe all patients on the same schedule regardless of skin condition or state of cleanliness, or rewrite assessments and care plans at specified intervals regardless of the patient's changes or stability? Often regulations and policies are developed under the assumption that, without them, the vital signs would never be taken, baths would not be given, and other facets of care would not be completed. Perhaps the time has come for nurses to aggressively convince others that nurses have the professional judgment to determine the need for and frequency of assessment, care planning, and care delivery.

Ensure safe care. The implementation of cost-containment efforts should be accompanied by concurrent studies of the impact on rates of complications; readmissions; incidents; consumer satisfaction; and staff turnover, absenteeism, and morale. Specific numbers and documented cases carry more weight than broad criticisms or complaints that care is suffering.

Advocate for older adults. The priorities of society and professions change. History shows us that at different times the spotlight has focused on various underserved groups, such as children, pregnant women, the mentally ill, the handicapped, substance abusers, and, most recently, the aged. As interests and priorities shift to new groups, gerontological nurses must make certain that the needs of the elderly are not forgotten or shortchanged.

As gerontological nursing continues to shed its obscure image of a less than *bona fide* specialty for less than competent nurses and fully emerges as the dynamic, multifaceted, and opportunity-filled form of nursing that it is, it will be seen that this is a specialty for the finest talent the profession has to offer. Gerontological nursing has just begun to show its true potential.

Appendix

APPENDIX MINIMUM DATA SET FOR NURSING HOME RESIDENT ASSESSMENT AND CARE SCREENING (MDS)

(Status in last 7 days, unless other time frame indicated)

SECTION A. IDENTIFICATION AND BACKGROUND INFORMATION

1.	ASSESSMENT DATE	Month — Day — Year
2.	RESIDENT NAME	(First) (Middle Initial) (Last)
3.	SOCIAL SECURITY NO.	— —
4.	MEDICAID NO. (if applicable)	
5.	MEDICAL RECORD NO.	
6.	REASON FOR ASSESS-MENT	1. Initial admission assess. 2. Hosp/Medicare reassess. 3. Readmission assessment 4. Annual assessment 5. Significant change in status 6. Other (e.g., UR)
7.	CURRENT PAYMENT SOURCE(S) FOR N.H. STAY	*(Billing Office to indicate; check all that apply)* Medicaid a. Medicare b. CHAMPUS c. VA d. Self pay/Private insurance e. Other f.
8.	RESPONSI-BILITY/ LEGAL GUARDIAN	*(Check all that apply)* Legal guardian a. Other legal oversight b. Durable power attrny./health care proxy c. Family member responsible d. Resident responsible e. *NONE OF ABOVE* f.
9.	ADVANCED DIRECTIVES	*(For those items with supporting documentation in the medical record, check all that apply)* Living will a. Do not resuscitate b. Do not hospitalize c. Organ donation d. Autopsy request e. Feeding restrictions f. Medication restrictions g. Other treatment restrictions h. *NONE OF ABOVE* i.
10.	DISCHARGE PLANNED WITHIN 3 MOS.	*(Does not include discharge due to death)* 0. No 1. Yes 2. Unknown/uncertain
11.	PARTICIPATE IN ASSESS-MENT	a. Resident 0. No 1. Yes a. b. Family 0. No 1. Yes 2. No family b.
12.	SIGNATURES	Signature of RN Assessment Coordinator Signatures of Others Who Completed Part of the Assessment

SECTION B. COGNITIVE PATTERNS

1.	COMATOSE	*(Persistent vegetative state/no discernible consciousness)* 0. No 1. Yes *(Skip to SECTION E)*
2.	MEMORY	*(Recall of what was learned or known)* a. Short-term memory OK—seems/appears to recall after 5 minutes 0. Memory OK 1. Memory problem a. b. Long-term memory OK—seems/appears to recall long past 0. Memory OK 1. Memory problem b.
3.	MEMORY/ RECALL ABILITY	*(Check all that resident normally able to recall during last 7 days)* Current season a. Location of own room b. Staff names/faces c. That he/she is in a nursing home d. NONE OF ABOVE are recalled e.
4.	COGNITIVE SKILLS FOR DAILY DECISION-MAKING	*(Made decisions regarding tasks of daily life)* 0. Independent—decisions consistent/reasonable 1. Modified independence—some difficulty in new situations only 2. Moderately impaired—decisions poor; cues/supervision required 3. Severely impaired—never/rarely made decisions
5.	INDICATORS OF DELIRIUM —PERIODIC DISORDERED THINKING/ AWARENESS	*(Check if condition over last 7 days appears different from usual functioning)* Less alert, easily distracted a. Changing awareness of environment b. Episodes of incoherent speech c. Periods of motor restlessness or lethargy d. Cognitive ability varies over course of day e. *NONE OF ABOVE* f.
6.	CHANGE IN COGNITIVE STATUS	Change in resident's cognitive status, skills, or abilities in last 90 days 0. No change 1. Improved 2. Deteriorated

SECTION C. COMMUNICATION/HEARING PATTERNS

1.	HEARING	*(With hearing appliances, if used)* 0. Hears adequately—normal talk, TV, phone 1. Minimal difficulty when not in quiet setting 2. Hears in special situations only—speaker has to adjust tonal quality and speak distinctly 3. Highly impaired/absence of useful hearing
2.	COMMUNI-CATION DEVICES/ TECHNIQUES	*(Check all that apply during last 7 days)* Hearing aid, present and used a. Hearing aid, present and not used b. Other receptive comm. techniques used (e.g., lip read) c. *NONE OF ABOVE* d.
3.	MODES OF EXPRESSION	*(Check all used by resident to make needs known)* Speech a. Writing messages to express or clarify needs b. Signs/gestures/sounds c. Communication board d. Other e. *NONE OF ABOVE* f.
4.	MAKING SELF UNDER-STOOD	*(Express information content—however able)* 0. Understood 1. Usually Understood—difficulty finding words or finishing thoughts 2. Sometimes Understood—ability is limited to making concrete requests 3. Rarely/Never Understood
5.	ABILITY TO UNDER-STAND OTHERS	*(Understanding verbal information content—however able)* 0. Understands 1. Usually Understands—may miss some part/intent of message 2. Sometimes Understands—responds adequately to simple, direct communication 3. Rarely/Never Understands
6.	CHANGE IN COMMUNI-CATION/ HEARING	Resident's ability to express, understand or hear information has changed over last 90 days 0. No change 1. Improved 2. Deteriorated

SECTION D. VISION PATTERNS

1.	VISION	*(Ability to see in adequate light and with glasses if used)* 0. Adequate—sees fine detail, including regular print in newspapers/books 1. Impaired—sees large print, but not regular print in newspapers/books 2. Highly impaired—limited vision; not able to see newspaper headlines; appears to follow objects with eyes 3. Severely impaired—no vision or appears to see only light, colors, or shapes
2.	VISUAL LIMITATIONS/ DIFFICULTIES	Side vision problems—decreased peripheral vision (e.g., leaves food on one side of tray, difficulty traveling, bumps into people and objects, misjudges placement of chair when seating self) a. Experiences any of following: sees halos or rings around lights; sees flashes of light; sees "curtains" over eyes b. *NONE OF ABOVE* c.
3.	VISUAL APPLIANCES	Glasses; contact lenses; lens implant; magnifying glass 0. No 1. Yes

▒ = Code the appropriate response ☐ = Check all the responses that apply

Source: Health Care Financing Administration

(Continued)

SECTION E. PHYSICAL FUNCTIONING AND STRUCTURAL PROBLEMS

1. ADL SELF-PERFORMANCE — *(Code for resident's PERFORMANCE OVER ALL SHIFTS during last 7 days—Not including setup)*

0. *INDEPENDENT* — No help or oversight — OR — Help/oversight provided only 1 or 2 times during last 7 days

1. *SUPERVISION* — Oversight, encouragement or cueing provided 3+ times during last 7 days — OR — Supervision plus physical assistance provided only 1 or 2 times during last 7 days

2. *LIMITED ASSISTANCE* — Resident highly involved in activity; received physical help in guided maneuvering of limbs or other nonweight bearing assistance 3+ times — OR — More help provided only 1 or 2 times during last 7 days

3. *EXTENSIVE ASSISTANCE* — While resident performed part of activity, over last 7-day period, help of following types(s) provided 3 or more times:
— Weight-bearing support
— Full staff performance during part (but not all) of last 7 days

4. *TOTAL DEPENDENCE* — Full staff performance of activity during entire 7 days

2. ADL SUPPORT PROVIDED — *(Code for MOST SUPPORT PROVIDED OVER ALL SHIFTS during last 7 days; code regardless of resident's self-performance classification)*

0. No setup or physical help from staff
1. Setup help only
2. One-person physical assist
3. Two+ persons physical assist

			(1) SELF-PERF.	(2) SUPPORT
a.	BED MOBILITY	How resident moves to and from lying position, turns side to side, and positions body while in bed		
b.	TRANSFER	How resident moves between surfaces—to/from: bed, chair, wheelchair, standing position (EXCLUDE to/from bath/toilet)		
c.	LOCO-MOTION	How resident moves between locations in his/her room and adjacent corridor on same floor. If in wheelchair, self-sufficiency once in chair		
d.	DRESSING	How resident puts on, fastens, and takes off all items of street clothing, including donning/removing prosthesis		
e.	EATING	How resident eats and drinks (regardless of skill)		
f.	TOILET USE	How resident uses the toilet room (or commode, bedpan, urinal); transfer on/off toilet, cleanses, changes pad, manages ostomy or catheter, adjusts clothes		
g.	PERSONAL HYGIENE	How resident maintains personal hygiene, including combing hair, brushing teeth, shaving, applying makeup, washing/drying face, hands, and perineum (EXCLUDE baths and showers)		

3. BATHING — How resident takes full-body bath/shower, sponge bath, and transfers in/out of tub/shower (EXCLUDE washing of back and hair. *Code for most dependent in self-performance and support*. Bathing Self-Performance codes appear below).

0. Independent—No help provided
1. Supervision—Oversight help only
2. Physical help limited to transfer only
3. Physical help in part of bathing activity
4. Total dependence

a.	b.

4. BODY CONTROL PROBLEMS — *(Check all that apply during last 7 days)*

Balance—partial or total loss of ability to balance self while standing	a.
Bedfast all or most of the time	b.
Contracture to arms, legs shoulders, or hands	c.
Hemiplegia/hemi-paresis	d.
Quadriplegia	e.
Arm—partial or total loss of voluntary movement	f.
Hand—lack of dexterity (e.g., problem using toothbrush or adjusting hearing aid)	g.
Leg—partial or total loss of voluntary movement	h.
Leg—unsteady gait	i.
Trunk—partial or total loss of ability to position, balance, or turn body	j.
Amputation	k.
NONE OF ABOVE	l.

5. MOBILITY APPLIANCES/DEVICES — *(Check all that apply during last 7 days)*

Cane/walker	a.	Other person wheeled	d.
Brace/prothesis	b.	Lifted (manually/ mechanically)	e.
Wheeled self	c.	NONE OF ABOVE	f.

6. TASK SEG-MENTATION — Resident requires that some or all of ADL activities be broken into a series of subtasks so that resident can perform them.

0. No.   1. Yes

7. ADL FUNCTIONAL REHABILI-TATION POTENTIAL

Resident believes he/she capable of increased independence in at least some ADLs	a.
Direct care staff believe resident capable of increased independence in at least some ADLs	b.
Resident able to perform tasks/activity but is very slow	c.
Major difference in ADL Self-Performance or ADL Support in mornings and evenings (at least a one category change in Self-Performance or Support in any ADL)	d.
NONE OF ABOVE	e.

8. CHANGE IN ADL FUNCTION — Change in ADL self-performance in last 90 days

0. No Change   1. Improved   2. Deteriorated

SECTION F. CONTINENCE IN LAST 14 DAYS

1. CONTINENCE SELF-CONTROL CATEGORIES *(Code for resident performance over all shifts)*

0. CONTINENT — Complete control
1. USUALLY CONTINENT — BLADDER, incontinent episodes once a week or less; BOWEL, less than weekly
2. OCCASIONALLY INCONTINENT — BLADDER, 2+ times a week but not daily; BOWEL, once a week
3. FREQUENTLY INCONTINENT — BLADDER, tended to be incontinent daily, but some control present (e.g., on day shift); BOWEL, 2-3 times a week.
4. INCONTINENT — Had inadequate control. BLADDER, multiple daily episodes; BOWEL, all (or almost all) of the time

a.	BOWEL CONTINENCE	Control of bowel movement, with appliance or bowel continence programs, if employed	
b.	BLADDER CONTINENCE	Control of urinary bladder function (if dribbles, volume insufficient to soak through underpants), with appliances (e.g., foley) or continence programs, if employed	

2. INCONTI-NENCE RELATED TESTING *(Skip if resident's bladder continence code equals 0 or 1 AND no catheter is used.)*

Resident has been tested for a urinary tract infection	a.
Resident has been checked for presence of a fecal impaction, or there is adequate bowel elimination	b.
NONE OF ABOVE	c.

3. APPLIANCES AND PROGRAMS

Any scheduled toileting plan	a.	Pads/briefs used	f.
External (condom) catheter	b.	Enemas/irrigation	g.
Indwelling catheter	c.	Ostomy	h.
Intermittent catheter	d.	NONE OF ABOVE	i.
Did not use toilet room/ commode/urinal	e.		

4. CHANGE IN URINARY CONTINENCE — Change in urinary continence/appliances and programs in last 90 days

0. No change   1. Improved   2. Deteriorated

SECTION G. PHYCHOSOCIAL WELL-BEING

1. SENSE OF INITIATIVE/ INVOLVE-MENT

At ease interacting with others	a.
At ease doing planned or structural activities	b.
At ease doing self-initiated activities	c.
Establishes own goals	d.
Pursues involvement in life of facility (e.g., makes/keeps friends; involved in group activities; responds positively to new activities; assists at religious services)	e.
Accepts invitations into most group activities	f.
NONE OF ABOVE	g.

2. UNSETTLED RELATION-SHIPS

Covert/open conflict with and/or repeated criticism of staff	a.
Unhappy with roommate	b.
Unhappy with residents other than roommate	c.
Openly expresses conflict/anger with family or friends	d.
Absence of personal contact with family/friends	e.
Recent loss of close family member/friend	f.
NONE OF ABOVE	g.

3. PAST ROLES

Strong identification with past roles and life status	a.
Expresses sadness/anger/empty feeling over lost roles/status	b.
NONE OF ABOVE	c.

SECTION H. MOOD AND BEHAVIOR PATTERNS

1.	SAD OR ANXIOUS MOOD	*(Check all that apply during last 30 days)*	
		VERBAL EXPRESSIONS of DISTRESS by resident (sadness, sense that nothing matters, hopelessness, worthlessness, unrealistic fears, vocal expressions of anxiety or grief)	a.
		DEMONSTRATED (OBSERVABLE) SIGNS of mental DISTRESS	
		—Tearfulness, emotional groaning, sighing, breathlessness	b.
		—Motor agitation such as pacing, handwringing or picking	c.
		—Failure to eat or take medications, withdrawal from self-care or leisure activities	d.
		—Pervasive concern with health	e.
		—Recurrent thoughts of death — e.g., believes he/she about to die, have a heart attack	f.
		—Suicidal thoughts/actions	g.
		NONE OF ABOVE	h.
2.	MOOD PER-SISTENCE	Sad or anxious mood intrudes on daily life over last 7 days — not easily altered, doesn't "cheer up" 0. No 1. Yes	
3.	PROBLEM BEHAVIOR	*(Code for behavior in last 7 days)* 0. Behavior not exhibited in last 7 days 1. Behavior of this type occurred less than daily 2. Behavior of this type occurred daily or more frequently	
		WANDERING (moved with no rational purpose, seemingly oblivious to needs or safety)	a.
		VERBALLY ABUSIVE (others were threatened, screamed at, cursed at)	b.
		PHYSICALLY ABUSIVE (others were hit, shoved, scratched, sexually abused)	c.
		SOCIALLY INAPPROPRIATE/DISRUPTIVE BEHAVIOR (made disrupting sounds, noisy, screams, self-abusive acts, sexual behavior or disrobing in public, smeared/ threw food/feces, hoarding, rummaged through others' belongings)	d.
4.	RESIDENT RESISTS CARE	*(Check all types of resistance that occurred in the last 7 days)*	
		Resisted taking medications/injection	a.
		Resisted ADL assistance	b.
		NONE OF ABOVE	c.
5.	BEHAVIOR MANAGE-MENT PROGRAM	Behavior problem has been addressed by clinically developed behavior management program. (Note: Do not include programs that involve only physical restraints or psychotropic medications in this category) 0. No behavior problem 1. Yes, addressed 2. No, not addressed	
6.	CHANGE IN MOOD	Change in mood in last 90 days 0. No change 1. Improved 2. Deteriorated	
7.	CHANGE IN PROBLEM BEHAVIOR	Change in problem behavioral signs in last 90 days 0. No change 1. Improved 2. Deteriorated	

4.	GENERAL ACTIVITY PREFER-ENCES (adapted to resident's current abilities)	*(Check all PREFERENCES whether or not activity is currently available to resident)*			
		Cards/other games	a.	Spiritual/religious activities	f.
		Crafts/arts	b.	Trips/shopping	g.
		Exercise/sports	c.	Walking/wheeling outdoors	h.
		Music	d.	Watch TV	i.
		Read/write	e.	*NONE OF ABOVE*	j.
5.	PREFERS MORE OR DIFFERENT ACTIVITIES	Resident expresses/indicates preference for other activities/ choices 0. No 1. Yes			

SECTION J. DISEASE DIAGNOSES

Check only those diseases present that have a relationship to current ADL status, cognitive status, behavior status, medical treatments, or risk of death. (Do not list old/ inactive diagnoses.)

1.	DISEASES	*(If none apply, CHECK the NONE OF ABOVE box)*				
		HEART/CIRCULATION		PSYCHIATRIC/MOOD		
		Arteriosclerotic heart disease (ASHD)	a.	Anxiety disorder	p.
		Cardiac dysrhythmias	b.	Depression	q.
		Congestive heart failure	c.	Manic depressive (bipolar disease)	r.
		Hypertension	d.	SENSORY	
		Hypotension	e.	Cataracts	s.
		Peripheral vascular disease	f.	Glaucoma	t.
		Other cardiovascular disease	g.	OTHER	
		NEUROLOGICAL		Allergies	u.
		Alzheimer's	h.	Anemia	v.
		Dementia other than Alzheimer's	i.	Arthritis	w.
		Aphasia	j.	Cancer	x.
		Cerebrovascular accident (stroke)	k.	Diabetes melitus	y.
		Multiple sclerosis	l.	Explicit terminal prognosis	z.
		Parkinson's disease	m.	Hypothyroidism	aa.
		PULMONARY		Osteoporosis	bb.
		Emphysemia/Asthma COPD	n.	Seizure disorder	cc.
		Pneumonia	o.	Septicemia	dd.
				Urinary tract infection — in last 30 days	ee.
				NONE OF ABOVE	ff.
2.	OTHER CURRENT DIAGNOSES AND ICD-9 CODES	a. _____ b. _____ c. _____ d. _____ e. _____ f. _____				

SECTION I. ACTIVITY PURSUIT PATTERNS

1.	TIME AWAKE	*(Check appropriate time periods over last 7 days)* Resident awake all or most of time (i.e., naps no more than one hour per time period) in the:			
		Morning	a.	Evening	c.
		Afternoon	b.	*NONE OF ABOVE*	d.
2.	AVERAGE TIME INVOLVED IN ACTIVITIES	0. Most — more than 2/3 of time 2. Little—less than 1/3 of time 1. Some — 1/3 to 2/3 of time 3. None			
3.	PREFERRED ACTIVITY SETTINGS	*(Check all settings in which activities are preferred)*			
		Own room	a.	Outside facility	d.
		Day/activity room	b.	*NONE OF ABOVE*	e.
		Inside NH/off unit	c.		

SECTION K. HEALTH CONDITIONS

1.	PROBLEM CONDITIONS	*(Check all problems that are present in last 7 days unless other time frame indicated)*			
		Constipation	a.	Pain — resident complains or shows evidence of pain daily or almost daily	j.
		Diarrhea	b.		
		Dizziness/vertigo	c.		
		Edema	d.	Recurrent lung aspirations in last 90 days	k.
		Fecal impaction	e.	Shortness of breath	l.
		Fever	f.	Syncope (fainting)	m.
		Hallucinations/ delusions	g.	Vomiting	n.
		Internal bleeding	h.	*NONE OF ABOVE*	o.
		Joint pain	i.		
2.	ACCIDENTS	Fell in past 30 days	a.	Hip fracture in last 180 days	c.
		Fell in past 31-180 days	b.	*NONE OF ABOVE*	d.

3.	STABILITY OF CONDITIONS	Conditions/diseases make resident's cognitive, ADL, or behavior status unstable — fluctuating, precarious, or deteriorating	a.
		Resident experiencing an acute episode or a flare-up of a recurrent/chronic problem	b.
		NONE OF ABOVE	c.

SECTION L. ORAL/NUTRITIONAL STATUS

1.	ORAL PROBLEMS	Chewing problem	a.
		Swallowing problem	b.
		Mouth pain	c.
		NONE OF ABOVE	d.

| 2. | HEIGHT AND WEIGHT | *Record height (a.) in inches and weight (b.) in pounds. Weight based on most recent status in last 30 days; measure weight consistently in accord with standard facility practice — e.g., in a.m. after voiding, before meal, with shoes off, and in nightclothes.* HT (in.) [a.] WT (lb.) [b.] | |
| | | c. Weight loss (i.e., 5%+ in last 30 days; or 10% in last 180 days)   0. No   1. Yes | c. |

3.	NUTRITIONAL PROBLEMS	Complains about the taste of many foods [a.]	Regular complaint of hunger	d.
		Insufficient fluid; dehydrated [b.]	Leaves 25%+ food uneaten at most meals	e.
		Did NOT consume all/almost all liquids provided during last 3 days [c.]	*NONE OF ABOVE*	f.

4.	NUTRITIONAL APPROACHES	Parenteral/IV [a.]	Dietary supplement between meals	f.
		Feeding tube [b.]	Plate guard, stabilized built-up utensil, etc.	g.
		Mechanically altered diet [c.]	*NONE OF ABOVE*	h.
		Syringe (oral feeding) [d.]		
		Therapeutic diet [e.]		

SECTION M. ORAL/DENTAL STATUS

1.	ORAL STATUS AND DISEASE PREVENTION	Debris (soft, easily movable substance) present in mouth prior to going to bed at night	a.
		Has dentures and/or removable bridge	b.
		Some/all natural teeth lost — does not have or does not use dentures (or partial plates)	c.
		Broken, loose, or carious teeth	d.
		Inflamed gums (gingiva); swollen or bleeding gums; oral abscesses, ulcers or rashes	e.
		Daily cleaning of teeth/dentures	f.
		NONE OF ABOVE	g.

SECTION N. SKIN CONDITION

1.	STASIS ULCER	(open lesion caused by poor venous circulation to lower extremities) 0. No 1. Yes	
2.	PRESSURE ULCERS	*(Code for highest stage of pressure ulcer)* 0. No pressure ulcers 1. Stage 1 A persistent area of skin redness (without a break in the skin) that does not disappear when pressure is relieved 2. Stage 2 A partial thickness loss of skin layers that presents clinically as an abrasion, blister, or shallow crater 3. Stage 3 A full thickness of skin is lost, exposing the subcutaneous tissues — presents as a deep crater with or without undermining adjacent tissue 4. Stage 4 A full thickness of skin and subcutaneous tissue is lost, exposing muscle and/or bone	
3.	HISTORY OF RESOLVED/ CURED PRESSURE ULCERS	Resident has had a pressure ulcer that was resolved/cured in last 90 days 0. No 1. Yes	

4.	SKIN PROBLEMS/ CARE	Open lesions other than statis or pressure ulcers (e.g., cuts)	a.
		Skin desensitized to pain, pressure, discomfort	b.
		Protective/preventive skin care	c.
		Turing/repositioning program	d.
		Pressure relieving beds, bed/chair pads (e.g., egg crate pads)	e.
		Wound care/treatment (e.g., pressure ulcer care, surgical wound)	f.
		Other skin care/treatment	g.
		NONE OF ABOVE	h.

SECTION O. MEDICATION USE

1.	NUMBER OF MEDI- CATIONS	*(Record the number of different medications used in the last 7 days; enter "0" if none used)*	
2.	NEW MEDI- CATIONS	Resident has received new medications during the last 90 days 0. No 1. Yes	
3.	INJECTIONS	*(Record the number of days injections of any type received during the last 7 days)*	
4.	DAYS RECEIVED THE FOLLOWING MEDICATION	*(Record the number of days during last 7 days; enter "0" if not used; enter "1" if long-acting meds. used less than weekly)*	
		Antipsychotics	a.
		Antianxiety/hypnotics	b.
		Antidepressants	c.
5.	PREVIOUS MEDICATION RESULTS	*(SKIP this question if resident currently receiving antipsy-chotics, antidepressants, or antianxiety/hypnotics — otherwise code correct response for last 90 days)* Resident has previously received psychoactive medications for a mood or behavior problem, and these medications were effective (without undue adverse consequences) 0. No, drugs not used 1. Drugs were effective 2. Drugs were not effective 3. Drug effectivenss unknown	

SECTION P. SPECIAL TREATMENT AND PROCEDURES

1.	SPECIAL TREATMENTS AND PROCE- DURES	SPECIAL CARE — *Check treatments received during the last 14 days*				
		Chemotherapy	a.	IV meds	f.
		Radiation	b.	Transfusions	g.
		Dialysis	c.	O₂	h.
		Suctioning	d.	Other _____	i.
		Trach. care	e.	*NONE OF ABOVE*	j.
		THERAPIES — *Record the number of days each of the following therapies was administered (for at least 10 minutes during a day) in the last 7 days:*				
		Speech — language pathology and audiology services			k.
		Occupational therapy			l.
		Physical therapy			m.
		Psychological therapy (any licensed professional)			n.
		Respiratory therapy			o.
2.	ABNORMAL LAB VALUES	Has the resident had any abnormal lab values during the last 90-days? 0. No 1. Yes 2. No tests performed	
3.	DEVICES AND RESTRAINTS	*Use the following codes for last 7 days:* 0. Not used 1. Used less than daily 2. Used daily	
		Bed rails	a.
		Trunk restraint	b.
		Limb restraint	c.
		Chair prevents rising	d.

MDS QUARTERLY REVIEW

A2.	RESIDENT NAME			
		(First)	(Middle Initial)	(Last)

A3.	SOCIAL SECURITY NO.	☐☐☐ — ☐☐ — ☐☐☐☐

QUARTERS

| 1 | 2 | 3 |

B2.	MEMORY	*(Recall of what was learned or known)*			
		a. Short-term memory OK — seems/appears to recall after 5 minutes			
		0. Memory OK 1. Memory problem			
		b. Long-term memory OK — seems/appears to recall long past			
		0. Memory OK 1. Memory problem			

B4.	COGNITIVE SKILLS FOR DAILY DECISION-MAKING	*(Made decisions regarding tasks of daily life)*			
		0. Independent — decisions consistent/reasonable			
		1. Modified independence — some difficulty in new situations only			
		2. Moderately impaired — decisions poor; cues/supervision required			
		3. Severely impaired — never/rarely made decisions			

C4.	MAKING SELF UNDER-STOOD	*(Express information content — however able)*			
		0. Understood			
		1. Usually Understood — difficulty finding words or finishing thoughts			
		2. Sometimes Understood — ability is limited to making concrete requests			
		3. Rarely/Never Understood			

C5.	ABILITY TO UNDER-STAND OTHERS	*(Understanding verbal information content — however able)*			
		0. Understands			
		1. Usually Understands — may miss some part/intent of message			
		2. Sometimes Understands — responds adequately to simple, direct communication			
		3. Rarely/Never Understands			

E1.	ADL SELF-PERFORMANCE — *(Code for resident's PERFORMANCE OVER ALL SHIFTS during last 7 days — Not including setup)*
	0. *INDEPENDENT* — No help or oversight — OR — Help/oversight provided only 1 or 2 times during last 7 days
	1. *SUPERVISION* — Oversight, encouragement or cueing provided 3+ times during last 7 days — OR — Supervision plus physical assistance provided only 1 or 2 times during last 7 days
	2. *LIMITED ASSISTANCE* — Resident highly involved in activity; received physical help in guided maneuvering of limbs or other nonweight bearing assistance 3+ times — OR — More help provided only 1 or 2 times during last 7 days
	3. *EXTENSIVE ASSISTANCE* — While resident performed part of activity, over last 7-day period, help of following type(s) provided 3 or more times:
	— Weight-bearing support
	— Full staff performance during part (but not all) of last 7 days
	4. *TOTAL DEPENDENCE* — Full staff performance of activity during entire 7 days

b.	TRANSFER	How resident moves between surfaces — to/from: bed, chair, wheelchair, standing position (EXCLUDE to/from bath/toilet)			
c.	LOCO-MOTION	How resident moves between locations in his/her room and adjacent corridor on same floor. If in wheelchair, self-sufficiency once in chair			
d.	DRESSING	How resident puts on, fastens, and takes off all items of street clothing, including donning/removing prosthesis			
e.	EATING	How resident eats and drinks (regardless of skill)			
f.	TOILET USE	How resident uses the toilet room (or commode, bedpan, urinal); transfer on/off toilet, cleanses, changes pad, manages ostomy or catheter, adjusts clothes			

E3.	BATHING	How resident takes full-body bath/shower, sponge bath, and transfers in/out of tub/shower (EXCLUDE washing of back and hair. *Code for most dependent in self-performance.*)			
		0. Independent — No help provided			
		1. Supervision — Oversight help only			
		2. Physical help limited to transfer only			
		3. Physical help in part of bathing activity			
		4. Total dependence			

F1.	CONTINENCE SELF-CONTROL CATEGORIES
	(Code for resident's performance over all shifts)
	0. *CONTINENT* — Complete control
	1. *USUALLY CONTINENT* — BLADDER, incontinent episodes once a week or less; BOWEL, less than weekly
	2. *OCCASIONALLY INCONTINENT* — BLADDER, 2+ times a week but not daily; BOWEL, once a week
	3. *FREQUENTLY INCONTINENT* — BLADDER, tended to be incontinent daily, but some control present (e.g., on day shift); BOWEL, 2-3 times a week
	4. *INCONTINENT* — Had inadequate control. BLADDER, multiple daily episodes; BOWEL, all (or almost all) of the time

a.	BOWEL CONTI-NENCE	Control of bowel movement, with appliance or bowel continence programs, if employed			
b.	BLADDER CONTI-NENCE	Control of urinary bladder function (if dribbles, volume insufficient to soak through underpants), with appliances (e.g., foley) or continence programs, if employed			

H2.	MOOD PER-SISTENCE	Sad or anxious mood intrudes on daily life over last 7 days — not easily altered, doesn't "cheer up"			
		0. No 1. Yes			

H3.	PROBLEM BEHAVIOR	*(Code for behavior in last 7 days)*			
		0. Behavior not exhibited in last 7 days			
		1. Behavior of this type occurred less than daily			
		2. Behavior of this type occurred daily or more frequently			
		a. WANDERING (moved with no rational purpose seemingly oblivious to needs or safety)			
		b. VERBALLY ABUSIVE (others were threatened, screamed at, cursed at)			
		c. PHYSICALLY ABUSIVE (others were hit, shoved, scratched, sexually abused)			
		d. SOCIALLY INAPPROPRIATE/DISRUPTIVE BEHAVIOR (made disrupting sounds, noisy, screams, self-abusive acts, sexual behavior or disrobing in public, smeared/threw food/feces, hoarding, rummaged through others' belongings)			

J2.	OTHER CURRENT DIAGNOSES AND ICD-9 CODES	*(Include only those diseases diagnosed in the last 90 days that have a relationship to current ADL status, behavior status, medical treatments, or risk of death)*
		FIRST QUARTER
		a. _____
		b. _____
		SECOND QUARTER
		c. _____
		d. _____
		THIRD QUARTER
		e. _____
		f. _____

L2. c.	WEIGHT LOSS	(i.e., 5%+ in last 30 days; or 10% in last 180 days)			
		0. No 1. Yes			

O4.	DAYS RECEIVED THE FOLLOWING MEDICATION	*(Record the number of days during last 7 days; enter "0" if not used; enter "1" if long-acting meds. used less than weekly)*			
		a. Antipsychotics			
		b. Antianxiety/hypnotics			
		c. Antidepressants			

P3.	DEVICES AND RESTRAINTS	*(Use the following codes for last 7 days)*			
		0. Not used			
		1. Used less than daily			
		2. Used daily			
		b. Trunk restraint			
		d. Chair prevents rising			

Index

Page numbers followed by *f* indicate figures; those followed by *t* indicate tabular material.